RAINBOWS AT THE SHADOWS OF COVID-19

Library of Congress Control Number: 2021924929
ISBN: Hardcover   978-1-6698-0318-8
               Softcover   978-1-6698-0317-1
               eBook   978-1-6698-0316-4

Scripture quotations marked KJV are from the Holy Bible, King James Version (Authorized Version). First published in 1611. Quoted from the KJV Classic Reference Bible, Copyright © 1983 by The Zondervan Corporation.

Scripture taken from the Holy Bible, New International Version®. Copyright © 1973, 1978, 1984 Biblica. Used by permission of Zondervan. All rights reserved.

Scripture taken from The Holy Bible, English Standard Version® (ESV®), copyright © 2001 by Crossway, a publishing ministry of Good News Publishers. Used by permission. All rights reserved.

Any people depicted in stock imagery provided by Getty Images are models, and such images are being used for illustrative purposes only.
Certain stock imagery © Getty Images.

Print information available on the last page.

Rev. date: 02/07/2022

To order additional copies of this book, contact:
Xlibris
844-714-8691
www.Xlibris.com
Orders@Xlibris.com
831720

RAINBOWS AT THE SHADOWS OF COVID-19

RAMSIS F. GHALY, MD

Neurosurgeon and Anesthesiologist
Professor of Neurological Surgery and Anesthesiology
American Fully Trained and Board Certified in Quadruple Medical Specialties

CONTENTS

SECTION 1: LET ME FREE LET ME FLY HIGH TO THE MOST HIGH......1

Let Me Free! Let Me Fly High to the Most High! Let Me be Out of My Body! Let Me Ascend So High To Be Out Of Reach! Let Me Up high Above The Clouds With My Most High! 3

The Nature Free of COVID Between Earth and Heaven!................................. 16

Divine Humanity is in These Neurons!.. 25

Disabled Yet Genius and Impaired Yet Brilliant... 28

The Ancient Human Brains were Superior to Modern Human Brains! Wake Up Call!! 47

Is the Human Subconscious Mind Intelligent? 49

Act of Kindness is a Spiritual Treasure in Human Journey for Salvwation!! ... 55

Snap Human Brain and Introduction to Snap Bypass Circuit! 59

Look at my gorgeous eyes!!!... 73

Visiting Greek Church Friday Night for Mother's Weekend Happy Mother's Day 77

The Secret of My Garden! 82

Happy Fathers Day 84

Ironman and Flying Superman!! 89

To Those Unrecognized and Hidden Out of Sight!...................................... 90

Keep Dreaming with my Soul Life In Heaven! A Beautiful Diary to Keep Daily While Living! 98

SECTION 2: FAITHFUL FRONT LINERS AND ESSENTIAL WORKERS 103

A Prayer from the Author... 105

Calling for You all to Join and Salute the Medical Front liners and Essential Workers! 107

Faithful Healthcare Worker and Essential Workers!.................................... 111

Gratitude to all the Essentials Thank You! 113

Early morning at the dawn as the week is starting!!!.................................... 114

Give Credit and Respect to those Credit and Respect are Due! In Fact, Do Good and Love Those Don't Do Good and Don't Love!......................... 116

SECTION 3: RETURN OF RAINBOWS 125

God Almighty Our Lord Jesus is in Control!... 127

Give the Glory to God the Almighty Jesus and not to the Foolish Science and Vaccine! 139

Heavenly Message of Lifting up the COVID Curse!.................................... 151

Let us not forget our Heavenly and Merciful Father in defeating the
most devastating virus affecting universally the human race worldwide!! 153

America Let Us Go New Page for America A Year Later Still True!! 155

Let us go America! 158

America Resume Your Life Back! Let us walk in the Vine! Let Us
Rise Up and Smell the Roses Once More! 160

As We Journey Together through COVID Unfolding In So Many Ways 164

Don't Be Fearful But Joyful! The Second Wave Isn't As Bad As The
First Wave! 166

Do Not Run Do Not Hid the Coronavirus Will Determine What to Do 171

Cascade of Human Life! 176

Even at the Time of Catastrophe such as COVID, There Always a Rose
Around Us 179

Colorful PPE for Sporadic COVID 186

What COVID Taught Me?? 188

Lessons learned from COVID-19 Pandemic! 191

Lessons Learned from the Pandemic of the Year in Preparation for
New Year 2021 Resolutions! 194

A Theortical Idea to combat the COVID Pandemic and Any Other
Viral Pandemic Developed by Ramsis Ghaly 197

What is wrong of keep faceMasking??? 200

Supreme COVID Scientists SCS a New Proposal to lead the COVID
Taskforce! 202

Thirteen Psalms to Pray for the Ongoing Curse of COVID and
Facemasks Bestowed Upon all People so that Our Savior may Lifted
them up from the Face of Earth During the Holy Passion Week!! 205

Human Life is Purely a Gift From God And Not From Man!!! 211

Still a Time to Keep Working Hard filling the World around with
Good Deeds!! Labor to Enter Unto Rest! 214

Welcome to My Post Covid Neurosurgery Clinic and Office!! 218

Sarcasm and Funny for an Era The World Wish to Go Away and be
Erased But What Remains Difficult Memories!! Here is my take about
Life after Corona and the future of face masks!! 221

Reform Ourselves Before Asking to Reform Our System! Reform
Interior Before Reforming the Exterior! 227

SECTION 4:   INSPIRING STORIES OF COVID SURVIVAL 233

A True Story and Real Miracle of our Lord Jesus Of Two COVID
Survival: They weren't sisters but they were together in the same
hospital dying from COVID-19 235

Do not give up in COVID Coma even if in ECMO and intubated for
three months in ICU!! 252

SECTION 5: SELECTED PATIENTS STORIES DURING COVID
RECOVERY 261

Archangel Michael and My Patient MF. March 12, 2021 263
What a gorgeous touching heartfelt beautiful diamond painting of our
Savior and myself in Surgery drawn by my patient RC! 272
Today in my clinic a Unity of the Son to His Mother! 277
Words of my Patient! 279
The Journey of Donald Sargent! 280

SECTION 6: JESUS LOVE DURING COVID 283

Jesus Love is my Thanksgivings 2020 and my Thanksgiving is Jesus
Love During COVID Second Surge! 285
Happy Valentine's Day 2021: Continue to Make a Difference! True
love never be Conquered by Pandemics, Sickness and Death! 292
Early Happy Valentine Day During COVID 2/1/2021 311
America the Country We Love! 317
In COVID 19 To Whom Shall my Little Soul Go to But You My Lord? 319

SECTION 7: CHRISTMAS DURING COVID DECLINE 327

Christmas During COVID Unfolding 329
My Meditation with my Savior for 2020 Christmas and 2021 New Year! 340
Virtual 2020 Christmas and New Year 348
My Christmas EVE PPE 354
My Hospital On Call Christmas Uniform Isn't lighting Up For Sure!!! 360
To Do List 2020 Christmas 362
Lavender Color in Christmas! 369
It Is Sunday Let Us Be Ready to Serve Our Savior Jesus as We
Approaching His Birth! 371
The 2020 Christmas Trees are lonely This Year 373
In Christmas Eve Mass in the Streets Respecting Distancing Away and
Socially Protected! 379
Merry Christmas and happy new year! 384
In the Post-Christmas Day I am for another day in the Service! 389
Christmas 2020 by the Mountains of the Lord! 391
It is That Time to Cry in Sorrows and Griefs by the 2020 Christmas Tree! ... 405
Roses for 2020 Christmas Would You All Join Me to Pick Up Roses
for the Newborn King!! 438

SECTION 8: GOOD FRIDAY AND EASTER DURING COVID-19 RECOVERY 443

Good Friday By the Monastery faraway to comply with COVID Restriction and Resurrection Feast 2021! Easter during COVID-19 Recovery 445
Good Friday and Easter of Christian Orthodoxy April 2021......................... 450
My Orthodox Easter with COVID Patients! 457
Easter 2021 with Victor and Gamal and Grandma 84 Years Old! 459

SECTION 9: TO THE VICTIMS AND VULNERABLE OF COVID 19 461

Through the Atrocities caused by COVID Surge and Political Unrest
You are NOT Forgotten O Bravery Soldier of the Freedom! 463
May I Enter unto thy Court O Lord my God! 468
As a Human Flesh Gets Older It Withers Away While the Spirit.................... 472
It Is Not Death But It is New Beginning! 488
America Acknowledged the Aremenian Christian Genocide 1915-1918......... 491
Let us remember the millions at least 34 million of Russian Mass
Causalities in the turn of 20 century between world war II and the
Dictator Joseph Stalin!! 492
Dedicated to My Patient Carmel Perino.. 494
They Took Away my Son, my Man and my Only Brother!!! 501
He Looked Up To Heaven Crying In Tears And Said: "O God Please
Help Me And Look After My Dying Soul! Have mercy on me!!" Then,
in the darkness of the night, he spend the entire night praying in tears
while no one was seeing him!! 505
In the Memory of Isabella! 511
A Chicagoan's Mother from a Latino Descend!... 514

SECTION 10: TIME TO LIVE OUTDOORS AND RUN TO THE MOUNTAINS! 523

A Spiritual life by the Desert Surpass a Physical Life in Babylon by the Zion.... 525
As There is No Coronavirus in the Mountains, There isn't also in the
freezing crispy snow mountains!! 531
But I prefer to Stay That Way!.. 533
Run Away for thy Life! The Divine Calling Following COVID-19 539
Even for Just Few! I Found Comfort Running Away to the Desert
During Unfolding of COVID! 555
I Found Comfort Running Away to the Desert During Unfolding of COVID 559
Sunday the Day of the Lord by the White Mountains!! 561

SECTION 11: AUTHOR AND COVID-19...............567

My God Brought me all the Way From Egypt 36 Years Ago to Care for
COVID Victims!...569

January 20, 2020 was My very first post to warm the world against the
imminent COVID -19 pandemic and called upon worldwide chain of
prayers —-...571

This Post of Mine about the Beginning of COVID in Chicago, is so
Close to my Heart!..579

COVID Mystery Revealed!...583

Nomination and Awarded Notable Healthcare Award hero In Crain's
Chicago March 8, 2021 Thank you Chicago's Crain's March 2021................584

Another Day in the Paradise taking appropriate caution with PPE and
multiple layers!!!...593

Early Morning Leaving my Place of Service the Famous JSH of Cook
County Hospital!...594

It is Not My Daily Adventure But Rather My Daily Joy!.....................595

Every Day Serving with Many Front liners Looking Forward for
Better Days Ahead!..605

My Medical Mission...607

America's Most Honored Doctors award 2021...................................608

Five Stars!!...615

The "Journey of no Return" from Egypt to America at the hope of
"Journey of Return": A story from the heart must tell to the second
generation and future generations...619

Can our Modern Cowboy Chairs accept my Candidacy to Join The
Cowboy Club of America??..634

Writing While Walking and Looking Around....................................641

What I Do at the End of My Clinic?...645

BOOK AUTHORED BY DR RAMSIS F. GHALY.............................646

SECTION 12: PERSONAL VIEWS ON COVID-19 653

A Nation Shall Mourn!...655

The Second Wave of COVID...659

The Year of 2021 Shall Be All About COVID 2021!!.........................693

Goodbye COVID19 and Welcome COVID20!...................................699

The Year of 2021 Shall Give Birth to a New Brutal World!!...............702

My First Monday of 2021 as COVID spread continues!.....................705

COVID as a Shark Ready to Bite You and a Lion About to Kill You!............707

COVID Overpower Human Cells and Finally Crush Human Life to Dust!....709

COVID the Darkest Evil Antihuman killer! Merciless Death....................714

Even Late at Night COVID is Around!...717

In hours, COVID patients' Oxygenation Get so Much Worse that We
Run Racing to Intubate and Assist Them in Ventilators as a Life-saving!.......718
This what I do when I get emergency call to intubate a COVID patient.
Put as much layers of PAPR & PPE So excited to help out and I run to
save in my Lord Jesus Name! 721
Not again Getting called to intubate It isn't Deja vu but is real Friends
be in the Watch!... 724
COVID is Surfacing the Poor Standards of Government Operated
Hospitals and Widespread of Poverty!! 726
Children And Unfolding COVID 728
The Coronavirus is sparing largely the babies children and pregnant
mothers, in my Observation! 737
Second Wave Is Here, Be in The Watch!! 738
Please Consider My Advice During COVID Second Wave Surge! 741
Be Ready to Put Your head and Face Sealed Inside Air Purifiers
Connected to Filters and Air Tanks.. 743
Persistent Fever in Early COVID Illness: Please listen to my advice!! 747
Ghaly Photos with PPE... 751

SECTION 13: CRITICAL LOOK AT COVID-19 753
COVID Pandemic My Critical Look! 755
Critical Look at the World Eleventh Pandemic!... 757
Looking Back at COVID Pandemic!! Deep Reflections 765
Emergency and isn't Emergency! The world is still A Good Place to
Live and God is in Control! 770
Eccentricity of Science and Researchers and lack of Realism! 776
Show me a Worldwide COVID Hotspot Map that Matches Poverty
Hotspot Map!! 777
Ramsis Ghaly Cascade for Man Destructions! 780
My Deep Reflection on Face Mask!!.. 781

SECTION 14: VACCINATION CONTROVERSY 785
Is COVID Vaccine is a "True" or a "False" Security for Immunity?.............. 787
COVID VACCINE 794
COVID Vaccine and Toxin Spike Protein in Blood stream!............................. 802
The Man took the COVID Vaccine and Died of COVID! 804
Mandatory Vaccine Consent 805
Antibody Testing Prior and After Vaccination Is Not Being Mandated
or Part of the Requirements! Why??? 811
Compensation for the Victims of COVID Vaccine Complications!!................816
Anti- COVID Coat!! 819
Discriminatory Treatment Based on Vaccinated and Unvaccinated!!............. 823

SECTION 15: MEDICAL ISSUES DURING COVID-19 825

COVID Should Never be an Excuse to Let our Beloved Old People Go
Prematurely! 827
Virtual Medical Management in Modern Post COVID Medicine.................. 831
Motorcycle Riders, during COVID: Did You Know!!! 834
My Chicago Thanksgiving Between COVID and Gun Victims 836
Patient Empowerment with Faith 839
Ghaly Novel Checklist in Anesthesia and Neurological Surgery:
Editorial Publication 841
Worse Days Ahead for Chicago Violence!! 844
HAIR SAMPLES 847

SECTION 16: FUTURE COVID 849

Coronavirus a Powerful Bioterrorism Please Stay Away! 851
Look Beyond the Surface of COVID Pandemic! 854
Two years later no Treatment for COVID 19!! 857
The Crises in Healthcare is not Caused by COVID Calling for
Worldwide Healthcare Reform!! 860

SECTION 17: SPIRITUAL PHILOSOPHY 863

Two Secrets of Life Where Lord Visitation to Earth Full of Holiness
and Blessing: Giving Birth to a Newborn and Taking a Faithful Human
Soul! Looking Deeper to Theological Aspect! 865
If You Just Live Long Enough!!! 874
Friends This How Days Pass By Quickly!!! 877
Please Do Not Look Down at My Age!! 881
Minority A Philosophical View... 884
Diversity in life! 889
Quality Before Quantity 899
"Quality Builds Team And That Team Enforces Quality" 901
Reforming Modern Definition of Corporate Professionalism! 903

SECTION 18: POLITICAL EVENTS DURING COVID DECLINE 907

Where was the Wise? Where was the Scribe? Where was the Disputer
of this world? 909
Voting During COVID Unfolding... 911
The Latest Events Both Parties Are To Be Blamed While Not Excusing
the President Trump!! 930
Sadness over the land and gloominess all around! Post During Riots
Before Washington DC Capitol 1/5/2021 936
Jesus Name During 2021 Presidential Inauguration! 938

Tribunal 942
Today I am Thinking about the Inauguration of my Beloved! 946
Trio Presidents Instead of Unio President System! 952
Guard against the Fallen America!! 954
A Christian Phone Call Biden-Trump Working Together!! 956
Do not you think a global warming is a better choice than the deadly
and dreadful freezing cold weather? 960
A Puzzle with dead end no one could figure to solve Palestine and Israel! 962

SECTION 19: WITH MY RESIDENTS AND STUDENTS DURING
COVID 19 965

My two wonderful residents Brian and Shaun surprised me today!!
Both bought my book: "A Christian from Egypt: a life story of a
neurosurgeon and quadruple boards" 967
With My Residents During COVID Unfolding 968
My new year Eve with my Residents serving COVID 19 Patients. 978
End of the Academic Year!! 982
Graduation Party in the Early PostCOVID-19 Era! 988

SECTION 20 993

Illness Journey Goodbye 2020 to my Patients! 995
My Patients during the Unfolding COVID 997

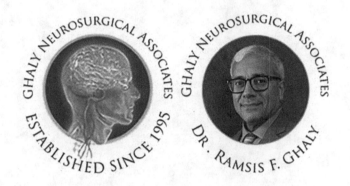

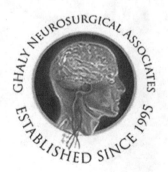

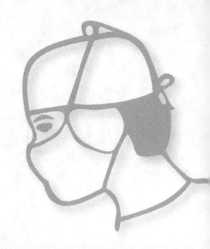

SECTION 1

Let Me Free Let Me Fly High to the Most High

Let Me Free! Let Me Fly High to the Most High! Let Me be Out of My Body! Let Me Ascend So High To Be Out Of Reach! Let Me be Up high Above The Clouds With My Most High!

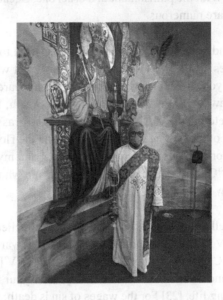

Let me go! Liberate my soul! I am jailed and confined! My soul is restrained and every season with a different type! My journey on earth hasn't been easy and I am in the hideout! To Whom I cry and whom shall reply! My cross is heaven and my heart is shut! My eyes are blind, my ears are deaf and mouth is mute! The darkness has wrapped me and restrained my soul with all kinds of harsh Mechanical handcuffs; leg shackles, ankle straps, straitjacket, and! I am dressed with vests and belts around my waist! I can't move as I am laying on restraint board at night and on restrained chairs during the day! Please Let me go! Liberate my soul!

I wish I am smart as a serpent and meek as a dove! But I am not!! I wish I have wings and the body of an eagle to fly! But I am not!! I wish I have the legs and the form of Giraffe or leopard or a tiger to run so fast! But I am not!! I wish I have the speed of cheetah, pronghorn, springbok, wildebeest, lion, blackbuck, kangaroo, or even ostrich or Africana wild dog! But I am not!!! I wish I am as strong as a lion with detriment will and spirit to win and succeed! But I am not!!

But who am I but nothing! I am a feeble soul within a weary body and a form of advanced in age!

Furthermore, I am a sinner and not worthy to be free or to set to fly high to the Most High as it is written: Psalm 14:3 They have all turned aside, together they have become corrupt; There is no one who does good, not even one. Romans 3:23 for all have sinned and fall short of the glory of God, Jeremiah 30:14 'All your lovers have forgotten you, They do not seek you; For I have wounded you with the wound of an enemy, With the punishment of a cruel one, Because your iniquity is great And your sins are numerous.

I am a vapor soon and soon vanishes away from this world to exist forever with the Most High! James 4:14 KJV [14] Whereas ye know not what shall be on the morrow. For what is your life? It is even a vapour, that appeareth for a little time, and then vanisheth away. Psalm 144:4 Man is like a breath; his days are like a passing shadow. 1 Peter 1:24 KJV[24] For all flesh is as grass, and all the glory of man as the flower of grass. The grass withereth, and the flower thereof falleth away: Psalm 102:3 For my days pass away like smoke, and my bones burn like a furnace. Psalm 39:4 "O Lord, make me know my end and what is the measure of my days; let me know how fleeting I am!

Yet, I am no longer fell unto despair since my soul is reconciled in my Savior and LordRomans 5:8 KJV 8] But God commendeth his love toward us, in that, while we were yet sinners, Christ died for us. Romans 6:22-23 KJV [22] But now being made free from sin, and become servants to God, ye have your fruit unto holiness, and the end everlasting life. [23] For the wages of sin is death; but the gift of God is eternal life through Jesus Christ our Lord.

Jesus is my King since He saved my soul to life eternity! Jesus is my Heavenly father since He bought me with His cherished blood! Jesus is my hope since He rescued my soul from damantion! Jesus is my Lord since He created me out of nothing and brought me to existence Jesus is my Lord of Glory since He conquered all the powers and overcome the ruler of this world!

There is no chance for my allied soul to set Free or to Fly! There is no way to live Out of My Body! I can't Ascend So High To Be Out Of Reach! It is impossible with my lowly soul to be Up high Above The Clouds With My Most High!

While my body was severely restrained and my soul was devastated and mind was constrained, I prayed to the Lord: O lord I don't have fifty million dollar to get a space bus and take a tour by the moon! Furthermore, My desire is You and not the glamorous universe Your hand made! But for now I shall continue to live the dream in hope that one day I shall be Free and Fly High to the Most High! I prayed to the Holy Spirit for my brain to dream for the impossible! I asked my mind to come out of the body and my mind to move out of the skull! I found my own light and flying out of space fantasizing unto the matters of the heaven and heavenly things! I was moved when I opened the holy book of God and impersonated the psalmist in his praises, the Song of Songs in the eternal Love and Revelations in the Almighty Pantacratour and the heavenly scenes!

+++

It is heaven and so heavenly standing in the Almighty Dome of the Pantacrator while holding a Shouria as a Thurifer (A Censor suspended from chains, the thurible where incense is burned using charcoal, censing the sweat aroma before God the prayers of His servants ascending up to heaven). The smoke of the Incense is the prayers of all His saints as it is written: "And another angel came and stood at the altar, having a golden censer; and there was given unto him much incense, that he should offer it with the prayers of all saints upon the golden altar which was before the throne. [4] And the smoke of the incense, which came with the prayers of the saints, ascended up before God out of the angel's hand." Revelation 8:3-4 KJV

It is my heavenly spot on earth in Alter, by the Dome of the Pantocrator, the Almighty, the Most High, the Creator of all things, the Ruler of the Universe, Christ the omnipotent lord of the universe, the all-powerful, by the bosom of God! When I stand by the Dome of the Pantocrator, I trembled in fear and I forgot all things! My heart ♥ fluttered, my eyes teared, I became tiny and I felt absolutely not worthy to be in the presence of His Majesty one to One. I sweated droplets of blood, gasping my breathe one after another, asking for forgiveness and I fell into prayers!!!! But soon I ran unto him as the prodigal son did and Knelt to Him saying from all my heart: "Father, I have sinned against heaven, and in thy sight, and am no more worthy to be called thy son." Luke 15:21 KJV Immediately my soul is exalted as the Holy Father as I was a great way off, had compassion, and ran, and fell on my neck, and kissed me! The Almighty Father took me to Himself, dressed me with the best robe and put a ring on my hand, and shoes on my feet: And brought hither the fatted calf, and dine with me in joy saying: "For this my son was dead, and is alive again; he was lost, and is found" Luke 15:20, 22-24 KJV

I felt I was indeed in heaven out of my body. And I knew such a man, (whether in the body, or out of the body, I cannot tell: God knoweth;) [4] How that he was caught up into paradise, and heard unspeakable words, which it is not lawful for a man to utter! Of such an one will I glory: yet of myself I will not glory, but in mine infirmities. [9]

5

And he said unto me, My grace is sufficient for thee: for my strength is made perfect in weakness! Most gladly therefore will I rather glory in my infirmities, that the power of Christ may rest upon me. [10] Therefore I take pleasure in infirmities, in reproaches, in necessities, in persecutions, in distresses for Christ's sake: for when I am weak, then am I strong! 2 Corinthians 12:3-5,9-10 KJV

Soon I felt rejuvenated and with full energy filled with Love ♥ and humility! My Lord opened my eyes to the unseen and let me hear the unspeakable! I open the books before the Lord the Pantacrator by the Almighty Dome, close my eyes while my own heart, mind and soul being lifted up to heaven, uttering the words of Revelations, Song of Songs and begin to sing with the Psalmist the praises of New Songs to the Lord!!! As I was absorbed I was taken up to heaven

As I was standing by the alter of the Most High, I fell at His feet as dead and He laid his right hand upon me, saying unto me, Fear not; "I am Alpha and Omega, the beginning and the ending, saith the Lord, which is, and which was, and which is to come, the Almighty. [17] And when I saw him, I fell at his feet as dead. And he laid his right hand upon me, saying unto me, Fear not; I am the first and the last: [18] I am he that liveth, and was dead; and, behold, I am alive for evermore, Amen; and have the keys of hell and of death." Revelation 1:8,17-18 KJV

O the Son of Man, the Holy Lamb of God in His glory in the midst of the seven candles—-"And in the midst of the seven candlesticks one like unto the Son of man, clothed with a garment down to the foot, and girt about the paps with a golden girdle. [14] His head and his hairs were white like wool, as white as snow; and his eyes were as a flame of fire; [15] And his feet like unto fine brass, as if they burned in a furnace; and his voice as the sound of many waters. [16] And he had in his right hand seven stars: and out of his mouth went a sharp twoedged sword: and his countenance was as the sun shineth in his strength." Revelation 1:13-16 KJV

I looked—"And immediately I was in the spirit: and, behold, a throne was set in heaven, and one sat on the throne. [3] And he that sat was to look upon like a jasper and a sardine stone: and there was a rainbow round about the throne, in sight like unto an emerald. [4] And round about the throne were four and twenty seats: and upon the seats I saw four and twenty elders sitting, clothed in white raiment; and they had on their heads crowns of gold. [5] And out of the throne proceeded lightnings and thunderings and voices: and there were seven lamps of fire burning before the throne, which are the seven Spirits of God. [6] And before the throne there was a sea of glass like unto crystal: and in the midst of the throne, and round about the throne, were four beasts full of eyes before and behind. [7] And the first

6

beast was like a lion, and the second beast like a calf, and the third beast had a face as a man, and the fourth beast was like a flying eagle. [8] And the four beasts had each of them six wings about him ; and they were full of eyes within: and they rest not day and night, saying, Holy, holy, holy, Lord God Almighty, which was, and is, and is to come. [9] And when those beasts give glory and honour and thanks to him that sat on the throne, who liveth for ever and ever, [10] The four and twenty elders fall down before him that sat on the throne, and worship him that liveth for ever and ever, and cast their crowns before the throne, saying, [11] Thou art worthy, O Lord, to receive glory and honour and power: for thou hast created all things, and for thy pleasure they are and were created." Revelation 4:2-11 KJV

I wept and wept much as I saw —, "—the four beasts and four and twenty elders fell down before the Lamb, having every one of them harps, and golden vials full of odours, which are the prayers of saints. And they sung a new song, saying, Thou art worthy to take the book, and to open the seals thereof: for thou wast slain, and hast redeemed us to God by thy blood out of every kindred, and tongue, and people, and nation; And hast made us unto our God kings and priests: and we shall reign on the earth. —And hast made us unto our God kings and priests: and we˙ shall reign on the earth. [11] And I beheld, and I heard the voice of many angels round about the throne and the beasts and the elders: and the number of them was ten thousand times ten thousand, and thousands of thousands; [12] Saying with a loud voice, Worthy is the Lamb that was slain to receive power, and riches, and wisdom, and strength, and honour, and glory, and blessing. [13] And every creature which is in heaven, and on the earth, and under the earth, and such as are in the sea, and all that are in them, heard I saying, Blessing, and honour, and glory, and power, be unto him that sitteth upon the throne, and unto the Lamb for ever and ever. [14] And the four beasts said, Amen. And the four and twenty elders fell down and worshipped him that liveth for ever and ever." Revelation 5:4-14 KJV

Under the alter I saw souls of them that were slain for the word of God, and for the testimony which they held: [10] And they cried with a loud voice, saying, How long, O Lord, holy and true, dost thou not judge and avenge our blood on them that dwell on the earth? [11] And white robes were given unto every one of them; and it was said unto them, that they should rest yet for a little season, until their fellowservants also and their brethren, that should be killed as they were, should be fulfilled. Soon and and behold a white horse: and he that sat on him had a bow; and a crown was given unto him: and he went forth conquering, and to conquer. Revelation 6:2,9-11 KJV

And cried with a loud voice, saying, Salvation to our God which sitteth upon the throne, and unto the Lamb. And all the angels stood round about the throne, and about the elders and the four beasts, and fell before the throne on their faces, and worshipped God, [12] Saying, Amen: Blessing, and glory, and wisdom, and thanksgiving, and honour, and power, and might, be unto our God for ever and ever. Amen. I saw four angels standing on the four corners of the earth, holding the four winds of the earth, that the wind should not blow on the earth, nor on the sea, nor on any tree. [9] After this I beheld, and, lo, a great multitude, which no man could number, of all nations, and kindreds, and people, and tongues, stood before the throne, and before the Lamb, clothed with white robes, and palms in their hands; [—15] Therefore are they before the throne of God, and serve him day and night in his temple: and he that sitteth on the throne shall dwell among them. [16] They shall hunger no more, neither thirst any more; neither shall the sun light on them, nor any heat. [17] For the Lamb which is in the midst of the throne shall feed them, and shall lead them unto living fountains of waters: and God shall wipe away all tears from their eyes. Revelation 7:1,9-12,15-17 KJV

I heard loud voice saying: Fear God, and give glory to him; for the hour of his judgment is come: and worship him that made heaven, and earth, and the sea, and the fountains of waters.

And I looked, and, lo, a Lamb stood on the mount Sion, and with him an hundred forty and four thousand, having his Father's name written in their foreheads. [2] And I heard a voice from heaven, as the voice of many waters, and as the voice of a great thunder: and I heard the voice of harpers harping with their harps: [3] And they sung as it were a new song before the throne, and before the four beasts, and the elders: and no man could learn that song but the hundred and forty and four thousand, which were redeemed from the earth. [4] These are they which were not defiled with women; for they are virgins. These are they which follow the Lamb whithersoever he goeth. These were redeemed from among men, being the firstfruits unto God and to the Lamb. [5] And in their mouth was found no guile: for they are without fault before the throne of God." Revelation 14:1-5,7 KJV

And after these things I heard a great voice of much people in heaven, saying, Alleluia; Salvation, and glory, and honour, and power, unto the Lord our God: [2] For true and righteous are his judgments: for he hath judged the great whore, which did corrupt the earth with her fornication, and hath avenged the blood of his servants at her hand. [3] And again they said, Alleluia. And her smoke rose up for ever and ever. [4] And the four and twenty elders and the four beasts fell down and worshipped God that sat on the throne, saying, Amen; Alleluia. [5] And a voice came out of the throne, saying, Praise our God, all ye his servants, and ye that fear him, both small and great. [6] And I heard as it were the voice of a great multitude, and as the voice of many waters, and as the voice of mighty

8

thunderings, saying, Alleluia: for the Lord God omnipotent reigneth. [7] Let us be glad and rejoice, and give honour to him: for the marriage of the Lamb is come, and his wife hath made herself ready. [8] And to her was granted that she should be arrayed in fine linen, clean and white: for the fine linen is the righteousness of saints." Revelation 19:1-8 KJV

His Name is The, KING OF KINGS, AND LORD OF LORDS: And I saw heaven opened, and behold a white horse; and he that sat upon him was called Faithful and True, and in righteousness he doth judge and make war. [12] His eyes were as a flame of fire, and on his head were many crowns; and he had a name written, that no man knew, but he himself. [13] And he was clothed with a vesture dipped in blood: and his name is called The Word of God. [14] And the armies which were in heaven followed him upon white horses, clothed in fine linen, white and clean. [15] And out of his mouth goeth a sharp sword, that with it he should smite the nations: and he shall rule them with a rod of iron: and he treadeth the winepress of the fierceness and wrath of Almighty God. [16] And he hath on his vesture and on his thigh a name written, KING OF KINGS, AND LORD OF LORDS." Revelation 19:11-16 KJV

It is done. I am Alpha and Omega, the beginning and the end. And I saw a new heaven and a new earth: for the first heaven and the first earth were passed away; and there was no more sea. [3] And I heard a great voice out of heaven saying, Behold, the tabernacle of God is with men, and he will dwell with them, and they shall be his people, and God himself shall be with them, and be their God. [4] And God shall wipe away all tears from their eyes; and there shall be no more death, neither sorrow, nor crying, neither shall there be any more pain: for the former things are passed away. [5] And he that sat upon the throne said, Behold, I make all things new. And he said unto me, Write: for these words are true and faithful. [6] And he said unto me, It is done. I am Alpha and Omega, the beginning and the end. I will give unto him that is athirst of the fountain of the water of life freely. [7] He that overcometh shall inherit all things; and I will be his God, and he shall be my son. Revelation 21:1,3-7 KJV

The New Jerusalem with twelve Pearls: And there came unto me one of the seven angels which had the seven vials full of the seven last plagues, and talked with me, saying, Come hither, I will shew thee the bride, the Lamb's wife. [10] And he carried me away in the spirit to a great and high mountain, and shewed me that great city, the holy Jerusalem, descending out of heaven from God, [11] Having the glory of God: and her light was like unto a stone most precious, even like a jasper stone, clear as crystal; [12] And had a wall great and high, and had twelve gates, and at the gates twelve angels, and names written thereon, which are the names of the twelve tribes of the children of Israel: [13] On the east three gates; on the north three gates; on the south three gates; and on the west three gates. [14] And the wall of the city had twelve foundations, and in them the names of the twelve apostles of the Lamb. [21] And the twelve gates were twelve pearls; every several gate was of one pearl: and the street of the city was pure gold, as it were transparent glass. [27] And there shall in no wise enter into it any thing that defileth, neither whatsoever worketh abomination, or maketh a lie: but they which are written in the Lamb's book of life. Revelation 21:9-14,21,27 KJV "And he shewed me a pure river of water of life, clear as crystal, proceeding out of the throne of God and of the Lamb. [2] In the midst of the street of it, and on either side of the river, was there the tree of life, which bare twelve manner of fruits, and yielded her fruit every month: and the leaves of the tree were for the healing of the nations. [3] And there shall be no more curse: but the throne of God and of the Lamb shall be in it; and his servants shall serve him: [4] And they shall see his face; and his name shall be in their foreheads. [5] And there shall be no night there; and they need no candle, neither light of the sun; for the Lord God giveth them light: and they shall reign for ever and ever." Revelation 22:1-5 KJV

And the Spirit and the bride say, Come. And let him that heareth say, Come. And let him that is athirst come. And whosoever will, let him take the water of life freely. Behold, I come quickly: blessed is he that keepeth the sayings of the prophecy of this book. [12] And, behold, I come quickly; and my reward is with me, to give every man according as his work shall be. [13] I am Alpha and Omega, the beginning and the end, the first and the last. [16] I Jesus have sent mine angel to testify unto you these things in the churches. I am the root and the offspring of David, and the bright and morning star. [20] He which testifieth these things saith, Surely I come quickly. Amen. Even so, come, Lord Jesus." Revelation 22:7,12-13,16-17,20 KJV

++++

In my Love, I screamed saying: Let Me Free! Let Me Fly! Let Me Ascend So High To Be Out Of Reach Up high To Be Above The Clouds With My Most High! In The Bosom Of My Heavenly Father I shall Live forever! By My Savior, All my Life! So Let Me Free1 Let Me Fly! Let Me Ascend So High To Be Out Of Reach Up high To Be Above The Clouds With My Most High!

Let me free let me fly let me ascend so high I am standing by my King of kings and Lord of lords! I can't come closer unless I die! All I want is You and no One else but You! My Beloved love me and I love my Beloved! Before You I stand in Your faith and I kneel by my soul saying My Father who art in Heaven,... my

Father which art in heaven, Hallowed be thy name. Thy kingdom come. Thy will be done in earth, as it is in heaven. Give me this day my daily bread. And forgive me my debts, as I forgive my debtors. And lead me not into temptation, but deliver me from evil: For thine is the kingdom, and the power, and the glory, for ever. Amen. ... Matthew 6:9-13 KJV

Let me kiss Him with the kisses—let me run unto thy draw me —"Let him kiss me with the kisses of his mouth: for thy love is better than wine. [4] Draw me, we will run after thee: the king hath brought me into his chambers: we will be glad and rejoice in thee, we will remember thy love more than wine: the upright love thee." Song of Songs 1:2,4 KJV "How fair is thy love, my sister, my spouse! how much better is thy love than wine! and the smell of thine ointments than all spices! [11] Thy lips, O my spouse, drop as the honeycomb: honey and milk are under thy tongue; and the smell of thy garments is like the smell of Lebanon." Song of Songs 4:10-11 KJV

My Beloved my Dove leaping upon the mountains skipping upon the hills—"The voice of my beloved! behold, he cometh leaping upon the mountains, skipping upon the hills. [9] My beloved is like a roe or a young hart: behold, he standeth behind our wall, he looketh forth at the windows, shewing himself through the lattice. [14] O my dove, that art in the clefts of the rock, in the secret places of the stairs, let me see thy countenance, let me hear thy voice; for sweet is thy voice, and thy countenance is comely. [16] My beloved is mine, and I am his: he feedeth among the lilies." Song of Songs 2:8-9,14,16 KJV

Thou art beautiful O my Love—Turn away thine eyes from me, for they have overcome me—: "I am my beloved's, and my beloved is mine: he feedeth among the lilies. [4] Thou art beautiful, O my love, as Tirzah, comely as Jerusalem, terrible as an army with banners. [5] Turn away thine eyes from me, for they have overcome me: thy hair is as a flock of goats that appear from Gilead." Song of Songs 6:3-5 KJV

My Beloved is pure white like snow—His eyes are the hes of doves—His mouth is most sweet—: "My beloved is white and ruddy, the chiefest among ten thousand. [11] His head is as the most fine gold, his locks are bushy, and black as a raven. [12] His eyes are as the eyes of doves by the rivers of waters, washed with milk, and fitly set. [13] His cheeks are as a bed of spices, as sweet flowers: his lips like lilies, dropping sweet smelling myrrh. [14] His hands are as gold rings set with the beryl: his belly is as bright ivory overlaid with sapphires. [15] His legs are as pillars of marble, set upon sockets of fine gold: his countenance is as Lebanon, excellent as the cedars. [16] His mouth is most sweet: yea, he is altogether lovely.

This is my beloved, and this is my friend, O daughters of Jerusalem." Song of Songs 5:10-16 KJV

My Love My Dove My only One— "My dove, my undefiled is but one; she is the only one of her mother, she is the choice one of her that bare her. The daughters saw her, and blessed her; yea, the queens and the concubines, and they praised her. [10] Who is she that looketh forth as the morning, fair as the moon, clear as the sun, and terrible as an army with banners?" Song of Songs 6:9-10 KJV

Come my Beloved — let Us get up early—-Let Us go forth to the field— let Us lodge in the villages— "I am my beloved's, and his desire is toward me. [11] Come, my beloved, let us go forth into the field; let us lodge in the villages. [12] Let us get up early to the vineyards; let us see if the vine flourish, whether the tender grape appear, and the pomegranates bud forth: there will I give thee my loves. [13] The mandrakes give a smell, and at our gates are all manner of pleasant fruits, new and old, which I have laid up for thee, O my beloved." Song of Songs 7:10-13 KJV

Make haste, my Beloved — Many waters cannot quench love, neither can the floods drown it—"Many waters cannot quench love, neither can the floods drown it: if a man would give all the substance of his house for love, it would utterly be contemned. [14] Make haste, my beloved, and be thou like to a roe or to a young hart upon the mountains of spices." Song of Songs 8:7,14 KJV

Let me touch the hem of my Master's garment! Let me drink from my Savior's Cup! Let me join Simon, the Cyrenian to bear the Cross after Jesus! Let me follow my Beloved to the Calvary, bewailed and lament with the great company of people, and of women! Let me be crucified with Him upside down as His disciple Peter and on the right hand with the malefactor the thief! Let the darkness be over all the earth and the sun hide its face and so is the moon and the stars! Let the veil of the temple be rented in the midst! Let me be buried with Him in the Golgotha! Let me take Him down with Joseph the Arimathaea, and wrap Him in linen and lay Him in a sepulchre that was hewn in stone, wherein never man before was laid! Let me return with the Marias with the prepared spices and ointments; and rest by His Body! Let me go the first day of the week, very early in the morning, unto the sepulchre, bringing the spices and see His glory! Let me run to the sepulchre with Mary Magdalene, and Joanna, and Mary the mother of James, and other women to see the Great stone rolled away and to hear the two angels with shining garments saying: "He is not here, but is risen: remember how he spake unto you when he was yet in Galilee, It was that were with them, which told these things unto the apostles." Let me go to the village named Emmaus, threescore furlongs from Jerusalem and walk Cleopas where I can find my Savior hear His voice and listen to His words! Let me enter to thy house and sit by His side and eat the blessed bread from His hand! Let me join the apostles by the Galilee waiting for my Beloved! Lead me to Bethany, bless me O Lord as You are carried up into heaven! And as thy disciples let me be continually in the temple, praising and blessing God. Amen! Luke 23:26-27,33, 44-45, 50, 53,55-56 Luke 24:1, 2,4,6,10, 18,30-32, 50-51,53 KJV

Let me stand at his feet behind and weep! Let me wash His feet with my tears and wipe them with the hairs of my head! Let me kiss His feet and anoint them with the ointment! Let me ask Him for forgiveness! Let me hear His voice: "Thy sins are forgiven! Thy faith hath saved thee; go in peace." Luke 7:38,48,50 KJV

The Lord is high but He regards the lowly! Though the Lord is up high but He loves ♥ me and I love ♥ Him endlessly! Though the Lord be high, yet hath he respect unto the lowly: but the proud he knoweth afar off. [7] Though I walk in the midst of trouble, thou wilt revive me: thou shalt stretch forth thine hand against the wrath of mine enemies, and thy right hand shall save me. [8] The Lord will perfect that which concerneth me: thy mercy, O Lord, endureth for ever: forsake not the works of thine own hands." Psalm 138:6-8 KJV

Look not upon me, because I am black—I am black, but comely—"I am black, but comely, O ye daughters of Jerusalem, as the tents of Kedar, as the curtains of Solomon. [6] Look not upon me, because I am black, because the sun hath looked upon me: my mother's children were angry with me; they made me the keeper of the vineyards; but mine own vineyard have I not kept." Song of Songs 1:5-6 KJV

I praise You my Lord and my Savior: Praise ye the Lord. Praise God in his sanctuary: praise him in the firmament of his power. Praise him for his mighty acts: praise him according to his excellent greatness. Praise him with the sound of the trumpet: praise him with the psaltery and harp. Praise him with the timbrel and dance: praise him with stringed instruments and organs. Praise him upon the loud cymbals: praise him upon the high sounding cymbals. Let every thing that hath breath praise the Lord. Praise ye the Lord. Psalm 150 Praise ye the Lord. Sing unto the Lord a new song, and his praise in the congregation of saints. [2] Let Israel rejoice in him that made him: let the children of Zion be joyful in their King. Let them praise his name in the dance: let them sing praises unto him with the timbrel and harp. For the Lord taketh pleasure in his people: he will beautify the meek with salvation. Let the saints be joyful in glory: let them sing aloud upon their beds. Let the high praises of God be in their mouth, and a twoedged sword in their hand; To execute vengeance upon the heathen, and punishments upon the people; To bind their kings with chains, and their nobles with fetters of iron; To execute upon them the judgment written: this honour have all his saints. Praise ye the Lord. Psalm 149 Praise ye the Lord. Praise ye the Lord from the heavens: praise him in the heights. [2] Praise ye him, all his angels: praise ye him, all his hosts. Praise ye him, sun and moon: praise him, all ye stars of light. Praise him, ye heavens of heavens, and ye waters that be above the heavens. [5] Let them praise the name of the Lord: for he commanded, and they were created. He hath also stablished them for ever and ever: he hath made a decree which shall not pass. Praise the Lord from the earth, ye dragons, and all deeps: Fire, and hail; snow, and vapour; stormy wind fulfilling his word: Mountains, and all hills; fruitful trees, and all cedars: Beasts, and all cattle; creeping things, and flying fowl: Kings of the earth, and all people; princes, and all judges of the earth: Both young men, and maidens; old men, and children: Let them praise the name of the Lord: for his name alone is excellent; his glory is above the earth and heaven. He also exalteth the horn of his people, the praise of all his saints; even of the children of Israel, a people near unto him. Praise ye the Lord. Psalm 148 Psalm Praise ye the Lord: for it is good to sing praises unto our God; for it is pleasant; and praise is comely. The Lord doth build up Jerusalem: he gathereth together the outcasts of Israel. He healeth the broken in heart, and bindeth up their wounds. He telleth the number of the stars; he calleth them all by their names. Great is our Lord, and of great power: his understanding is infinite. The Lord lifteth up the meek: he casteth the wicked down to the ground. Sing unto the Lord with thanksgiving; sing praise upon the harp unto our God: Who covereth the heaven with clouds, who prepareth rain for the earth, who maketh grass to grow upon the mountains. He giveth to the beast his food, and to the young ravens which cry. Praise the Lord, O Jerusalem; praise thy God, O Zion. For he hath strengthened the bars of thy gates; he hath blessed thy children within thee. He maketh peace in thy borders, and filleth thee with the finest of the wheat. He sendeth forth his commandment upon earth: his word runneth very swiftly. He giveth snow like wool: he scattereth the hoarfrost like ashes. He casteth forth his ice like morsels: who can stand before his cold? He sendeth out his word, and melteth them: he causeth his wind to blow, and the waters flow. He sheweth his word unto Jacob, his statutes and his judgments unto Israel. He hath not dealt so with any nation: and as for his judgments, they have not known them. Praise ye the Lord. Psalm 147 Praise ye the Lord. Praise the Lord, O my soul. While I live will I praise the Lord: I will sing praises unto my God while I have any being. Put not your trust in princes, nor in the son of man, in whom there is no help. His breath goeth forth, he returneth to his earth; in that very day his thoughts perish. Happy is he that hath the God of Jacob for his help, whose hope is in the Lord his God: Which made heaven, and earth, the sea, and all that therein is: which keepeth truth for ever: Which executeth judgment for the oppressed: which giveth food to the hungry. The Lord looseth the prisoners: The Lord openeth the eyes of the blind: the Lord raiseth them that are bowed down: the Lord loveth the righteous: The Lord preserveth the strangers; he relieveth

14

the fatherless and widow: but the way of the wicked he turneth upside down. The Lord shall reign for ever, even thy God, O Zion, unto all generations. Praise ye the Lord. Psalm 146 I will extol thee, my God, O king; and I will bless thy name for ever and ever. Every day will I bless thee; and I will praise thy name for ever and ever. Great is the Lord, and greatly to be praised; and his greatness is unsearchable. One generation shall praise thy works to another, and shall declare thy mighty acts. I will speak of the glorious honour of thy majesty, and of thy wondrous works. And men shall speak of the might of thy terrible acts: and I will declare thy greatness. They shall abundantly utter the memory of thy great goodness, and shall sing of thy righteousness. The Lord is gracious, and full of compassion; slow to anger, and of great mercy. The Lord is good to all: and his tender mercies are over all his works. All thy works shall praise thee, O Lord ; and thy saints shall bless thee. They shall speak of the glory of thy kingdom, and talk of thy power; To make known to the sons of men his mighty acts, and the glorious majesty of his kingdom. Thy kingdom is an everlasting kingdom, and thy dominion endureth throughout all generations. The Lord upholdeth all that fall, and raiseth up all those that be bowed down. The eyes of all wait upon thee; and thou givest them their meat in due season. Thou openest thine hand, and satisfiest the desire of every living thing. The Lord is righteous in all his ways, and holy in all his works. The Lord is nigh unto all them that call upon him, to all that call upon him in truth. He will fulfil the desire of them that fear him: he also will hear their cry, and will save them. The Lord preserveth all them that love him: but all the wicked will he destroy. My mouth shall speak the praise of the Lord: and let all flesh bless his holy name for ever and ever. Psalm 145

Let Me Free! Let Me Fly High to the Most High! Let Me be Out of My Body! Let Me Ascend So High To Be Out Of Reach! Let Me be Up high Above The Clouds With My Most High!

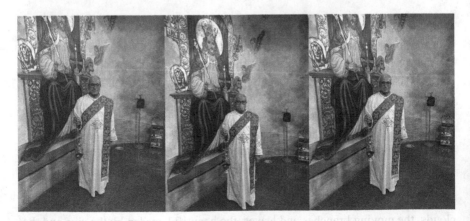

The Nature Free of COVID Between Earth and Heaven!

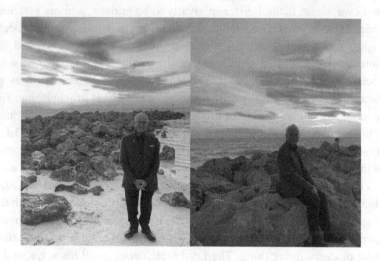

As I reflect in life change as a result of COVID-19 while the second year is rolling and almost coming to an end with no cure of this horrific pandemic and continue to threaten mankind and humanity risking the world's peace and prosperity!!

I found in the world 🌍, there is no longer comfort but only the nature and the world 🌍 has no truth but the nature! It is time to move to the very original and untouched nature leaving COVID-19 behind and all its siblings of waves and mutations! There is no reason to struggle and suffer being subjected to man-made disasters and pollutions leading to self-destruction!

I ran away to escape from the world 🌍 to be with my Savior by the nature! Yes walking in native land and living by the nature as it was created mingling with the nature and take oneself away by the waters and the seaside, between the sun ☀ rise and sunset 🌄, between the seas and sky, between the heaven and earth, between the sun rise and sun set, between the day and the night, between the daylight and the nighttime, between the smooth breeze and the high winds, between the flat ground and the rocks, between the sands and the rocks, between the earthquakes and and the erupted volcanos, —-. One day I sat by the sands, other days I sat over the rocks and many other days, I pulled a chair made of tree wood and looked around praising the Lord of nature thanking His Majesty and praising His Name! My eyes never got tired looking at the sky and the clouds, the moving branches and leaves, the beautiful garden by the rive and the grass and the fruits. My ears never got sick hearing the birds, the parrots, crow, hummingbirds, columbidea, owls, dove, sparrows, peacock, pigeon, goose, stark, seagull, flamingo, robin, ostrich, and eagle.

Looking around, the eyes sea the fingers of God and the power of His Almighty Hand. The sky has no end so is God creation! My joy of the nature is endless. It turns on my mind to meditate in my Lord and His creation more and more! My thoughts do not stop ⬤ pouring so is my pen ✏ not stop ⬤ writing ✍. Being in nature, my space is unlimited since the sky is my roof and the church is made of the woods of expensive trees and the covers are made of leaves and the church full of prayers and praises! The atmosphere around is Peace and quiescence.

The universe and the earth planet 🌍 are full of so much beauty and always they are cheer givers. Many are cyclic and predictor for now and many others are unpredictable. These are only few I remember and at the tip of my tongue including: the Sunset 🌆 and the Sunrise 🌄, the Earth and the Heaven, the Sand and the Waters, the Dry Land and the Seas, the Land and the Clouds, the Fields and the Mountains, the Desert and the Grass, the Harsh Waves and the Soft Breeze, the Tornados and Sunny Clear Sky, the Earthquakes and Stability, the Volcanos and the Quiescence, the City Noise and the Tranquility, the Disruption and Production, Nightmares and Deep Sleep, Yellow Dry Leaves and Green Healthy Trees, Famine and Rains, Polluted Air and Fresh Air, Sadness and Joy, Failure and Success, Violence and Harmony, Wars and Peace, Irritability and Calmness, Negative Energy and Positive Energy, Poverty and Richness, Scarce and Abundance, Emptiness and Wealth, Ruddiness and Polity,

Living is in serenity and solitude governed by Nature. Time spend is in breathing fresh air and pure of all viruses. At times be in hand manual laboring and other times in walking, hiking, climbing, and swimming! Having innumerable hours in reflection, meditation with praises and prayers. I find constant blessing, rejuvenation and descending gifts with renewed energy as God renew His promises every morning! Furthermore, because of the God given plasticity and adaptation, my body acquired strength, natural senses, clear eyes, sharp ears and echoic voice!

COVID made me renew my vows to God created nature and the unlimited Universe staying far away from all man-made tools, self-centered industry and self absorbed creation. Indeed, mankind always find his refuge in the God created nature! And this is still hold true in the era of increased knowledge, artificial intelligence, wireless technology, data acquisition, informatics and robats!!! Even if man formed the higher tower of Babylon or living under the undefeated Roman empire, or protected by the Spanish colony, no matter what generation man live in, empire ruled by, kings and queens, decades and centuries, it is a reminder to the grandiose ego of human-being, from dust was formed and to dust shall return!! taken: for dust thou art, and unto dust shalt thou return: from nature came and to nature shall wander all his life. As it is written:

"And unto Adam he said, Because thou hast hearkened unto the voice of thy wife, and hast eaten of the tree, of which I commanded thee, saying, Thou shalt not eat of it: cursed is the ground for thy sake; in sorrow shalt thou eat of it all the days of thy life; [18] Thorns also and thistles shall it bring forth to thee; and thou shalt eat the herb of the field; [19] In the sweat of thy face shalt thou eat bread, till thou return unto the ground; for out of it wast thou taken: for dust thou art, and unto dust shalt thou return." Genesis 3:17-19 KJV

Perhaps the early days of our father Adam and mother Eve return back. The world 🌍 will be the new garden of Eden and the Heavenly Father in its midst. There will be no more man-made troubles, disasters and destruction!! God and His untouched universe should rule over me! I shall walk among the trees, rivers, greens, flying birds, creeping beasts and living creatures under the seas!! I am going away to the nature and I don't mind the harshness of the universe. I carry the Holy Bible knowing with tribulations there are blessing and joy. I would rather escape with Jonah in the big fish and be swallowed by the whales for three days. I would rather go camping barefeeted with my father Moses unto the desert of Siani for forty years and climb with my father Moses up to the mountain. I remember the days of God appearances in the clouds with holiness of His Tabernacle in the midst of the desert! What about the natural food of Mana and waters emanating from the rocks full of minerals and nutrients,

In those very early days, there was no viruses 💊 illness and sickness never existed! What a joy to drift with imagination and slip to dream the early days of creation of mankind as it is described: "And God created great whales, and every living creature that moveth, which the waters brought forth abundantly, after their kind, and every winged fowl after his kind: and God saw that it was good. [22] And God blessed them, saying, Be fruitful, and multiply, and fill the waters in the seas, and let fowl multiply in the earth. [23] And the evening and the morning were the fifth day. [24] And God said, Let the earth bring forth the living creature after his kind, cattle, and creeping thing, and beast of the earth after his kind: and it was so. [25] And God made the beast of the earth after his kind, and cattle after their kind, and every thing that creepeth upon the earth after his kind: and God saw that it was good. [26] And God said, Let us make man in our image, after our likeness: and let them have dominion over the fish of the sea, and over the fowl of the air, and over the cattle, and over all the earth, and over every creeping thing that creepeth upon the earth. [27] So God created man in his own image, in the image of God created he him; male and female created he them. [28] And God blessed them, and God said unto them, Be fruitful, and multiply, and replenish the earth, and subdue it: and have dominion over the fish of the sea, and over the fowl of the air, and over every living thing that moveth upon the earth. [29] And God said, Behold, I have given you every herb bearing seed, which is upon the face of all the earth, and every tree, in the which is the fruit of a tree yielding seed; to you it shall be for meat. [30] And to every beast of the earth, and to every fowl of the air, and to every thing that creepeth upon the earth, wherein there is life, I have given every green herb for meat: and it was so. [31] And God saw every thing that he had made, and, behold, it was very good. And the evening and the morning were the sixth day." Genesis 1:21-31 KJV

"And the Lord God planted a garden eastward in Eden; and there he put the man whom he had formed. [9] And out of the ground made the Lord God to grow every tree that is pleasant to the sight, and good for food; the tree of life also in the midst of the garden, and the tree of knowledge of good and evil. [10] And a river went out of Eden to water the garden; and from thence it was parted, and became into four heads. [11] The name of the first is Pison: that is it which compasseth the whole land of Havilah, where there is gold; [12] And the gold of that land is good: there is bdellium and the onyx stone. [13] And the name of the second river is Gihon: the same is it that compasseth the whole land of Ethiopia. [14] And the name of the third river is Hiddekel: that is it which goeth toward the east of Assyria. And the fourth river is Euphrates. [15] And the Lord God took the man, and put him into the garden of Eden to dress it and to keep it." Genesis 2:8-15 KJV

God the Almighty is in control regardless of man doing!! While evolving from the nightmares of COVID-19 and escaping to find the Lord in the mountains, the seas and the virgin lands all alone, it is good to remember the words in Laminations: "This I recall to my mind, therefore have I hope. [22] It is of the Lord's mercies that we are not consumed, because his compassions fail not. [23] They are new every morning: great is thy faithfulness. [24] The Lord is my portion, saith my soul; therefore will I hope in him. [25] The Lord is good unto them that wait for him, to the soul that seeketh him. [26] It is good that a man should both hope and quietly wait for the salvation of the Lord. [27] It is good for a man that he bear the yoke in his youth. [28] He sitteth alone and keepeth silence, because he hath borne it upon him. [29] He putteth his mouth in the dust; if so be there may be hope. [30] He giveth his cheek to him that smiteth him: he is filled full with reproach. [31] For the Lord will not cast off for ever: [32] But though he cause grief, yet will he have compassion according to the multitude of his mercies." Lamentations 3:21-32 KJV

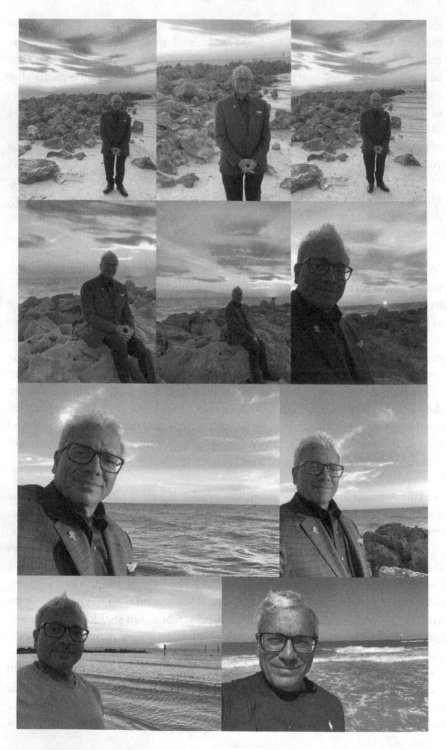

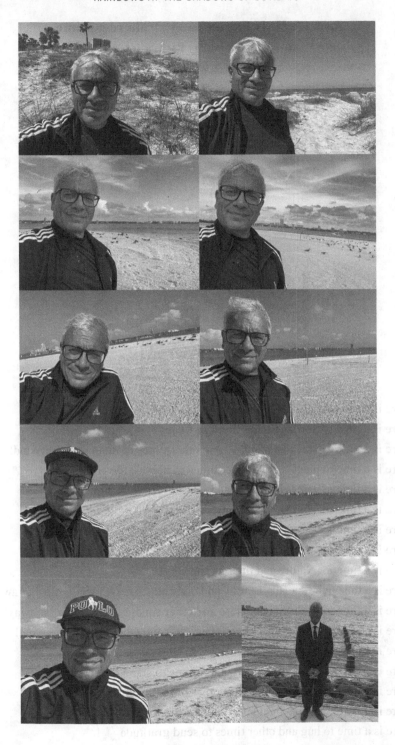

As COVID is fading away: "There is Time to—-and Other Times to—"
Written by Ramsis Ghaly

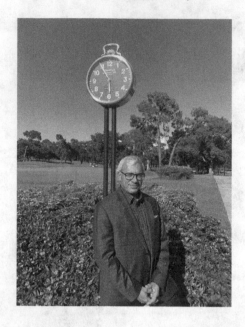

There is a time for virtual zoom in and other times for In-Person!
There is a time to Sow and other times to Reap!
There is a time to Sow the Wind 🌱 and other times to Reap the whirlwind!
There is a time to plant 🌱 and other times to harvest the crop!
There is a time to gather in groups and other times for solitudes!
There is a time to labor and other times to rest!
There is a time for the self and other times for the other-selves!
There is a time to put on face mask and other times to take out face mask!
There is a time for Nature and time for the City!
There is a time to be socially near by and other times to be socially further away!
There is a time to be distancing close and other times to distancing far away!
There is a time to keep things to your heart 💜 and other times to vent out!
There is a time to step in and other times to step out!
There is a time to stand up 🆙 and other times to stand back!
There is a time for sunrise 🌅 and another time for sunset 🌆!
There is a time to for daylight and another time for night time!
There is a time to hug and other times to send gratitude 🙏!

22

There is a time to kiss the lips 👄 and other times to send the kisses!

There is a time to laugh 😄 and others times to cry!

There is a time for joy and other times for sorrows!

There is a time to joke and other times to be serious!

There is a time to think and meditate and other times perform and do!

There is a time to speak out and other times to be silent!

There is a time to talk and other times to listen!

There is a time to study and other times to go out!

There is a time to learn and other times to be taught!

There is a time to be a student and other times to be a teacher!

There is a time to lead and other times to be lead!

There is a time to be in the drive seat and other times to be in the passenger seat!

There is a time to walk and other times to race!

There is a time to climb 🧗 and other times to make foot steps!

There is a time to cruise 🚢 and others times to fly above the clouds!

There is a time to land and other times to fly!

There is a time to be in the waters and other times to walk by shore side!

There is a time to fast and other times to eat!

There is a time to play and other times to work!

There is a time to host and other times to be a guest!

There is a tine to dress VIP suit and other times to put on heavy labor cloth!

There is a time to sit at the head of the table and other times to sit at the foot of the table!

There is a time to be on the power seat and others times to be on the regular seat!

There is a time to render love 🖤 to another and other times to be loved!

Nonetheless

There are All the times to Love 🖤 and to Pray!

There is always a time to do good and to serve!

There always a time to help, reach out and be cheerful giver!

There is all the time to appreciate life and living!

There is all the time to be thankful and praise the Heavenly Father!

There is no time to be unfaithful, unloving, unforgiving, lose hope, lose control, do evil 😈 or join the darkness!

Respectfully

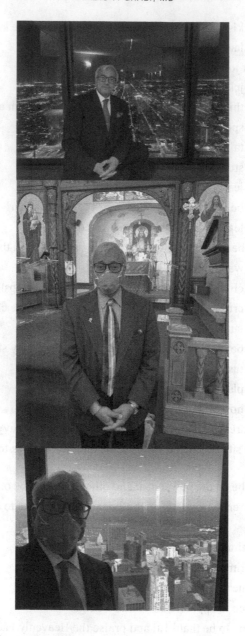

CG. Great words!

Divine Humanity is in These Neurons!

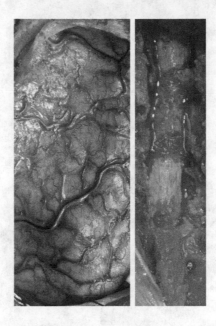

As a Neurosurgeon, I get the honor and privilege to be in God's territory of the most entrust core of Divine Humanity!

The secret of God to mankind is in the invisible human brain and spinal cord!

Divine Humanity is within these Neurons and the soul of the spirit!

They are in order, invisible, inseparable and connects the human soul with the Spirit!

All the connections and communications are wireless, unseen and virtual between earth and heaven!

Ramsis Ghaly
Www.ghalyneurosurgeon.com

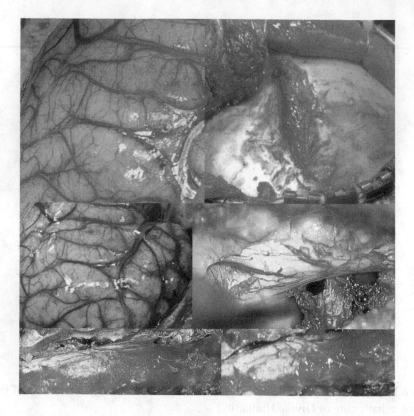

JJ. Wow! That's amazing to see.

MP. Speak truth brother! Thank you.

LR. I remember those "crani's" well. My mother had 3 very long ones during her lifetime. My OR nursing friends in surgery took excellent care of her during each one. I found the brain fascinating each time I had been assigned a "crani"

SK. Amazing!

CC. Amazing!

MR. Amazing

BV. May God bless you

AB. Amazing!!

RH. How complicated

SJ. That was beautifully expressed

AE. Beautiful 🤩

JU. Amazing!

DB. God bless you daily in His miracles!

LG. Everything about the human body is a miracle-every second of every day.

AOP. Looking at those pictures I see God at work

KE. If all doctors had true relationships with Jesus and truly loved their work/ career then our health and world would a better place. May God continue to bless you and your healing hands!

JD. You are a special, gifted Doctor; my friend!

CL. You are one of God's miracles. Thank you for helping so many people have better lives. 😇🙏😊

CT. Awesome

CS. God Bless you!

GS. Many blessings brother 👋

Disabled Yet Genius and Impaired Yet Brilliant

Written by Ramsis Ghaly

It is subject close to my heart and I feel I can describe and discuss very well. This isn't I am a genius but I am much below average. But some of the gifts have raised so much troubles for me throughout my years since I was a small baby in all stages of life!

Impaired and physically disabled yet with genius brain and brilliant mind. But why people with major disability and handicapped can have genius brain with superhuman gifts and exceptional brilliance in certain tasks?

Many of those are living among us and made the schools and community around them puzzled and shocked in the same time. But not their parents since they have seen their distinguished gifts and watered them as young as few months and years of age to grow and flourish all the way. Examples are as recent as such Patrick Henry Hughes(multi instrumental musician born without eyes and very defective limbs, Jacob Barnett (born with severe mutism, genius in physics, mathematics computational mind and Kim Peek (exceptional memory born with defective brain lacking corpus callosum and cerebellum). Adam Riess. He was always unusually creative and skipped a grade in school, she says. In 2011, he became one of the youngest people to ever win Nobel prize in physics for his work universe is expanding at an accelerated rate. Benacerraf struggled on standardized tests. She was more successful absorbing information by studying charts and graphs than by reading the text, a gift in imaging and pattern recognition like you have. It's uncanny," She could see something that other people could not see on the visual-spatial perspective, and things jumps out in a way that almost seems like magic. Stephen Hawking, one of the most accomplished physicists of our time, who happens to suffer from amyotrophic lateral sclerosis, or ALS. What you may not know is that Hawking isn't the only brilliant mind who has refused to be defined by his physical limitations. John Forbes Nash: Nash's thinking was inspirational in business and political strategizing, and he won a Nobel Prize in 1994 for his efforts based on a simple, one-page explanation of his theories. But Nash was also a diagnosed schizophrenic. Thomas Edison: One of our great fathers of electricity and the owner of over 1000 patents, Edison was a quantifiable genius. But a bout of scarlet fever as a youth had left him almost entirely deaf in both ears. Temple Grandin, Animal behaviorist and autism activist, who was diagnosed with autism as a child, received her master's in animal science and was as an inspiration for multiple changes to the livestock industry, including how animals are cared for at meat processing plants. Albert Einstein, dyslexic, yet If he's not the most famous intellectual in American history, he's certainly close. But Einstein's achievements in the fields of mathematics and physics didn't come without challenges. Suffering from a learning disability, that Einstein did not learn to talk until age four and was often confronted by teachers for his inability to grasp concepts as fast as other students. Ralf Braun, was diagnosed with muscular dystrophy. Braun was inventor and helped pioneer a series of revolutionary mobility-assistance devices, the world's first battery-powered scooter and wheelchair lift. Thanks to Braun, millions of physically-impaired individuals have been able to chart their own path in life. Geerat Vermeij, diagnosed with glaucoma as a child and blind since age 3, Paleontology a renowned expert on the history of life whose research has led to how fossils once interacted with the world at large. Vermeij's inspection of relics is by tactile feel: insight into evolution, absorbing detail of layers and shapes that might otherwise go unnoticed. Edwin Krebs, hearing impaired since childhood, Nobel prize-winning biochemist Krebs made a sensational discovery in the 1950s about cellular activity in the human body that led to know about hormones, cell life spans, and even how the body can reject transplanted organs. Leonardo Da Vinci, dyslexic, obtained a master of art, mathematics, astronomy, and dozens of other pursuits, da Vinci's inventions went on to inspire hundreds of years' worth of ingenuity. Much of his handwriting was composed in reverse. Richard Leaky A notable paleontologist, Leakey is famous for his discovery of near-complete bone sets and his conservationist efforts in his native Kenya. He was involved in a crash led to the cutting of both his legs below the knee. After recovering, Leakey resumed efforts to rework Kenya's constitution in order to better serve its people. Gustav Kirchhoff, Physicist Kirchhoff's work in the 1800s is to our understanding of electricity today. Born with unknown disability that restricted his movement to a wheelchair or crutches for most of his life. Later, Kirchhoff's of the sun's spectrum contributed to new discoveries in astronomy. Farida Bedwei, cerebral palsy at one years old, Software engineer has been hailed as one of South Africa's most important figures in financial technology, pioneering cloud platforms that have helped make small loan decisions available to consumers across the world immediately. Charles German-born Steinmetz made pioneering contributions to electrical engineering, with theories about power loss how direct and alternating currents were developed. Steinmetz was also afflicted with kyphosis, a congenital curvature of the spine.

The known list go on and the unknowns are so many and remained buried in their societies.

Prodigy child has a brain of an adult expert brain! Before the first decade, the child brain ready for college! The prodigy brain can comprehend, process and retain adult textbooks in no time. Yet, the prodigy brain autistic and has limited social skills, no desire for social gathering or make friends, lacking nonverbal communication, and being clumsy (Asperger's syndrome). The community reviewed the prodigy child as eccentric genius with bright human brain, mentally disordered with high intelligence Isaac Newton, Michelangelo, George Orwell, Jan Austen, Mozart and Beethoven —

Fourteen per cent of intellectually gifted children may also have a learning disability, compared to four per cent of the general population! It is usually heartbreaking when the parents get to know that their child is called by legal and medical terminology disabled and handicapped. Many parents get a very and done start to blame each other for the reason why their child became handicapped! Who fault is this and the anger continues pointing fingers. Yet most of the time the love of the parents particularly the mothers overshadow all these shortcoming!

However some parents may entertain thoughts of getting rid of the handicapped children, ignoring, neglecting, and torture the disabled child. As if it is their faults! This article and post remind these parents and the society that these children are gifts and never look down at them, treat them like all other children, be conscious they are sensitive kids! Don't ever think once to get ride of those named disabled child. These children are the sons and daughters of Adam and Eve with the same human rights as all other human being!

The prodigy children are exposed to bullying by other children. They are perceived by their the other children so called "normal" as vulnerable and handicapped. So the Prodigy children may get harm, intimidate, or coerced. It almost considered incompatible when you have minds of extreme gab put them in one class under the roof of one school. Friction, jealousy and unease will eveolve. As if they are from different planet! Since the prodigy children are genius in certain subjects, the other children become jealous of them. The prodigy children are much mature and adult in their thought! They almost feel choked and restrained to sit or be part of immature kids!

However the so called normal kids. The normal children won't understand them and vice verse. The children don't know any better and the struggle and bullying between each other. They are then pulled out of the school to private tutoring and psychotherapy!

What about those among us but unknown and their potentials were buried and lived undiscovered until they departed from our world without acknowledging their superb potentials. The end result, the world lost what they could have offered mankind. These talented individuals come scarce and all over the world. They are in the richest regions as well as in the poorest regions of the world equally distributed! They are being ignored, neglected, rejected and oppressed, partly because of the overwhelming disability and handicapped and partly because of their ignorance, lack of knowledge and limited resources and increase cost. Furthermore, these prodigy children and young adults, because of their genius status, over achievers and brilliance, can be a source of intimidation, jealousy and threatening among the norms. They are in constant need of protection and surveillance. Education and Awareness and ensure awareness and elevated awareness are the keys to address these issues. In fact, it is not their fault to be genius and it isn't under their control! The world owe to reach out to them! All those individuals worldwide, among us, unknown, undiscovered. Let us search for them! let the world and other countries take them and host them in a better environment with much respect and dignity!

DISCUSSION

Perhaps one of the best verses describes those individuals categorized as disabled in the eyes of men yet their human brains are genius in other aspects with brilliant gifts is: "And he said unto me, My grace is sufficient for thee: for my strength is made perfect in weakness. Most gladly therefore will I rather glory in my infirmities, that the power of Christ may rest upon me." 2 Corinthians 12:9 KJV. Indeed God glory appears in the weakness of man and lowly. The impossible of man is possible of God. As it is written: "And he said, The things which are impossible with men are possible with God." Luke 18:27 KJV God can raise up new human brains out of stones as said: "And think not to say within yourselves, We have Abraham to our father: for I say unto you, that God is able of these stones to raise up children unto Abraham." Matthew 3:9 KJV

In fact perhaps man is wrong and science is foolish to define them as disabled. It is written: "Let no man deceive himself. If any man among you seemeth to be wise in this world, let him become a fool, that he may be wise. [19] For the wisdom of this world is foolishness with God. For it is written, He taketh the wise in their own craftiness. [20] And again, The Lord knoweth the thoughts of the wise, that they are vain." 1 Corinthians 3:18-20 KJV

31

Indeed science thus far failed to explain exactly how the prodigy brains being transformed and achieve superhuman function status. The psychologists came up with assumptions and various theories based in close observations. Yet to find a diagnostic test or ways to study their brains microscopically and at the cell level. Even autopsy and section their brains at the laboratory after their death revealed minimal information! The reason and the way, how, why —- for **Disabled Yet Genius and Impaired Yet Brilliant, remain largely hidden and unknown. Science isn't there yet and these individuals are not being accepted and looked upon as odd, strange, unique, not normal,—-**

But it shouldn't be so among us. Not knowing the process during which their brains become brilliance such as matt and music prodigy, isn't excuse to be frustrated and not recognize them as part of us and they are also regular human being, the sons and daughters of Adam and Eve. But also God choose those disabled individual at the eyes of the world to confound the wise, to confound the things which are mighty by men. God made in us: God is made unto us wisdom, and righteousness, and sanctification, and redemption: [31] That, according as it is written, He that glorieth, let him glory in the Lord. As it is written: "Because the foolishness of God is wiser than men; and the weakness of God is stronger than men. [26] For ye see your calling, brethren, how that not many wise men after the flesh, not many mighty, not many noble, are called: [27] But God hath chosen the foolish things of the world to confound the wise; and God hath chosen the weak things of the world to confound the things which are mighty; [28] And base things of the world, and things which are despised, hath God chosen, yea, and things which are not, to bring to nought things that are: [29] That no flesh should glory in his presence. [30] But of him are ye in Christ Jesus, who of God is made unto us wisdom, and righteousness, and sanctification, and redemption: [31] That, according as it is written, He that glorieth, let him glory in the Lord." 1 Corinthians 1:25-31 KJ

Being genius in the world means mentally disabled. Perhaps the reasons of being genius is faulty developed or impaired development as examined by the normal human so called scientists! Indeed the uncontrolled capacity of glows within the neural network produce flow of ideas ... divergent ideas, unusual ideas" that can lead to creativity and innovation, and much more. These supernatural gifts can't be measured with normal human scales or assessed by normal human brain. They are extraordinary human brains and the man-made society any extraordinary or odd behaviors are considered illness, impairment and disability. Those exceptional qualities and abilities including remarkable memory, recall, power house of talents, matt and science prodigy, genius, mastermind, creative, innovative, —-

Those impaired individuals with genius gifts are usually struggling with standard schooling and testing and living in matters similar to the so called norms. And when they are asked, they don't know why they are superhuman in their own gifts other than: these fluency and extraordinary ways just jump out in a way that almost seems like magic, indescribable and unspeakable. It almost appear Spiritual words and unusual Spiritual gifts from above outside the physical brain within the skull!!

It isn't normal to be genius! It isn't decent to be highly intelligent! It isn't socially accepted to be superhuman! It is considered to be so odd to be above everyone else in knowledge, understanding and achievement! Those with mental health disorders, learning disability, dyslexia, autism, schizophrenia, cerebral palsy and physical infirmity somehow transformed to brilliance and many became overachiever greatest authors, artists and figures in history, such as Albert Einstein, Ernest Hemingway and Charles Darwin.

But why a physically impaired and disabled human being become genius, brilliant and superhuman in the same time?? Perhaps the quick answer because is because we don't know and science and behavior health judge them wrongly since there isn't any known measurable quantitate scale fir their genius mental abilities! Simply they are off the human chart! Since they are out of normal standard deviation, human scale therefore call them odd, disabled!

Some of my theories of these genius human brains and brilliance are as follows:

1) Brain potentials to survive in the harsh world and sharpen the existing talents and their related circuits while taking the energy away from the list circuits!!
2) Create new high speed bypasses and generate high ways and free ways to absorb, process, retain and execute genius tasks
3) Inherited Human brain plasticity at the early years of life with unlimited plasticity, reformation and creation for superhuman potentials
4) Human brain and human body can be disabled in certain aspects, underdeveloped in others but over developed in the few developed task oriented!
5) The infantile human brain had the capacity to suppress the disabled circuits and use them for the new developed circuits to the Benefits of ongoing developed superhuman gifts! So the human brain exert majority of efforts of exploring and enhancing strengths but not in the negative shortcoming. It almost appear such a human brain bridge from the physical brain capacity to

the spiritual partner of the disabled physical human brain and accelerate in gaining the spiritual unseen talents!

6) Stealing phenomenon of the nutrients and the genetic inherited stem cells of the disabled circuits and redirect them with unique features to the newly formed seeds! The end result aberrant but very fast neuronal network to process and execute with storage capacity of unlimited information

7) Develop early on not the physical impaired brain within the skull but the invisible unseen outside the skull. And take the wireless outside network all the way up high where the sky is the limit!

8) God looks from heaven to lowly and disabled and search for those with infirmity and so called disabilities in the human eyes and breath upon them superhuman creation as Jesus did to all those born with disabilities when He was in the flesh! In fact the Holy Spirit is always connected to the human brain and can enter and dine and the human brain becomes hone to the holy Spirit supernatural gifts and talents once the human subject let the Spirit!

It won't be the first time to change the course of the human brain after being born. For instance the Holy Spirit raised Solomon human brain to supernatural brain with absolutely no human brain like Solomon's brain. Solomon brain without going to new schooling or training or tutoring instantly inherited wisdom and honor and much more than any brain on the face of earth from the beginning to the end of ages as it is described: "I have given thee a wise and an understanding heart; so that there was none like thee before thee, neither after thee shall any arise like unto thee. [13] And I have also given thee that which thou hast not asked, both riches, and honour: so that there shall not be any among the kings like unto thee all thy days. "It is written: "In Gibeon the Lord appeared to Solomon in a dream by night: and God said, Ask what I shall give thee. [6] And Solomon said, Thou hast shewed unto thy servant David my father great mercy, according as he walked before thee in truth, and in righteousness, and in uprightness of heart with thee; and thou hast kept for him this great kindness, that thou hast given him a son to sit on his throne, as it is this day. [7] And now, O Lord my God, thou hast made thy servant king instead of David my father: and I am but a little child: I know not how to go out or come in. [8] And thy servant is in the midst of thy people which thou hast chosen, a great people, that cannot be numbered nor counted for multitude. [9] Give therefore thy servant an understanding heart to judge thy people, that I may discern between good and bad: for who is able to judge this thy so great a people? [10] And the speech pleased the Lord, that Solomon had asked this thing. [11] And God said unto him, Because thou hast asked this thing, and hast not asked for thyself long life; neither hast asked riches for thyself, nor hast asked the life of thine enemies; but hast asked for thyself understanding to discern judgment; [12] Behold, I have done according to thy words: lo, I have given thee a wise and an understanding heart; so that there was none like thee before thee, neither after thee shall any arise like unto thee. [13] And I have also given thee that which thou hast not asked, both riches, and honour: so that there shall not be any among the kings like unto thee all thy days. [14] And if thou wilt walk in my ways, to keep my statutes and my commandments, as thy father David did walk, then I will lengthen thy days." 1 Kings 3:5-14 KJV

What about Jesus disciples and all those were in house when the Holy Ghost descended upon them and instantly their human brains were speaking tongues and marvelous wonders prophecy and dream dreams as described: they were all filled with the Holy Ghost, and began to speak with other tongues, as the Spirit gave them utterance— I will pour out of my Spirit upon all flesh: and your sons and your daughters shall prophesy, and your young men shall see visions, and your old men shall dream dreams: [18] And on my servants and on my handmaidens I will pour out in those days of my Spirit; and they shall prophesy: [19] And I will shew wonders in heaven above, and signs in the earth beneath; blood, and fire, and vapour of smoke—It is written; "And suddenly there came a sound from heaven as of a rushing mighty wind, and it filled all the house where they were sitting. [3] And there appeared unto them cloven tongues like as of fire, and it sat upon each of them. [4] And they were all filled with the Holy Ghost, and began to speak with other tongues, as the Spirit gave them utterance. [7] And they were all amazed and marvelled, saying one to another, Behold, are not all these which speak Galilaeans? [11] Cretes and Arabians, we do hear them speak in our tongues the wonderful works of God. [13] Others mocking said, These men are full of new wine. [16] But this is that which was spoken by the prophet Joel; [17] And it shall come to pass in the last days, saith God, I will pour out of my Spirit upon all flesh: and your sons and your daughters shall prophesy, and your young men shall see visions, and your old men shall dream dreams: [18] And on my servants and on my handmaidens I will pour out in those days of my Spirit; and they shall prophesy: [19] And I will shew wonders in heaven above, and signs in the earth beneath; blood, and fire, and vapour of smoke: [20] The sun shall be turned into darkness, and the moon into blood, before that great and notable day of the Lord come: [21] And it shall come to pass, that whosoever shall call on the name of the Lord shall be saved." Acts 2:2-4,7,11,13,16-21 KJV

Notice that the superhuman gifts were implemented unto the human brain instantly without tutoring or learning or schooling! The superhuman gifts weren't physical or made of matters or has limited capacity but wireless boundless, go through boundaries transparent —-. The Spiritual gifts are unutterable and inexplainable with diversities of gifts and operations as it is written: "Now concerning spiritual gifts, brethren, I would not have you ignorant. [4] Now there are diversities of

35

gifts, but the same Spirit. [6] And there are diversities of operations, but it is the same God which worketh all in all. [8] For to one is given by the Spirit the word of wisdom; to another the word of knowledge by the same Spirit; [9] To another faith by the same Spirit; to another the gifts of healing by the same Spirit; [10] To another the working of miracles; to another prophecy; to another discerning of spirits; to another divers kinds of tongues; to another the interpretation of tongues: [11] But all these worketh that one and the selfsame Spirit, dividing to every man severally as he will."1 Corinthians 12:1,4,6,8-11 KJV

These gifts are immeasurable and can't be traced or explained. It is all brain function and isn't other physical organs such as heart, lung, liver or skeletal muscles. They are purely intellectual originated from the human brain. Jesus said: "For the Holy Ghost shall teach you in the same hour what ye ought to say." Luke 12:12 KJV. In fact the Holy Spirit bring what is fir God to the Human brain, the Spirit of Truth, whom the world can't receive, and dwells in the human brain of the faithful and see Him and know Him but the world won't. It will teach, bring to remembrance, —as it is described: "And I will pray the Father, and he shall give you another Comforter, that he may abide with you for ever; [17] Even the Spirit of truth; whom the world cannot receive, because it seeth him not, neither knoweth him: but ye know him; for he dwelleth with you, and shall be in you. [26] But the Comforter, which is the Holy Ghost, whom the Father will send in my name, he shall teach you all things, and bring all things to your remembrance, whatsoever I have said unto you." John 14:16-17,26 KJV

The Unknowns Disabled but Brilliant Human Brains:

The fear is those individuals who are handicapped yet brilliant remain unknown. I guess those **unknowns are so many and remained buried in their societies.** What about those among us but unknown and their potentials were buried and lived undiscovered until they departed from our world without acknowledging their superb potentials. The end result, the world lost what they could have offered mankind. These talented individuals come scarce and all over the world. They are in the richest regions as well as in the poorest regions of the world equally distributed! They are being ignored, neglected, rejected and oppressed, partly because of the overwhelming disability and handicapped and partly because of their ignorance, lack of knowledge and limited resources and increase cost. Furthermore, these prodigy children and young adults, because of their genius status, over achievers and brilliance, can be a source of intimidation, jealousy and threatening among the norms. They are in constant need of protection and surveillance. Education and Awareness and ensure awareness and elevated awareness are the keys to address these issues. In fact, it is not their fault to be genius and it isn't under their control! The world owe to reach out to them! All those individuals worldwide, among us, unknown, undiscovered. Let us search for them! let the world and other countries take them and host them in a better environment with much respect and dignity!

The Unknowns Disabled but Brilliant Human Brains:

The concern is those individuals who are handicapped yet brilliant remain unknown. I guess those **unknowns are so many and remained buried in their societies.** What about those among us but unknown and their potentials were buried and lived undiscovered until they departed from our world without acknowledging their superb potentials. The end result, the world lost what they could have offered mankind. These talented individuals come scarce and all over the world. They are in the richest regions as well as in the poorest regions of the world equally distributed! They are being ignored, neglected, rejected and oppressed, partly because of the overwhelming disability and handicapped and partly because of their ignorance, lack of knowledge and limited resources and increase cost. Furthermore, these prodigy children and young adults, because of their genius status, over achievers and brilliance, can be a source of intimidation, jealousy and threatening among the norms. They are in constant need of protection and surveillance. Education and Awareness and ensure awareness and elevated awareness are the keys to address these issues. In fact, it is not their fault to be genius and it isn't under their control! The world owe to reach out to them! All those individuals worldwide, among us, unknown, undiscovered. Let us search for them! let the world and other countries take them and host them in a better environment with much respect and dignity!

Ancient Brains

Ancient Human Brains were Naturally Talented and inherited Brilliant Compared to Modern Brains!!

As the disabled individuals challenge their brains to maximum and earn brilliance so were the ancient human brains! The earlier ancient human brains must have been of magnificent talents with superb unlimited potentials! At that time, the ancient man was dependent in his brain to navigate through the hard times of primitive years. At that time the human brain was independent and challenged to maximum. There was no artificial intelligence, calculators, or GPS, or digital technology or informactics to rely on. The labor was manual and nature was harsh and risky in those days. In contrary nowadays, the human brain is dependent in technology and other resources with no much of challenging times as in the ancient years. For instance, how brilliant the ancient human brains were, look into the Pyramids, the unsolved mystery. Out of nothing the Egyptian pharaoh were able to built the three genius pyramids of Giza over centuries and until today the modern human brain cannot explain. The modern brains are becoming stagnant status quo with not exposed to constant challenges, imposed demands and stimulation.

If this topic is teaching us a lesson, it is the unbelievable brilliance and potentials of the smallest organ in body 1500 gram human brain, hidden and protected from the outside by the rigid and stiff armed skull!! The human brain has unlimited potentials and isn't utilized to maximum capacity. In fact, the process of brain development is being hindered by technology and artificial intelligence. The human brain has inherited creativity and autonomy beyond imagination and isn't used. Subsequently, the modern human brain ⊘ is inferior to the Ancient Human Brain. The society must put stop ⬤ at converting human brains with great potentials to stagnant brains. The human brains must be challenged, used to maximum potentials and stimulated. Zoom in unto each brain gifts and let it grow to the unlimited capacity at early age and as early as it is discovered. Mothers know their babies so well and they are usually the very first individuals to diagnose, support, encourage and open the doors to promote their children unlimited brilliance! The schools, the churches and the society should do the same!

My Advice to the World:

Please never ever look down at your child and don't judge the human brain with human scale. Many are gifted human brains were send from God to make the world better place for all others including so called normal. The society should accept them and open the doors wide open to each of them to flourish and spread their gifts freely!

The schools and churches must recognize those children with extraordinary gifts, not to suppress them or medicate them but rather bring them close, love them, adore their gifts and cultivate the talents by supplying the good fertile ground! They are sent from above as gifts to the world!!

Being different with external features of retardation because of lack of social engagement and not being friendly, shouldn't be foundation of naming them socially unacceptable and mentally disabled with learning disability. It is harmful profiling!

Most importantly, the parents should never reject them, or refuse them, or belittle them, or disrespect them, or demean them or ignore them! But rather, the parents must hug them, accept them and surround them with love ♥! The parents must recognize, help them with workarounds for whatever the difficult issues are, and by utilizing their strength along with those workarounds, they are giving their child the opportunity to be highly successful! And the world shall watch the geniuses of God upon the human brain since they all are created the image of God and the Heavenly Father blessed them disabled and not disabled as it is written: "So God created man in his own image, in the image of God created he him; male and female created he them. [28] And God blessed them, and God said unto them, Be fruitful, and multiply, and replenish the earth, and subdue it: and have dominion over the fish of the sea, and over the fowl of the air, and over every living thing that moveth upon the earth." Genesis 1:27-28 KJV

God doesn't discriminate and send His gifts to all human brains in all the corners of the earth. As God taught us, He also make the sun rise over the just and unjust brains and the good and evil brains as it is written: "That ye may be the children of your Father which is in heaven: for he maketh his sun to rise on the evil and on the good, and sendeth rain on the just and on the unjust." Matthew 5:45 KJV

The world must open the doors wide open and bring them to their existence. Self-identity is crucial to nourish them and flourish their gifts. They are God sent to teach us, to bring what is for Him to us and they can explain His mysteries to His people! They can read the signs and interpret dreams as He previously gifted Joseph and Elijah. Joseph genius brain from God interpret the unsolved dreams as follows: "And Joseph said unto him, This is the interpretation of it: The three branches are three days: [13] Yet within three days shall Pharaoh lift up thine head, and restore thee unto thy place: and thou shalt deliver Pharaoh's cup into his hand, after the former manner when thou wasn't his butler." Genesis 40:12-13 KJV it was used to prepare Joseph for much important Divine message later on. And indeed, Joseph saved the earth for seven years through the genius gift from above given to him by God to send the Divine messages as follows: "And Joseph said unto Pharaoh, The dream of Pharaoh is one: God hath shewed Pharaoh what he is about to do. [26] The seven good kine are seven years; and the seven good ears are seven years: the dream is one. [27] And the seven thin and ill favoured kine that came up after them are seven years; and the seven empty ears blasted with the east wind shall be seven years of famine. [28] This is the thing which I have spoken unto Pharaoh: What God is about to do he sheweth unto Pharaoh. [29] Behold, there come seven years of great plenty throughout all the land of Egypt: [30] And there shall arise after them seven years of famine; and all the plenty shall be forgotten in the land of Egypt; and the famine shall consume the land; [31] And the plenty shall not be known in the land by reason of that famine following; for it shall be very grievous. [32] And for that the dream was doubled unto Pharaoh twice; it is because the thing is established by God, and God will shortly bring it to pass. [33] Now therefore let Pharaoh look out a man discreet and wise, and set him over the land of Egypt. [34] Let Pharaoh do this, and let him appoint officers over the land, and take up the fifth part of the land of Egypt in the seven plenteous years. [35] And let them gather all the food of those good years that come, and lay up corn under the hand of Pharaoh, and let them keep food in the cities. [36] And that food shall be for store to the land against the seven years of famine, which shall be in the land of Egypt; that the land perish not through the famine." Genesis 41:25-36 KJV

And similarly God gifted Daniel human brain with genius superhuman gifts as it is described: "As for these four children, God gave them knowledge and skill in all learning and wisdom: and Daniel had understanding in all visions and dreams." Daniel 1:17 KJV Daniel then interpreted the unsolved king's Nebuchadnezzar dream as follows: "Thou, O king, art a king of kings: for the God of heaven hath given thee a kingdom, power, and strength, and glory. [38] And wheresoever the children of men dwell, the beasts of the field and the fowls of the heaven hath he given into thine hand, and hath made thee ruler over them all. Thou art this head of gold. [39] And after thee shall arise another kingdom inferior to thee, and another third kingdom of brass, which shall bear rule over all the earth. [40] And the fourth kingdom shall be strong as iron: forasmuch as iron breaketh in pieces and subdueth all things: and as iron that breaketh all these, shall it break in pieces and bruise. [41] And whereas thou sawest the feet and toes, part of potters' clay, and part of iron, the kingdom shall be divided; but there shall be in it of the strength of the iron, forasmuch as thou sawest the iron mixed with miry clay. [42] And as the toes of the feet were part of iron, and part of clay, so the kingdom shall be partly strong, and partly broken. [43] And whereas thou sawest iron mixed with miry clay, they shall mingle themselves with the seed of men: but they shall not cleave one to another, even as iron is not mixed with clay. [44] And in the days of these kings shall the God of heaven set up a kingdom, which shall never be destroyed: and the kingdom shall not be left to other people, but it shall break in pieces and consume all these kingdoms, and it shall stand for ever. [45] Forasmuch as thou sawest that the stone was cut out of the mountain without hands, and that it brake in pieces the iron, the brass, the clay, the silver, and the gold; the great God hath made known to the king what shall come to pass hereafter: and the dream is certain, and the interpretation thereof sure. [46] Then the king Nebuchadnezzar fell upon his face, and worshipped Daniel, and commanded that they should offer an oblation and sweet odours unto him. [47] The king answered unto Daniel, and said, Of a truth it is, that your God is a God of gods, and a Lord of kings, and a revealer of secrets, seeing thou couldest reveal this secret." Daniel 2:37-47 KJV and "This is the interpretation, O king, and this is the decree of the most High, which is come upon my lord the king: [25] That they shall drive thee from men, and thy dwelling shall be with the beasts of the field, and they shall make thee to eat grass as oxen, and they shall wet thee with the dew of heaven, and seven times shall pass over thee, till thou know that the most High ruleth in the kingdom of men, and giveth it to whomsoever he will. [26] And whereas they commanded to leave the stump of the tree roots; thy kingdom shall be sure unto thee, after that thou shalt have known that the heavens do rule. [27] Wherefore, O king, let my counsel be acceptable unto thee, and break off thy sins by righteousness, and thine iniquities by shewing mercy to the poor; if it may be a lengthening of thy tranquillity." Daniel 4:24-27 KJV

Discrimination Against Prodigy Children

Those children aren't having it easy at all. Both the society and their immediate families tend to name them, profile them and be derogatory. This should never be permissible or allowed. This behavior must stop. They feel not appreciated, recognized and source of the surrounding of shame. It is usually heartbreaking when the parents get to know that their child is called by legal and medical terminology disabled and handicapped. Many parents get a very and done start to blame each other fur the reason why their child became handicapped! Who fault is this and the anger continues pointing fingers. Yet most of the time the love of the parents particularly the mothers overshadow all these shortcoming!

However some parents may entertain thoughts of getting rid of the handicapped children, ignoring, neglecting, and torture the disabled child. As if it is their faults! This article and post remind these parents and the society that these children are gifts and never look down at them, treat them like all other children, be conscious they are sensitive kids! Don't ever think once to get rid of those named disabled child. These children are the sons and daughters of Adam and Eve with the same human rights as all other human being!

Protect Prodigy Children From Bullying

The prodigy children are exposed to bullying by other children. They are perceived by their the other children so called "normal" as vulnerable and handicapped. So the Prodigy children may get harm, intimidate, or coerced. It almost considered incompatible when you have minds of extreme gab put them in one class under the roof of one school. Friction, jealousy and unease will evolve. As if they are from different planet! Since the prodigy children are genius in certain subjects, the other children become jealous of them. The prodigy children are much mature and adult in their thought! They almost feel choked and restrained to sit or be part of immature kids!

However the so called normal kids. The normal children won't understand them and vice verse. The children don't know any better and the struggle and bullying between each other. They are then pulled out of the school to private tutoring and psychotherapy!

Unknown Impaired Yet Genius

The Unknowns Disabled but Brilliant Human Brains:

The fear is those individuals who are handicapped yet brilliant remain unknown. I guess those **unknowns are so many and remained buried in their societies.** What about those among us but unknown and their potentials were buried and lived undiscovered until they departed from our world without acknowledging their superb potentials. The end result, the world lost what they could have offered mankind. These talented individuals come scarce and all over the world. They are in the richest regions as well as in the poorest regions of the world equally distributed! They are being ignored, neglected, rejected and oppressed, partly because of the overwhelming disability and handicapped and partly because of their ignorance, lack of knowledge and limited resources and increase cost. Furthermore, these prodigy children and young adults, because of their genius status, over achievers and brilliance, can be a source of intimidation, jealousy and threatening among the norms. They are in constant need of protection and surveillance. Education and Awareness and ensure awareness and elevated awareness are the keys to address these issues. In fact, it is not their fault to be genius and it isn't under their control! The world owe to reach out to them! All those individuals worldwide, among us, unknown, undiscovered. Let us search for them! let the world and other countries take them and host them in a better environment with much respect and dignity!

They are among us but unknown and their potentials were buried and lived undiscovered until they departed from our world without acknowledging their superb potentials. The end result, the world lost what they could have offered mankind. These talented individuals come scarce and all over the world. What about those born in poverty in remote villages and has no means to come out in the world! What about those born in countries with no opportunity but doctrine of oppression and no recognition or resources to manifest their talents and let them grow. Or they were discriminated against them and buried all their gifts. The answer is clear open the border and open the doors to receive them and give them the opportunity to grow!! Furthermore, elevate the Awareness awareness awareness worldwide to those exist among us yet remain unknown, undiscovered and oppressed. The developed rich country should reach out and gather those talents. The number of those impaired yet with extraordinary talents and brilliance are limited worldwide and their potential contribution is huge to serve mankind worldwide. Let us search for them and let the world and other countries take them and host them in a better environment with much respect and freedom, courage and love and they shall produce, thirty, sixty and hundred folds of those with so called normal brains: "But other fell into good ground, and brought forth fruit, some an hundredfold, some sixtyfold, some thirtyfold." Matthew 13:8 KJV

They were visitors born among us, profiled as disabled and they proof us wrong and became legends, contributors and extraordinary scientists. Their lifetime spent to serve and give and they were able to solve many mysteries while making our world for so called "normal people" much better place! The final result the world is much better place and much closer to the Divine Nature that visited and lived with us during the incarnation of the Son of God Jesus the Lord!

They come and go and gift our world with so much and bless our humanity and enforce the human brilliance even when they are considered

If this topic is teaching us a lesson, it is the unbelievable brilliance and potentials of the smallest organ in body 1500 gram human brain, hidden and protected from the outside by the rigid and stiff armed skull!! The human brain has unlimited potentials and isn't utilized to maximum capacity. In fact, the process of brain development is being hindered by technology and artificial intelligence. The human brain has inherited creativity and autonomy beyond imagination and isn't used. Subsequently, the modern human brain 🧠 is inferior to the Ancient Human Brain. The society must put stop ⬣ at converting human brains with great potentials to stagnant brains. The human brains must be challenged, used to maximum potentials and stimulated. Zoom in unto each brain gifts and let it grow to the unlimited capacity at early age and as early as it is discovered. Mothers know their babies so well and they are usually the very first individuals to diagnose, support, encourage and open the doors to promote their children unlimited brilliance! The schools, the churches and the society should do the same!

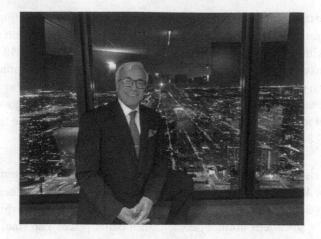

LW. The pictures are great! And so true. I had a brain tumor fixed by cyber knife in 2006. I had a large black spot they said would never fill in again. I also lost almost all the creative thinking. BUT the left side compensated. I started college (finished the 10th grade) maintained 4.0, homeschooling my kids and working full time. I started with first responder, EMT, Paramedic, registered nurse, BSN, and last year finished my masters and now an nurse practitioner. Oh and the black spot, it's filled in and I'm painting again. Also, maybe if you are disabled maybe your brain doesn't have to control the other parts and it just works on being a genius

JM. love your writings

LA. 🖤 AMEN and 🖤 AME!!N

Angels among us.... Angels among us.

⌐■♡☞.
(ˉOˉ)
./|. *
./|\\ .☆,.°*"~~"*°•.☆•.°*"~~"*°•. ♥

"Be not forgetful to entertain strangers:
for thereby some have entertained angels unawares."
~ Hebrews 13:2

AS. I love it

MH. You make an awesome Superman.

MH. Love 🐿 this picture of you. which building are you sitting in with this awesome view of the city?

BL. AMEN! Everyone could learn much necessary information from your article. I wish they would and pay heed.

Thank you for an insightful message.

You are such a wonderful blessing. This article is written by such an amazing man, neurosurgeon, teacher, writer, lover of mankind...he is an phenomenal blessing

Julian visited my office today. Genius child yet blind since birth. He loves Jesus so much. He and Renee Colosi read my post. I prayed with Julian and I told him about new research to restore sight for blind. He sat with me by our Lord Jesus framed. And he will start to use his geniuses into restoring sight for the blind children

Julian prayers with me and Renee, his words: "I believe Jesus the Lord can heal the blind and hep me to find a cure for the blind children in Jesus might name. Amen"

Ramsis Ghaly

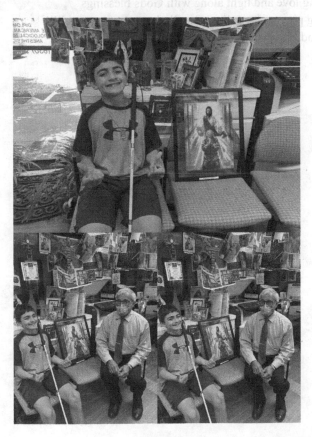

Julian Ellis
Dr Ghaly this Julián thank you for praying with me today. I listened to your
message using voiceover. I can't wait to study the new research to restore sight
and see what I can do to help make this happen faster.

JM. Just "Sensational"!!!

RC. Lovely. Best of all. Julian and you!

CG. What a lovely boy! I pray with you both that his sight can be restored someday
soon. Bless him and you for caring about him and giving him hope. 🖤🙏

KO. That would be so awesome, best to all

AV. Thank u so much Dr Ghaly for this wonderful information! Our God is so
good! Praying for Julian! Such a great young boy! God Bless u both! 😊💚🙏

KG. How wonderful Dr. Ghaly. Hope you can help this sweet boy see!!!!

JK. If the lord wants it it will happen!!! & if the lord give the great lord a gift to
Dr. Ghaly to help give the boy sight than it's the lord's well!!!

LM. Sending love and light along with Gods blessings 🙏🙏🙏🖤

LM. Sending love and light along with Gods blessings 🙏🙏🙏🖤

BB. Sending prayers for Julian! Dr. Ghaly, you at an angel!!!!

AS. May God bless you. You are a very special person. 🖤

The Ancient Human Brains were Superior to Modern Human Brains! Wake Up Call!!

Written by <u>Ramsis Ghaly</u>

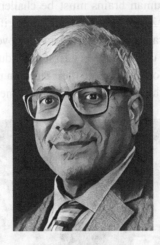

Ancient Human Brains were Naturally Talented and inherited Brilliant Compared to Modern Brains!!

As the disabled individuals challenge their brains to maximum and earn brilliance so were the ancient human brains! The earlier ancient human brains must have been of magnificent talents with superb unlimited potentials! At that time, the ancient man was dependent in his brain to navigate through the hard times of primitive years. At that time the human brain was independent and challenged to maximum. There was no artificial intelligence, calculators, or GPS, or digital technology or informactics to rely on. The labor was manual and nature was harsh and risky in those days. In contrary nowadays, the human brain is dependent in technology and other resources with no much of challenging times as in the ancient years. For instance, how brilliant the ancient human brains were, look into the Pyramids, the unsolved mystery. Out of nothing the Egyptian pharaoh were able to built the three genius pyramids of Giza over centuries and until today the modern human brain cannot explain. The modern brains are becoming stagnant status quo with not exposed to constant challenges, imposed demands and stimulation.

If this topic is teaching us a lesson, it is the unbelievable brilliance and potentials of the smallest organ in body 1500 gram human brain, hidden and protected from the outside by the rigid and stiff armed skull!! The human brain has unlimited potentials and isn't utilized to maximum capacity. In fact, the process of brain development is being hindered by technology and artificial intelligence. The human brain has inherited creativity and autonomy beyond imagination and isn't used. Subsequently, the modern human brain 🧠 is inferior to the Ancient Human Brain. The society must put stop ⬤ at converting human brains with great potentials to stagnant brains. The human brains must be challenged, used to maximum potentials and stimulated. Zoom in unto each brain gifts and let it grow to the unlimited capacity at early age and as early as it is discovered. Mothers know their babies so well and they are usually the very first individuals to diagnose, support, encourage and open the doors to promote their children unlimited brilliance! The schools, the churches and the society should do the same!

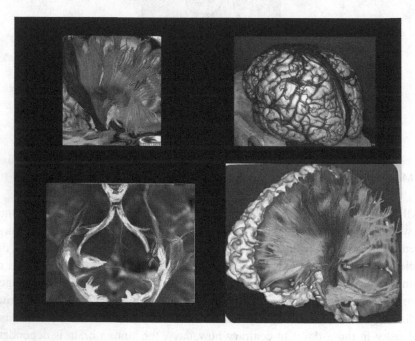

SC. Absolutely amazing

RC. Great post! We gave to learn so much of this

Jm. Yes Great article

JC. amen to that, thank you for sharing, interesting!! 🌸

JM. Yes

CL. Amazing! Thank you for sharing.

JE. well said, Dr. Ghaly!

I am as guilty as anyone. Instead of building on our knowledge with study, we just Google the answer.

CG. Another amazing informative article. Thank you for sharing.

Is the Human Subconscious Mind Intelligent?

Written by Ramsis Ghaly

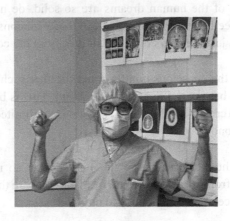

The Spiritual visions come as dreams at night!

But the regular day to day dreams have long been known to come from the human Subconscious Mind!

But the human subconscious mind isn't creative enough but rather a follower center and not a leader center!

Yet the subconscious mind is still considered the main source of human dreams!

From where then the human dreams originate? We have been told from the stored and already processed data cumulated over the years in the Subconscious Mind!

Furthermore, the subconscious mind has in its store so much experiences, emotions and hidden thoughts and desires and ambitions and various feelings associated with the persona and previous events! These opens up as well in the form of dreams at night ...and various feelings associated with the persona and previous events! These opens up as well in the form of dreams at night as well!

So does this mean that the human Subconscious Mind is able to think, process and form independently generating intelligent stories together without the conscious mind!

Can the human Subconscious Mind go outside the human skull and get sources from the outside world through wireless networking!

Many times these human dreams are kind of fabricated as if they are made in a fantasy Hollywood store!

Nonetheless, Some of the human dreams are so solid, de novo, complex and ordered to the degree it is very hard to believe that a subconscious mind create them all alone from just the years of stored of data from the conscious mind!

On the other hand, the conscious mind can put together such a fantastic highly intellectual dreams but not the Subconscious Mind! This is because the human conscious mind had creative ability and in addition to unlimited intelligence with completely free autonomy!

Many times these human dreams are left behind with so much unanswered questions? Not just from where they come from but what are their interpretations and their significance to our human day to day life!

But if the human subconscious mind is also independent and intelligent and is connected freely with higher sources including the conscious mind inside the skull and the outside spiritual networking, then indeed the subconscious mind can manufacture and produce genius human dreams! Many of those from the realistic world we live in and make much sense and many others from the futuristic world we shall live in!

But also within human dreams there are conversations taking place and dialogues between minds putting together plans and establishing rationales to the purpose and the cause of such dreams! In fact a dream usually is finished once a conclusion is inferred and an end had been reached between these invisible minds!! Otherwise, the dream transformed to a nightmare as a result of unsettled arguments between the minds and scary end!

So the human mind searches for its own dream source and meaning and usually gets no answer but theories and thoughts!

++Biblical Verses of Human Dreams

15 Samuel said to Saul, "Why have you disturbed me by bringing me up?" "I am in great distress," Saul said. "The Philistines are fighting against me, and God has

departed from me. He no longer answers me, either by prophets or by dreams. So I have called on you to tell me what to do." 1Samuel: 28:15

17 " 'In the last days, God says, I will pour out my Spirit on all people. Your sons and daughters will prophesy, your young men will see visions, your old men will dream dreams. Acts 2:17

17 To these four young men God gave knowledge and understanding of all kinds of literature and learning. And Daniel could understand visions and dreams of all kinds. Daniel 1:17

7 Much dreaming and many words are meaningless. Therefore fear God. Ecclesiastes 5:7

3 But God came to Abimelek in a dream one night and said to him, "You are as good as dead because of the woman you have taken; she is a married woman. Genesis 20:3

8 "We both had dreams," they answered, "but there is no one to interpret them." Then Joseph said to them, "Do not interpretations belong to God? Tell me your dreams. Genesis 40:8

8 In the morning his mind was troubled, so he sent for all the magicians and wise men of Egypt. Pharaoh told them his dreams, but no one could interpret them for him. 9 Then the chief cupbearer said to Pharaoh, "Today I am reminded of my shortcomings. 10 Pharaoh was once angry with his servants, and he imprisoned me and the chief baker in the house of the captain of the guard. 11 Each of us had a dream the same night, and each dream had a meaning of its own. 12 Now a young Hebrew was there with us, a servant of the captain of the guard. We told him our dreams, and he interpreted them for us, giving each man the interpretation of his dream. Genesis 41:8-12

14 For God does speak—now one way, now another— though no one perceives it. 15 In a dream, in a vision of the night, when deep sleep falls on people as they slumber in their beds, 16 he may speak in their ears and terrify them with warnings, 17 to turn them from wrongdoing and keep them from pride, 18 to preserve them from the pit, their lives from perishing by the sword. Job 33:14-18

9 Then he remembered his dreams about them and said to them, "You are spies! You have come to see where our land is unprotected." Genesis 42: 9

25 Then Joseph said to Pharaoh, "The dreams of Pharaoh are one and the same. God has revealed to Pharaoh what he is about to do. 26 The seven good cows are seven years, and the seven good heads of grain are seven years; it is one and the same dream. 27 The seven lean, ugly cows that came up afterward are seven years, and so are the seven worthless heads of grain scorched by the east wind: They are seven years of famine. Genesis 41:25-27

32 Indeed, I am against those who prophesy false dreams," declares the LORD. "They tell them and lead my people astray with their reckless lies, yet I did not send or appoint them. They do not benefit these people in the least," declares the LORD. Jeremiah 23:32

6 he said, "Listen to my words: "When there is a prophet among you, I, the LORD, reveal myself to them in visions, I speak to them in dreams. Numbers 12:6

2 The idols speak deceitfully, diviners see visions that lie; they tell dreams that are false, they give comfort in vain. Therefore the people wander like sheep oppressed for lack of a shepherd. Zechariah 10:2.

28 "And afterward, I will pour out my Spirit on all people. Your sons and daughters will prophesy, your old men will dream dreams, your young men will see visions. Joel 2:28

7 Then the hordes of all the nations that fight against Ariel, that attack her and her fortress and besiege her, will be as it is with a dream, with a vision in the night— 8 as when a hungry person dreams of eating, but awakens hungry still; as when a thirsty person dreams of drinking, but awakens faint and thirsty still. So will it be with the hordes of all the nations that fight against Mount Zion. Isiah 29: 7-8

1 In the first year of Belshazzar king of Babylon, Daniel had a dream, and visions passed through his mind as he was lying in bed. He wrote down the substance of his dream. 2 Daniel said: "In my vision at night I looked, and there before me were the four winds of heaven churning up the great sea. 3 Four great beasts, each different from the others, came up out of the sea. Daniel 7:1-3

1 If a prophet, or one who foretells by dreams, appears among you and announces to you a sign or wonder, 2 and if the sign or wonder spoken of takes place, and the prophet says, "Let us follow other gods" (gods you have not known) "and let us worship them," 3 you must not listen to the words of that prophet or dreamer. The LORD your God is testing you to find out whether you love him with all your heart and with all your soul. Deuteronomy 13:1-3

Acts 2:17 - And it shall come to pass in the last days, saith God, I will pour out of my Spirit upon all flesh: and your sons and your daughters shall prophesy, and your young men shall see visions, and your old men shall dream dreams:

Joel 2:28 - And it shall come to pass afterward, [that] I will pour out my spirit upon all flesh; and your sons and your daughters shall prophesy, your old men shall dream dreams, your young men shall see visions:

Amos 3:7 - Surely the Lord GOD will do nothing, but he revealeth his secret unto his servants the prophets.

1 John 4:1 - Beloved, believe not every spirit, but try the spirits whether they are of God: because many false prophets are gone out into the world.

Daniel 1:17 - As for these four children, God gave them knowledge and skill in all learning and wisdom: and Daniel had understanding in all visions and dreams.

Proverbs 29:18 - Where [there is] no vision, the people perish: but he that keepeth the law, happy [is] he.

Numbers 12:6 - And he said, Hear now my words: If there be a prophet among you, [I] the LORD will make myself known unto him in a vision, [and] will speak unto him in a dream.

20 But after he had considered this, an angel of the Lord appeared to him in a dream and said, "Joseph son of David, do not be afraid to take Mary home as your wife, because what is conceived in her is from the Holy Spirit. 21 She will give birth to a son, and you are to give him the name Jesus, because he will save his people from their sins." 22 All this took place to fulfill what the Lord had said through the prophet: 23 "The virgin will conceive and give birth to a son, and they will call him Immanuel" (which means "God with us"). Matthew 1:20-23

13 When they had gone, an angel of the Lord appeared to Joseph in a dream. "Get up," he said, "take the child and his mother and escape to Egypt. Stay there until I tell you, for Herod is going to search for the child to kill him." Matthew 2:13

19 After Herod died, an angel of the Lord appeared in a dream to Joseph in Egypt. Matthew 2:19

RH. This photograph should be titled "Success". Or" By Jove I've got It". 😄👍
🙏 Praise God amen

KE. Brilliant

ML. You're amazing Dr. Ghaly!

GR. God bless you

SJ. Yes, our dreams can connect us to God and can be prophetic. I love it when I have these days 🖤
Are you back to normal operating attire?.

PR. Good weekend to YOU.

MH. That is definitely a yes! God Bless you & keep you safe.

Cg. I believe dreams are as you said. Fabricated from things we see everyday or our stored memories. Excellent article! 🖤🙏

Act of Kindness is a Spiritual Treasure in Human Journey for Salvwation!!

As I look back to my fruitful years of my upbringing and decades in my career, I worked with so many and I came across many more!

They all gone but the memories last ranged of good and no so good experiences!

One thing is common among all was that each had to play his own game and his or her self was in its midst!

Nonetheless, what is still standing is the act of kindness and the self denial!

Indeed, if I rewind my days back, I would have focused my working days in those unselfish act of kindness!

My soul remember our Lord Jesus words: "Then shall the King say unto them on his right hand, Come, ye blessed of my Father, inherit the kingdom prepared for you from the foundation of the world: [35] For I was an hungred, and ye gave me meat: I was thirsty, and ye gave me drink: I was a stranger, and ye took me in: [36] Naked, and ye clothed me: I was sick, and ye visited me: I was in prison, and ye came unto me. [37] Then shall the righteous answer him, saying, Lord, when saw we thee an hungred, and fed thee ? or thirsty, and gave thee drink? [38] When saw we thee a stranger, and took thee in? or naked, and clothed thee ? [39] Or when saw we thee sick, or in prison, and came unto thee? [40] And the King shall answer and say unto them, Verily I say unto you, Inasmuch as ye have done it unto one of the least of these my brethren, ye have done it unto me." Matthew 25:34-40 KJV

The shameful memories were those spent in disputes, arguments and negativism!

The results of those day, I continue to ripe until today and perhaps until I die!

The other deeds carved in my memories those deeds I did eye for eye and teeth fir teeth!

I thought at that time I am doing good, being smart and outsmart the others taking advantage of the world the best I can do how!!! My daily mission, go after the powers and the wealth, don't stop cumulate more richness and boost up the ego!

I was blind, deaf and mute throughout those years! Now I criticize myself and past as I result the painful fact of life: O my soul naked to came to earth and naked you shall depart as my father Job said: "And said, Naked came I out of my mother's womb, and naked shall I return thither: the Lord gave, and the Lord hath taken away; blessed be the name of the Lord." Job 1:21 KJV

At those years, I was as a publicans and I wished I would have listened to my Master words: "Ye have heard that it hath been said, An eye for an eye, and a tooth for a tooth: [39] But I say unto you, That ye resist not evil: but whosoever shall smite thee on thy right cheek, turn to him the other also. [40] And if any man will sue thee at the law, and take away thy coat, let him have thy cloke also. [41] And whosoever shall compel thee to go a mile, go with him twain. [42] Give to him that asketh thee, and from him that would borrow of thee turn not thou away. [43] Ye have heard that it hath been said, Thou shalt love thy neighbour, and hate thine enemy. [44] But I say unto you, Love your enemies, bless them that curse you, do good to them that hate you, and pray for them which despitefully use you, and persecute you; [45] That ye may be the children of your Father which is in heaven: for he maketh his sun to rise on the evil and on the good, and sendeth rain on the just and on the unjust. [46] For if ye love them which love you, what reward have ye? do not even the publicans the same? [47] And if ye salute your brethren only, what do ye more than others ? do not even the publicans so? [48] Be ye therefore perfect, even as your Father which is in heaven is perfect." Matthew 5:38-48 KJV

When I was young, I had huge interest to be rich and famous so fast stepping in the others' shoulders! I didn't care about their feeling and what negative impact I left on each of them!

The words of the bible you ripe what you saw, they were just words that I didn't believe I had to listen to! I wish I did!!! As it is written: Galatians 6:7 - "Be not deceived; God is not mocked: for whatsoever a man soweth, that shall he also reap." 2 Corinthians 9:6 - "But this [I say], He which soweth sparingly shall reap also sparingly; and he which soweth bountifully shall reap also bountifully." Proverbs 16:18 - "Pride [goeth] before destruction, and an haughty spirit before a fall." Proverbs 14:14 - "The backslider in heart shall be filled with his own ways: and a good man [shall be satisfied] from himself." Luke 6:38 - "Give, and it shall be given unto you; good measure, pressed down, and shaken together, and running over, shall men give into your bosom. For with the same measure that ye mete withal it shall be measured to you again.". "Ecclesiastes 11:4-6 - He that observeth the wind shall not sow; and he that regardeth the clouds shall not reap."

One evening in the community councilor meeting, I raised my hand: "Why aren't we educating the younger generations to compete for the act of kindness and not just how to be successful business man and woman entrepreneur and rich??

So to my soul what I should say to my aged soul: "It isn't never too late do an act of kindness no matter how small and how many! Just go ahead and do it and my Lord shall give the strength now and rewards at the Judgment day!

Don't be like that rich fool who stored all the worldly fruits, goods and earthly bags and alms,

in the parable: "And he spake a parable unto them, saying, The ground of a certain rich man brought forth plentifully: [17] And he thought within himself, saying, What shall I do, because I have no room where to bestow my fruits? [18] And he said, This will I do: I will pull down my barns, and build greater; and there will I bestow all my fruits and my goods. [19] And I will say to my soul, Soul, thou hast much goods laid up for many years; take thine ease, eat, drink, and be merry. [20] But God said unto him, Thou fool, this night thy soul shall be required of thee: then whose shall those things be, which thou hast provided? [21] So is he that layeth up treasure for himself, and is not rich toward God. [33] Sell that ye have, and give alms; provide yourselves bags which wax not old, a treasure in the heavens that faileth not, where no thief approacheth, neither moth corrupteth. [34] For where your treasure is, there will your heart be also."

If you are young starting to bright years learn from those like me elders with silver gray hairs! Lessons aren't written in book and aren't taught in the schools!

It should have never been playing games, or outsmart others, or take advantage of so many! Life isn't about comfort and convenience! Life isn't about powers, money and lusts! Life indeed is Being a faithful Christian Stewart about act of kindness and unselfishness and everything else follows in our Lord Jesus Name, Love and glory!

Work for the Spiritual dollars and treasures that treasure in the heavens that "— faileth not, where no thief approacheth, neither moth corrupteth. [34] For where your treasure is, there will your heart be also."

Remember my sons and daughters as I currently tell my soul at my dying bed, the words of our Savior and the Judge: "For whosoever will save his life shall lose it: and whosoever will lose his life for my sake shall find it. [26] For what is a man profited, if he shall gain the whole world, and lose his own soul? or what shall a man give in exchange for his soul? [27] For the Son of man shall come in the glory of his Father with his angels; and then he shall reward every man according to his works. [28] Verily I say unto you, There be some standing here, which shall not taste of death, till they see the Son of man coming in his kingdom." Matthew 16:25-28 KJV

I kneel in humility and tears for how much I have wished, throughout my journey of salvation, to do the good works throughout my life so for my Savior to be glorified as He said: "Let your light so shine before men, that they may see your good works, and glorify your Father which is in heaven." Matthew 5:16 KJV

I should have done, during my salvation journey, the works that glorify God in every deed I have done and to do act of kindness for my Savior to be glorified and when my time comes I can say: "— I finished the work which thou gavest me to do": John 17:4 KJV "I have glorified thee on the earth: I have finished the work which thou gavest me to do."

Indeed, let us spread Act of Kindness Through Human Journey of Salvation!!

Amen 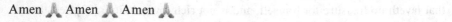 Amen 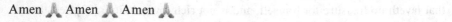 Amen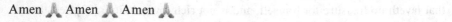

Snap Human Brain and Introduction to Snap Bypass Circuit!

Developed by Ramsis Ghaly

This represents my own theory and philosophy in the topic. By all means my explanation to the snap does not justify the snap or used to qualify the snap brain! A man is responsible for his brain ☺!

Over years, I get so surprised to individuals without external notice, they snap and do the worse mistake ever that will cost them fortune including their lives. Those individuals on the other hand were completely normal, smart and very successful. They were able to control themselves and rational everything they did except that one time. Unfortunately that snap resulted in irreparable damages and cannot be erased or fixed forever.

So many examples, I have seen and some I witnessed such as a very accomplished and well liked fourth year surgery resident commit suicidal by hanging all of a sudden.

I am always wonder regarding the exact mechanism of the act of sudden "snap", impulsive without reasoning or thinking. And this is my theory as follows:

A snap judgment done or taken on the spur of the moment. A sudden break split apart

Normal the human brain ☺ gets all kind of ideas and thoughts from within. The human brain, in turn filter them all and reason among them all the good, the bad, the reasonable and the unreasonable, the silly, the foolish, sense and no sense, smart and stupid and so forth—

All those inputs get to process in the Rational station within the heart of the human brain. The inhibitory circuits compete with excitatory circuits and process keep going under tight directions and controlled condition. Yes, no, reject, accept, do and don't do, wait and rush—-and so on.

The subconscious together the conscious proceed to a plan and once an agreement has reached and a decision be made, the task is executed and the details are formed in an order fashion according to the heart of the brain.

However, it appears that during the snap, the entire neural system is bypassed and a snap decision made in the same time as its execution with much in thinking or getting it passed by the rational!

But snap does not occur de novo and the human brain 🐢 just snap of no where. Over time, repeated bombardments, arguments, disagreements and clashes occur within the brain 🐢 and continues to be unsettled. The product of these repeated clashes is creation of bypass circuit that takes a sudden idea originate from within immediately to an action without going through the normal process. Many of those snaps are recalculated and premeditated but suppressed, not liked and not encouraged. Until such a time where the undesirable and not encouraged super-pass the inhibitory circuits and bypass the rational center and hence jump to execute the snap!!!

You can imagine the end result could be devastating such as self harm or harm others or it will cost the person divorce, a job, a degree, a gain, —-. Some of these snaps are ranging from minor such as wrong decision to much serious such as suicidals, crimes, lose control, cheating, ——

Early diversion from the snap bypass circuits may prevent the snap itself especially if get caught early. There is no early monitor of such a signal but high suspicion and frequent engagement to converse directly to that snap human brain 🐢.

Many of those interventions we already do such as start dialogue, stress relievers, relaxation techniques, distraction measures, de-escalate maneuvers, change environment, frequent breaks, —-small glass of wine—— anxiolytics medications such as benzodiazepines—or even temporary brain shock such as electroconvulsive therapy——etc

In fact, in the practice of medicine and anesthesia, hostility, panics and many others could be controlled by medications. Does this tell us that if the snap brains get pre-medicated, they may not snap!!!

Obviously, the most important is early recognition and intervention. Reach out, be available, provide easy access, be jn the watch——No one will ever know who will snap. Be vigilant to spoken words and odd but calculable steps. Pay attention to your intuition, Those snap brains aren't easy to figure out.

Perhaps in the future functional imaging can visualize or detect the snap bypass or even the neurochemical analysis in certain regions of the brain along these circuits can determine the exact disorderly managed and erroneous calculations that mislead the subject and provide instant convincing argument to commit the irrational snap. Furthermore, perhaps specific pharmaceutical medications or intervention to target the snap bypass circuits and interrupt the distorted neural circuity.

Four Biblical Snaps

1) Cain slew his brother Abel. God accepted Abel offering and not Cain. In turn, Cain Brain snapped, rose instantly and slew his brother: "If thou doesn't well, shalt thou not be accepted? and if thou doesn't not well, sin lieth at the door. And unto thee shall be his desire, and thou shalt rule over him. [8] And Cain talked with Abel his brother: and it came to pass, when they were in the field, that Cain rose up against Abel his brother, and slew him." Genesis 4:7-8 KJV

Cain snap brain didn't calculate that God is watching and if he commit such an evil, he does so against God. In turn, Cain Brain snapped, rose instantly and slew his brother for which he paid the price and all his descendants. "And the Lord said unto Cain, Where is Abel thy brother? And he said, I know not: Am I my brother's keeper? [10] And he said, What hast thou done? the voice of thy brother's blood crieth unto me from the ground. [11] And now art thou cursed from the earth, which hath opened her mouth to receive thy brother's blood from thy hand; [12] When thou tillest the ground, it shall not henceforth yield unto thee her strength; a fugitive and a vagabond shalt thou be in the earth. [13] And Cain said unto the Lord, My punishment is greater than I can bear." Genesis 4:9-13 KJV

2) David brain snapped and commit adultery with Bath-sheba wife of Uriah: "And it came to pass in an eveningtide, that David arose from off his bed, and walked upon the roof of the king's house: and from the roof he saw a woman washing herself; and the woman was very beautiful to look upon. [3] And David sent and enquired after the woman. And one said, Is not this Bath-sheba, the daughter of Eliam, the wife of Uriah the Hittite? [4] And David sent messengers, and took her; and she came in unto him, and he lay with her; for she was purified from her uncleanness: and she returned unto her house. [5] And the woman conceived, and sent and told David, and said, I am with child." 2 Samuel 11:2-5

David brain with his holiness and righteousness, yet in an eveningtide, David brain snapped and commit such an evil before the Lord for which his brain miscalculated and snapped irrationally.

61

3) David brain was about to snap and kill Nabal if not for Abigail: "And Nabal answered David's servants, and said, Who is David? and who is the son of Jesse? there be many servants now a days that break away every man from his master. [11] Shall I then take my bread, and my water, and my flesh that I have killed for my shearers, and give it unto men, whom I know not whence they be ? [12] So David's young men turned their way, and went again, and came and told him all those sayings. [13] And David said unto his men, Gird ye on every man his sword. And they girded on every man his sword; and David also girded on his sword: and there went up after David about four hundred men; and two hundred abode by the stuff." 1 Samuel 25:10-13 KJV Abigail was able to rational with the snap brain of David and prevented david from snapping and committing irreparable bloodshed: "Then Abigail made haste, and took two hundred loaves, and two bottles of wine, and five sheep ready dressed, and five measures of parched corn, and an hundred clusters of raisins, and two hundred cakes of figs, and laid them on asses. [20] And it was so, as she rode on the ass, that she came down by the covert of the hill, and, behold, David and his men came down against her; and she met them. [21] Now David had said, Surely in vain have I kept all that this fellow hath in the wilderness, so that nothing was missed of all that pertained unto him: and he hath requited me evil for good. [22] So and more also do God unto the enemies of David, if I leave of all that pertain to him by the morning light any that pisseth against the wall. [23] And when Abigail saw David, she hasted, and lighted off the ass, and fell before David on her face, and bowed herself to the ground, [24] And fell at his feet, and said, Upon me, my lord, upon me let this iniquity be: and let thine handmaid, I pray thee, speak in thine audience, and hear the words of thine handmaid. [25] Let not my lord, I pray thee, regard this man of Belial, even Nabal: for as his name is, so is he; Nabal is his name, and folly is with him: but I thine handmaid saw not the young men of my lord, whom thou didst send. [26] Now therefore, my lord, as the Lord liveth, and as thy soul liveth, seeing the Lord hath withholden thee from coming to shed blood, and from avenging thyself with thine own hand, now let thine enemies, and they that seek evil to my lord, be as Nabal. [27] And now this blessing which thine handmaid hath brought unto my lord, let it even be given unto the young men that follow my lord. [28] I pray thee, forgive the trespass of thine handmaid: for the Lord will certainly make my lord a sure house; because my lord fighteth the battles of the Lord, and evil hath not been found in thee all thy days. [29] Yet a man is risen to pursue thee, and to seek thy soul: but the soul of my lord shall be bound in the bundle of life with the Lord thy God; and the souls of thine enemies, them shall he sling out, as out of the middle of a sling. [30] And it shall come to pass, when the Lord shall have done to my lord according to all the good that he hath spoken concerning thee, and shall have appointed thee ruler over Israel; [31] That this shall be no

grief unto thee, nor offence of heart unto my lord, either that thou hast shed blood causeless, or that my lord hath avenged himself: but when the Lord shall have dealt well with my lord, then remember thine handmaid. [32] And David said to Abigail, Blessed be the Lord God of Israel, which sent thee this day to meet me: [33] And blessed be thy advice, and blessed be thou, which hast kept me this day from coming to shed blood, and from avenging myself with mine own hand. [34] For in very deed, as the Lord God of Israel liveth, which hath kept me back from hurting thee, except thou hadst hasted and come to meet me, surely there had not been left unto Nabal by the morning light any that pisseth against the wall. [35] So David received of her hand that which she had brought him, and said unto her, Go up in peace to thine house; see, I have hearkened to thy voice, and have accepted thy person." 1 Samuel 25:18,20-35 KJV

4) Herod brain snapped and give an order to kill all the children 2 years old and younger after he learned the wisemen didn't return to him after visiting with the King. Herod brain instantly got angry, miscalculated and commit mass murder of all young children in Bethlehem: "Then Herod, when he saw that he was mocked of the wise men, was exceeding wroth, and sent forth, and slew all the children that were in Bethlehem, and in all the coasts thereof, from two years old and under, according to the time which he had diligently enquired of the wise men. [17] Then was fulfilled that which was spoken by Jeremy the prophet, saying, [18] In Rama was there a voice heard, lamentation, and weeping, and great mourning, Rachel weeping for her children, and would not be comforted, because they are not." Matthew 2:16-18 KJV

Judah brain snapped after he betrayed innocent blood his Master and hanged himself: "Then Judas, which had betrayed him, when he saw that he was condemned, repented himself, and brought again the thirty pieces of silver to the chief priests and elders, [4] Saying, I have sinned in that I have betrayed the innocent blood. And they said, What is that to us? see thou to that. [5] And he cast down the pieces of silver in the temple, and departed, and went and hanged himself. [6] And the chief priests took the silver pieces, and said, It is not lawful for to put them into the treasury, because it is the price of blood." Matthew 27:3-6 KJV

Biblical verses

Psalm 46:9 He causes wars to cease all over the earth, he causes the bow to break, the spear to snap, the chariots to ignite and burn.

63

Isaiah 33:20 Look at Zion, the city where we hold religious festivals! You will see Jerusalem, a peaceful settlement, a tent that stays put; its stakes will never be pulled up; none of its ropes will snap in two.

Jeremiah 30:8 "On that day"—this is the declaration of the Lord of Hosts—"I will break his yoke from your neck and tear off your chains so strangers will never again enslave him.

Amos 3:5 Does a bird fall into a snare on the ground without any bait in the trap? Will a trap snap shut when there is nothing to catch?

Nahum 1:13 And now, I will break his yoke from upon you; I will snap your bonds."

Matthew 12:20 He will not snap off a broken reed or snuff out a smoldering wick until he has brought justice through to victory.

Luke 8:29 For He had commanded the unclean spirit to come out of the man. Many times it had seized him, and though he was guarded, bound by chains and shackles, he would snap the restraints and be driven by the demon into deserted places.

Be Careful Think First

Ephesians 5:15-17 ESV Look carefully then how you walk, not as unwise but as wise, making the best use of the time, because the days are evil. Therefore do not be foolish, but understand what the will of the Lord is.

1 John 4:1 ESV Beloved, do not believe every spirit, but test the spirits to see whether they are from God, for many false prophets have gone out into the world.

James 4:17 ESV So whoever knows the right thing to do and fails to do it, for him it is sin.

Proverbs 14:16 ESV One who is wise is cautious and turns away from evil, but a fool is reckless and careless.

Colossians 2:8 ESV See to it that no one takes you captive by philosophy and empty deceit, according to human tradition, according to the elemental spirits of the world, and not according to Christ.

2 Timothy 3:16 ESV All Scripture is breathed out by God and profitable for teaching, for reproof, for correction, and for training in righteousness,

Proverbs 22:3 ESV The prudent sees danger and hides himself, but the simple go on and suffer for it.

Proverbs 12:26 ESV One who is righteous is a guide to his neighbor, but the way of the wicked leads them astray.

Galatians 5:16 ESV But I say, walk by the Spirit, and you will not gratify the desires of the flesh.

Deuteronomy 8:1 ESV "The whole commandment that I command you today you shall be careful to do, that you may live and multiply, and go in and possess the land that the Lord swore to give to your fathers.

Revelation 13:8 ESV And all who dwell on earth will worship it, everyone whose name has not been written before the foundation of the world in the book of life of the Lamb who was slain.

Ephesians 6:17 ESV And take the helmet of salvation, and the sword of the Spirit, which is the word of God,

Luke 16:10 ESV "One who is faithful in a very little is also faithful in much, and one who is dishonest in a very little is also dishonest in much.

1 Corinthians 10:12 ESV Therefore let anyone who thinks that he stands take heed lest he fall.

Hebrews 4:12 ESV For the word of God is living and active, sharper than any two-edged sword, piercing to the division of soul and of spirit, of joints and of marrow, and discerning the thoughts and intentions of the heart.

2 Timothy 1:1-18 ESV Paul, an apostle of Christ Jesus by the will of God according to the promise of the life that is in Christ Jesus, To Timothy, my beloved child: Grace, mercy, and peace from God the Father and Christ Jesus our Lord. I thank God whom I serve, as did my ancestors, with a clear conscience, as I remember you constantly in my prayers night and day. As I remember your tears, I long to see you, that I may be filled with joy. I am reminded of your sincere faith, a faith that dwelt first in your grandmother Lois and your mother Eunice and now, I am sure, dwells in you as well. ...

1 Timothy 2:4 ESV Who desires all people to be saved and to come to the knowledge of the truth.

Philippians 4:6 ESV Do not be anxious about anything, but in everything by prayer and supplication with thanksgiving let your requests be made known to God.

John 8:44 ESV You are of your father the devil, and your will is to do your father's desires. He was a murderer from the beginning, and has nothing to do with the truth, because there is no truth in him. When he lies, he speaks out of his own character, for he is a liar and the father of lies.

John 3:18 ESV Whoever believes in him is not condemned, but whoever does not believe is condemned already, because he has not believed in the name of the only Son of God.

John 3:16 ESV "For God so loved the world, that he gave his only Son, that whoever believes in him should not perish but have eternal life.

Matthew 24:1-51 ESV Jesus left the temple and was going away, when his disciples came to point out to him the buildings of the temple. But he answered them, "You see all these, do you not? Truly, I say to you, there will not be left here one stone upon another that will not be thrown down." As he sat on the Mount of Olives, the disciples came to him privately, saying, "Tell us, when will these things be, and what will be the sign of your coming and of the close of the age?" And Jesus answered them, "See that no one leads you astray. For many will come in my name, saying, 'I am the Christ,' and they will lead many astray. ...

Luke 16:19-31 ESV "There was a rich man who was clothed in purple and fine linen and who feasted sumptuously every day. And at his gate was laid a poor man named Lazarus, covered with sores, who desired to be fed with what fell from the rich man's table. Moreover, even the dogs came and licked his sores. The poor man died and was carried by the angels to Abraham's side. The rich man also died and was buried, and in Hades, being in torment, he lifted up his eyes and saw Abraham far off and Lazarus at his side. ...

Exodus 3:14 ESV God said to Moses, "I am who I am." And he said, "Say this to the people of Israel, 'I am has sent me to you.'"

Isaiah 43:18 ESV "Remember not the former things, nor consider the things of old.

Joshua 1:7-8 ESV Only be strong and very courageous, being careful to do according to all the law that Moses my servant commanded you. Do not turn from it to the right hand or to the left, that you may have good success wherever you go. This Book of the Law shall not depart from your mouth, but you shall meditate on it day and night, so that you may be careful to do according to all that is written in it. For then you will make your way prosperous, and then you will have good success.

Numbers 35:34 ESV You shall not defile the land in which you live, in the midst of which I dwell, for I the Lord dwell in the midst of the people of Israel."

Hebrews 1:3 ESV He is the radiance of the glory of God and the exact imprint of his nature, and he upholds the universe by the word of his power. After making purification for sins, he sat down at the right hand of the Majesty on high,

John 1:13 ESV Who were born, not of blood nor of the will of the flesh nor of the will of man, but of God.

Hebrews 4:1 ESV Therefore, while the promise of entering his rest still stands, let us fear lest any of you should seem to have failed to reach it.

Proverbs 13:16 ESV In everything the prudent acts with knowledge, but a fool flaunts his folly.

Colossians 3:17 ESV And whatever you do, in word or deed, do everything in the name of the Lord Jesus, giving thanks to God the Father through him.

Ecclesiastes 12:6-8,13-14 KJV

Be Wise

James 1:5 - If any of you lack wisdom, let him ask of God, that giveth to all [men] liberally, and upbraideth not; and it shall be given him.

Proverbs 1:7 - The fear of the LORD [is] the beginning of knowledge: [but] fools despise wisdom and instruction.

Proverbs 2:1-22 - My son, if thou wilt receive my words, and hide my commandments with thee;

Psalms 111:10 - The fear of the LORD [is] the beginning of wisdom: a good understanding have all they that do [his commandments]: his praise endureth for ever.

Ecclesiastes 7:12 - For wisdom [is] a defence, [and] money [is] a defence: but the excellency of knowledge [is, that] wisdom giveth life to them that have it.

Isaiah 11:2 - And the spirit of the LORD shall rest upon him, the spirit of wisdom and understanding, the spirit of counsel and might, the spirit of knowledge and of the fear of the LORD;

Colossians 2:8 - Beware lest any man spoil you through philosophy and vain deceit, after the tradition of men, after the rudiments of the world, and not after Christ.

1 Timothy 2:4 - Who will have all men to be saved, and to come unto the knowledge of the truth.

Matthew 7:7-8 - Ask, and it shall be given you; seek, and ye shall find; knock, and it shall be opened unto you:

1 Corinthians 3:19-20 - For the wisdom of this world is foolishness with God. For it is written, He taketh the wise in their own craftiness.

Proverbs 4:1-27 - Hear, ye children, the instruction of a father, and attend to know understanding.

Romans 1:22-25 - Professing themselves to be wise, they became fools,

James 3:15-18 - This wisdom descendeth not from above, but [is] earthly, sensual, devilish.

2 Chronicles 1:7-12 - In that night did God appear unto Solomon, and said unto him, Ask what I shall give thee.

Proverbs 29:11 ESV A fool gives full vent to his spirit, but a wise man quietly holds it back.

Ephesians 5:15 ESV Look carefully then how you walk, not as unwise but as wise,

James 3:13-14 ESV Who is wise and understanding among you? By his good conduct let him show his works in the meekness of wisdom. But if you have bitter jealousy and selfish ambition in your hearts, do not boast and be false to the truth.

Proverbs 21:23 ESV Whoever keeps his mouth and his tongue keeps himself out of trouble.

Proverbs 14:12 ESV There is a way that seems right to a man, but its end is the way to death.

Proverbs 13:20-21 ESV Whoever walks with the wise becomes wise, but the companion of fools will suffer harm. Disaster pursues sinners, but the righteous are rewarded with good.

Proverbs 12:15 ESV The way of a fool is right in his own eyes, but a wise man listens to advice.

Proverbs 4:26-27 Ponder the path of your feet; then all your ways will be sure. Do not swerve to the right or to the left; turn your foot away from evil.

Jeremiah 9:23-24 ESV Thus says the Lord: "Let not the wise man boast in his wisdom, let not the mighty man boast in his might, let not the rich man boast in his riches, but let him who boasts boast in this, that he understands and knows me, that I am the Lord who practices steadfast love, justice, and righteousness in the earth. For in these things I delight, declares the Lord."

Proverbs 21:29-31 ESV A wicked man puts on a bold face, but the upright gives thought to his ways. No wisdom, no understanding, no counsel can avail against the Lord. The horse is made ready for the day of battle, but the victory belongs to the Lord.

Proverbs 3:26-27 ESV For the Lord will be your confidence and will keep your foot from being caught. Do not withhold good from those to whom it is due, when it is in your power to do it.

Proverbs 2:6-15 ESV For the Lord gives wisdom; from his mouth come knowledge and understanding; he stores up sound wisdom for the upright; he is a shield to those who walk in integrity, guarding the paths of justice and watching over the way of his saints. Then you will understand righteousness and justice and equity, every good path; for wisdom will come into your heart, and knowledge will be pleasant to your soul; ....

Psalm 94:11-13 ESV The Lord—knows the thoughts of man, that they are but a breath. Blessed is the man whom you discipline, O Lord, and whom you teach out of your law, to give him rest from days of trouble, until a pit is dug for the wicked.

Psalm 41:1-3 ESV Blessed is the one who considers the poor! In the day of trouble the Lord delivers him; the Lord protects him and keeps him alive; he is called blessed in the land; you do not give him up to the will of his enemies. The Lord sustains him on his sickbed; in his illness you restore him to full health.

Psalm 39:1 ESV I said, "I will guard my ways, that I may not sin with my tongue; I will guard my mouth with a muzzle, so long as the wicked are in my presence."

Psalm 34:11-14 ESV Come, O children, listen to me; I will teach you the fear of the Lord. What man is there who desires life and loves many days, that he may see good? Keep your tongue from evil and your lips from speaking deceit. Turn away from evil and do good; seek peace and pursue it.

Psalm 32:1-5 ESV Blessed is the one whose transgression is forgiven, whose sin is covered. Blessed is the man against whom the Lord counts no iniquity, and in whose spirit there is no deceit. For when I kept silent, my bones wasted away through my groaning all day long. For day and night your hand was heavy upon me; my strength was dried up as by the heat of summer. Selah I acknowledged my sin to you, and I did not cover my iniquity; I said, "I will confess my transgressions to the Lord," and you forgave the iniquity of my sin. Selah

Job 5:12-14 ESV He frustrates the devices of the crafty, so that their hands achieve no success. He catches the wise in their own craftiness, and the schemes of the wily are brought to a quick end. They meet with darkness in the daytime and grope at noonday as in the night.

1 John 4:4-6 ESV Little children, you are from God and have overcome them, for he who is in you is greater than he who is in the world. They are from the world; therefore they speak from the world, and the world listens to them. We are from God. Whoever knows God listens to us; whoever is not from God does not listen to us. By this we know the Spirit of truth and the spirit of error.

1 John 1:8-10 ESV If we say we have no sin, we deceive ourselves, and the truth is not in us. If we confess our sins, he is faithful and just to forgive us our sins and to cleanse us from all unrighteousness. If we say we have not sinned, we make him a liar, and his word is not in us.

James 3:16-18 ESV For where jealousy and selfish ambition exist, there will be disorder and every vile practice. But the wisdom from above is first pure, then peaceable, gentle, open to reason, full of mercy and good fruits, impartial and sincere. And a harvest of righteousness is sown in peace by those who make peace.

James 1:4-8 ESV And let steadfastness have its full effect, that you may be perfect and complete, lacking in nothing. If any of you lacks wisdom, let him ask God, who gives generously to all without reproach, and it will be given him. But let him ask in faith, with no doubting, for the one who doubts is like a wave of the sea that is driven and tossed by the wind. For that person must not suppose that he will receive anything from the Lord; he is a double-minded man, unstable in all his ways.

Hebrews 10:38-39 ESV / 8 helpful votes Helpful Not Helpful

But my righteous one shall live by faith, and if he shrinks back, my soul has no pleasure in him." But we are not of those who shrink back and are destroyed, but of those who have faith and preserve their souls.

Hebrews 10:21-24 ESVAnd since we have a great priest over the house of God, let us draw near with a true heart in full assurance of faith, with our hearts sprinkled clean from an evil conscience and our bodies washed with pure water. Let us hold fast the confession of our hope without wavering, for he who promised is faithful. And let us consider how to stir up one another to love and good works,

1 Thessalonians 5:17-19 ESV Pray without ceasing, give thanks in all circumstances; for this is the will of God in Christ Jesus for you. Do not quench the Spirit.

Philippians 2:3-8 ESV Do nothing from rivalry or conceit, but in humility count others more significant than yourselves. Let each of you look not only to his own interests, but also to the interests of others. Have this mind among yourselves, which is yours in Christ Jesus, who, though he was in the form of God, did not count equality with God a thing to be grasped, but made himself nothing, taking the form of a servant, being born in the likeness of men. ...

2 Corinthians 6:14-15 ESV Do not be unequally yoked with unbelievers. For what partnership has righteousness with lawlessness? Or what fellowship has light with darkness? What accord has Christ with Belial? Or what portion does a believer share with an unbeliever?

2 Corinthians 5:7 For we walk by faith, not by sight.

John 9:39-41 ESV Jesus said, "For judgment I came into this world, that those who do not see may see, and those who see may become blind." Some of the Pharisees near him heard these things, and said to him, "Are we also blind?" Jesus said to them, "If you were blind, you would have no guilt; but now that you say, 'We see,' your guilt remains.

Isaiah 40:28-31 ESV Have you not known? Have you not heard? The Lord is the everlasting God, the Creator of the ends of the earth. He does not faint or grow weary; his understanding is unsearchable. He gives power to the faint, and to him who has no might he increases strength. Even youths shall faint and be weary, and young men shall fall exhausted; but they who wait for the Lord shall renew their strength; they shall mount up with wings like eagles; they shall run and not be weary; they shall walk and not faint.

James 1:5 ESV If any of you lacks wisdom, let him ask God, who gives generously to all without reproach, and it will be given him.

"Or ever the silver cord be loosed, or the golden bowl be broken, or the pitcher be broken at the fountain, or the wheel broken at the cistern. [7] Then shall the dust return to the earth as it was: and the spirit shall return unto God who gave it. [8] Vanity of vanities, saith the preacher; all is vanity. [13] Let us hear the conclusion of the whole matter: Fear God, and keep his commandments: for this is the whole duty of man. [14] For God shall bring every work into judgment, with every secret thing, whether it be good, or whether it be evil." Ecclesiastes 12:6-7, 13-14

"Blessed is the man that walketh not in the counsel of the ungodly, nor standeth in the way of sinners, nor sitteth in the seat of the scornful. [2] But his delight is in the law of the Lord ; and in his law doth he meditate day and night. [3] And he shall be like a tree planted by the rivers of water, that bringeth forth his fruit in his season; his leaf also shall not wither; and whatsoever he doeth shall prosper. [4] The ungodly are not so: but are like the chaff which the wind driveth away. [5] Therefore the ungodly shall not stand in the judgment, nor sinners in the congregation of the righteous. [6] For the Lord knoweth the way of the righteous: but the way of the ungodly shall perish." Psalm 1:1-6 KJV

Look at my gorgeous eyes!!!

Dedicated to Baby Liam grandson of Father Jeff Freeman
Written by Ramsis Ghaly

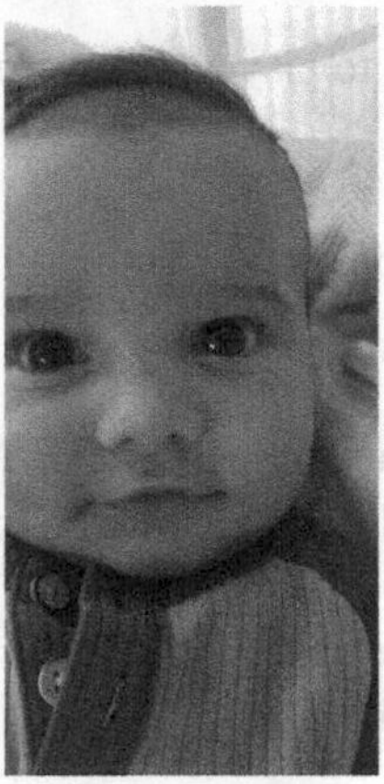

My name is Liam and few months of age! I am a baby boy, petite and sweet with a small mouth but with cute smile, little but with big beautiful eyes, tiny feet but with good kicks and soft and snoozy but with loud voice! I love to play and watch, sing and smile and the happiest child in the bosom of my mommy!

My parents brought me here and my Heavenly Father put a breath of life upon my soul! I am cute and I have His bright look and meekness!!

Look at my gorgeous eyes: they will make you speechless and lose thy self in them! My eyes are world ready to be discovered!!

I am full of love 🖤, precious and innocent! Come and taste my purity!

I can't talk yet but my eyes are gorgeous, attractive and magic! Come and give me a kiss 😘 and a hug, hold me and lift me up! I am full of energy and ready to play!!

I am new in this world 🌎 and eager to learn as much! Simple in my ways and I love people! Beautiful lil guy!

I am fascinated as I am crawling around to find my fortune! Look at me adorable, pretty and famous and I have so many followers!

I am growing every day and although I have nothing to offer you but a heart felt
♥ smile and hug!

My God brought me to her to bring you all hope! Come and visit me, you won't
regret! I am a beautiful Gift ready to share! Tell me more about you and I will
certainly tell you all about me!!

I am joyful child 🙂 and ready to play and run around and the Heaven is when I
am with mom and dad!

But my I love to be with grandma and grandpa! I feel the world is all mine the
earth below and the heaven above!

I laugh so much and my joy when they lift me up in their arms!
So look at my eyes and you will fell in love with me instantly!

Wonders and rivers of thoughts shall run as all could learn from looking at me
and the Heavenly Father's newborns!

Grandma come and give me a kiss and tell me a story! Grandpa come put me to
sleep and teach me how to pray to Our Father who art in heaven—-"

"And said, Verily I say unto you, Except ye be converted, and become as little
children, ye shall not enter into the kingdom of heaven. [4] Whosoever therefore
shall humble himself as this little child, the same is greatest in the kingdom of
heaven. [5] And whoso shall receive one such little child in my name receiveth
me. [6] But whoso shall offend one of these little ones which believe in me, it
were better for him that a millstone were hanged about his neck, and that he were
drowned in the depth of the sea. [10] Take heed that ye despise not one of these
little ones; for I say unto you, That in heaven their angels do always behold the
face of my Father which is in heaven." Matthew 18:3-6,10 KJV

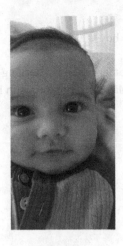

Jeff Freeman

I just signed on to Facebook, and discovered these AMAZING words from my dear friend, Dr. Ramsis Ghaly in honor of our new grandson Liam. WOW!!!! Thank you, Dr. Ghaly! I must share this with everyone!!!!!!!!!!!!! Thank you! Thank you! Thank you!

-- DR. GHALY is ABSOLUTELY PRECIOUS!!!!!!!!! (As you all know!!!!) What a wonderful gift to us!!!

TM.

Jeff Freeman

what a blessing to know Dr. Ramsis Ghaly. He is truly given his his power in the operating room, by God. And how true about Liam's eyes, like sparkling pools. One can lose oneself in them. God bless Ramsis, God bless you and Cecilia, and may God bless Liam, surrounded by love 🖤

VG. Such a beautiful little blessing! 🖤🖤🖤
KR. same hair pattern as grandpa!

Jeff Freeman

what a blessing to know Dr. Ramsis Ghaly. He is truly given his his power in the operating room, by God. And how true about Liam's eyes, like sparkling pools. One can lose oneself in them. God bless Ramsis, God bless you and Cecilia, and ...

CF. Love this...Ramsis, thank you for this holy blessing on Liam

75

ST. Such a beautiful blessing 🖤

JC. Absolutely beautiful little boy 🖤

PW. Precious ❤️

HH. Such a beautiful face another of Gods Blessing 🙏🖤

MW. Love it!!!! Adorable!!! Maybe commercials in his future??

AT. Beautiful boy!!

LM. Adorable

AT. So neat!!

CS. Just beautiful! 🖤

JM. Precious

DC. A beautiful child!!! 🖤

CB. So cute 🌷💕

KH. Wow he's so beautiful!

JC. Beautiful baby 💕

MA. So cute God bless

JB. What a beautiful little boy!!! 👏👏

KE. Beautiful baby

MS. So cute

JU. Precious present from God!

KG. Sweetness 🖤

CG. What a beautiful baby boy! Bless him.

MC. Gorgeous face ad look at those eyes!! Precious.

JJ. Beautiful lil guy!

DS. Loooooooveeeeeeeee this picture! Gorgeous.

AB. Praise God!

RC. Beutifull baby!

KB. Beautiful baby.

VG. Prelepa beba!

BV. Beautiful baby boy 💕

MH. Cute

JPF. Well said! I do hope to "Come visit me."

EH. Is that your relative

NV. Such adorable baby with beautiful eyes and a cute smile 💕

MN. You are a handsome little ham everyone stay safe

MH. The Perfect Face For Gerber Babyfood. Send That One In, It Will Definitely
Be A Winner 🏆👏😄😎🙈

Visiting Greek Church Friday Night for Mother's Weekend Happy Mother's Day

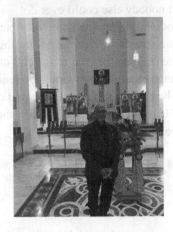

There was no church service and the doors were closed!

I found a church servant named Tony to open the church door!

Tony was kind to open the church door for a stranger like myself originally from Egypt and not from Greece!

I entered and prayed for my mother in heaven and to all the mothers on earth and heaven, received the special Friday blessing and concluded with "Our Father Who art in heaven—"

"For we are His workmanship, created in Christ Jesus for good works, which God prepared beforehand that we should walk in them" (Ephesians 2:10)

Happy Mother's Day
- Mother's Love 💜 no other love can come close!
- Mother's sacrifice can never be measured by human scale!
- Mother's care much more than anybody else could do!
- Mother's bond to humanity so strong that nothing exist to breaks it!
- Mother's blessing to her children super pass many saints!
- Mother's protection to her children is immeasurable!
- Mothers give life, nourish and gather her children together as a hen doth gather her brood under her wings as the Heavenly Father with his children:

"O Jerusalem, Jerusalem, which killest the prophets, and stonest them that are sent unto thee; how often would I have gathered thy children together, as a hen doth gather her brood under her wings, and ye would not! Luke 13:34

- Mothers do what nobody else could ever do!
- Mothers have mothers and mothers can trace back to their mothers from generation to generation and from the beginning to the first mother Eve of human race the daughter of God to the end of the world until the end comes to the human race and the wombs be sealed!
- There is a day when all the mothers living and dead from all corners of earth when the Heavenly Father shall award them for the life and love 🖤 that they have given to mankind!!!

Happy Mother's Day! 🖤🖤🖤

Biblical Verses

"When Jesus therefore saw his mother, and the disciple standing by, whom he loved, he saith unto his mother, Woman, behold thy son! Then saith he to the disciple, Behold thy mother! And from that hour that disciple took her unto his own home." – John 19:26-27

"And Mary said, 'My soul magnifies the Lord, and my spirit rejoices in God my Savior, for he has looked on the humble estate of his servant. For behold, from now on all generations will call me blessed.'" – Luke 1:46-48

Honor your father and your mother, that your days may be long in the land that the Lord your God is giving you." – Exodus 20:12

"Her children rise up and call her blessed; her husband also, and he praises her: 'Many women have done excellently, but you surpass them all.'" – Proverbs 31:28-31

"Every one of you shall revere his mother and his father." – Leviticus 19:3

Isaiah 66:13: "As one whom his mother comforts, so I will comfort you."

Isaiah 49:15: "Can a mother forget her nursing child? Can she feel no love for the child she has borne?"

Proverbs 31:25: "She is clothed with strength and dignity; she can laugh at the days to come."

Proverbs 31:26: "She opens her mouth with wisdom, and the teaching of kindness is on her tongue."

Proverbs 31:28–29: "Her children rise up and call her blessed; her husband also, and he praises her: 'Many women have done excellently, but you surpass them all.'"

"Strength and dignity are her clothing, and she laughs at the time to come. She opens her mouth with wisdom, and the teaching of kindness is on her tongue. She looks well to the ways of her household and does not eat the bread of idleness." – Proverbs 31:25-28

"A gracious woman gets honor…" – Proverbs 11:16

"Hear, my son, your father's instruction, and forsake not your mother's teaching, for they are a graceful garland for your head and pendants for your neck." – Proverbs 1:8-9

"Only take care, and keep your soul diligently, lest you forget the things that your eyes have seen, and lest they depart from your heart all the days of your life. Make them known to your children and your children's children…" – Deuteronomy 4:9

Deuteronomy 6:6–7: "And these words that I command you today shall be on your heart. You shall teach them diligently to your children, and shall talk of them when you sit in your house, and when you walk by the way, and when you lie down, and when you rise."

Proverbs 31:31: "Honor her for all that her hands have done, and let her works bring her praise at the city gate."

Psalm 139:13-14: "For you formed my inward parts; you knitted me together in my mother's womb. I praise you, for I am fearfully and wonderfully made. Wonderful are your works; my soul knows it very well."

Genesis 3:20: "The man called his wife's name Eve, because she was the mother of all living."

1 Peter 3:4: "You should be known for the beauty that comes from within, the unfading beauty of a gentle and quiet spirit, which is so precious to God."

Deuteronomy 4:9: "Only be careful, and watch yourselves closely so that you do not forget the things your eyes have seen or let them fade from your heart as long as you live. Teach them to your children and to their children after them."

Luke 2:51: "And his mother treasured up all these things in her heart."

Happy Mother's Day! Happy Mother's Day

Ramsis Ghaly

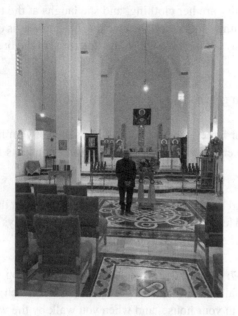

FA. Dr Ghaly ... the Surgeon with a heart of 🤍 God bless you. 🙏
RL: God bless u. 🤍🙏
DT. God Bless you Doc. 👍🤍
SJThank you God bless you Doc. 🙏🙏🙏
CG. You are such a blessing to all! 🤍🙏
KG. God Bless you, Dr Ghaly! Blessings from Egypt.
HH. Beautiful Church.. glad you were able to go in & pray 🤍 God Bless You!
BK. God bless you, Dr. Ghaly.
YR: God Bless you Dr Ghaly. 🙏 👣 🤍
MS. You are a good soul 🌷 💕
BM. Thank you! God Bless!
RC: Blessings for your mother, your family and for you!
DS. Always in my prayers, Dr. Ghaly. 🙏🤍
MW: Beautiful 🤍🤍🤍

MH: Thank You & May God Bless 🙏 you 💜 on this special day.
JC: Bless you Dr, sending 🙏🙏🙏 Blessings to you 💜
MD. Thank you and may God bless you always.
BL. Thank you for your prayers. God's blessings for you and your loved ones. 🤗
GB. Love how God allowed your encounter with Tony.
KE: Exceptional Doctor Amen

The Secret of My Garden!

So many years ago, my patients began to bring me gifts of lively planets and I promised myself that as much as I can, I will water them keeping them alive!

Over the years, not only the joy to see indoor planets in my office growing but also the blessing of each patient brought me the plant. I wrote the patients names by each plant and after few years the garden was huge and God blessed my office indoor garden by His grace and the blessing and prayers of my patients.

My wonderful patient came for her visit only two month from surgery and doing great. Thank you Lord

Tricia brought me a new addition to my garden, a flowering house planet and Brandon her nephew was able to look it up Kalanchoe blossfeldiana. So proud of Tricia and her mom and nephew and Daniel for helping out.

Speed recovery in our Lord healing hands

Ghaly neurosurgeon is a landscaping architect

Congratulations Tricia
Respectfully

Www.ghalyneurosurgeon.com

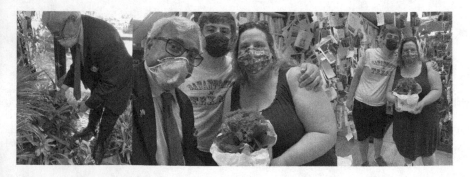

AV. Great photos & Praise God for her healing! 😊 💜 🙏

CG, So happy she is healing! What a wonderful gift. Dr. you are going to have to move if your beautiful garden keeps growing. 🪴

JC. Love to such great news Tricia!! 💜

TB. You went WAY above the call of duty and u did it while working. You were with me every spare moment you had. You really are the best. I love you!

Happy Fathers Day

Written by Ramsis Ghaly

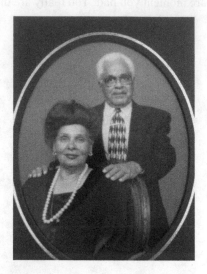

Happy Father's Day. Thank you all for who you are and all what you do

🌾🌾🌾🌾🌾🌾🌾🌾

It is a journey where it begins it shall end,
But the life you endure, the love you give, the heroic steps you undertake, and the
sacrifice you leave behind, it will all last forever and ever more

🌾🌾🌾🌾🌾🌾🌾🌾

It is a journey where it begins it shall end,
But the life you endure, the love you give, the heroic steps you undertake, and the
sacrifice you leave behind, it will all last forever and ever more

🌾🌾🌾🌾🌾🌾🌾🌾

Happy Father's Day. Thank you all for who you are and all what you do
With my Father: FARID FAHMY GHALY
When I was a child, my eyes followed my dad,
By the door, I waited for him knocking in my door,

In the morning, my dad hugged me before I went to school, In the afternoon, my
dad helped me with my homework, When he left me, I used to cry until I realized
he is working to raising me! I did not close my eyes to sleep before I said "good

84

night dad" As I grew up, my dad was my mentor, I mastered my labor hands from my dad! My dad became my best friend, Together with my dad, nothing we could not do, During my upbringing, my demands increased, he had to work day and night, As he moved from one job to another, so I moved with him, He was an innocent prisoner of war in 1967 and could not see him for 9 months, Prayers and tears, cries and cries were not enough, My dad was a teacher and artist, in love and sacrifice he never stopped working,

For his eight children, he made sure our foundation was as strong and even much more! To each child, he did not hesitate to do more and even more, There was no question, he did not know the answer, He kept in order all our memories, As we got older, he shared the memories, so much I did not understand, but years later I did, He was our refuge and safety, In his bosom, I always felt protected, As I held his hand I always felt special, I ran to him every time I saw him, In his heart, I was there, He carried my load and with a smile he lifted up my burden, I cried when he had to tell me goodbye, He started to prepare me for the early departure, Before long, it happened, All of a sudden, I lost my dad and appreciated him much more, So much he had done for me that i never knew, I should have been much more to you dad, I am sorry I was not, Soon before his death, my mother passed away, I should have known the love between my dad and mom, there was no more life for either without being together, Now, I am deeply saddened with memories, so much I wished I had been different, I pray every day for my father to rest in peace as i follow his steps and regret of my shortcoming, I miss you dad and i know you love me, soon I will be with you.

THE FATHERS:

Fathers first existed in the creation of human race,

From the breathe of life, man became, Direct from the Heavenly Father, first man was created! From God and from man's flesh, first woman was created, Together a father and a mother, a child was born, A man and a woman, happy family was established, From a family, another family was born, From families, generations and generations followed! In a strange land, human race preserved, protected and blessed, From the evil and darkness, the Cross of Our Father Jesus saved the human inheritance from eternal damnation! In eternity, the human race will live forever! The Son of Man, the Father of all fathers, is the exemplary image for fathers

WHAT FATHERS DO?

As Jesus was, so fathers do, As first Adam shared life with his children, so fathers do, As Noah build the Arc of wood and took his entire family to safety, so fathers do, As first Abraham sacrificed his the so best of him, Isaac, so fathers do, As Isaac love spread on earth, so fathers do, As Jacob became fathers of Israel twelve tribes, so fathers do, As Joseph was thrown in the prison in strange land, so fathers do, As Sheppard and Hunters, so fathers do, As farmers and cattle raisers, so fathers do, As the strength and prayers of Elijah and Elisha, so fathers do, As the leadership of Samuel, so fathers do, As David ruled the wars of God, so fathers do! As the cornerstone of the family, so fathers do! As refuge to the children, so fathers do! As David played the instruments and sang the psalms, so fathers do! As the men of tribes labored day and nights with sweats, so fathers do! As Job endured the extreme suffering and loss, so fathers do! As Joseph in the Dawn, took his wife and child to Egypt away from his home town, so fathers do! As Simpson muscular and hidden power protected his people, so fathers do! As the twelve Apostles of Jesus breach the faith of our Lord Jesus and shed their blood for Him, so fathers do! As Our Father Jesus lay His life for others, so fathers do! As Warriors in the frontiers of the battles, so fathers do! As the Martyrs die day and night for the good cause, so fathers do! As Peace negotiators, so fathers do! As Deal breakers and committee leaders, so fathers do! As Scientists explore our universe, so fathers do! As Teachers educate the coming generations, so fathers do! As Sailors, so fathers do! As Pilots and drivers, so fathers do! As Bridge builders and high rise workers, so fathers do! As st Luke the Physician and healer, so fathers do! As lessons learned and shared, so fathers do! As Moses had the children of Israel in his heart, so fathers do! As Moses carried the burden of Israel in his shoulder, so fathers do, As Moses cared for the coming generations after his death, so fathers do! As st John saw the vision of the end of days, so fathers do!

FOR OUR FATHERS WE PRAY

In these days of hardship and persecution, we pray for you fathers, In these days of famine and hunger, we pray for you fathers In these days of wars and darkness, we pray for you fathers! In these days of competition and unrest, we pray for you fathers, In these days of uprising and killing, we pray for you fathers,

Fathers Come and Go:

So many times not appreciated enough,

Please take the time to pay your gratitude! Tomorrow you will be a father or a mother! So life continues and their names will be written! May the Lord keep you all safe! For the departed fathers, may the Lord repose your souls and comfort your families and friends. Today fathers, we are children saying thank you, Today fathers we celebrating you: alleluia, alleluia and alleluia.

Happy Father's Day. Thank you all for who you are and all what you do.

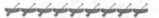

It is a journey where it begins it shall end,
But the life you endure, the love you give, the heroic steps you undertake, and the sacrifice you leave behind, it will all last forever and ever more

It is a journey where it begins it shall end,
But the life you endure, the love you give, the heroic steps you undertake, and the sacrifice you leave behind, it will all last forever and ever more

Happy Father's Day. Thank you all for who you are and all what you do

Respectfully
Ramsis Ghaly

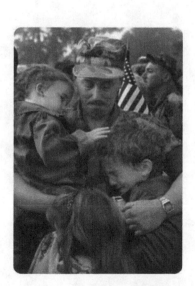

CG. This writing tugs at my heartstrings. What wonderful memories you share with us. Blessings. 🙏❤️
BL. Another insightful, wonder writing by Dr Ramsis Ghaly.

DK. Very touching and true. Im sure your parents know how much you love them. Just remember how much they love you and you can release your guilt. What wouldnt we do or forgive or hold back from our children?! Think upon the good times and one day we can all reunite in heaven and never part. Your parents want you to be happy like all good parents do. 💜⚖ Bask in the love of your heavenly father and may he fill your voids and give you peace and comfort! Thank you for touching so many hearts and lives!!

NC. Wonderful tribute to your father and others!

RC. Lovely thougths, memories. I hope you recibe all your love too! Happy father's day!

RH. Happy Father's Day Dr. . You have made so many fathers days come true for so many people. God bless you you are deeply loved by all of us that means your paper

CS. Feliz dia del padre. bendiciones

MA. Happy Father day God Bless

PR, Happy Father's Day beloved.

RP. Happy Father's Day Ramsis Ghaly.

JE. and thank you for helping me see my Father's Day. God bless.

MM. Happy Father's Day Doctor Ghaly

Er. Happy Fathers Day Doctor Ramsis Ghaly!

Ironman and Flying Superman!!

A Jet Suit

Soon the sky will be crowded with people flying to commute!! But also people may enter through the windows or balconies or land on the roofs! As long as no fear of height!!!

The British Royal Navy and Royal Marines have tested out a jet suit developed by the company Gravity Industries. Gravity says its suit can fly up to 80 mph and climb to 12,000 feet in the air.

This would be amazing for paramedic response, mountain rescue and sea transportation—-! But it is also as a new way of daily transportation and also traveling! This is especially true for high traffic cities!

What about developing a flying car or flying mini-bus or mini-aeroplane or even mini-Carriage for outdoor activities and entertainments!!

But also the sky can be used for run away and falling accidents and hiding the beauty of clear skies!!

What else the future will hold!!!
https://youtu.be/gtvCnZqZnxc
https://youtu.be/suHOLFhbwsM

Ramsis Ghaly
Professor

To Those Unrecognized and Hidden Out of Sight!

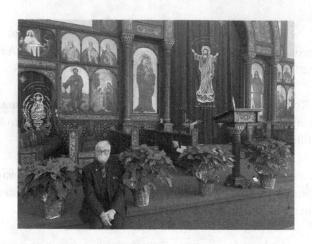

To Those Unrecognized and Hidden Out of Sight!
Written by <u>Ramsis Ghaly</u>

To Those Unrecognized: Don't Be Afraid! Thou aren't Forgotten But Known to the Lord! Thou Very Much Appreciated on Earth as in Heaven! Be Patient God Knows thou Deed and thou Labor! Behold, Jesus is Coming Quickly and His Reward is with Him to Give Every Man According as His Work!

"Fear them not therefore: for there is nothing covered, that shall not be revealed; and hid, that shall not be known. [27] What I tell you in darkness, that speak ye in light: and what ye hear in the ear, that preach ye upon the housetops." Matthew 10:26-27 KJV "For nothing is secret, that shall not be made manifest; neither any thing hid, that shall not be known and come abroad." Luke 8:17 KJV

To those the least
To those the last among the first!

"So the last shall be first, and the first last: for many be called, but few chosen." Matthew 20:16 KJV at

"And the King shall answer and say unto them, Verily I say unto you, Inasmuch as ye have done it unto one of the least of these my brethren, ye have done it unto me." Matthew 25:40 KJV

++

To those light candles under the table soon thy soul be lifted up above the table in heaven!

To those under the bushel soon be on a candlestick to give light unto all!

"Ye are the light of the world. A city that is set on an hill cannot be hid. [15] Neither do men light a candle, and put it under a bushel, but on a candlestick; and it giveth light unto all that are in the house. [16] Let your light so shine before men, that they may see your good works, and glorify your Father which is in heaven." Matthew 5:14-16 KJV

++

To those Pelican in the wilderness!
To those sparrows alone upon the house top!
"I am like a pelican of the wilderness: I am like an owl of the desert. [7] I watch, and am as a sparrow alone upon the house top." Psalm 102:6-7 KJV
To those like drops 💧 in the oceans!
To those minority among the majority!
To those disabled among the healed!
To those impaired among the wholeness!
To those bruised reeds!
To those smoking flax!
"A bruised reed shall he not break, and smoking flax shall he not quench, till he send forth judgment unto victory." Matthew 12:20 KJV

++

To those little birds 🐦 among the serpents!
To those tiny doves 🕊 among the snakes 🐍!
To those small nostril babies among the giant wolves 🐺!
To those small fishes among the whales 🐋 and Octopus 🐙!
To those swallowed in the fish's belly for three days
To those unto the deep, in the midst of the seas
To those submerged by the floods
To those covered under the great waves
To those cast out of sight
To those at the bottom of mountains and at the dungeon pit
To those honest among immortals and corruption!
To those thrown unto the darkness!
"Then Jonah prayed unto the Lord his God out of the fish's belly, [3] For thou hadst cast me into the deep, in the midst of the seas; and the floods compassed me

about: all thy billows and thy waves passed over me. [4] Then I said, I am cast out of thy sight; yet I will look again toward thy holy temple. [6] I went down to the bottoms of the mountains; the earth with her bars was about me for ever: yet hast thou brought up my life from corruption, O Lord my God. [7] When my soul fainted within me I remembered the Lord: and my prayer came in unto thee, into thine holy temple. [10] And the Lord spake unto the fish, and it vomited out Jonah upon the dry land." Jonah 2:1,3-4,6-7,10 KJV

++

To those tiny rosaries among the large impressive stones!
To those lost silver coins among the saved ancient gold coins!
"Either what woman having ten pieces of silver, if she lose one piece, doth not light a candle, and sweep the house, and seek diligently till she find it ? [9] And when she hath found it, she calleth her friends and her neighbours together, saying, Rejoice with me; for I have found the piece which I had lost. [10] Likewise, I say unto you, there is joy in the presence of the angels of God over one sinner that repenteth." Luke 15:8-10 KJV

++

To those Denarii among the costly Roman Denarius!
To those tribute pennies among the heavy silver shekels!
To those mites among the bronzes!
To those penury poor widows with mites among the rich men with abundant gifts
"And he looked up, and saw the rich men casting their gifts into the treasury. [2] And he saw also a certain poor widow casting in thither two mites. [3] And he said, Of a truth I say unto you, that this poor widow hath cast in more than they all: [4] For all these have of their abundance cast in unto the offerings of God: but she of her penury hath cast in all the living that she had." Luke 21:1-4 KJV

++

To those sheep among the wolves!
"Behold, I send you forth as sheep in the midst of wolves: be ye therefore wise as serpents, and harmless as doves." Matthew 10:16 KJV
To those little ones among the principalities!
To those lost among the royals!
To those went astray among the righteous sheep!
"And if thine eye offend thee, pluck it out, and cast it from thee: it is better for thee to enter into life with one eye, rather than having two eyes to be cast into hell fire. [10] Take heed that ye despise not one of these little ones; for I say unto you, That in heaven their angels do always behold the face of my Father which

is in heaven. [11] For the Son of man is come to save that which was lost. [12] How think ye? if a man have an hundred sheep, and one of them be gone astray, doth he not leave the ninety and nine, and goeth into the mountains, and seeketh that which is gone astray? [13] And if so be that he find it, verily I say unto you, he rejoiceth more of that sheep, than of the ninety and nine which went not astray. [14] Even so it is not the will of your Father which is in heaven, that one of these little ones should perish." Matthew 18:9-14 KJV

++

To those poor in the Spirit among the spoken tongues!
To those mourning among the mockers and laughable!
To those powerless among army warriors!
Yo those troubled among the joyful!
To those distressed among the reckless!
To those despair among the established!
To those rejected among those accepted!
To those despised among the popular!
"But we have this treasure in earthen vessels, that the excellency of the power may be of God, and not of us. [8] We are troubled on every side, yet not distressed; we are perplexed, but not in despair; [9] Persecuted, but not forsaken; cast down, but not destroyed; [10] Always bearing about in the body the dying of the Lord Jesus, that the life also of Jesus might be made manifest in our body." 2 Corinthians 4:7-10 KJV

++

To those persecuted and degraded for righteousness by the hands of unbelieving!
"Blessed are the poor in spirit: for theirs is the kingdom of heaven. [4] Blessed are they that mourn: for they shall be comforted. [5] Blessed are the meek: for they shall inherit the earth. [6] Blessed are they which do hunger and thirst after righteousness: for they shall be filled. [10] Blessed are they which are persecuted for righteousness' sake: for theirs is the kingdom of heaven. [11] Blessed are ye, when men shall revile you, and persecute you, and shall say all manner of evil against you falsely, for my sake. [12] Rejoice, and be exceeding glad: for great is your reward in heaven: for so persecuted they the prophets which were before you." Matthew 5:3-6,10-12 KJV

++

To those fallen in tribulation among those aren't!
"And not only so, but we glory in tribulations also: knowing that tribulation worketh patience; [4] And patience, experience; and experience, hope: [5]

And hope maketh not ashamed; because the love of God is shed abroad in our hearts by the Holy Ghost which is given unto us." Romans 5:3-5 KJV

To those fallen into temptations among those aren't!

"My brethren, count it all joy when ye fall into divers temptations; [3] Knowing this, that the trying of your faith worketh patience. [4] But let patience have her perfect work, that ye may be perfect and entire, wanting nothing." James 1:2-4 KJV

++

To those hungered among the filled!

To those thirst among the drunken!

To those strangers among the natives!

To those uncommon among the common!

To those naked among those dressed with luxury clothes!

To those sick among the wholeness crowd!

To those jailed among those living free!

"For I was an hungred, and ye gave me meat: I was thirsty, and ye gave me drink: I was a stranger, and ye took me in: [36] Naked, and ye clothed me: I was sick, and ye visited me: I was in prison, and ye came unto me. [37] Then shall the righteous answer him, saying, Lord, when saw we thee an hungred, and fed thee ? or thirsty, and gave thee drink? [38] When saw we thee a stranger, and took thee in? or naked, and clothed thee ? [39] Or when saw we thee sick, or in prison, and came unto thee? [40] And the King shall answer and say unto them, Verily I say unto you, Inasmuch as ye have done it unto one of the least of these my brethren, ye have done it unto me." Matthew 25:35-40 KJV

++

To those unrecognized souls yet they do most of the work!

To those in the Front Line yet they aren't appreciated!

To those the unknowns and thought to be few yet they are so many!

To those laboring in silence and not being rewarded according to their deeds!

To those in the harms way and battlefield and are forgotten!

To those heroes and not appreciated!

To those soldiers remained unknown!

To those hidden patriots and aren't elevated!

To those out of sight hardworking and considered unworthy to sit at the king's table!

To those invisible doers and not being acknowledged!

To those suppressed angels and not freed!

To those cornerstones and considered left over!

To those oppressed and not released!

To those slaved and not liberated!
To those fatherless and motherless and not adopted!
To those lonely defending the Nobel cause and not supported!
To those with no advocate or defense and remained unprotected!
To those powerless and pushed around and coerced!
To those feeble and weary and not nourished!
To those aged and not cared for!
To those in the closet and not in prominence or corners of the streets!
To those who fast in secret and pray in silence and neglected!

Biblical Verses

"And, behold, I come quickly; and my reward is with me, to give every man according as his work shall be. [13] I am Alpha and Omega, the beginning and the end, the first and the last. [14] Blessed are they that do his commandments, that they may have right to the tree of life, and may enter in through the gates into the city." Revelation 22:12-14 KJV

"I know thy works, and thy labour, and thy patience, and how thou canst not bear them which are evil: and thou hast tried them which say they are apostles, and are not, and hast found them liars: [3] And hast borne, and hast patience, and for my name's sake hast laboured, and hast not fainted." Revelation 2:2-3 KJV

"I know thy works, and charity, and service, and faith, and thy patience, and thy works; and the last to be more than the first." Revelation 2:19 KJV

"I know thy works: behold, I have set before thee an open door, and no man can shut it: for thou hast a little strength, and hast kept my word, and hast not denied my name." Revelation 3:8 KJV

"Therefore remember from where you have fallen, and repent and do the deeds you did at first; or else I am coming to you and will remove your lampstand out of its place—unless you repent." Revelations 2:5

"And I heard a voice from heaven, saying, "Write, 'Blessed are the dead who die in the Lord from now on!'" "Yes," says the Spirit, "so that they may rest from their labors, for their deeds follow with them." Revelation 14:13

"And when thou prayest, thou shalt not be as the hypocrites are: for they love to pray standing in the synagogues and in the corners of the streets, that they may be seen of men. Verily I say unto you, They have their reward. [6] But thou, when thou prayest, enter into thy closet, and when thou hast shut thy door, pray to thy Father which is in secret; and thy Father which seeth in secret shall reward thee openly." Matthew 6:5-6 KJV

"Moreover when ye fast, be not, as the hypocrites, of a sad countenance: for they disfigure their faces, that they may appear unto men to fast. Verily I say unto you, They have their reward. [17] But thou, when thou fastest, anoint thine head, and wash thy face; [18] That thou appear not unto men to fast, but unto thy Father which is in secret: and thy Father, which seeth in secret, shall reward thee openly." Matthew 6:16-18 KJV

"And I say unto you, That many shall come from the east and west, and shall sit down with Abraham, and Isaac, and Jacob, in the kingdom of heaven. [12] But the children of the kingdom shall be cast out into outer darkness: there shall be weeping and gnashing of teeth." Matthew 8:11-12 KJV

"each man's work will become evident; for the day will show it because it is to be revealed with fire, and the fire itself will test the quality of each man's work." 1 Corinthians 3:13

"But prove yourselves doers of the word, and not merely hearers who delude themselves." James 1:22

To Those Unrecognized: Don't Be Afraid! Thou aren't Forgotten But Known to the Lord! Thou Very Much Appreciated on Earth as in Heaven! Be Patient God Knows thou Deed and thou Labor! Behold, Jesus is Coming Quickly and His Reward is with Him to Give Every Man According as His Work!

Psalm 102:1-28 KJV
[1] Hear my prayer, O Lord, and let my cry come unto thee. [2] Hide not thy face from me in the day when I am in trouble; incline thine ear unto me: in the day when I call answer me speedily. [3] For my days are consumed like smoke, and my bones are burned as an hearth. [4] My heart is smitten, and withered like grass; so that I forget to eat my bread. [5] By reason of the voice of my groaning my bones cleave to my skin. [6] I am like a pelican of the wilderness: I am like an owl of the desert. [7] I watch, and am as a sparrow alone upon the house top. [8] Mine enemies reproach me all the day; and they that are mad against me are sworn against me. [9] For I have eaten ashes like bread, and mingled my drink with weeping, [10] Because of thine indignation and thy wrath: for thou hast lifted me up, and cast me down. [11] My days are like a shadow that declineth; and I am withered like grass. [12] But thou, O Lord, shalt endure for ever; and thy

remembrance unto all generations. [13] Thou shalt arise, and have mercy upon Zion: for the time to favour her, yea, the set time, is come. [14] For thy servants take pleasure in her stones, and favour the dust thereof. [15] So the heathen shall fear the name of the Lord, and all the kings of the earth thy glory. [16] When the Lord shall build up Zion, he shall appear in his glory. [17] He will regard the prayer of the destitute, and not despise their prayer. [18] This shall be written for the generation to come: and the people which shall be created shall praise the Lord. [19] For he hath looked down from the height of his sanctuary; from heaven did the Lord behold the earth; [20] To hear the groaning of the prisoner; to loose those that are appointed to death; [21] To declare the name of the Lord in Zion, and his praise in Jerusalem; [22] When the people are gathered together, and the kingdoms, to serve the Lord. [23] He weakened my strength in the way; he shortened my days. [24] I said, O my God, take me not away in the midst of my days: thy years are throughout all generations. [25] Of old hast thou laid the foundation of the earth: and the heavens are the work of thy hands. [26] They shall perish, but thou shalt endure: yea, all of them shall wax old like a garment; as a vesture shalt thou change them, and they shall be changed: [27] But thou art the same, and thy years shall have no end. [28] The children of thy servants shall continue, and their seed shall be established before thee.

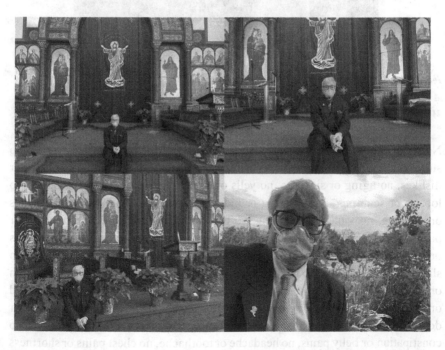

Keep Dreaming with my Soul Life In Heaven! A Beautiful Diary to Keep Daily While Living!

Written by Ramsis Ghaly

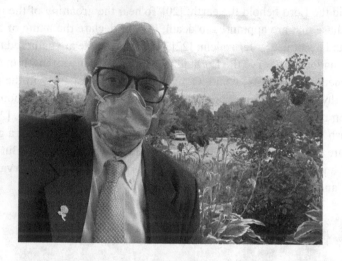

Keep Dreaming with my Soul, Life In Heaven!
A Beautiful Diary to Keep Daily While Living!
What else you wish you no longer see in Heaven??

No more death 💀 or departure, No sorrows or sadness, no tears or cries, no suffering or tiredness, no worries or fears, no cruelty or harshness, no hates or dislikes, no aging or sickness, no yells or screams, no thief or perpetrators, no looters or scammers, no stealing or kidnapping, no lies or cursing, no crimes or stabbing, no violence or killing, no persecution or prejudice, no injustice or partiality, no death or separation, no funeral or demonstrations, no need for favors or man help, no need for meeting or conferences, to begging or demeaning, no slavery or impartiality, no need to eat or drink, no hunger or thirst, no starvation or deprivation, no need to sleep or take breaks, no need to cloth or to cover, no cold or sun burn, no darkness or gloominess m, no need to labor or to farm, no need for doctors or medicine, no pain and no aches, no need for vaccines or injections, no constipation or belly pains, no headache or toothache, no chest pains or shortness of breath, no heart attack or pneumonia, no gangrene or stroke, no flue or COVID, no wounds or broken bones, no need for healthcare or government, no courts or town hall whining, no need to work or sweat, no yearly election or president nomination, no need for money or cash, no need for credit card or money orders, no need for scale or appeal, no need to save or store, no need to walk or run, no need for taxi cabs or Uber or Lyft, no need for trains or aero planes, no need for wires or cables, no need for radio or television, no need for Cinemas or large screens, no need for capital or big cities, no need to moping or cleaning, no need for painting or watering the plants, no need to snow shoveling or mowing, no need for washers or dryers, no need for fishing or grilling, no need to read or study, no ridicule or unprofessionalism, no need to be concern or matters, no lines or waiting, no noise or peeps, no rings or distraction, no depression or anxiety, no computers or robots, no conspirators or betrayals, no politicians or golfing, no Republicans or Democrats and all in between, no need for covers or umbrellas, no need for a clock or watch, no need to sign in or sign out, no need for toxiscreen or hair samples, no need for ceiling or high rise, no need for renting or shopping , no need to repair or fixing, no need to buy cars or bicycles, no crashing or destruction, no need for insurance or security, no Costco or Walmart's, no Lowe or groceries, no Amazon or Facebook, no googles or Twitters, no need for silicon valley or Wall Street, no need fir walk street or stocks and trades, no wars or concerns of bioterrorism, no unrest or uprise of any source, no snap chats or Skype, no computers or Laptops, no Macy's or hardware stores, no drowning or car accidents, no drinking or smoking, no loses or hard feeling, no disability or infirmity, no deafness or mutism, no blindness or paralysis, no autism or psychiatry illnesses, no surgeries or malnourishment,, no pregnancies or deliveries, no more births or new comers, no hills or wickedness, no typing or texting, no phones or Bluetooth, no fingerprints or footsteps, no drought or fames, no East's or garbage collectors, no sewage back up or street holes, no bridges or stairs, no struggles or downs, no homeless or shortage, no orphans or shelters, no passwords or E-mails, no messages or texting, no heart beating or air gasping, no snoring or irritability, no nausea or vomiting, no sitting or standing, no racing or competition, no ugliness or poverty, no uncleanliness or dirt, no pollution or disputes, no falling or condescending, no need to fast or donate, no need to give up or be exhausted, no thinking or searching, no need to gravity or universe, no need to United Nation or WHO, no White House or Supreme Court, no sixth circuit or seventh Appellate Court, no delta variant or Epsilon variant to come, no infection or invasions, no serpents or dominance, no hostility or fights, no arguments or uncomforted, no temptation or tribulations, no days, months, years, or calendars, no seasons or snows or rains, no nightmares or wrinkles, no grievances or inequities, no enemies or shames, no distress or stumbling, no oppression or restrains, no foolishness or slumbering, no selling or buying, no misleading or fooling, no manipulation or taking advantage, no disrespect or unfairness, no bylaws or policies, no procedure Manuel or reference book, no offenders or adversaries, no controversies or defilement, no sins of evilness, no jealousy of oppression, no obsession or greediness, no need or shortage, no affliction or sojourning, no de Novo or memory lapse, no trembling or freezing, no great waves of storms, no global warming or global cooling, no earthquakes or tornados, no nuclear station or mining, no tsunamis or volcanoes, no under-developing or developing, no corruption or moth, no unbelievers or atheists, no trespasses or mistakes, no drunkenness or elusion, no need to smart phones or new Apps, no need for passport or new ID, no need for visas or permissions, no need to renew licenses or cross traffic intersections, no federal or state taxes, no allowances or wages, No strangers or invaders, no need to race or compete, no need to cook or bake, no need to clean or decontaminate,—————-

What else you wish you no longer see in Heaven??

KEEP DREAMING UNTIL THAT DAY WHEN TAKING LAST BREATH SND HEART BEAT THE LAST!!

Biblical Verses

"For I reckon that the sufferings of this present time are not worthy to be compared with the glory which shall be revealed in us. [19] For the earnest expectation of the creature waiteth for the manifestation of the sons of God. [36] As it is written, For thy sake we are killed all the day long; we are accounted as sheep for the slaughter. [37] Nay, in all these things we are more than conquerors through him that loved us. [38] For I am persuaded, that neither death, nor life, nor angels, nor principalities, nor powers, nor things present, nor things to come, [39] Nor height, nor depth, nor any other creature, shall be able to separate us from the love of God, which is in Christ Jesus our Lord." Romans 8:18-19,36-39 KJV

"And he shewed me a pure river of water of life, clear as crystal, proceeding out of the throne of God and of the Lamb. [2] In the midst of the street of it, and on either side of the river, was there the tree of life, which bare twelve manner of fruits, and yielded her fruit every month: and the leaves of the tree were for the healing of the nations. [3] And there shall be no more curse: but the throne of God and of the Lamb shall be in it; and his servants shall serve him: [4] And they shall see his face; and his name shall be in their foreheads. [5] And there shall be no night there; and they need no candle, neither light of the sun; for the Lord God giveth them light: and they shall reign for ever and ever. [7] Behold, I come quickly: blessed is he that keepeth the sayings of the prophecy of this book." Revelation 22:1-5,7 KJV

Keep Dreaming with my Soul Life In Heaven! A Beautiful Diary to Keep Daily While Living!

100

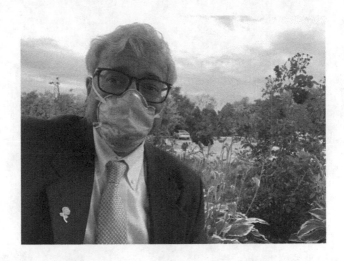

CG. Great article! I believe you have covered everything that we no longer wish to see in heaven. 🖤🙏

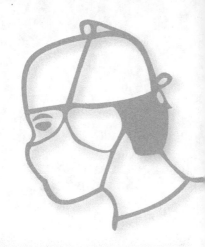

SECTION 2

Faithful Front Liners and Essential Workers

A Prayer from the Author

To You All, I Pray for: "A New breath of fresh air, a smell of sweet aroma and a new sun rise with daylight full of hope, In Jesus Name we shall be blessed in His Grace and be healed in His renewed promises to His children!"

Written by Ramsis F Ghaly

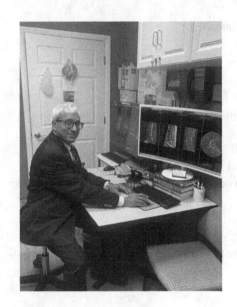

KO. Amen dear Lord,

SJ. Amen

CB. Amen

RP. Amén 🙏

LW. SP. 🙏❤️🙏

EV. Amen. 🙏❤️

RC. Amen!

LB. Amen. 🙏

YH. Amen

MD. Amen

LL. Amen. 💜

JM. Amen

NC. Amen

TG. Amen dear Lord, 🙏❤️

MO. Amen. 💜
VP. 🙏 amén
CG. Praise be to God! 🙏
SS. Amen.
JU. Amen
VG. Amen
BLM. Amen and Amen 🙏
KS. Amen
DS. Amen. 🙏💜
YF. Amen
NC. God bless dr. Ramsis
VFA. Amen 💯 💜
AP. Amen
LG. Amen.
JM. To you too dear friend 💕
BH. The same to you dear man!! Amen
BS. Amen
RC. Let pray for all!
AT. Well said. Amen
EH. Sing Praises to our Beloved Jesus!!!
KH. Amen
MM. Amen 🙏
RS. Amen 🙏🙏🙏
MN. I wish the same to you Dr.Ghaly stay safe.
TJ. AMEN!

Calling for You all to Join and Salute the Medical Front liners and Essential Workers!

Written by Ramsis Ghaly

A Poem Dedicated To our Heroes 👪👪👪 Front-liners and Essential workers combating against COVID-19!

Our planet 🌍 is being attacked with flying inhalant lethal particles spreading all over targeting every human being as the primary target. The victims are buried and the living are disabled as human life became covered with gloominess! The loss and the tears could be seen even by the blind eyes and could be heard by the deaf and the mute are screaming. The world 🌍 is in a hopeless state reaching out with helpless hands and the dire to outcry to the Lord and Its Creator!

While they were caring for the ill, they themselves attracted the virus!

While they were reaching out to the sick, they got infected with the same lethal coronavirus!

I just saw them laying in the hospital beds in isolation and intubated! They were struggling with breathing gasping for air until they couldn't do it no more! Now they are connected to breathing ventilators heavily sedated in high PEEP pressure struggling for their lives!

It is my turn to reach out to them those the silent angels of the Lord servants to His Name whose the earth aren't worthy of them! They sacrificed all what they had, their own lives for others!

My heart 💜 is broken! My soul is torn apart! I cried in tears and I kneeled praying for each of them! I begged my Lord and Savior to come down and heal them soon! Those are the true children of God, the disciples of the Most High!

Let us show kindness to those Front-liners! Let us pray for them day and night! They are the silent soldiers in our times against the evil COVID-19!

The Medical Frontliners and Essential Workers are precious! Indeed they are priceless! There is no word to express our gratitude! Our hates off for each of

107

them! Let us do what we can to help them, to support them and lift up their souls up High! Indeed their angels are standing before the face of the Lord!

In these times, the true heroes 🦸🦸🦸 become visible and distinguish themselves from those serving only with their lips!

O friends, perhaps one day, our nation will Commemorate those known and unknown fighters against Coronavirus Pandemic! Let us designate a day to celebrate those frontlines, medical care givers and Essential workers one by one! All say Amen and Amen! 🙏🙏🙏

Let us remember the words of Love 💜 from Our Master and Savior said: "This is My commandment, that you love one another as I have loved you. 13 Greater love has no one than this, than to lay down one's life for his friends." (John 15:12-13)

Let us make a day to commemorate all the lives laid down for others! Let us have that day to pay respect for all those who sacrificed their gift of life to save lives, to heal the souls, to care for the sick and to defeat the human pandemic of the century!

When it is over, however, millions and millions will be sick, many lives in the thousands will be lost, and many others will continue to suffer from so many complications!!

Sorrowfully 😞😞😞, every home will have a COVID story to tell their children and grandchildren! It shall never be forgotten! Sadness will affect all people; a house with no father, a home with no mother, a wife with no husband, a woman with no man, a family with cousins or aunts, children with no grandma and grandma!

COVID-19 will ever change the way we live and shall be named the world human enemy September 11, 2019 -2021!

Amen 🙏 to you al, The Bible said:

"And I looked, and, lo, a Lamb stood on the mount Sion, and with him an hundred forty and four thousand, having his Father's name written in their foreheads. [12] Here is the patience of the saints: here are they that keep the commandments of God, and the faith of Jesus. [13] And I heard a voice from heaven saying unto me, Write, Blessed are the dead which die in the Lord from henceforth: Yea, saith the Spirit, that they may rest from their labours; and their works do follow them." Revelation 14:1,12-13 KJV

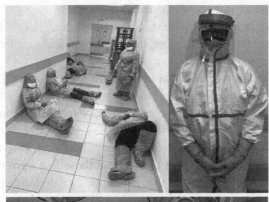

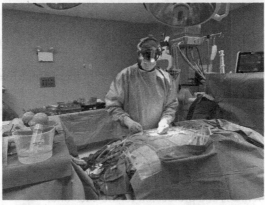

CG. This is so special. Prayers are always a great healer and helper so, many prayers for you and all the front liners. Bless you all! ❤️🙏

SC. Please everyone do your part to help people that have weakened immune systems. The mask helps protect OTHERS. This is why surgeons wear a mask during surgery. Not to protect themselves but the patient!

AV. Thank you for sharing this! Lord help us not to take anything for granted! We are so Blessed! And it's a good idea to dedicate a day to honor all those who are on the front line! We don't have any idea what you & all your coworkers are doing to save the sick! So sorry to hear that many are getting sick as well! 😢 Love & praying for the Lord's protection upon all of you! God Bless you all! 😊💚🙏🇺🇸

RB. As someone who is currently struggling to regain my wellness back, while I'm dealing with the many symptoms of COVID 😷😷, I am in prayer for all front liners. I want to thank y'all for being there to help those who get extremely ill and they find themselves being admitted to the hospitals. I thank you for what you do on a daily basis!! May God Bless each and every one of you. 🙏

MD. Written by our friend, Dr. Ghaly G-D bless all the Front Line Workers 🙏🙏

GK. May God protect you and all the front liners.

KO. Lord hear our prayers for those front line workers, 🙏🙏❤️

TN. You all amaze me! Day after day, the mental toll and sacrifice it must take. May God Bless you all.

YC. We are praying for you and your colleagues! Thank you for your dedication and sacrifice.

VE. You are all in our continued prayers. May God bless and protect you. 🙏❤️

SC. be safe my friend sadly only getting worse

CY. Lord cover our front liners. Give them strength to fight each day as they do what you have called for them to do. Heal those that have contracted this deadly virus. Bring an end to this pandemic swiftly Lord. In Jesus name. Amen.

VG. Prayers for you all 🙏🙏 💕

JC. Saying 🙏🙏🙏 for all the front liners and you Dr, thank you for all you do 🌷

GH. Prayers

JC. Bless the whole world o Almighty especially those front line workers keep them in all name of danger....... Amen

HD. Dear Heavenly Father please hear these prayers for those on the front line, bring healing, and peace to this world. We are humbling ourselves, oh Lord, as we are nothing without you. 🙏❤️ Amen

CA. AMEM

RC, Thanks for the things to do for the ill people, you ate de hralt héroes and we pray for de wellness and protección forma each one!

AM. May God bless you all

RH. My heart is with yours in Prayer and tears.

JP. Father God, we know you see all. You see your servants exhausted. You see your children suffering. Please ABBA, place your healing hands on this broken world. I ask this in Jesus's name, Amen 🙏

MF. Bendiciones y agradecimiento a todos estos ángeles terrenales 🙏🙏🙏

AR. Thank you for you sacrifice

God give them the strength so they can carry on in their job. God bless you all frontliners and thank you so much for all the sacrifices.

JB. Prayers, blessings and protection for our caregivers!! We must thank them, care for them and appreciate them. 💜

JM. May God Protect All Of You AMEN

KG. Our hearts and prayers go out to these heroes on the front line!

JB. May God watch over all of you and protect you doctor..Lord please have Mercy on all of us....please bring an end to this nightmare I am praying daily for all of you. 💜

CL. God, please protect and bless all their souls. 🙏😌 💜

Faithful Healthcare Worker and Essential Workers!

Indeed much blessing to those unselfish healthcare workers whom care from hearts, dedicated sincerely to save lives, sincerely committed fully to rescue the sick, sacrificing to the last breath and consider their jobs sacred and holy and never ever business! Those faithful workers shall ripe grace and blessing from the Most High and miracles shall be performed through their hands saving lives, curing illnesses and bringing smiles and hopes upon the face of earth 🌍 and nothing shall be impossible for them in Jesus Name, Amen 🙏!

Our Savior Promise to those workers: "And he said unto them, Go ye into all the world, and preach the gospel to every creature. [16] He that believeth and is baptized shall be saved; but he that believeth not shall be damned. [17] And these signs shall follow them that believe; In my name shall they cast out devils; they shall speak with new tongues; [18] They shall take up serpents; and if they drink any deadly thing, it shall not hurt them; they shall lay hands on the sick, and they shall recover." Mark 16:15-18 KJV

Ramsis Ghaly
Www.ghalyneurosurgeon.com

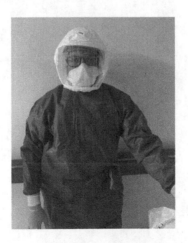

AV. Thank you for sharing this wonderful scripture verse! God continue to
Bless & watch over u & all our health-care workers! Also our Policemen &
Women!! 🇺🇸🙏🇺🇸

CG. What would we do without you and all the healthcare workers. Everyday
they go to the hospital put on their PPE attire and work endless ours. We are
so grateful for you all. Bless you all. 🙏❤️

Gratitude to all the Essentials Thank You!

Through this political heat and disputes, we must recognize in action and appreciate the continuing hardworking frontlines since February 2020 and ongoing tremendous sacrifice to do their work in person exposing themselves in the harm's way.

Instead, many of the essentials received demotion, cut benefits and salaries and none was awarded or got raises despite repeated promises!

We can't thank you enough all essentials including but not limited to healthcare as nurses, paramedics, physicians and hospitals, teachers and schools and colleges and universities, law enforcement, military troops, navy, homeland, FBI, CIA, Cyber Security and all other security agents, food and grocery, farmers, Restaurants, construction workers, plumbing and repairs, manufacturers, businesses, IT informatics,——-and many others! Thank you 🙏, thank you 🙏 thank you! 🙏 from our hearts and souls!!

Ramsis Ghaly
Www.ghalyneurosurgeon.com

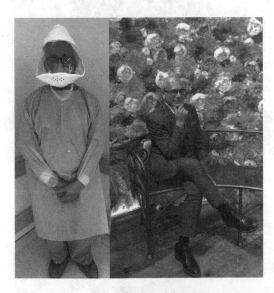

CT. Well put my Friend, and Awesome picture, so distinguished. ✨👍✨
AR. Thank you
RA. Great photo and a loving doctor.

Early morning at the dawn as the week is starting!!!

Help is needed for a COVID patient and here I went serving My Lord child!

In my way back, a dear nurse with COVID laying in the bed in darkness with high glow oxygen in her Belly in a closed well ventilated room crying 😭 and fearing death with difficult breathing and coughing. Broke my heart.

I said to here. O Maria, O my wonderful soul and loving nurse, my Lord shall soon heal you, don't be afraid! We pray.

Ramsis Ghaly

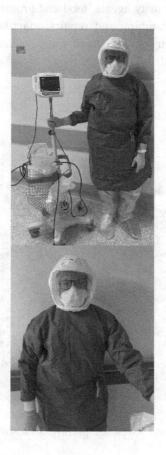

DM. I pray for healing

CY. Lord God we pray for covering for Dr Ghaly and all the nurses and residents and other doctors that are serving the community. Keep them safe God. Bring healing to those that have contracted the virus. Heal our nation and bring relief quickly Lord. In Jesus name. Amen.

LS. Thank you Dr. Ghaly for what you do your bravery, your spirituality and your expertise. You are a Saint. God bless you and may the Lord keep you, your staff, and all who you care for in the palm of his hand. 🙏🙏🙏

CY. amen.

DR. thank you 🙏

May God Bless You & All who are sick 🤍.

ML. Praying for her and for you!

CC. For all of the people with this horrible virus

KO, Good Lord hear our prayers for all the people. 🙏🙏🙏🙏

SM. Stay safe my friend!!! The world needs you!!! 👍👍👍

CY. May she gets healed, prayers to her and God bless ur work doctor

AV. Praying for you Dr Ghaly! 🙏

EM. Strong prayers to pull her through!

ML. Our loving Dr. Ghaly, please pray that he stays healthy so that he is able to help those seriously ill with Covid in the ICU. He gives so much of himself. 🙏

AB. Stay safe!

KP. Prayers

JB. This man is a saint

RC. Pray for the lovely nurse abd for all who need blessings!

MB. Many prayers to all of you working tirelessly to care for the ill. 🙏❤️

Give Credit and Respect to those Credit and Respect are Due! In Fact, Do Good and Love Those Don't Do Good and Don't Love!

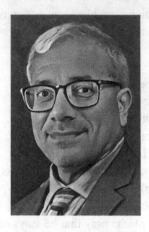

"Give her of the fruit of her hands; and let her
own works praise her in the gates."
Proverbs 31:31 KJV

A man liveth like a husbandman takes over the vineyard and kills the householder and the lord of the vineyard!! As it is explained in this parable: "Hear another parable: There was a certain householder, which planted a vineyard, and hedged it round about, and digged a winepress in it, and built a tower, and let it out to husbandmen, and went into a far country: [34] And when the time of the fruit drew near, he sent his servants to the husbandmen, that they might receive the fruits of it. [35] And the husbandmen took his servants, and beat one, and killed another, and stoned another. [36] Again, he sent other servants more than the first: and they did unto them likewise. [37] But last of all he sent unto them his son, saying, They will reverence my son. [38] But when the husbandmen saw the son, they said among themselves, This is the heir; come, let us kill him, and let us seize on his inheritance. [39] And they caught him, and cast him out of the vineyard, and slew him. [40] When the lord therefore of the vineyard cometh, what will he do unto those husbandmen?" Matthew 21:33-40 KJV

++Treasure comes as an entire packages 🗋 (owner)!
A man or a woman will dig deeply and peal layer by layer until he finds the pearl
As soon as he hold the pearl in his hand, he threw the entire package (owner) away!

116

A man may indeed run away with the pearl and destroy the package (owner)! Another perhaps, take credit of the pearl and cast out the package(owner)! Does a man know that Whoever made the inside made the outside?

++Many times, a man or a woman picks up the fruit and ignores the tree 🌳? While pulling the fruit out of the tree 🌳, a man doesn't think at all about the tree 🌳! It isn't uncommon that a man won't even acknowledge the existence of the tree? In fact, a man cares about the fruits much more than the tree produces the fruits! Does the man ever thought that the tree gives the fruit and the fruit can't exist without the Tree 🌳?

A man picks up the seeds and never acknowledge the plant 🌱 that gave rise to the seeds!

"Ye shall know them by their fruits. Do men gather grapes of thorns, or figs of thistles? [17] Even so every good tree bringeth forth good fruit; but a corrupt tree bringeth forth evil fruit. [18] A good tree cannot bring forth evil fruit, neither can a corrupt tree bring forth good fruit. [19] Every tree that bringeth not forth good fruit is hewn down, and cast into the fire. [20] Wherefore by their fruits ye shall know them." Matthew 7:16-20 KJV

+ A man gathers all the fruits and credit himself and never acknowledge or reward the laborers that worked day and night to produce!

+ A man picks up the eggs and never made consideration to the mother that gave birth to the eggs!

+ A man picks up the newborn and does not appreciate the mother that gave birth to the child!

+ A father as soon as a child is born, he takes total ownership of the child, becomes rude to the mother of the baby, his wife and drop her and divorce her!

+ A grown up child look only at the wellbeing of himself and ignore his parents and grandparents and their wellbeing!

+ A student takes credit to his schooling grades and doesn't acknowledge the school that taught him much!

117

+ A successful profession makes it all about himself and never once pay tributes to his household and teachers!

+ A well-disciplined young adult give himself credit for his good manners and success and doesn't give tribute to his parents and upbringing!

+ A man borrows loans and make huge profits, he takes all the credit and run away with the profits and forgets totally all about the loaners and those helped him!

+ A business man takes credit sole for his fortunate and not to his advisory (s)!

+ A man takes advantage of his master and attributes all earning and degrees to himself alone!

+ A man takes credit for his good gifts and talents and not God that gave him the gifts and talents! "Do not err, my beloved brethren. [17] Every good gift and every perfect gift is from above, and cometh down from the Father of lights, with whom is no variableness, neither shadow of turning. [18] Of his own will begat he us with the word of truth, that we should be a kind of first fruits of his creatures." James 1:16-18 KJV

+ A man bites the hands that feed him!

+ A man destroy the house that raised him!

+ A man bad mouth the hospital and doctors and staff that provided him with excellent medical care!

+ A man deny those stood by him at the time of need!

+ A man gives credit to himself for the prosperity, opportunity and freedom he enjoys and not to America US and the heroes the brave!

+ A patient attribute his good recovery based in his strength and doesn't give credit to his doctor and medical team that treated him thoroughly!

+ A man enjoys life and being living in good health attributing all to himself and not to his home, his country and his church!

+ A man gives credit to himself for being born and exist in the world fruitful and blessed without giving credit to the Creator!

+ A man attribute his Christian faith and Christianity to his good will and not to the Holy Spirit!

+ A man gives credit to his salvation without recognize that all the credit goes to the Savior that came down in the flesh and died for him in the cross to save his soul! "Blessed be the God and Father of our Lord Jesus Christ, who hath blessed us with all spiritual blessings in heavenly places in Christ: [4] According as he hath chosen us in him before the foundation of the world, that we should be holy and without blame before him in love: [5] Having predestinated us unto the adoption of children by Jesus Christ to himself, according to the good pleasure of his will, [6] To the praise of the glory of his grace, wherein he hath made us accepted in the beloved. [7] In whom we have redemption through his blood, the forgiveness of sins, according to the riches of his grace;" Ephesians 1:3-7 KJV "For when we were yet without strength, in due time Christ died for the ungodly. [7] For scarcely for a righteous man will one die: yet peradventure for a good man some would even dare to die. [8] But God commendeth his love toward us, in that, while we were yet sinners, Christ died for us. [9] Much more then, being now justified by his blood, we shall be saved from wrath through him. [10] For if, when we were enemies, we were reconciled to God by the death of his Son, much more, being reconciled, we shall be saved by his life. [11] And not only so, but we also joy in God through our Lord Jesus Christ, by whom we have now received the atonement. [12] Wherefore, as by one man sin entered into the world, and death by sin; and so death passed upon all men, for that all have sinned: [13] (For until the law sin was in the world: but sin is not imputed when there is no law." Romans 5:6-13 KJV

+ A man believes he deserves the kingdom of God because of him alone and nobody else!

+ **A man doesn't own himself but owned by God:**[19] What? know ye not that your body is the temple of the Holy Ghost which is in you, which ye have of God, and ye are not your own? [20] For ye are bought with a price: therefore glorify God in your body, and in your spirit, which are God's."1 Corinthians 6:19-20 KJV And: "[16] Know ye not that ye are the temple of God, and that the Spirit of God dwelleth in you? [17] If any man defile the temple of God, him shall God destroy; for the temple of God is holy, which temple ye are." 1 Corinthians 3:16-17 KJV

+ **A man shall give credit to the Lord of the servants and give all the credit to Whom He created him and His talents as it is explained in the parable:** "For the kingdom of heaven is as a man travelling into a far country, who called his own servants, and delivered unto them his goods. [15] And unto one he gave five talents, to another two, and to another one; to every man according to his several ability; and straightway took his journey. [16] Then he that had received the five talents went and traded with the same, and made them other five talents. [17] And likewise he that had received two, he also gained other two. [18] But he that had received one went and digged in the earth, and hid his lord's money. [19] After a long time the lord of those servants cometh, and reckoneth with them. [20] And so he that had received five talents came and brought other five talents, saying, Lord, thou deliveredst unto me five talents: behold, I have gained beside them five talents more. [21] His lord said unto him, Well done, thou good and faithful servant: thou hast been faithful over a few things, I will make thee ruler over many things: enter thou into the joy of thy lord. [22] He also that had received two talents came and said, Lord, thou deliveredst unto me two talents: behold, I have gained two other talents beside them. [23] His lord said unto him, Well done, good and faithful servant; thou hast been faithful over a few things, I will make thee ruler over many things: enter thou into the joy of thy lord. [24] Then he which had received the one talent came and said, Lord, I knew thee that thou art an hard man, reaping where thou hast not sown, and gathering where thou hast not strawed: [25] And I was afraid, and went and hid thy talent in the earth: lo, there thou hast that is thine. [26] His lord answered and said unto him, Thou wicked and slothful servant, thou knewest that I reap where I sowed not, and gather where I have not strawed: [27] Thou oughtest therefore to have put my money to the exchangers, and then at my coming I should have received mine own with usury. [28] Take therefore the talent from him, and give it unto him which hath ten talents. [29] For unto every one that hath shall be given, and he shall have abundance: but from him that hath not shall be taken away even that which he hath. [30] And cast ye the unprofitable servant into outer darkness: there shall be weeping and gnashing of teeth." Matthew 25:14-30 KJV

+ A man not only give credit and respect to those credit and respect are due but also, a Christian man should do good to those no good and love those with more love as it is written: "Give to every man that asketh of thee; and of him that taketh away thy goods ask them not again. [31] And as ye would that men should do to you, do ye also to them likewise. [32] For if ye love them which love you, what thank have ye? for sinners also love those that love them. [33] And if ye do good to them which do good to you, what thank have ye? for sinners also do even the same. [34] And if ye lend to them of whom ye hope to receive, what thank have ye? for sinners also lend to sinners, to receive as much again. [35] But love ye your enemies, and do good, and lend, hoping for nothing again; and your reward shall be great, and ye shall be the children of the Highest: for he is kind unto the unthankful and to the evil. [36] Be ye therefore merciful, as your Father also is merciful." Luke 6:30-36 KJV

Biblical Verses

"And they came unto John, and said unto him, Rabbi, he that was with thee beyond Jordan, to whom thou barest witness, behold, the same baptizeth, and all men come to him. [27] John answered and said, A man can receive nothing, except it be given him from heaven. [28] Ye yourselves bear me witness, that I said, I am not the Christ, but that I am sent before him. [29] He that hath the bride is the bridegroom: but the friend of the bridegroom, which standeth and heareth him, rejoiceth greatly because of the bridegroom's voice: this my joy therefore is fulfilled. [30] He must increase, but I must decrease. [31] He that cometh from above is above all: he that is of the earth is earthly, and speaketh of the earth: he that cometh from heaven is above all. [32] And what he hath seen and heard, that he testifieth; and no man receiveth his testimony. [33] He that hath received his testimony hath set to his seal that God is true. [34] For he whom God hath sent speaketh the words of God: for God giveth not the Spirit by measure unto him. [35] The Father loveth the Son, and hath given all things into his hand. [36] He that believeth on the Son hath everlasting life: and he that believeth not the Son shall not see life; but the wrath of God abideth on him." John 3:26-36 KJV

"Who then is Paul, and who is Apollos, but ministers by whom ye believed, even as the Lord gave to every man? [6] I have planted, Apollos watered; but God gave the increase. [7] So then neither is he that planteth any thing, neither he that watereth; but God that giveth the increase. [8] Now he that planteth and he that watereth are one: and every man shall receive his own reward according to his own labour. [9] For we are labourers together with God: ye are God's husbandry, ye are God's building. [10] According to the grace of God which is given unto me, as a wise masterbuilder, I have laid the foundation, and another buildeth thereon. But let every man take heed how he buildeth thereupon. [11] For other foundation can no man lay than that is laid, which is Jesus Christ. [12] Now if any man build upon this foundation gold, silver, precious stones, wood, hay, stubble; [13] Every man's work shall be made manifest: for the day shall declare it, because it shall be revealed by fire; and the fire shall try every man's work of what sort it is." 1 Corinthians 3:5-13 KJV

"Having then gifts differing according to the grace that is given to us, whether prophecy, let us prophesy according to the proportion of faith; [7] Or ministry, let us wait on our ministering: or he that teacheth, on teaching; [8] Or he that exhorteth, on exhortation: he that giveth, let him do it with simplicity; he that ruleth, with diligence; he that sheweth mercy, with cheerfulness."

Romans 12:6-8 KJV
"From whom the whole body fitly joined together and compacted by that which every joint supplieth, according to the effectual working in the measure of every part, maketh increase of the body unto the edifying of itself in love. [17] This I say therefore, and testify in the Lord, that ye henceforth walk not as other Gentiles walk, in the vanity of their mind, [18] Having the understanding darkened, being alienated from the life of God through the ignorance that is in them, because of the blindness of their heart:" Ephesians 4:16-18 KJV

"Wherefore comfort yourselves together, and edify one another, even as also ye do. [12] And we beseech you, brethren, to know them which labour among you, and are over you in the Lord, and admonish you; [13] And to esteem them very highly in love for their work's sake. And be at peace among yourselves. [14] Now we exhort you, brethren, warn them that are unruly, comfort the feebleminded, support the weak, be patient toward all men." 1 Thessalonians 5:11-14 KJV

"Bear ye one another's burdens, and so fulfil the law of Christ. [3] For if a man think himself to be something, when he is nothing, he deceiveth himself. [4] But let every man prove his own work, and then shall he have rejoicing in himself alone, and not in another. [5] For every man shall bear his own burden. [6] Let him that is taught in the word communicate unto him that teacheth in all good things. [7] Be not deceived; God is not mocked: for whatsoever a man soweth, that shall he also reap. [8] For he that soweth to his flesh shall of the flesh reap corruption; but he that soweth to the Spirit shall of the Spirit reap life everlasting. [9] And let us not be weary in well doing: for in due season we shall reap, if we faint not. [10] As we have therefore opportunity, let us do good unto all men, especially unto them who are of the household of faith." Galatians 6:2-10 KJV

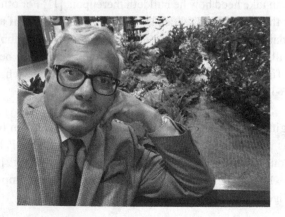

KG. Beautiful, Dr Ghaly. All is possible ...with God. No matter what the name we know HIM by. God is good if we but believe even the tiniest bit.

Like a mustard seed. God is good all the time. God Bless you Always

BL. Thank you Dr. Ghaly for another excellent lesson.

My prayer for Dr Ghaly:

Numbers 6:24-26 NIV

"The Lord bless you and keep you; the Lord make his face to shine upon you and be gracious to you; the Lord lift up his countenance upon you and give you peace."

SK. Amen

KE. Tremendous insight TY

MP. Judas was self-reliant and carried out his own plans perfectly, to what end?

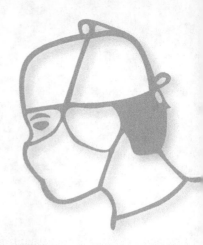

SECTION 3

Return of Rainbows

God Almighty Our Lord Jesus is in Control!

Written by Ramsis Ghaly

In the midst of the widespread tribulation and fears, let us remember that God Almighty Our Lord Jesus is in Control!

Neither man nor virus is but Lord Jesus is In Control!

Neither Coronavirus nor Pandemic nor epidemic nor illnesses nor sickness is but Lord Jesus is In Control!

Neither Kings nor Queens, Presidents nor Prime Minister nor Rulers, nor Leaders nor Commanders nor Giants are but Lord Jesus is In Control!

Neither Doctrine nor Supreme Court nor Court nor Law nor worldly Orders nor Regulations are but Lord Jesus is In Control!

Neither political party nor COVID virus is but Lord Jesus is In Control!

Neither Chinese High Tech Virology Lab nor the scientists are but Lord Jesus is In Control!

Neither the wise of this world nor the rich but Lord Jesus is In Control!

Neither the haters of mankind nor the haters of good are but Lord Jesus is In Control!

Neither the opportunistic nor the wicked is but Lord Jesus is In Control!

Neither the anti-godly nor the ungodly is but Lord Jesus is In Control!

Neither Facebook nor Twitter nor Google nor Linkin nor Wikipedia or any social media is but Lord Jesus is In Control!

Neither CNN nor FOX nor MSNBC nor CNBC nor Bloomberg nor Headline nor ABC nor BBC nor any News is but Lord Jesus is In Control!

Neither Washington Post nor Wall Street nor New York Times, USA Today nor Herald nor Tribune nor any Newspapers are but Lord Jesus is In Control!

127

Neither the millionaires nor the Billionaires nor the most affluent but Lord Jesus is In Control!

Neither Satan nor darkness is but Lord Jesus is In Control!

Neither wars nor earthquakes or hurricanes are but Lord Jesus is In Control!

Neither global warming nor flooding are but Lord Jesus is In Control!

Neither bioweapons nor terrors nor army nor machine guns nor sonic bombs nor explosives nor any weapon of evils are but Lord Jesus is In Control!

Biblical Verses

Isaiah 35:4 say to those with fearful hearts, "Be strong, do not fear; your God will come, he will come with vengeance; with divine retribution he will come to save you."

Isaiah 43:1 But now, this is what the LORD says— he who created you, Jacob, he who formed you, Israel: "Do not fear, for I have redeemed you; I have summoned you by name; you are mine.

Joshua 1:9 Have I not commanded you? Be strong and courageous. Do not be afraid; do not be discouraged, for the LORD your God will be with you wherever you go."

Matthew 6:34 Therefore do not worry about tomorrow, for tomorrow will worry about itself. Each day has enough trouble of its own.

John 14:27 Peace I leave with you; my peace I give you. I do not give to you as the world gives. Do not let your hearts be troubled and do not be afraid.

Psalm 23:4 Even though I walk through the darkest valley, I will fear no evil, for you are with me; your rod and your staff, they comfort me.

Psalm 34:4 I sought the LORD, and he answered me; he delivered me from all my fears.

Psalm 94:19 When anxiety was great within me, your consolation brought me joy.

Romans 8:38-39 For I am convinced that neither death nor life, neither angels nor demons, neither the present nor the future, nor any powers, neither height nor depth, nor anything else in all creation, will be able to separate us from the love of God that is in Christ Jesus our Lord.

Psalm 27:1 The LORD is my light and my salvation— whom shall I fear? The LORD is the stronghold of my life— of whom shall I be afraid?

1 Peter 5:6-7 Humble yourselves, therefore, under God's mighty hand, that he may lift you up in due time. Cast all your anxiety on him because he cares for you.

Psalm 118:6 The LORD is with me; I will not be afraid. What can mere mortals do to me?

Psalm 115:11 You who fear him, trust in the LORD— he is their help and shield.

Romans 8:28 ESV And we know that for those who love God all things work together for good, for those who are called according to his purpose.

Isaiah 41:10 ESV Fear not, for I am with you; be not dismayed, for I am your God; I will strengthen you, I will help you, I will uphold you with my righteous right hand.

Proverbs 19:21 ESV Many are the plans in the mind of a man, but it is the purpose of the Lord that will stand.

Proverbs 16:9 ESV The heart of man plans his way, but the Lord establishes his steps.

1 Corinthians 10:13 ESV No temptation has overtaken you that is not common to man. God is faithful, and he will not let you be tempted beyond your ability, but with the temptation he will also provide the way of escape, that you may be able to endure it.

Joshua 1:9 ESV Have I not commanded you? Be strong and courageous. Do not be frightened, and do not be dismayed, for the Lord your God is with you wherever you go."

Matthew 6:34 ESV "Therefore do not be anxious about tomorrow, for tomorrow will be anxious for itself. Sufficient for the day is its own trouble.

Jeremiah 29:11 ESV For I know the plans I have for you, declares the Lord, plans for welfare and not for evil, to give you a future and a hope.

Ephesians 1:11 ESV In him we have obtained an inheritance, having been predestined according to the purpose of him who works all things according to the counsel of his will,

Psalm 27:1 ESV Of David. The Lord is my light and my salvation; whom shall I fear? The Lord is the stronghold of my life; of whom shall I be afraid?

Psalm 115:3 ESV Our God is in the heavens; he does all that he pleases.

Matthew 19:26 ESV But Jesus looked at them and said, "With man this is impossible, but with God all things are possible."

2 Timothy 1:7 ESV For God gave us a spirit not of fear but of power and love and self-control.

Isaiah 45:6-7 ESV That people may know, from the rising of the sun and from the west, that there is none besides me; I am the Lord, and there is no other. I form light and create darkness, I make well-being and create calamity, I am the Lord, who does all these things.

Isaiah 45:7 ESV I form light and create darkness, I make well-being and create calamity, I am the Lord, who does all these things.

Isaiah 14:24 ESV The Lord of hosts has sworn: "As I have planned, so shall it be, and as I have purposed, so shall it stand,

Proverbs 21:1 ESV The king's heart is a stream of water in the hand of the Lord; he turns it wherever he will.

Psalm 94:19 ESV When the cares of my heart are many, your consolations cheer my soul.

Psalm 46:1 ESV To the choirmaster. Of the Sons of Korah. According to Alamoth. A Song. God is our refuge and strength, a very present help in trouble.

John 14:27 ESV Peace I leave with you; my peace I give to you. Not as the world gives do I give to you. Let not your hearts be troubled, neither let them be afraid.

Philippians 4:6-7 ESV Do not be anxious about anything, but in everything by prayer and supplication with thanksgiving let your requests be made known to God. And the peace of God, which surpasses all understanding, will guard your hearts and your minds in Christ Jesus.

Psalm 22:28 ESV For kingship belongs to the Lord, and he rules over the nations.

Proverbs 16:4 ESV The Lord has made everything for its purpose, even the wicked for the day of trouble.

Luke 12:22-26 ESV And he said to his disciples, "Therefore I tell you, do not be anxious about your life, what you will eat, nor about your body, what you will put on. For life is more than food, and the body more than clothing. Consider the ravens: they neither sow nor reap, they have neither storehouse nor barn, and yet God feeds them. Of how much more value are you than the birds! And which of you by being anxious can add a single hour to his span of life? If then you are not able to do as small a thing as that, why are you anxious about the rest?

Isaiah 55:8-11 ESV For my thoughts are not your thoughts, neither are your ways my ways, declares the Lord. For as the heavens are higher than the earth, so are my ways higher than your ways and my thoughts than your thoughts. "For as the rain and the snow come down from heaven and do not return there but water the earth, making it bring forth and sprout, giving seed to the sower and bread to the eater, so shall my word be that goes out from my mouth; it shall not return to me empty, but it shall accomplish that which I purpose, and shall succeed in the thing for which I sent it.

Job 12:10 ESV In his hand is the life of every living thing and the breath of all mankind.

1 Peter 5:6-7 ESV Humble yourselves, therefore, under the mighty hand of God so that at the proper time he may exalt you, casting all your anxieties on him, because he cares for you.

1 John 4:18 ESV There is no fear in love, but perfect love casts out fear. For fear has to do with punishment, and whoever fears has not been perfected in love.

1 Chronicles 29:11-12 ESV Yours, O Lord, is the greatness and the power and the glory and the victory and the majesty, for all that is in the heavens and in the earth is yours. Yours is the kingdom, O Lord, and you are exalted as head above

all. Both riches and honor come from you, and you rule over all. In your hand are power and might, and in your hand it is to make great and to give strength to all.

Psalm 118:6-7 ESV The Lord is on my side; I will not fear. What can man do to me? The Lord is on my side as my helper; I shall look in triumph on those who hate me.

Revelation 1:17 ESV When I saw him, I fell at his feet as though dead. But he laid his right hand on me, saying, "Fear not, I am the first and the last,

Psalm 23:4 ESV Even though I walk through the valley of the shadow of death, I will fear no evil, for you are with me; your rod and your staff, they comfort me.

Psalm 56:3 ESV When I am afraid, I put my trust in you.

Psalm 23:1-6 ESV A Psalm of David. The Lord is my shepherd; I shall not want. He makes me lie down in green pastures. He leads me beside still waters. He restores my soul. He leads me in paths of righteousness for his name's sake. Even though I walk through the valley of the shadow of death, I will fear no evil, for you are with me; your rod and your staff, they comfort me. You prepare a table before me in the presence of my enemies; you anoint my head with oil; my cup overflows. ...

Psalm 103:19 ESV The Lord has established his throne in the heavens, and his kingdom rules over all.

1 Timothy 6:15 ESV Which he will display at the proper time—he who is the blessed and only Sovereign, the King of kings and Lord of lords,

Jeremiah 32:27 ESV "Behold, I am the Lord, the God of all flesh. Is anything too hard for me?

Hebrews 1:3 ESV He is the radiance of the glory of God and the exact imprint of his nature, and he upholds the universe by the word of his power. After making purification for sins, he sat down at the right hand of the Majesty on high,

Genesis 50:20 ESV As for you, you meant evil against me, but God meant it for good, to bring it about that many people should be kept alive, as they are today.

Psalm 55:22 ESV Cast your burden on the Lord, and he will sustain you; he will never permit the righteous to be moved.

Philippians 4:13 ESV I can do all things through him who strengthens me.

Daniel 4:35 ESV All the inhabitants of the earth are accounted as nothing, and he does according to his will among the host of heaven and among the inhabitants of the earth; and none can stay his hand or say to him, "What have you done?"

2 Chronicles 20:6 ESV And said, "O Lord, God of our fathers, are you not God in heaven? You rule over all the kingdoms of the nations. In your hand are power and might, so that none is able to withstand you.

Job 42:2 ESV "I know that you can do all things, and that no purpose of yours can be thwarted.

Lamentations 3:37 ESV Who has spoken and it came to pass, unless the Lord has commanded it?

1 Peter 5:7 ESV Casting all your anxieties on him, because he cares for you.

Psalm 135:6 ESV Whatever the Lord pleases, he does, in heaven and on earth, in the seas and all deeps.

Matthew 10:29 ESV Are not two sparrows sold for a penny? And not one of them will fall to the ground apart from your Father.

John 16:33 ESV I have said these things to you, that in me you may have peace. In the world you will have tribulation. But take heart; I have overcome the world."

Isaiah 14:27 ESV For the Lord of hosts has purposed, and who will annul it? His hand is stretched out, and who will turn it back?

Psalm 34:7 ESV The angel of the Lord encamps around those who fear him, and delivers them.

Psalm 46:10 ESV "Be still, and know that I am God. I will be exalted among the nations, I will be exalted in the earth!"

Mark 6:50 ESV For they all saw him and were terrified. But immediately he spoke to them and said, "Take heart; it is I. Do not be afraid."

Revelation 1:1-20 ESV The revelation of Jesus Christ, which God gave him to show to his servants the things that must soon take place. He made it known by sending his angel to his servant John, who bore witness to the word of God and to the testimony of Jesus Christ, even to all that he saw. Blessed is the one who reads aloud the words of this prophecy, and blessed are those who hear, and who keep what is written in it, for the time is near. John to the seven churches that are in Asia: Grace to you and peace from him who is and who was and who is to come, and from the seven spirits who are before his throne, and from Jesus Christ the faithful witness, the firstborn of the dead, and the ruler of kings on earth. To him who loves us and has freed us from our sins by his blood ...

Isaiah 43:1 ESV But now thus says the Lord, he who created you, O Jacob, he who formed you, O Israel: "Fear not, for I have redeemed you; I have called you by name, you are mine.

Zephaniah 3:17 ESV The Lord your God is in your midst, a mighty one who will save; he will rejoice over you with gladness; he will quiet you by his love; he will exult over you with loud singing.

Amos 3:6 ESV Is a trumpet blown in a city, and the people are not afraid? Does disaster come to a city, unless the Lord has done it?

Mark 5:36 ESV But overhearing what they said, Jesus said to the ruler of the synagogue, "Do not fear, only believe."

Genesis 1:1 ESV In the beginning, God created the heavens and the earth.

Psalm 34:4 ESV I sought the Lord, and he answered me and delivered me from all my fears.

Romans 8:38-39 ESV For I am sure that neither death nor life, nor angels nor rulers, nor things present nor things to come, nor powers, nor height nor depth, nor anything else in all creation, will be able to separate us from the love of God in Christ Jesus our Lord.

Daniel 2:21 ESV He changes times and seasons; he removes kings and sets up kings; he gives wisdom to the wise and knowledge to those who have understanding;

1 Peter 3:14 ESV But even if you should suffer for righteousness' sake, you will be blessed. Have no fear of them, nor be troubled,

Proverbs 16:33 ESV The lot is cast into the lap, but its every decision is from the Lord.

Isaiah 41:2 ESV Who stirred up one from the east whom victory meets at every step? He gives up nations before him, so that he tramples kings underfoot; he makes them like dust with his sword, like driven stubble with his bow.

Isaiah 43:9 ESV All the nations gather together, and the peoples assemble. Who among them can declare this, and show us the former things? Let them bring their witnesses to prove them right, and let them hear and say, It is true.

Psalm 24:1 ESV A Psalm of David. The earth is the Lord's and the fullness thereof, the world and those who dwell therein,

2 Timothy 1:6 ESV For this reason I remind you to fan into flame the gift of God, which is in you through the laying on of my hands,

Isaiah 35:4 ESV Say to those who have an anxious heart, "Be strong; fear not! Behold, your God will come with vengeance, with the recompense of God. He will come and save you."

John 14:5 ESV Thomas said to him, "Lord, we do not know where you are going. How can we know the way?"

Psalm 91:4 ESV He will cover you with his pinions, and under his wings you will find refuge; his faithfulness is a shield and buckler.

Deuteronomy 31:6 ESV Be strong and courageous. Do not fear or be in dread of them, for it is the Lord your God who goes with you. He will not leave you or forsake you."

1 Chronicles 29:11 ESV Yours, O Lord, is the greatness and the power and the glory and the victory and the majesty, for all that is in the heavens and in the earth is yours. Yours is the kingdom, O Lord, and you are exalted as head above all.

Psalm 66:7 ESV Who rules by his might forever, whose eyes keep watch on the nations— let not the rebellious exalt themselves. Selah

Ephesians 1:11-12 ESV In him we have obtained an inheritance, having been predestined according to the purpose of him who works all things according to the counsel of his will, so that we who were the first to hope in Christ might be to the praise of his glory.

Romans 13:1 ESV Let every person be subject to the governing authorities. For there is no authority except from God, and those that exist have been instituted by God.

Matthew 6:12 ESV And forgive us our debts, as we also have forgiven our debtors.

Ephesians 1:4 ESV Even as he chose us in him before the foundation of the world, that we should be holy and blameless before him. In love

Zechariah 4:6 ESV Then he said to me, "This is the word of the Lord to Zerubbabel: Not by might, nor by power, but by my Spirit, says the Lord of hosts.

Revelation 1:8 ESV "I am the Alpha and the Omega," says the Lord God, "who is and who was and who is to come, the Almighty."

1 Corinthians 13:12 ESV For now we see in a mirror dimly, but then face to face. Now I know in part; then I shall know fully, even as I have been fully known.

John 6:37 ESV All that the Father gives me will come to me, and whoever comes to me I will never cast out.

Psalm 27:14 ESV Wait for the Lord; be strong, and let your heart take courage; wait for the Lord!

John 13:7 ESV Jesus answered him, "What I am doing you do not understand now, but afterward you will understand."

Romans 3:23 ESV For all have sinned and fall short of the glory of God,

Hebrews 11:1-40 ESV Now faith is the assurance of things hoped for, the conviction of things not seen. For by it the people of old received their commendation. By faith we understand that the universe was created by the word of God, so that what is seen was not made out of things that are visible. By faith Abel offered to God a more acceptable sacrifice than Cain, through which he was commended as righteous, God commending him by accepting his gifts. And through his faith, though he died, he still speaks. By faith Enoch was taken up so that he should not see death, and he was not found, because God had taken him. Now before he was taken he was commended as having pleased God. ...

Philippians 4:19 ESV And my God will supply every need of yours according to his riches in glory in Christ Jesus.

Psalm 91:1-16 ESV He who dwells in the shelter of the Most High will abide in the shadow of the Almighty. I will say to the Lord, "My refuge and my fortress, my God, in whom I trust." For he will deliver you from the snare of the fowler and from the deadly pestilence. He will cover you with his pinions, and under his wings you will find refuge; his faithfulness is a shield and buckler. You will not fear the terror of the night, nor the arrow that flies by day, ...

Revelation 1:1 ESV The revelation of Jesus Christ, which God gave him to show to his servants the things that must soon take place. He made it known by sending his angel to his servant John,

Romans 9:21 ESV Has the potter no right over the clay, to make out of the same lump one vessel for honorable use and another for dishonorable use?

Isaiah 8:1-22 ESV Then the Lord said to me, "Take a large tablet and write on it in common characters, 'Belonging to Maher-shalal-hash-baz.' And I will get reliable witnesses, Uriah the priest and Zechariah the son of Jeberechiah, to attest for me." And I went to the prophetess, and she conceived and bore a son. Then the Lord said to me, "Call his name Maher-shalal-hash-baz; for before the boy knows how to cry 'My father' or 'My mother,' the wealth of Damascus and the spoil of Samaria will be carried away before the king of Assyria." The Lord spoke to me again: ...

John 3:16-17 ESV "For God so loved the world, that he gave his only Son, that whoever believes in him should not perish but have eternal life. For God did not send his Son into the world to condemn the world, but in order that the world might be saved through him.

Hebrews 11:3 ESV By faith we understand that the universe was created by the word of God, so that what is seen was not made out of things that are visible.

John 19:11 ESV Jesus answered him, "You would have no authority over me at all unless it had been given you from above. Therefore he who delivered me over to you has the greater sin."

Acts 17:10-11 ESV The brothers immediately sent Paul and Silas away by night to Berea, and when they arrived they went into the Jewish synagogue. Now these Jews were more noble than those in Thessalonica; they received the word with all eagerness, examining the Scriptures daily to see if these things were so.

Genesis 8:22 ESV While the earth remains, seedtime and harvest, cold and heat, summer and winter, day and night, shall not cease."

Jonah 1:4 ESV But the Lord hurled a great wind upon the sea, and there was a mighty tempest on the sea, so that the ship threatened to break up.

James 1:13 ESV Let no one say when he is tempted, "I am being tempted by God," for God cannot be tempted with evil, and he himself tempts no one.

Romans 8:29-30 ESV For those whom he foreknew he also predestined to be conformed to the image of his Son, in order that he might be the firstborn among many brothers. And those whom he predestined he also called, and those whom he called he also justified, and those whom he justified he also glorified.

Psalm 9:10 ESV And those who know your name put their trust in you, for you, O Lord, have not forsaken those who seek you.

VW. Amen!
VG. Amin!
MY. God bless you Dr Ramses Amen

Give the Glory to God the Almighty Jesus and not to the Foolish Science and Vaccine!

If Science is so good and Pharmaceuticals are so smart where were they when at least 80 million confirmed infected and 1.7 million confirmed dead worldwide! And of those 18 million in USA confirmed infected and 315 thousands died!

The virus is fading away and much weaker not because of wisdom science and pharmaceuticals but because the natural immunity God created in each human being as a self-defense mechanism!

For almost a year science and pharmaceuticals only given us foolishness house arrest, face mask, social isolation, curfews and physical separation! And governments and politicians blaming the people but themselves never secured real scientists to eradicate a virus before spread and build more hospital beds and staff and resources!

Let us give glory to God the Lord Jesus and not to Pfizer or any pharmaceuticals or science!

Next time if science or pharmaceuticals need to take credit please step up and have treatment and vaccine ready from day one before the world get infected! O foolish science and scientists and incompetent medicine and advisory boards!

The Truth is furious in seeing images of people praising not God but pharmaceuticals counterparts and their countries are taking away the credit from God who created natural immunity and already weakened the man made virus! The images are evil these pharmaceuticals and their countries present themselves as God sent salvation and mercy to the world. It is absolutely fake and they do not deserve credit but reproach and accountability for their incompetence and inability to produce treatment of vaccine for a year before the entire world got infected!

God wrath on those whom are taking the Glory from Him as He did to Herod and the worms ate his flesh: "And upon a set day Herod, arrayed in royal apparel, sat upon his throne, and made an oration unto them. [22] And the people gave a shout, saying, It is the voice of a god, and not of a man. [23] And immediately the angel of the Lord smote him, because he gave not God the glory: and he was eaten of worms, and gave up the ghost." Acts 12:21-23 KJV

"I am the Lord: that is my name: and my glory will I not give to another, neither my praise to graven images." Isaiah 42:8 KJV

"For mine own sake, even for mine own sake, will I do it: for how should my name be polluted? and I will not give my glory unto another. [12] Hearken unto me, O Jacob and Israel, my called; I am he; I am the first, I also am the last." Isaiah 48:11-12 KJV

"As concerning therefore the eating of those things that are offered in sacrifice unto idols, we know that an idol is nothing in the world, and that there is none other God but one. [5] For though there be that are called gods, whether in heaven or in earth, (as there be gods many, and lords many,) [6] But to us there is but one God, the Father, of whom are all things, and we in him; and one Lord Jesus Christ, by whom are all things, and we by him."1 Corinthians 8:4-6 KJV

"What if God, wanting to show His wrath and to make His power known, endured with much longsuffering the vessels of wrath prepared for destruction," Romans 9:22

For the Scripture says to Pharaoh, "For this very purpose I have raised you up, that I might show my power in you, and that my name may be proclaimed in all the earth." (Romans 9:17)

Please give credit to God and not to man! Let us rise and give glory to God and not to man!

In Christmas 🎄 remember to give the glory yo no one but God and to Him only Thanksgiving!

Amen 🙏 thank you lord Jesus to thine is the Power, the Glory and the Kingdom for ever and ever Amen 🙏

Biblical Verses

And my God will meet all your needs according to the riches of his glory in Christ Jesus. To our God and Father be glory for ever and ever. Amen. - Philippians 4:19-20

+ Yet he did not waver through unbelief regarding the promise of God, but was strengthened in his faith and gave glory to God. - Romans 4:20

+ For God, who said, "Let light shine out of darkness," made his light shine in our hearts to give us the light of the knowledge of God's glory displayed in the face of Christ. - 2 Corinthians 4:6

+ The Word became flesh and made his dwelling among us. We have seen his glory, the glory of the one and only Son, who came from the Father, full of grace and truth. - John 1:14

+ The heavens declare the glory of God; the skies proclaim the work of his hands. - Psalm 19:1

+ So whether you eat or drink or whatever you do, do it all for the glory of God. - 1 Corinthians 10:31

+ I pray that out of his glorious riches he may strengthen you with power through his Spirit in your inner being. - Ephesians 3:16

+ All this is for your benefit, so that the grace that is reaching more and more people may cause thanksgiving to overflow to the glory of God. - 2 Corinthians 4:15

+ "Glory to God in the highest heaven, and on earth peace to those on whom his favor rests." - Luke 2:14

+ That at the name of Jesus every knee should bow, in heaven and on earth and under the earth, and every tongue acknowledge that Jesus Christ is Lord, to the glory of God the Father. - Philippians 2:10-11

1 Corinthians 10:31 ESV So, whether you eat or drink, or whatever you do, do all to the glory of God.

1 Corinthians 6:20 ESV For you were bought with a price. So glorify God in your body.

Hebrews 13:15 ESV Through him then let us continually offer up a sacrifice of praise to God, that is, the fruit of lips that acknowledge his name.

John 1:14 ESV And the Word became flesh and dwelt among us, and we have seen his glory, glory as of the only Son from the Father, full of grace and truth.

Matthew 5:16 ESV In the same way, let your light shine before others, so that they may see your good works and give glory to your Father who is in heaven.

Psalm 69:30 ESV I will praise the name of God with a song; I will magnify him with thanksgiving.

Hebrews 1:3 ESV He is the radiance of the glory of God and the exact imprint of his nature, and he upholds the universe by the word of his power. After making purification for sins, he sat down at the right hand of the Majesty on high,

Philippians 2:11 ESV And every tongue confess that Jesus Christ is Lord, to the glory of God the Father.

Romans 11:36 ESV For from him and through him and to him are all things. To him be glory forever. Amen.

John 3:16 ESV "For God so loved the world, that he gave his only Son, that whoever believes in him should not perish but have eternal life.

Isaiah 43:7 ESV Everyone who is called by my name, whom I created for my glory, whom I formed and made."

Psalm 86:12 ESV I give thanks to you, O Lord my God, with my whole heart, and I will glorify your name forever.

Psalm 50:23 ESV The one who offers thanksgiving as his sacrifice glorifies me; to one who orders his way rightly I will show the salvation of God!"

Revelation 14:7 ESV And he said with a loud voice, "Fear God and give him glory, because the hour of his judgment has come, and worship him who made heaven and earth, the sea and the springs of water."

1 Peter 2:9 ESV But you are a chosen race, a royal priesthood, a holy nation, a people for his own possession, that you may proclaim the excellencies of him who called you out of darkness into his marvelous light.

Romans 1:21 ESV For although they knew God, they did not honor him as God or give thanks to him, but they became futile in their thinking, and their foolish hearts were darkened.

Luke 2:14 ESV "Glory to God in the highest, and on earth peace among those with whom he is pleased!"

Psalm 22:23 ESV You who fear the Lord, praise him! All you offspring of Jacob, glorify him, and stand in awe of him, all you offspring of Israel!

1 Peter 4:11 ESV Whoever speaks, as one who speaks oracles of God; whoever serves, as one who serves by the strength that God supplies—in order that in everything God may be glorified through Jesus Christ. To him belong glory and dominion forever and ever. Amen.

Colossians 3:23 ESV Whatever you do, work heartily, as for the Lord and not for men,

Colossians 3:17 ESV And whatever you do, in word or deed, do everything in the name of the Lord Jesus, giving thanks to God the Father through him.

Colossians 1:27 ESV To them God chose to make known how great among the Gentiles are the riches of the glory of this mystery, which is Christ in you, the hope of glory.

Ephesians 5:19 ESV Addressing one another in psalms and hymns and spiritual songs, singing and making melody to the Lord with your heart,

2 Corinthians 4:16-18 ESV So we do not lose heart. Though our outer self is wasting away, our inner self is being renewed day by day. For this light momentary affliction is preparing for us an eternal weight of glory beyond all comparison, as we look not to the things that are seen but to the things that are unseen. For the things that are seen are transient, but the things that are unseen are eternal.

2 Corinthians 3:18 ESV And we all, with unveiled face, beholding the glory of the Lord, are being transformed into the same image from one degree of glory to another. For this comes from the Lord who is the Spirit.

1 Corinthians 15:57 ESV But thanks be to God, who gives us the victory through our Lord Jesus Christ.

Romans 15:7 ESV Therefore welcome one another as Christ has welcomed you, for the glory of God.

Romans 8:28 ESV And we know that for those who love God all things work together for good, for those who are called according to his purpose.

Romans 1:1-32 ESV Paul, a servant of Christ Jesus, called to be an apostle, set apart for the gospel of God, which he promised beforehand through his prophets in the holy Scriptures, concerning his Son, who was descended from David according to the flesh and was declared to be the Son of God in power according to the Spirit of holiness by his resurrection from the dead, Jesus Christ our Lord, through whom we have received grace and apostleship to bring about the obedience of faith for the sake of his name among all the nations, ...

John 21:19 ESV (This he said to show by what kind of death he was to glorify God.) And after saying this he said to him, "Follow me."

John 15:8 ESV By this my Father is glorified, that you bear much fruit and so prove to be my disciples.

Luke 17:15 ESV Then one of them, when he saw that he was healed, turned back, praising God with a loud voice;

Daniel 2:23 ESV To you, O God of my fathers, I give thanks and praise, for you have given me wisdom and might, and have now made known to me what we asked of you, for you have made known to us the king's matter."

Isaiah 42:8 ESV I am the Lord; that is my name; my glory I give to no other, nor my praise to carved idols.

Psalm 118:28 ESV You are my God, and I will give thanks to you; you are my God; I will extol you.

Psalm 106:1 ESV Praise the Lord! Oh give thanks to the Lord, for he is good, for his steadfast love endures forever!

Psalm 101:1 ESV A Psalm of David. I will sing of steadfast love and justice; to you, O Lord, I will make music.

Psalm 100:4 ESV Enter his gates with thanksgiving, and his courts with praise! Give thanks to him; bless his name!

Psalm 97:12 ESV Rejoice in the Lord, O you righteous, and give thanks to his holy name!

Psalm 95:2 ESV Let us come into his presence with thanksgiving; let us make a joyful noise to him with songs of praise!

Psalm 92:1 ESV A Psalm. A Song for the Sabbath. It is good to give thanks to the Lord, to sing praises to your name, O Most High;

Psalm 71:14 ESV But I will hope continually and will praise you yet more and more.

Psalm 50:15 ESV And call upon me in the day of trouble; I will deliver you, and you shall glorify me."

Psalm 19:1 ESV To the choirmaster. A Psalm of David. The heavens declare the glory of God, and the sky above proclaims his handiwork.

Revelation 15:4 ESV Who will not fear, O Lord, and glorify your name? For you alone are holy. All nations will come and worship you, for your righteous acts have been revealed."

Revelation 11:17 ESV Saying, "We give thanks to you, Lord God Almighty, who is and who was, for you have taken your great power and begun to reign.

Revelation 7:12 ESV Saying, "Amen! Blessing and glory and wisdom and thanksgiving and honor and power and might be to our God forever and ever! Amen."

Revelation 5:13 ESV And I heard every creature in heaven and on earth and under the earth and in the sea, and all that is in them, saying, "To him who sits on the throne and to the Lamb be blessing and honor and glory and might forever and ever!"

Revelation 4:11 ESV "Worthy are you, our Lord and God, to receive glory and honor and power, for you created all things, and by your will they existed and were created."

Revelation 1:1-20 ESV The revelation of Jesus Christ, which God gave him to show to his servants the things that must soon take place. He made it known by sending his angel to his servant John, who bore witness to the word of God and to the testimony of Jesus Christ, even to all that he saw. Blessed is the one who reads aloud the words of this prophecy, and blessed are those who hear, and who keep what is written in it, for the time is near. John to the seven churches that are in

Asia: Grace to you and peace from him who is and who was and who is to come, and from the seven spirits who are before his throne, and from Jesus Christ the faithful witness, the firstborn of the dead, and the ruler of kings on earth. To him who loves us and has freed us from our sins by his blood ...

1 John 2:6 ESV Whoever says he abides in him ought to walk in the same way in which he walked.

2 Peter 3:9 ESV The Lord is not slow to fulfill his promise as some count slowness, but is patient toward you, not wishing that any should perish, but that all should reach repentance.

1 Peter 5:1 ESV So I exhort the elders among you, as a fellow elder and a witness of the sufferings of Christ, as well as a partaker in the glory that is going to be revealed:

1 Peter 4:16 ESV Yet if anyone suffers as a Christian, let him not be ashamed, but let him glorify God in that name.

1 Peter 4:8 ESV Above all, keep loving one another earnestly, since love covers a multitude of sins.

1 Peter 2:12 ESV Keep your conduct among the Gentiles honorable, so that when they speak against you as evildoers, they may see your good deeds and glorify God on the day of visitation.

1 Timothy 2:11-15 ESV Let a woman learn quietly with all submissiveness. I do not permit a woman to teach or to exercise authority over a man; rather, she is to remain quiet. For Adam was formed first, then Eve; and Adam was not deceived, but the woman was deceived and became a transgressor. Yet she will be saved through childbearing—if they continue in faith and love and holiness, with self-control.

1 Timothy 2:1 ESV First of all, then, I urge that supplications, prayers, intercessions, and thanksgivings be made for all people,

1 Timothy 1:17 ESV To the King of ages, immortal, invisible, the only God, be honor and glory forever and ever. Amen.

1 Thessalonians 5:18 ESV Give thanks in all circumstances; for this is the will of God in Christ Jesus for you.

Colossians 3:15 ESV And let the peace of Christ rule in your hearts, to which indeed you were called in one body. And be thankful.

Colossians 3:4 ESV When Christ who is your life appears, then you also will appear with him in glory.

Philippians 4:13 ESV I can do all things through him who strengthens me.

Philippians 4:6 ESV Do not be anxious about anything, but in everything by prayer and supplication with thanksgiving let your requests be made known to God.

Philippians 2:13 ESV For it is God who works in you, both to will and to work for his good pleasure.

Philippians 1:11 ESV Filled with the fruit of righteousness that comes through Jesus Christ, to the glory and praise of God.

Ephesians 3:21 ESV To him be glory in the church and in Christ Jesus throughout all generations, forever and ever. Amen.

Ephesians 1:18 ESV Having the eyes of your hearts enlightened, that you may know what is the hope to which he has called you, what are the riches of his glorious inheritance in the saints,

Ephesians 1:3 ESV Blessed be the God and Father of our Lord Jesus Christ, who has blessed us in Christ with every spiritual blessing in the heavenly places,

Galatians 6:14 ESV But far be it from me to boast except in the cross of our Lord Jesus Christ, by which the world has been crucified to me, and I to the world.

Galatians 5:22-23 ESV But the fruit of the Spirit is love, joy, peace, patience, kindness, goodness, faithfulness, gentleness, self-control; against such things there is no law.

2 Corinthians 9:13 ESV By their approval of this service, they will glorify God because of your submission flowing from your confession of the gospel of Christ, and the generosity of your contribution for them and for all others,

2 Corinthians 4:15 ESV For it is all for your sake, so that as grace extends to more and more people it may increase thanksgiving, to the glory of God.

147

2 Corinthians 4:7 ESV But we have this treasure in jars of clay, to show that the surpassing power belongs to God and not to us.

2 Corinthians 4:6 ESV For God, who said, "Let light shine out of darkness," has shone in our hearts to give the light of the knowledge of the glory of God in the face of Jesus Christ.

2 Corinthians 1:20 ESV For all the promises of God find their Yes in him. That is why it is through him that we utter our Amen to God for his glory.

1 Corinthians 14:34-36 ESV The women should keep silent in the churches. For they are not permitted to speak, but should be in submission, as the Law also says. If there is anything they desire to learn, let them ask their husbands at home. For it is shameful for a woman to speak in church. Or was it from you that the word of God came? Or are you the only ones it has reached?

1 Corinthians 1:2 ESV To the church of God that is in Corinth, to those sanctified in Christ Jesus, called to be saints together with all those who in every place call upon the name of our Lord Jesus Christ, both their Lord and ours:

Romans 9:4 ESV They are Israelites, and to them belong the adoption, the glory, the covenants, the giving of the law, the worship, and the promises.

Romans 8:30 ESV And those whom he predestined he also called, and those whom he called he also justified, and those whom he justified he also glorified.

Romans 8:29 ESV For those whom he foreknew he also predestined to be conformed to the image of his Son, in order that he might be the firstborn among many brothers.

Romans 8:1-39 ESV There is therefore now no condemnation for those who are in Christ Jesus. For the law of the Spirit of life has set you free in Christ Jesus from the law of sin and death. For God has done what the law, weakened by the flesh, could not do. By sending his own Son in the likeness of sinful flesh and for sin, he condemned sin in the flesh, in order that the righteous requirement of the law might be fulfilled in us, who walk not according to the flesh but according to the Spirit. For those who live according to the flesh set their minds on the things of the flesh, but those who live according to the Spirit set their minds on the things of the Spirit. ...

Romans 5:2 ESV Through him we have also obtained access by faith into this grace in which we stand, and we rejoice in hope of the glory of God.

Romans 4:20 ESV No distrust made him waver concerning the promise of God, but he grew strong in his faith as he gave glory to God,

Romans 3:23 ESV For all have sinned and fall short of the glory of God,

Romans 3:21-26 ESV But now the righteousness of God has been manifested apart from the law, although the Law and the Prophets bear witness to it— the righteousness of God through faith in Jesus Christ for all who believe. For there is no distinction: for all have sinned and fall short of the glory of God, and are justified by his grace as a gift, through the redemption that is in Christ Jesus, whom God put forward as a propitiation by his blood, to be received by faith. This was to show God's righteousness, because in his divine forbearance he had passed over former sins. ...

Romans 1:18-23 ESV For the wrath of God is revealed from heaven against all ungodliness and unrighteousness of men, who by their unrighteousness suppress the truth. For what can be known about God is plain to them, because God has shown it to them. For his invisible attributes, namely, his eternal power and divine nature, have been clearly perceived, ever since the creation of the world, in the things that have been made. So they are without excuse. For although they knew God, they did not honor him as God or give thanks to him, but they became futile in their thinking, and their foolish hearts were darkened. Claiming to be wise, they became fools, ...

Acts 16:25 ESV About midnight Paul and Silas were praying and singing hymns to God, and the prisoners were listening to them,

John 17:22 ESV The glory that you have given me I have given to them, that they may be one even as we are one,

John 17:5 ESV And now, Father, glorify me in your own presence with the glory that I had with you before the world existed.

John 17:4 ESV I glorified you on earth, having accomplished the work that you gave me to do.

John 15:18-21 ESV "If the world hates you, know that it has hated me before it hated you. If you were of the world, the world would love you as its own; but because you are not of the world, but I chose you out of the world, therefore the world hates you. Remember the word that I said to you: 'A servant is not greater than his master.' If they persecuted me, they will also persecute you. If they kept

149

my word, they will also keep yours. But all these things they will do to you on account of my name, because they do not know him who sent me.

John 14:6 ESV Jesus said to him, "I am the way, and the truth, and the life. No one comes to the Father except through me.

John 11:40 ESV Jesus said to her, "Did I not tell you that if you believed you would see the glory of God?"

John 10:10 ESV The thief comes only to steal and kill and destroy. I came that they may have life and have it abundantly.

John 8:54 ESV Jesus answered, "If I glorify myself, my glory is nothing. It is my Father who glorifies me, of whom you say, 'He is our God.'

John 3:16-17 ESV "For God so loved the world, that he gave his only Son, that whoever believes in him should not perish but have eternal life. For God did not send his Son into the world to condemn the world, but in order that the world might be saved through him.

John 2:11 ESV This, the first of his signs, Jesus did at Cana in Galilee, and manifested his glory. And his disciples believed in him

VA Love what you write. God should be given the glory for everything...my mom used to tell us, thank God for all things good and bad. We asked why bad, because things could be worse, and God chastises whom he loves. God watches all of us.

DE. Amen good doctor. Well written from the heart. Bless you and Happy Holidays! 🙏🌲

Heavenly Message of Lifting up the COVID Curse!

As COVID was started by in the forty days Lent 2020, so it shall be lifted up in the Lent of 2021!

God has remembered mankind His handmade creation: His children-"-God made a wind to pass over the earth, and the waters asswaged;"

O people of the entire world 🌍, God is sending His Heavenly dove in the evening; and, lo, in her mouth shall be an olive leaf pluckt off: as in Noah time and at that time you all should know because of God's mercy and love 💜 and not man, the earth is once more a life to return!

The message from heaven came loud and clear; God the Almighty our Savior is lifting up the curse from the world 🌍 and COVID is over soon! Let us sing with the multitudes: Hosanna to the Son of David: Blessed is he that cometh in the name of the Lord; Hosanna in the highest." Matthew 21:9 And with the Psalmist: "Bless the Lord, O my soul: and all that is within me, bless his holy name. [2] Bless the Lord, O my soul, and forget not all his benefits:-" Psalm 103

LORD smelled a sweet savour; and the LORD said in his heart, I will not again curse the ground any more for man's sake;

God set His bow in the cloud ☁ once more, and it shall be for a token of a covenant between God and the earth. And God shall remember His covenant between Him and us and every living creature of all flesh;—

Soon the healing for thy people and peace upon the face of the earth 🌍 as it shall be a memorials for all the lives were taken and the victims of the wrath of the century!!!

"And God remembered Noah, and every living thing, and all the cattle that was with him in the ark: and God made a wind to pass over the earth, and the waters asswaged; [6] And it came to pass at the end of forty days, that Noah opened the window of the ark which he had made: [11] And the dove came in to him in the evening; and, lo, in her mouth was an olive leaf pluckt off: so Noah knew that the waters were abated from off the earth. [15] And God spake unto Noah, saying, [16] Go forth of the ark, thou, and thy wife, and thy sons, and thy sons' wives with thee.

[17] Bring forth with thee every living thing that is with thee, of all flesh, both of fowl, and of cattle, and of every creeping thing that creepeth upon the earth; that they may breed abundantly in the earth, and be fruitful, and multiply upon the earth. [18] And Noah went forth, and his sons, and his wife, and his sons' wives with him: [19] Every beast, every creeping thing, and every fowl, and whatsoever creepeth upon the earth, after their kinds, went forth out of the ark. [20] And Noah builded an altar unto the Lord ; and took of every clean beast, and of every clean fowl, and offered burnt offerings on the altar. [21] And the Lord smelled a sweet savour; and the Lord said in his heart, I will not again curse the ground any more for man's sake; for the imagination of man's heart is evil from his youth; neither will I again smite any more every thing living, as I have done. [22] While the earth remaineth, seedtime and harvest, and cold and heat, and summer and winter, and day and night shall not cease." Genesis 8:1,6,11,15-22 KJV

"And God said, This is the token of the covenant which I make between me and you and every living creature that is with you, for perpetual generations: [13] I do set my bow in the cloud, and it shall be for a token of a covenant between me and the earth. [14] And it shall come to pass, when I bring a cloud over the earth, that the bow shall be seen in the cloud: [15] And I will remember my covenant, which is between me and you and every living creature of all flesh; and the waters shall no more become a flood to destroy all flesh. [16] And the bow shall be in the cloud; and I will look upon it, that I may remember the everlasting covenant between God and every living creature of all flesh that is upon the earth. [17] And God said unto Noah, This is the token of the covenant, which I have established between me and all flesh that is upon the earth." Genesis 9:12-17 KJV

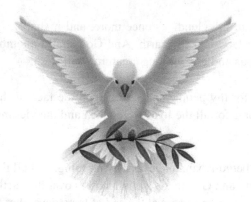

CG. Always sending beautiful hopeful thoughts our way. Bless you!
RH. I pray. 🙏 😌
CR. Praise the Lord for herd immunity!
BCD. Great message

Let us not forget our Heavenly and Merciful Father in defeating the most devastating virus affecting universally the human race worldwide!!

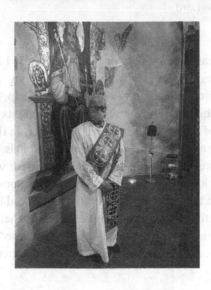

Let us praise and thank our Lord Jesus! He provided the best ever natural human immunity to mankind!

Seven billion six hundred seventy million five hundred thousand spared from dying from COVID-19!

And seven billion five hundred twenty-one million spared from getting infected from COVID-19!

Thus far out of 7.674 billion worldwide populations and only 3.5 million worldwide died from coronavirus COVID-19!

The percent of death rate is 0.00041699244

And percent of infection rate (153 million) is 0.01993745113!

Let us care about the billions of people and help them and care for them and not to be forgotten!!

Psalm 150

[1] Praise ye the Lord. Praise God in his sanctuary: praise him in the firmament of his power. [2] Praise him for his mighty acts: praise him according to his excellent greatness. [3] Praise him with the sound of the trumpet: praise him with the psaltery and harp. [4] Praise him with the timbrel and dance: praise him with stringed instruments and organs. [5] Praise him upon the loud cymbals: praise him upon the high sounding cymbals. [6] Let every thing that hath breath praise the Lord. Praise ye the Lord.

Psalm 146

Praise ye the Lord. Praise the Lord, O my soul. [2] While I live will I praise the Lord: I will sing praises unto my God while I have any being. [3] Put not your trust in princes, nor in the son of man, in whom there is no help. [4] His breath goeth forth, he returneth to his earth; in that very day his thoughts perish. [5] Happy is he that hath the God of Jacob for his help, whose hope is in the Lord his God: [6] Which made heaven, and earth, the sea, and all that therein is: which keepeth truth for ever: [7] Which executeth judgment for the oppressed: which giveth food to the hungry. The Lord looseth the prisoners: [8] The Lord openeth the eyes of the blind: the Lord raiseth them that are bowed down: the Lord loveth the righteous: [9] The Lord preserveth the strangers; he relieveth the fatherless and widow: but the way of the wicked he turneth upside down. [10] The Lord shall reign for ever, even thy God, O Zion, unto all generations. Praise ye the Lord.

Ramsis Ghaly

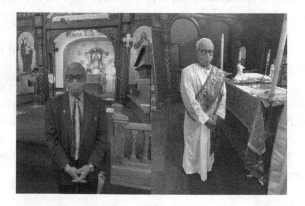

KG. God Bless you, Dr Ghaly. Blessings from Egypt.
RC. Thanks! Blessings!
AV. Beautiful message & photos Dr. Ghaly! Hope u had a blessed Easter! 🐣🙏
JB. Praise God forever for all His goodness and love to mankind 🙌🙌🙌
CG. Praise our Lord and Bless you. ❤️🙏

America Let Us Go New Page for America A Year Later Still True!!

Written by Ramsis Ghaly
May 5, 2020

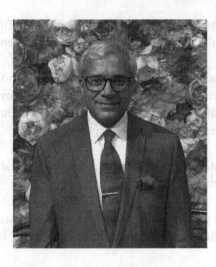

America let us use the time to rebuild America for the coming generations! —let us go America. Do not surrender and wait for what tomorrow will bring but instead make tomorrow!

The most logic thing to do is do not look back at the past, learn from it and be wise: Rrise and rebuild America in such away that won't surrender to future biochemical threats whereas life won't stop!

"And Jesus said unto him, No man, having put his hand to the plough, and looking back, is fit for the kingdom of God." Luke 9:62 and "Brethren, I count not myself to have apprehended: but this one thing I do, forgetting those things which are behind, and reaching forth unto those things which are before, 14I press toward the mark for the prize of the high calling of God in Christ Jesus. 15Let us therefore, as many as be perfect, be thus minded: and if in any thing ye be otherwise minded, God shall reveal even this unto you." Philippians 3: 13-16

American engineers and construction workers rise up to the task and reform shops, malls, businesses and entertainment industry for people while to protecting the people and the crowd from the future biochemical terrorism!

Las Vegas, the Entertainment City of the world and so is the Orlando Disney world rise up, use the opportunity and be innovative: rebuild your entire structure to entertain the public of all ages from everywhere while adapting to the new era that always will carry the threats of more Biochemicals warfare!

America Department of Defense, let us Reform and make America No longer be threatened to the new threats of biochemical weapons!

Let us all use the time to rebuild America to combat the future enemies while enjoying freedom again and quality social life among all people!

Smart businesses, schools, universities, factories——will modify their firms to be digital technology spread into spacious multi-floor structures! No more clustered closets! So are Entertainments to rebuild in such a way avoiding compact cubicles such as wide Bars, Restaurants, outdoors cinemas, ——!

Wall Street and investors put your money in the new innovations and encourage novelty for restructuring the new world!!

New generations and youngsters stand up and start to create the new world 🌍 for you all to fit the threats and be much better than ours!

New companies, new ideas, new minds, new ways,——let us go America! Let us start open-minded manufactures! Do not surrender and wait for what tomorrow will bring but instead make tomorrow!

What a great opportunity of a lifetime to Rebuild the World again!! So now answer your calling and let us run the race all run to transform the world to a new spectacular world with new minds, solidarity and strength of steel against all the new threats, yet won't ever stop our life ever again!

America, you must lead the world to the next phase and help to conquer the new threats in a world of evil and terrorism. We must not stop living and surrender to the destruction of the devil and be helpless in a house arrest any longer!

Return to Jesus and have America again under one God, do what it takes, get ride of the bureaucracy, fake scientists, talkers, staggers and evil doers scientists, Stock your vaccine laboratories and line up true swellheaded skilled and caring staff.

Romans 14:8 KJV For whether we live, we live unto the Lord; and whether we die, we die unto the Lord: whether we live therefore, or die, we are the Lord's.

Amen 🙏

Ramsis Ghaly www.ghalyneurosurgeon.com

CG. This is all true today! Great photo! 🖤🙏

SP. Your spot on, now we need people to wake up and go back to normalcy instead of being afraid of one another, go out and live life and bring life to this great world again!

NC. Praying for your friend! 🙏🙏🙏🙏

Let us go America!

Prior to Inauguration 1/13/2021
Written by Ramsis Ghaly

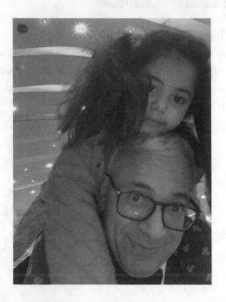

Let us go America 🇺🇸! Let us renew our vows as one country and one people! Let us build America 🇺🇸 for our children!

Let us go America 🇺🇸! Let us move on and run fast carrying the Olympic Flame 🔥 to lead the globe 🌍 to a new page!

Let us go America 🇺🇸 to the other aisle! Let us walk and shake hands! We are much better country than this!

Let us go America 🇺🇸 and look to your future for the sake of our children and generations to come!

Let us go America 🇺🇸! No riots and no demonstrations and no destruction but love!

Let us go America 🇺🇸 and take the first step!

Let us go America 🇺🇸 in open mind in love and faith!

Let us go America 🇺🇸 to make peace and extend our hands to call for Unity!

Let us go America 🇺🇸 and bring our hearts 💜 and commitment!

Let us go America 🇺🇸 to share what you have with what they have and make the best out of both world!

Let us go America 🇺🇸 and move forward, the past is past the present is present that soon leads to the near future!

Let us go America 🇺🇸 and let it sink in your mind one country one constitution in one God, Amen!

Let us go America 🇺🇸 get washed and start clean in a new page the Day of the Lord Jesus our Savior is Near!

Ramsis Ghaly

Mk. I will never unite with the Demon. party.
Tj. Absolutely beautiful! I pray that God will restore UNITY to this country. God, help us all!
Ab. Amen praise God!
Sc. cute
Ko. Amen let's go America beautiful children
Cg. I wish all these could happen but I am afraid to many people are angry and not ready to move on. All we can do is pray that our country will someday be united again. 💜🙏🇺🇸
Sj. You are such a natural with kids 💜
Sa. She is adorable!
Jm. Yes for families
Rn. Beautiful 😊💜🙏✝️🙏
Nc. Can't we just accept the election?
Rc. Cute, good thougs! Buenos Pensamientos! Go for beauty
Bl. We are to love one another even in politics. We are adults and should behave as such. I see so much hate and evil actions directed towards our fellow man for the purpose of destroying them. How is it people can claim they love God while at the same time behaving so ungodly? 😫

God please heal our country.

America Resume Your Life Back! Let us walk in the Vine! Let Us Rise Up and Smell the Roses Once More!

Written by Ramsis Ghaly

America 🏴 2020 was a nightmare dream and envy of satanism! Come out of your homes and hidden places America 🏴! Start to walk in the light 💡 in daytime before the darkness takes away and swallow you alive!

Our Lord Jesus words to you America 🏴 and the World 🌍 today: "Are there not twelve hours in the day? If any man walk in the day, he stumbleth not, because he seeth the light of this world. [10] But if a man walk in the night, he stumbleth, because there is no light in him." John 11:9-10 KJV

The Coronavirus is not as strong and the caysakitues aren't as bad!

America 🏴 take hold of yourself and stand up and begin to run the global race as you used to be leading the world in success!

The COVID numbers are up but the critical Intensive Care Unit is not as used to be!

The COVID is much weaker and the symptomatic patients aren't as sick!

America 🏴 start to normalize your life cautiously and enough surrender your precious life!

It will take much for you America 🏴 to recondition yourself!

It won't easy because leaving your homes, your nest and your remote hid out aren't that simple!

To return back and expose yourself to the outside world and start to interact with people in person isn't that trivial!

To resume Ore-COVID era, it will need years!

Furthermore wireless jobs and technologies may not be of help in the transition or supporting change!

In fact, the existing state of affairs and status quo is very attractive to continue since there is no much of hardworking, sweeting, accountability and much of exposure with no more excuses of cover up!!!

America 🏴 Take your first step, wash 🧼🧼 out the past and cheer, fear not be of good courage!

Matthew 14:27 But straightway Jesus spake unto them, saying, Be of good cheer; it is I; be not afraid.

Psalm 31:24 ESV Be strong, and let your heart take courage, all you who wait for the Lord!

Psalm 27:14 ESV Wait for the Lord; be strong, and let your heart take courage; wait for the Lord!

Joshua 1:9 ESV Have I not commanded you? Be strong and courageous. Do not be frightened, and do not be dismayed, for the Lord your God is with you wherever you go."

Acts 23:11 ESV The following night the Lord stood by him and said, "Take courage, for as you have testified to the facts about me in Jerusalem, so you must testify also in Rome."

Isaiah 40:31 ESV But they who wait for the Lord shall renew their strength; they shall mount up with wings like eagles; they shall run and not be weary; they shall walk and not faint.

America 🏴 Resume Your Life Back! Let us walk in the Vine! Let Us Rise Up and Smell the Roses 🌹 🌹 Once More!

Psalm 68:1-35
Let God arise, let his enemies be scattered: let them also that hate him flee before him. [2] As smoke is driven away, so drive them away: as wax melteth before the fire, so let the wicked perish at the presence of God. [3] But let the righteous be glad; let them rejoice before God: yea, let them exceedingly rejoice. [4] Sing unto God, sing praises to his name: extol him that rideth upon the heavens by his name Jah, and rejoice before him. [5] A father of the fatherless, and a judge of

the widows, is God in his holy habitation. [6] God setteth the solitary in families: he bringeth out those which are bound with chains: but the rebellious dwell in a dry land. [7] O God, when thou wentest forth before thy people, when thou didst march through the wilderness; Selah: [8] The earth shook, the heavens also dropped at the presence of God: even Sinai itself was moved at the presence of God, the God of Israel. [9] Thou, O God, didst send a plentiful rain, whereby thou didst confirm thine inheritance, when it was weary. [10] Thy congregation hath dwelt therein: thou, O God, hast prepared of thy goodness for the poor. [11] The Lord gave the word: great was the company of those that published it. [12] Kings of armies did flee apace: and she that tarried at home divided the spoil. [13] Though ye have lien among the pots, yet shall ye be as the wings of a dove covered with silver, and her feathers with yellow gold. [14] When the Almighty scattered kings in it, it was white as snow in Salmon. [15] The hill of God is as the hill of Bashan; an high hill as the hill of Bashan. [16] Why leap ye, ye high hills? this is the hill which God desireth to dwell in; yea, the Lord will dwell in it for ever. [17] The chariots of God are twenty thousand, even thousands of angels: the Lord is among them, as in Sinai, in the holy place. [18] Thou hast ascended on high, thou hast led captivity captive: thou hast received gifts for men; yea, for the rebellious also, that the Lord God might dwell among them. [19] Blessed be the Lord, who daily loadeth us with benefits, even the God of our salvation. Selah. [20] He that is our God is the God of salvation; and unto God the Lord belong the issues from death. [21] But God shall wound the head of his enemies, and the hairy scalp of such an one as goeth on still in his trespasses. [22] The Lord said, I will bring again from Bashan, I will bring my people again from the depths of the sea: [23] That thy foot may be dipped in the blood of thine enemies, and the tongue of thy dogs in the same. [24] They have seen thy goings, O God; even the goings of my God, my King, in the sanctuary. [25] The singers went before, the players on instruments followed after; among them were the damsels playing with timbrels. [26] Bless ye God in the congregations, even the Lord, from the fountain of Israel. [27] There is little Benjamin with their ruler, the princes of Judah and their council, the princes of Zebulun, and the princes of Naphtali. [28] Thy God hath commanded thy strength: strengthen, O God, that which thou hast wrought for us. [29] Because of thy temple at Jerusalem shall kings bring presents unto thee. [30] Rebuke the company of spearmen, the multitude of the bulls, with the calves of the people, till every one submit himself with pieces of silver: scatter thou the people that delight in war. [31] Princes shall come out of Egypt; Ethiopia shall soon stretch out her hands unto God. [32] Sing unto God, ye kingdoms of the earth; O sing praises unto the Lord; Selah: [33] To him that rideth upon the heavens of heavens, which were of old; lo, he doth send out his voice, and that a mighty voice. [34] Ascribe ye strength unto God: his excellency is over Israel, and his strength is in the clouds. [35] O God, thou art terrible out of thy holy places: the God of Israel is he that giveth strength and power unto his people. Blessed be God.

America 🇺🇸 Resume Your Life Back! Let us walk in the Vine! Let Us Rise Up and Smell the Roses 🌹 🕯 Once More!

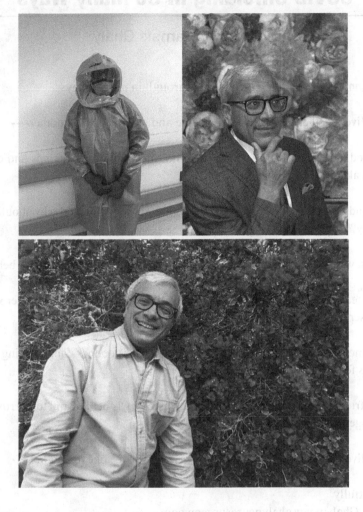

AV. Thank u so much Dr Ghaly for these wonderful verses of truth & encouragement!

SC. You prayers fill me with hope and tears of joy!

SC. You prayers fill me with hope and tears of joy!

As We Journey Together through COVID Unfolding In So Many Ways

Written By Ramsis Ghaly

In so many ways, we share what we go through in our journeys.

Let us live together the life worthy in love and service one to another----

The good that we do, the bad that we do not mean to do and the ups and downs that we always face in our days.

Our minds wonders of when we began, where are we going and why should it be this way???

Friends, what matters are what we do for others and the fruits we leave behind.

In the meanwhile, we continue living, learning from the past and stronger we get and wiser we become.

In the morning, we renew our vows to the God of goodness and looking up to heavens for a better day ahead.

So my friends, today is coming to an end, yesterday is behind and tomorrow is at hand together we shall share.

Let us live together the life worthy in love and service one to another----

Respectfully
Ramsis Ghaly www.ghalyneurosurgeon.com

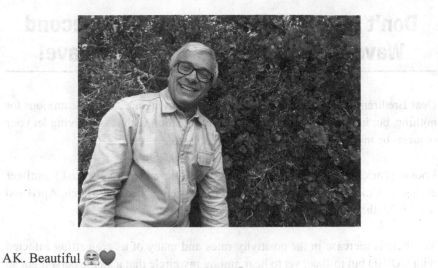

AK. Beautiful 😂💜
JC. You look very happy there, nice smile 🙏
KM. Keep smiling & shinning 💚🙏
MR. Great picture Dr.Ghaly! It shows your inner light!
LB. Looking very dapper!!!
RC. This is wonderful. Can I share it? Love your smile!
MS. Beautiful flowers behind you.
KC. Great picture!
CG. Such beautiful thoughts! Bless you! Nice picture. Miss that smile!
AB. Amen praise God
MN. Dr Ghaly your write as aways you have a great day and stay safe.
SW. Beautiful heart, Beautiful smile. ☺
SC. Yes!
RN. Beautiful 💜💜
KO. Amen, what we do for others, without asking for anything in return, is what really counts in life.

Don't Be Fearful But Joyful! The Second Wave Isn't As Bad As The First Wave!

Dear Brethren: St Paul is sending you all the following message: "Be anxious for nothing, but in everything by prayer and supplication with thanksgiving let your requests be made known to God." Philippians 4:6

Looking back as a since the very beginning until the end as a Very First Frontliner caring for Chicagoans and Illinoisans COVID victims back on March, April and May 2020, there is no comparison and not even close!

Yes there is increase in the positivity rates and many of us are getting infected with COVID but to-date, yet to hear among my circle that a single person got so sick and needed an ICU bed or getting intubated!

Don't Be Fearful But Joyful! Let us Help Each Other in This Tough Time and Support One Another!

The Second Wave Isn't As Bad As The First Wave!

Brethren, Stay Strong Against the Second Wave and Arm Yourself with Faith and Mask to Defeat it as You Defeated the First Wave!

The Second Wave Isn't As Bad As The First Wave! Praise Lord Jesus but praise neither man made vaccine nor treatment nor Medicine nor Science nor intellectual intelligence nor Modern Frontiers nor vaccine research Lab nor WHO nor NIH nor CDC nor Google nor Microsoft nor Facebook nor Twitter nor Linkin nor so called "Experts"! But Who to praise is Lord Jesus and his creation to human Natural Immunity that stood thousands of years against all kind of human enemies!

Therefore, Be Vigilant and Put your Mask and Keep Going:

1) *Don't surrender!*
2) *Don't lose hope!*
3) *Don't hid in the dark!*
4) *Don't be gloomy!*
5) *Don't isolate yourself!*
6) *Don't burden yourself!*
7) *Don't overwhelm yourself!*

8) *Don't tangle yourself in the mud—-!*
9) *Don't stop ● living!*
10) *Don't let it intimidate you!*
11) *Don't trust everything you hear!*
12) *Don't be pessimistic and look at half full!*
13) *Don't lose faith in God the Lord of earth and heaven!*
14) *Don't lose focus!*
15) *Don't be down in ourselves!*
16) *Don't overcome by evil!*
17) *Don't cry 😱 or she'd any tears!*
18) *Don't Be Fearful but Joyful!*

The Second Wave Isn't As Bad As The First Wave!

Brethren, Stay Strong Against the Second Wave and Arm Yourself with Faith and Mask to Defeat it as You Defeated the First Wave!

The Almighty provided His children with Natural Vaccine called "Autoimmunity" within our flesh and blood to combat viruses, weaken them and ultimately kill them!

God knows our weak nature and the grandiose fake minds of our scientists and the powerless so called "Modern Medicine", and the clueless of so called "Artificial Intelligence" and stupidity of so called "Digital Informatics"

In fact God laughs at them saying; "He that sitteth in the heavens shall laugh: the Lord shall have them in derision. Then shall he speak unto them in his wrath, and vex them in his sore displeasure. Yet have I set my king upon my holy hill of Zion. I will declare the decree: the Lord hath said unto me, Thou art my Son; this day have I begotten thee. Ask of me, and I shall give thee the heathen for thine inheritance, and the uttermost parts of the earth for thy possession. Thou shalt break them with a rod of iron; thou shalt dash them in pieces like a potter's vessel. Be wise now therefore, O ye kings: be instructed, ye judges of the earth. Serve the Lord with fear, and rejoice with trembling-"

As it is written: *"Why do the heathen rage, and the people imagine a vain thing? [2] The kings of the earth set themselves, and the rulers take counsel together, against the Lord, and against his anointed, saying, [3] Let us break their bands asunder, and cast away their cords from us. [4] He that sitteth in the heavens shall laugh: the Lord shall have them in derision. [5] Then shall he speak unto them in his wrath, and vex them in his sore displeasure. [6] Yet have I set my king upon my holy hill of Zion. [7] I will declare the decree: the Lord hath said unto me, Thou art my Son; this day have I begotten thee. [8] Ask of me, and I shall give thee the heathen for thine inheritance, and the uttermost parts of the earth for thy possession. [9] Thou shalt break them with a rod of iron; thou shalt dash them in pieces like a potter's vessel. [10] Be wise now therefore, O ye kings: be instructed, ye judges of the earth. [11] Serve the Lord with fear, and rejoice with trembling. [12] Kiss the Son, lest he be angry, and ye perish from the way, when his wrath is kindled but a little. Blessed are all they that put their trust in him."*

Psalm 2:1-12 KJV
Therefore, Don't Be Fearful but Joyful! The Second Wave Isn't As Bad As The First Wave! Stay Strong Against the Second Wave and Arm with Faith and Mask to Defeat it as the First Wave was Conquered!

Now let us all praise our Lord Jesus the Conquer of all our enemies and the True Healer against all pandemics singing increase the praises to Christ with our tongues, lift up Jesus with our hearts and sing to our savior with our tunes saying with those Middle East Arabic Christians:

https://www.facebook.com/WheyJeremiah/videos/629162931062183/?vh=
e&d=n

Our Savior has triumphed over the darkness and it's authority and lit up our days and give them joyful colors and the light of day is increasing:

https://www.facebook.com/WheyJeremiah/videos/629162931062183/?vh=
e&d=n

Psalm 147
Praise ye the Lord: for it is good to sing praises unto our God; for it is pleasant; and praise is comely. The Lord doth build up Jerusalem: he gathereth together the outcasts of Israel. He healeth the broken in heart, and bindeth up their wounds. He telleth the number of the stars; he calleth them all by their names. Great is our Lord, and of great power: his understanding is infinite. The Lord lifteth up the meek: he casteth the wicked down to the ground. Sing unto the Lord with thanksgiving; sing praise upon the harp unto our God: Who covereth the heaven with clouds, who prepareth rain for the earth, who maketh grass to grow upon the mountains. He giveth to the beast his food, and to the young ravens which cry. [10] He delighteth not in the strength of the horse: he taketh not pleasure in the legs of a man. The Lord taketh pleasure in them that fear him, in those that hope in his mercy. Praise the Lord, O Jerusalem; praise thy God, O Zion. For he

hath strengthened the bars of thy gates; he hath blessed thy children within thee. He maketh peace in thy borders, and filleth thee with the finest of the wheat. He sendeth forth his commandment upon earth: his word runneth very swiftly. He giveth snow like wool: he scattereth the hoarfrost like ashes. He casteth forth his ice like morsels: who can stand before his cold? He sendeth out his word, and melteth them: he causeth his wind to blow, and the waters flow. He sheweth his word unto Jacob, his statutes and his judgments unto Israel. He hath not dealt so with any nation: and as for his judgments, they have not known them. Praise ye the Lord.

Psalm 148

Praise ye the Lord. Praise ye the Lord from the heavens: praise him in the heights. Praise ye him, all his angels: praise ye him, all his hosts. Praise ye him, sun and moon: praise him, all ye stars of light. Praise him, ye heavens of heavens, and ye waters that be above the heavens. Let them praise the name of the Lord: for he commanded, and they were created. He hath also stablished them for ever and ever: he hath made a decree which shall not pass. Praise the Lord from the earth, ye dragons, and all deeps: Fire, and hail; snow, and vapour; stormy wind fulfilling his word: Mountains, and all hills; fruitful trees, and all cedars: Beasts, and all cattle; creeping things, and flying fowl: Kings of the earth, and all people; princes, and all judges of the earth: Both young men, and maidens; old men, and children: Let them praise the name of the Lord: for his name alone is excellent; his glory is above the earth and heaven. He also exalteth the horn of his people, the praise of all his saints; even of the children of Israel, a people near unto him. Praise ye the Lord.

We must move forward as a nation to learn from the fatal mistakes and shortcoming in order to recruit the true Doers and scientists to combat Bioweapons and Bioterrorism using such viruses and other danger species to humanity. The failure is huge to prevent early on and to find prompt treatment in the beginning of pandemic before the spread of COVID!

Amen

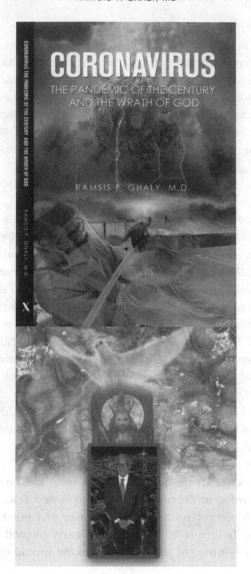

JM: Thank you

SA. ربنا يفرحك د. رمسيس ويبارك حياتك 🌷🌷

CG. You always offer positive words and thoughts in a troubled world. Thank you! Bless you always! 🖤🙏

SC. Thank you, Dr. Ghaly.

Do Not Run Do Not Hid the Coronavirus Will Determine What to Do

Don't Run and Don't Hid! The Coronavirus ✹✹✹ Will Determine What To Do! It Is No Longer Who Won Or Who Lost Since Coronavirus Particle Has Won! We All Lost And No One Has a Cure!

Written by Ramsis Ghaly

The wrath of God upon the wickedness of the world and the corruption of man! Your voice is no longer count nor your demonstrations, coronavirus ✹✹✹ is running the show!

O man, Don't Run and Don't Hid! The Corona virus ✹ Will Determine What To Do! We All Lost And No One Has a Cure!

O man save your energy and redirect your ways before Coronavirus ✹✹✹ rule over you! Give it up! It is no longer who won and who lost, repent and reform and call your Savior Jesus the Lord!

It isn't important any longer for who shall lead our nation since it appears that Coronavirus ✹✹✹ shall do so! We All Lost And No One Has a Cure!

The kings and queens and the leaders of the earth 🌍 have no more dominion as Coronavirus ✹✹✹ has!

The people 🌍 can't say a word as they are running away from the smallest monster 👹👹👹 known to man!

It is no longer what people wish for or want, Coronavirus ✹✹✹ shall impose upon their ways!

Coronavirus ✹✹✹ was sent to stay and to surface the ongoing worldwide corruption!

COVID is overpowering the world 🌍 and not stopping as mankind dreaming for the return of the early Pre-COVID days!

The leaders of all nations have no longer authority but Coronavirus 🦠🦠🦠 does! We All Lost And No One Has a Cure!

Let us not deceive ourselves, It Is No Longer Who Won Or Who Lost Since Coronavirus 🦠🦠🦠 Particle Has Won!

Let us in pure Love and Faith casting away the evil among us and unit all together as a nation and as world, fast and pray to the Lord God of Earth 🌍 and Heaven Jesus Christ our Savior to have mercy upon His people and the world whom He descended down in Christmas and saved!

The kings, queens, leaders and all people need to rise from their thrones and lay their robes and cover themselves with sackcloths and sit in ashes fasting anc praying unceasing as the people of Nineveh had done in order for our merciful God lift up thd COVID plague 🦠🦠🦠!

"For word came unto the king of Nineveh, and he arose from his throne, and he laid his robe from him, and covered him with sackcloth, and sat in ashes. [7] And he caused it to be proclaimed and published through Nineveh by the decree of the king and his nobles, saying, Let neither man nor beast, herd nor flock, taste any thing: let them not feed, nor drink water: [8] But let man and beast be covered with sackcloth, and cry mightily unto God: yea, let them turn every one from his evil way, and from the violence that is in their hands. [9] Who can tell if God will turn and repent, and turn away from his fierce anger, that we perish not? [10] And God saw their works, that they turned from their evil way; and God repented of the evil, that he had said that he would do unto them; and he did it not." Jonah 3:6-10 KJV

If my people, who are called by my name, will humble themselves and pray and seek my face and turn from their wicked ways, then I will hear from heaven, and I will forgive their sin and will heal their land.

2 Chronicles 7:14
If we confess our sins, he is faithful and just and will forgive us our sins and purify us from all unrighteousness.

1 John 1:9
Repent, then, and turn to God, so that your sins may be wiped out, that times of refreshing may come from the Lord.

Repent, then, and turn to God, so that your sins may be wiped out, that times of refreshing may come from the Lord.

Acts 3:19
Whoever conceals their sins does not prosper,
but the one who confesses and renounces them finds mercy.
Proverbs 28:13sin confession mercy
Produce fruit in keeping with repentance.

Matthew 3:8conversion life fruitfulness
For the Lord your God is gracious and compassionate. He will not turn his face
from you if you return to him.

2 Chronicles 30:9
The Lord is not slow in keeping his promise, as some understand slowness. Instead
he is patient with you, not wanting anyone to perish, but everyone to come to
repentance.

2 Peter 3:9
But go and learn what this means: 'I desire mercy, not sacrifice.' For I have not
come to call the righteous, but sinners.

Matthew9:13
From that time on Jesus began to preach, "Repent, for the kingdom of heaven has
come near."

Matthew 4:17
Come near to God and he will come near to you. Wash your hands, you sinners,
and purify your hearts, you double-minded.

James 4:8
Rend your heart
and not your garments.
Return to the Lord your God,
for he is gracious and compassionate,
slow to anger and abounding in love,
and he relents from sending calamity.

Joel 2:13
Those whom I love I rebuke and discipline. So be earnest and repent.

Revelation 3:19 love life punishment
I tell you that in the same way there will be more rejoicing in heaven over one sinner
who repents than over ninety-nine righteous persons who do not need to repent.

173

Luke 15:7
For I take no pleasure in the death of anyone, declares the Sovereign Lord. Repent and live!

Ezekiel 18:32
In the past God overlooked such ignorance, but now he commands all people everywhere to repent.

Acts 17:30
The time has come," he said. "The kingdom of God has come near. Repent and believe the good news!"

Mark 1:15
I have not come to call the righteous, but sinners to repentance.

Luke 5:32
Return to me,' declares the Lord Almighty, 'and I will return to you,' says the Lord Almighty.

Zechariah 1:3bconversion reliability obedience
Peter replied, "Repent and be baptized, every one of you, in the name of Jesus Christ for the forgiveness of your sins. And you will receive the gift of the Holy Spirit."

Acts 2:38
In the same way, I tell you, there is rejoicing in the presence of the angels of God over one sinner who repents.

Luke 15:10
I tell you, no! But unless you repent, you too will all perish.

Luke 13:3
Repent at my rebuke!
Then I will pour out my thoughts to you,
I will make known to you my teachings.

Proverbs 1:23conversion wisdom Spirit
If your brother or sister sins against you, rebuke them; and if they repent, forgive them. Even if they sin against you seven times in a day and seven times come back to you saying 'I repent,' you must forgive them.

Luke 17:3b-4

O man m, don't run don't hid! Don't Run and Don't Hid! We All Lost And No One Has a Cure! The Coronavirus 🦠🦠🦠🦠🦠 Will Determine What To Do! O man save your energy and redirect your ways before Coronavirus rule over you! Give it up! It is no longer who won and who lost, repent and reform and call your Savior Jesus the Lord!

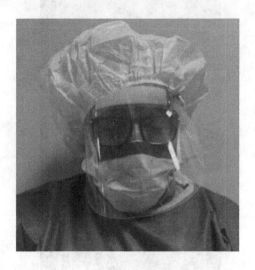

MM. Amen and Amen!

PH. Amen!!!

HD. Amen

GG. Amen

CS. Amen it is time to repent and look past men and turn back to God

VG. Amen!

AR. Amen

JS. Amen

MN. Amen

CG. This writing expresses exactly what I believe. The world needs to connect with God again. To show him our love and remorse and ask forgiveness. Through him we can get strength to get through this pandemic. Be safe! 🖤🙏

KO. Amen to this

Cascade of Human Life!

Written by Ramsis Ghaly

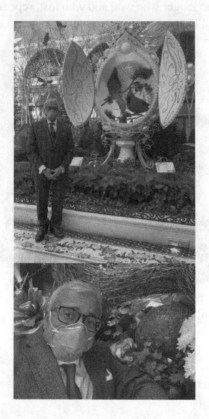

Newborn Life starts rightly so with a cry 😭 and ends with a cry 😭!

Indeed life journey is nourished with tears and matures in sorrows!

However, behind the scene is a joy and deep with is a spirit preparing for life eternal with her Savior!

Jesus said to the human soul: "Verily, verily, I say unto you, That ye shall weep and lament, but the world shall rejoice: and ye shall be sorrowful, but your sorrow shall be turned into joy. [21] A woman when she is in travail hath sorrow, because her hour is come: but as soon as she is delivered of the child, she remembereth no more the anguish, for joy that a man is born into the world. [22] And ye now therefore have sorrow: but I will see you again, and your heart shall rejoice, and your joy no man taketh from you." John 16:20-22 KJV

And He also explained saying: "Let not your heart be troubled: ye believe in God, believe also in me. [2] In my Father's house are many mansions: if it were not so, I would have told you. I go to prepare a place for you. [3] And if I go and prepare a place for you, I will come again, and receive you unto myself; that where I am, there ye may be also. [4] And whither I go ye know, and the way ye know." John 14:1-4 KJV

I thought the depth of human cascade as follows:

With Heavenly Father comes Love!
With Love comes Jesus Christ!
With Jesus Christ comes Son of Man!
With Son of Man comes Salvation!
With salvation comes Life!
With life comes Children of God!
With children of God comes Promise!
With promise comes Living!
With living comes Seniority!
with seniority comes Experience!
With experience comes Wisdom!
With wisdom comes Maturity!
With maturity comes Dues!
With dues comes Aging!
With aging comes Decline!
With decline comes Illness!
With illness comes Suffering!
With suffering comes Loss!
With loss comes Sadness!
With sadness comes Grieving!
With grieving comes Cries!
With cries comes Tears!
With tears comes Life Again!
With life again comes Memories!
With memories comes Inheritance!
With inheritance comes Wealth!
With wealth comes Prosperity!
With prosperity comes Enrichment!
With enrichment comes Abundance!

With abundance comes Fruitfulness!
With fruitfulness comes Spirituality!
With spirituality comes Eternity!
With eternity comes Heaven!
With heaven comes Kingdom!
With kingdom comes Jesus!
With Jesus comes Life eternity!

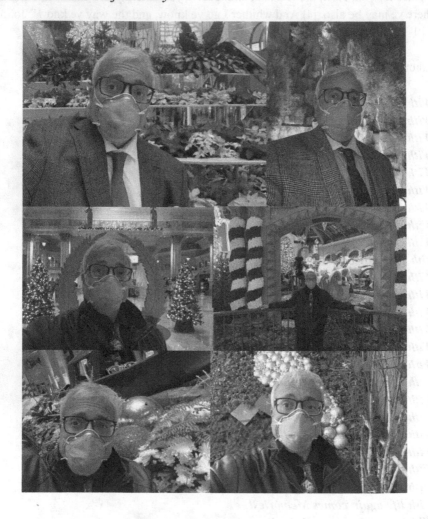

Even at the Time of Catastrophe such as COVID, There Always a Rose Around Us

Even at the Time of Catastrophe such as COVID, There Always a Rose 🌷 Around Us! There always a Rose 🌷 in Everything! Let us look for that Rose 🌷 keeping our eyes at the Rose among Thorns! The Heavenly Rose 🌷 is our Ultimate Eternal Rose 🌷!

Written by
Ramsis Ghaly

Even at the Time of Catastrophe such as COVID and at the time of darkness and horrific gravity, there always a Mighty Rose 🍁 around us coming from above!

For every Rose 🌹, there is a trunk branched in leaves 🍁 with spikes deep rooted in mud, dark ground underneath and spikes in the leaves 🍁

Do not let the surrounding mud and underground dirt and the spikes in the leaves 🍁 take the joy away from you

When you care about a patient, do not let the surrounding bureaucracy take the patient Rose 🌷 away from you

In everything around, there is a Rose 🌷 to find and do not let the mud and darkness around take you away from the Rose 🌷

The Roses 🌷 are usually hidden in the fields, hard to find, covered with many things, but they worth the pearls of everlasting treasures

The Rose 🌷 is waiting for you to find it, to uncover it, to discover it. The Rose 🌷 🌹 🌸 has so much to give you, so please strive to find the Rose 🌷 and do not let the bureaucracy around to distract you or take away

O my soul, let us strive to find the Roses 🌷 and ignore the dirts, the spikes and bureaucracy all around

Remember, the most joy is when you find that Rose 🌷 among the mud, with the Rose comes the ultimate blessing and true everlasting treasure:

179

Jesus our Master represent the Rose 🌹 with the treasure hidden in a field and the Pearl of Great Price for His Kingdom:

"44 Again, the kingdom of heaven is like treasure hidden in a field, which a man found and hid; and for joy over it he goes and sells all that he has and buys that field. 45 "Again, the kingdom of heaven is like a merchant seeking beautiful pearls, 46 who, when he had found one pearl of great price, went and sold all that he had and bought it." (Matthew 13:44-45)

It is meant for the human soul for all the days to find the Rose 🌹 in everything, your spirit is your guide as the Holy Spirit open the eyes of your brain 🧠 and the gate to your heart,

THE HUMAN SOUL WITH THE ROSES 🌹

Our Heavenly Father gives the strength and all what the human soul needs to is to pick up the Roses 🌹 🥀 🌹

The smell of it's incense and the holiness, the Lord will not miss. The Roses 🌹 🌹 that He places in your journey for you destiny,

The Father of the Harvest is calling upon your soul yo harvest these Roses, they are reaped and ready to be picked up,

The Roses are truly plenteous, the laborers are few, do pray therefore for the Lord of the harvest to send you as a laborer into His harvest:

"when he saw the multitudes, he was moved with compassion on them, because they fainted, and were scattered abroad, as sheep having no shepherd. 37Then saith he unto his disciples, The harvest truly is plenteous, but the labourers are few; 38Pray ye therefore the Lord of the harvest, that he will send forth labourers into his harvest." (Matthew 9:36-38)

My Heavenly Rose 🌹

The Heavenly Rose 🌹 is my ultimate Rose 🌹 I want! My Savior is the Rose 🌹 of Sharon and the Lily of the valleys! My Beloved is the only Rose 🌹 among thorns! My eyes are steadfast at the Rose of Sharon! "I am the rose of Sharon, and the lily of the valleys.

2 As the lily among thorns, so is my love among the daughters." (Song of Songs 2:1-2)

My Heavenly Rose 🌹 is mine and I am His! My Rose is my Beloved, feeders among the lilies: "My beloved is mine, and I am his: he feedeth among the lilies." (Song of Songs 2:16)

My Heavenly Rose 🌹 hears me and I hear Him, He is the Rose 🌹 of my heart 💜 from far. My Rose 🌹 cometh leaping upon the mountains, skipping upon the hills: "The voice of my beloved! behold, he cometh leaping upon the mountains, skipping upon the hills." (Song of Songs 2:8)

My Heavenly Rose 🌹 is my Love and my fair One tender and give a good smell: "The fig tree putteth forth her green figs, and the vines with the tender grape give a good smell. Arise, my love, my fair one, and come away."

My Heavenly Rose 🌹 is my Dove, sweet and Comely: "O my dove, that art in the clefts of the rock, in the secret places of the stairs, let me see thy countenance, let me hear thy voice; for sweet is thy voice, and thy countenance is comely." (Song of Songs 2:14)

My Heavenly Rose 🌹 is coming out of the wilderness Who is this that cometh out of the wilderness like pillars of smoke, perfumed with myrrh and frankincense, with all powders of the merchant: "Who is this that cometh out of the wilderness like pillars of smoke, perfumed with myrrh and frankincense, with all powders of the merchant?" (Song of Songs 3:6)

My Heavenly Rose 🌹 is mine: a garden inclosed is my sister, my spouse; a spring shut up, a fountain sealed: "A garden inclosed is my sister, my spouse; a spring shut up, a fountain sealed." (Song of Songs: 4:12)

My Heavenly Rose 🌹 is an Orchard full of pleasant fruits frankincense; myrrh and aloes, with all the chief spices: "Thy plants are an orchard of pomegranates, with pleasant fruits; camphire, with spikenard,14 Spikenard and saffron; calamus and cinnamon, with all trees of frankincense; myrrh and aloes, with all the chief spices:" (Song of Songs 4:13-14)

My Heavenly Rose 🌹 is a fountain of gardens, a well of living waters, and streams from Lebanon: "A fountain of gardens, a well of living waters, and streams from Lebanon." (Song of Songs4:15)

My Heavenly Rose 🌹 is all together lovely, head, eyes, cheeks, mouth, hands, belly, legs—His head is as the most fine gold- His eyes are as the eyes of doves by the rivers of waters, washed with milk, and fitly set—His cheeks are as a bed of spices, as sweet flowers: his lips like lilies, dropping sweet smelling myrrh—His hands are as gold rings set with the beryl—his belly is as bright ivory overlaid with sapphires—-His legs are as pillars of marble, set upon sockets of fine gold—his countenance is as Lebanon, excellent as the cedars—His mouth is most sweet: —My Beloved all together a Lovely: "My beloved is white and ruddy, the chiefest among ten thousand.11 His head is as the most fine gold, his locks are bushy, and black as a raven.12 His eyes are as the eyes of doves by the rivers of waters, washed with milk, and fitly set.13 His cheeks are as a bed of spices, as sweet flowers: his lips like lilies, dropping sweet smelling myrrh.14 His hands are as gold rings set with the beryl: his belly is as bright ivory overlaid with sapphires.15 His legs are as pillars of marble, set upon sockets of fine gold: his countenance is as Lebanon, excellent as the cedars.16 His mouth is most sweet: yea, he is altogether lovely. This is my beloved, and this is my friend, O daughters of Jerusalem." (Song of Songs 5:10-16)

My Heavenly Rose 🌹 is My dove, my undefiled is but one; a fair as the moon and clear as the sun, the only one and all the daughters of Jerusalem bless her and praise her: "My dove, my undefiled is but one; she is the only one of her mother, she is the choice one of her that bare her. The daughters saw her, and blessed her; yea, the queens and the concubines, and they praised her.10 Who is she that looketh forth as the morning, fair as the moon, clear as the sun, and terrible as an army with banner?" (Song of Songs 6: 9-10)

My Heavenly Rose 🌹 is my Love and Many waters cannot quench love, neither can the floods drown it: "Many waters cannot quench love, neither can the floods drown it: if a man would give all the substance of his house for love, it would utterly be contemned." (Song of Songs 8:7)

Let me kiss my Heavenly Rose 🌹 with the kisses of His mouth for thy love is better than wine, thy good ointments thy name is as ointment poured forth, therefore do the virgins love thee—

"Let him kiss me with the kisses of his mouth: for thy love is better than wine.3 Because of the savour of thy good ointments thy name is as ointment poured forth, therefore do the virgins love thee." (Song of Sobgs 1:2-3)

O my Lord and Savior open my eyes 👀 to see thou Rose among the daughters of Jerusalem. O my Heavenly Rose Draw me, we will run after thee: the king hath brought me into his chambers: we will be glad and rejoice in thee, we will remember thy love more than wine: the upright love thee: "4 Draw me, we will run after thee: the king hath brought me into his chambers: we will be glad and rejoice in thee, we will remember thy love more than wine: the upright love thee." (Song of Songs 1:4)

The Mini Roses 🌹🌹🌹 are

The Roses 🌹 are the lambs and the children of God are the Roses among the wolves 🦊: "Go your ways: behold, I send you forth as lambs among wolves." (Luke 10:3)

The mini Roses 🕯🌹 are the oil of your virgin soul that will Light your soul at the time of Jesus second coming in His glory after a brief drowsiness while falling asleep,

The mini Roses 🕯🌹 you have harvested, are what you need when you hear the midnight cry, the sign of the arrival of the Bridegroom as you wake up to dress your soul to be worthy to enter the Wedding Banquet of my Lord at the marriage ceremony of the Lamb of God in His Kingdom,

The Heavenly door ⬛ will never shut to the human souls with the Roses 🌹🕯 🌺. The Roses are your labors during the earthly journey that will make your soul ready as soon as the Bridegroom cometh, your soul will join Him and enter into His Wedding Banguet in the New Jerusalem,

"At that time the kingdom of heaven will be like ten virgins who took their lamps and went out to meet the bridegroom. 2 Five of them were foolish and five were wise. 3 The foolish ones took their lamps but did not take any oil with them. 4 The wise ones, however, took oil in jars along with their lamps. 5 The bridegroom was a long time in coming, and they all became drowsy and fell asleep.6 "At midnight the cry rang out: 'Here's the bridegroom! Come out to meet him!' 7 "Then all the virgins woke up and trimmed their lamps. 8 The foolish ones said to the wise, 'Give us some of your oil; our lamps are going out.' 9 "'No,' they replied, 'there may not be enough for both us and you. Instead, go to those who sell oil and buy some for yourselves.' 10 "But while they were on their way to buy the oil, the bridegroom arrived. The virgins who were ready went in with him to the wedding banquet. And the door was shut." (Matthew 25:5-10)

Let us enter His marriage with the bouquet 🌺 of Roses you have worked hard to collect that the Bridegroom accept it and find you worthy to His eternal Feast

May our Lord Jesus give us the spiritual eyes to see the Rose 🌹🌹 in everything around and the divine brain 🧠 to recognize the Rose 🌹🌹 in the darkness and the mud of the current world. The Roses 🌹🌹 are all the good deeds your soul had done. The Rose 🌹 is the oil for the lamb of the human soul to lighten it's figure and be visible to the Holy Spirit. The Rose will allow the human soul to enter and not to shut the Heavenly gate forever before the human soul with the Roses 🌹🌹🌹🌹. The Roses 🌹🌹 are what mankind needs to enter into the Coming Wedding Banquet of Our Lord Jesus,

There always a Rose 🌹 around us! There always a Rose 🌹 in Everything! Let us look for that Rose keeping our eyes at the Rose 🌹 among Thorns! The Heavenly Rose 🌹 is our Ultimate Eternal Rose!

Even at the Time of Catastrophe such as COVID, There Always a Rose 🌹 Around Us! There always a Rose 🌹 in Everything! Let us look for that Rose keeping our eyes at the Rose 🌹 among Thorns! The Heavenly Rose 🌹 is our Ultimate Eternal Rose 🌹!

Respectfully
Ramsis Ghaly

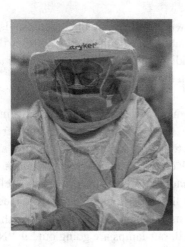

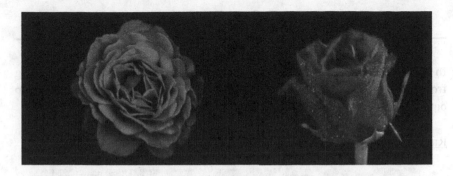

ml. Beautiful!
KG. Thank you for that reminder Dr Ghaly
CG. Another beautiful writing!
This is a great reminder that the rose is a symbol of Gods love. Bless you! 🖤🙏

Colorful PPE for Sporadic COVID

In the way to intubate a COVID patient with my PPE uniform with much blessing from my residents. Today I put on colorful PPE!! So ready and so prepared to help out and serve and be always in the frontline!!

Ramsis Ghaly

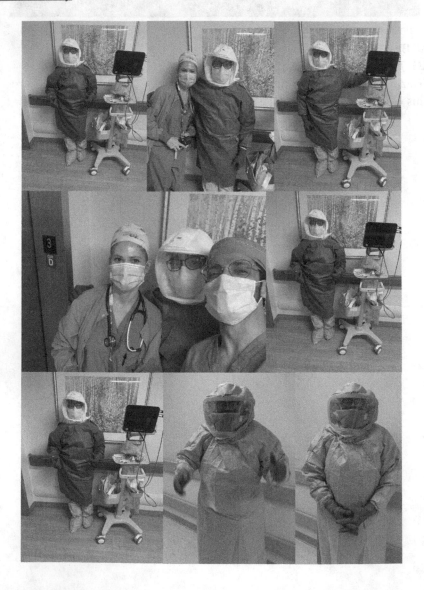

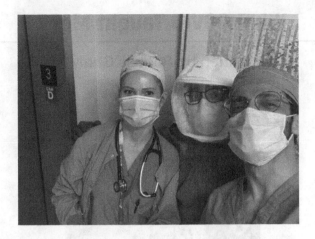

Another Day in the Paradise taking appropriate caution with PPE and multiple layers!!!

Ramsis Ghaly

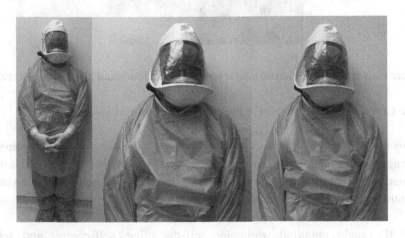

Awesome 🖤
CG. Be safe! 🖤🙏
CB. You are the instrument of God. May the Lord cover you with His precious blood.....
ML. Thank you Dr. **Ramsis Ghaly** and residents for all that you do.
FA. Stay safe Dr Ghaly God bless you the doctor with a heart of gold 🤍.

What COVID Taught Me??

Written by Ramsis Ghaly

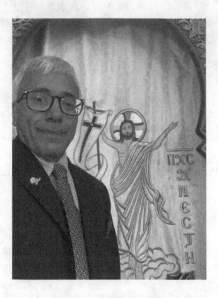

There is always resurrection no matter how dark the clouds and gloomy things are!!!

Post COVID is a Resurrection in itself!! Thank you Lord Jesus!!!!

Jesus the Lord with us forever and ever more and will always keep His promise and never ever change as it is written: "So that we may boldly say, The Lord is my helper, and I will not fear what man shall do unto me. [8] Jesus Christ the same yesterday, and to day, and for ever." Hebrews 13:6,8 KJV

COVID taught mankind worldwide self-discipline, self-control and self-abstinence! COVID gave us a lesson, yes we can do it!! As during COVID, a man was able to force himself all of a sudden to change his life and custom radically against his wishes and wore a mask, distance away and be socially isolated, a man can do the same and even more to earn his soul and save his life! A man can elect in Jesus sack to live in an abstinence life and cut down many of the lusts and desires and luxury when it comes down to for self discipline and salvation to life eternity!!!

Love!
Compassion!

Service!
Sadness and sorrows!
Hope and cheers!
Value life and reach out!

Patience and perseverance and Lird Jesus never slack: "The Lord is not slack concerning his promise, as some men count slackness; but is longsuffering to us-ward, not willing that any should perish, but that all should come to repentance. [15] And account that the longsuffering of our Lord is salvation; even as our beloved brother Paul also according to the wisdom given unto him hath written unto you; [18] But grow in grace, and in the knowledge of our Lord and Saviour Jesus Christ. To him be glory both now and for ever. Amen."2 Peter 3:9,15,18 KJV

Be of good courage and do not be afraid: Isaiah 41:10 So do not fear, for I am with you; do not be dismayed, for I am your God. I will strengthen you and help you; I will uphold you with my righteous right hand. Isaiah 41:13 For I am the LORD, your God, who takes hold of your right hand and says to you, Do not fear; I will help you. Matthew 10:28 And do not fear those who kill the body but cannot kill the soul. But rather fear Him who is able to destroy both soul and body in hell. 1 Corinthians 16:13 Be on your guard; stand firm in the faith; be men of courage; be strong. Philippians 1:12-14 Now I want you to know, brothers, that what has happened to me has really served to advance the gospel. As a result, it has become clear throughout the whole palace guard and to everyone else that I am in chains for Christ. Because of my chains, most of the brothers in the Lord have been encouraged to speak the word of God more courageously and fearlessly. Hebrews 13:5-6 For He Himself has said, "I will never leave you nor forsake you." So we may boldly say: "The LORD is my helper; I will not fear. What can man do to me?" Deuteronomy 31:6 Be strong and of good courage, do not fear nor be afraid of them; for the LORD your God, He is the One who goes with you. He will not leave you nor forsake you. Psalm 27:1 The LORD is my light and my salvation; Whom shall I fear? The LORD is the strength of my life; Of whom shall I be afraid? 2 Timothy 1:7 For God has not given us a spirit of fear and timidity, but of power, love, and self-discipline. 1 John 4:18 There is no fear in love. But perfect love drives out fear, because fear has to do with punishment. The one who fears is not made perfect in love. Psalm 56:3-4 When I am afraid, I will trust in you. In God, whose word I praise, in God I trust; I will not be afraid. What can mortal man do to me? 1 Chronicles 28:20 David also said to Solomon his son, "Be strong and courageous, and do the work. Do not be afraid or discouraged, for the LORD God, my God, is with you. He will not fail you or forsake you until all the work for the service of the temple of the LORD is finished.

Do not trust the news blindly!
Stay away from politics and politicians!
Examine everything and do not trust blindly!!

Some officials are suffering from major BIPOLAR Disorder!!! Crazy crazy, one week, they are afraid of mutations and various strains and just overnight everything is open and in between nothing was done to explain this bipolar behavior of manic depressive disorder!!

I realized and I was told "I am so irreplaceable and if I do not like it leave, and do repeatedly I was told why I am still working, make a space to the new comer"

Physicians all over America had it, they are having fun making more money in stocks, gambling, outing in golfing and buying real estate!!

No one like to work anymore and this is the bottom line!!

No need to dress up, Bahamas are good enough as long as the face and upper chest looks professional!!

No need for mental assessment test as long as you keep up with so many passwords and hit correct bottoms of next —, it is good enough!!

I became a Prime Amazon Member and Executive Costco member for life!! Drive through for Starbucks coffee is win-win!

I bought George Foramen grill and air fryer and forget about good cuisine just put whatever you wish and it will taste great at the end of day especially if you so hungry!!!

Ramsis Ghaly

CG. Your thoughts and words are always so honest and truthful. Although I am a prime member of Amazon and Costco also I will never give up cooking. I love to cook new and interesting food. Bless you! 🖤🙏
RH. Amen
KB. Amen
AB. Good words
TG. Good words. your thoughts and words always truthful God Bless you 🙏

Lessons learned from COVID-19 Pandemic!

The pendulum swings hourly between the truth and false and yet sometimes stuck in between!

Written by
Ramsis Ghaly

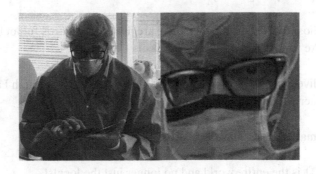

Human life vanishes away in no time! And human body can recover from any illness but it takes long time and perseverance!

We learned to examine facts since nothing written on a steel or engraved in a stone! The pendulum swings hourly between the truth and false and yet sometimes stuck in between! It is not to be trusted since nothing is perfect and so much incompetence running around!

The world is becoming an experimental laboratory 🔬🔪🍽 for human adventures!

Modern man pushed humanity to work under artificial intelligence and robotic arms and minds And made Wireless technology and virtual communications our new world 🌐!

Living under Emergency conditions and executive orders are the new way of life!

Medicine and Science are not the holy Bible and have mislead the public and continued to be severely limited!

Animal eaters and using animals for experiments and experimenting with viruses and gene cloning are invitation for future disasters and playing with fires 🔥!

Church, family and friends are much more valuable than wealth of stocks and bank savings!

Self-prevention, healthy living and hygiene basics learned from forefather are the best medicine!

Politics, greediness and self-interest are the enemies of the sovereign society!

Modern technology and human ambition come with significant cost to mankind and have major impact globally!

Man's grandiose and ego to conquer alone are just empty words full of hot air and evaporate like vapors!

The way to live through the pandemic and post pandemic is through Faith! Love ♥! Care! Sacrifice! Endurance! And Patience!

Everything matters even thousands of miles away!

Our world 🌏 is the entire world and no longer just the locals!

Fresh and clean air is priceless! Nature and Outdoors are essential to rejuvenate the Human souls! It is okay to live in a distant environment and always keeping a distance!

During the pandemic, although physical separation and social isolation become prominent yet cohesiveness and service to one another are essentials! Live to serve and reach out to next door neighbors and to others!

While Facing pandemic, be fearless and courageous and believe you can do it! Look up for tomorrow! Nothing be taken for granted!

Always remember: God our Lord is in Control!

You may wish to add!!!

Respectfully

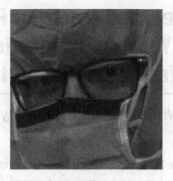

RH. This I will treasure every day. I'm going to try to copy it and save it. Is it sad and me and lifted me. Thank you thank you doctor. You are deeply appreciated and loved. And I pray for you and your team. Godspeed amen

CG. Always the great thinker and the conveyor of those thoughts. Wonderful! Bless you! 🙏❤️

AV. Thank you Dr. Ghaly for your insight! 🐋🙏

Lessons Learned from the Pandemic of the Year in Preparation for New Year 2021 Resolutions!

Written by Ramsis Ghaly

It isn't only in no time be hooked to ventilator and never be seen by loved ones no more but also many other lessons moving forward for 2021 New Year Eve Resolutions—!

As 2020 soon coming to an end, let me share with you my deep thoughts of lessons learned from the COVID Pandemic of the Century!

All is vanity as it is written: *"Vanity of vanities, saith the Preacher, vanity of vanities; all is vanity. [3] What profit hath a man of all his labour which he taketh under the sun? [4] One generation passeth away, and another generation cometh: but the earth abideth for ever. [11] There is no remembrance of former things ; neither shall there be any remembrance of things that are to come with those that shall come after. [18] For in much wisdom is much grief: and he that increaseth knowledge increaseth sorrow." Ecclesiastes 1:2-4,11,18 KJV*

Human body is so fragile and in no time a human soul can get ill 😔 and in no time, a strong man or strong woman can end in a ventilator and never be seen by loved ones no more!!!

Therefore, value every minute of thy life! Remember every day is precious! Do good and spread love 💜! Serve multitudes and never be part of drama negativism!

But more deep Lessons Learned as follows:

It isn't the outward hope but the genuine faith seated and rooted deeply in the inner the soul!

It isn't the exuberant exterior of a person but the interior Truth within that person!

It isn't the visible flesh of the human soul but the invisible spirit of that soul!

It isn't the degrees and ranks that a person has beside the name but the true Love 💜 and humility within the heart of that person!

It isn't the master and teacher at the desk but the servant in the field in person with the students!

It isn't the commander at the office but the serviceman and servicewoman in the Frontline!

It isn't the fame of a person that recognizes a person but the willingness to lay down the soul and sacrifice for others!

It isn't the prestige of the title a person hold makes that person distinguished but the actual sacrifice made in the front line by that person!

It isn't the alloy of the chain that carries the value but the invisible Spirit what the chain actually represent!

It isn't the science to enter the space and reach out the moon, solar system and the Mars that count but having the actual science to develop an immediate vaccine to combat to the pandemic before any human causality!

It isn't arrogance and influence of a person but empathy and down to earth sharing with the common!

It isn't the net wealth of a society but the treasures of its people!

It isn't the sophisticated military tanks but the ability to save thy own people!

It isn't how fast a man can run but how fast a man can give!

It isn't what does a human soul consider oneself but what the Lord considers a human soul!

It isn't what does a human soul think about oneself but rather what the Heavenly Father think of a human soul!

It isn't how much a human soul valued but it is how much Jesus Love a human soul!

"I have planted, Apollos watered; but God gave the increase. [7] So then neither is he that planteth any thing, neither he that watereth; but God that giveth the increase. [8] Now he that planteth and he that watereth are one: and every man shall receive his own reward according to his own labour. [9]

For we are labourers together with God: ye are God's husbandry, ye are God's building. [10] According to the grace of God which is given unto me, as a wise masterbuilder, I have laid the foundation, and another buildeth thereon. But let every man take heed how he buildeth thereupon. [11] For other foundation can no man lay than that is laid, which is Jesus Christ. [12] Now if any man build upon this foundation gold, silver, precious stones, wood, hay, stubble; [13] Every man's work shall be made manifest: for the day shall declare it, because it shall be revealed by fire; and the fire shall try every man's work of what sort it is. [14] If any man's work abide which he hath built thereupon, he shall receive a reward. [15] If any man's work shall be burned, he shall suffer loss: but he himself shall be saved; yet so as by fire. [16] Know ye not that ye are the temple of God, and that the Spirit of God dwelleth in you? [17] If any man defile the temple of God, him shall God destroy; for the temple of God is holy, which temple ye are. [18] Let no man deceive himself. If any man among you seemeth to be wise in this world, let him become a fool, that he may be wise. [19] For the wisdom of this world is foolishness with God. For it is written, He taketh the wise in their own craftiness. [20] And again, The Lord knoweth the thoughts of the wise, that they are vain. [21] Therefore let no man glory in men. For all things are yours; [22] Whether Paul, or Apollos, or Cephas, or the world, or life, or death, or things present, or things to come; all are yours; [23] And ye are Christ's; and Christ is God's." 1 Corinthians 3:6-23 KJV

Respectfully

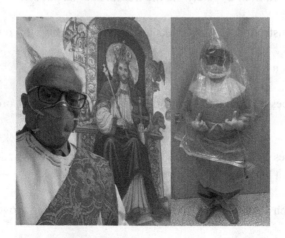

- Thank you for sharing these lessons with us. We can all learn to live life to its fullest and to be grateful for what we have. Bless you! ♥🙏

KG. We all need to live our faith from within 🙏. Stay safe, Dr. Ghaly!

A Theortical Idea to combat the COVID Pandemic and Any Other Viral Pandemic Developed by Ramsis Ghaly

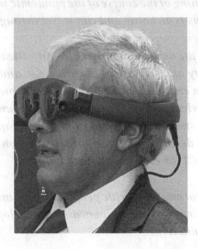

I have been praying 🙏 to my Savior to give me the way that I should have handled the pandemic back in January 2020 when I predicted about the coming wrath and put a stop 🛑 to COVID-19 back when it was erupting!!

I have been closely monitoring, thinking, working and never stopped searching and dreaming of "out of box" ideas!!

I just got this genius theoretical idea and if turn out to be true, It will prevent the second surge and open up early on and shorten the time to close. If it proved much effective, it will put the so called "follow the science" was absolutely wrong and we shouldn't ever had to suffer another surge!!!

! If it worked it will have radically changed the course and minimized the second surge and the curfew and lockdown-

It won't need any pharmaceuticals to be involved!!

I am certain there are so many ideas not just mine but they have been suppressed. Or because they aren't part of the main stream "old boy club", the "establishment" and so called "Science"

Thank you 🙏 dear Lord!!!

Idea as follows

Release and Spread low virulent strain of virus in the air not unto people or their arms in the beginning of the course of the pandemic in every state. It takes advantage that the virus is airborne and can travel through air and droplets.

So the art is to develop the most benign particle that will stimulate each person immunity to the fatality and severity of the virus 🦠 and elevate the defense against the pandemic in each region. Choose the least protein harmful particles of the sequence in the virus and released to air without any additional vehicle to take it to the blood stream. The human lungs will capture these particles and process low grade defense to kill the particle yet won't severely infect the individual or require ICU or even hospitalization.

It encourages living normal, mix with people and no mask when immunity developed. It kills the virus early on by immediately developing mega immunity in the public Indiscriminately.

Restricting the spread early on is a disaster and does not give chance to develop necessary immunity.

There is a reason that God created natural immunity and there is a reason why such pandemic didn't wipe out poor unhygienic and crowded populations!

GHALYNEUROSURGEON.COM

Neurosurgeon | Brain surgery, spine surgery | Treating carpal tunnel symptoms, spinal stenosis, sciatica in Aurora, Il

Facebook post

Ramsis Ghaly
1h · 1pm 2/2/21
Shared with Public

I have been praying 🙏 to my Savior to give me the way that I should have handled the pandemic back in January 2020 when I predicted about the coming wrath and put a stop ⏺ to COVID-19 back when it was erupting!!

I have been closely monitoring, thinking, working and never stopped searching and dreaming of "out of box" ideas!!

I just got this genius idea and if turn out to be true and much effective, it will put the so called "follow the science" was absolutely wrong and we shouldn't ever had to suffer another surge!!!

It won't need any pharmaceuticals to be involved!!

I am certain there are so many ideas not just mine but they have been suppressed because they aren't part of the "old boy club", the "establishment" and so called "Science"

Thank you 🙏 dear Lord!!!

My Original email with time and date of the idea that came to my mind while driving to Illinois Masonic hospital from Mt Practice in aurora:

-----Original Message-----
From: RAMSIS GHALY <rfghaly@aol.com>
To: Ramsis Ghaly <rfghaly@aol.com>
Sent: Tue, Feb 2, 2021 1:19 pm
Subject: Ghaly idea

Release and Spread low virulent strain of virus in the beginning of the course of the pandemic in every state

So the art is to develop the most benign particle that will stimulate each person immunity to the fatality and severity of the virus 🔴 and elevate the defense against the pandemic in each region

Restricting the spread early on is a disaster and does not give chance to develop necessary immunity.

Here you go so called "Science" wrong wrong

What is wrong of keep faceMasking???

I love 💜 my facemask! And the only time I shall take off my facemask is when I am all alone with my Lord Jesus, in His company and grace!

I am used to my facemask!
My facemask likes me and I like my facemask!
I get to smell my own and breath my own!
I feel protected from the outside breath!
No one can read my lips or hear my soft voice!
My lipsticks 💋 are hidden from the outsiders so are my shiny teeth!

After all, I have collected so many of facemasks in my closets and many of those are fashionable! Therefore, I am not throwing my colorful facemasks away!

By wearing my facemask, I am in my own and not worrying about the breath of others!! Furthermore, I should be prepared of what the evil will do next!! Bioweapon and bio terrorizing unfortunately is here to stay!!

If the facemasks were important back then, in my book, it is still important today and tomorrow! I am keeping my facemasks since I don't know what is circulating in the air and the pollution outside!!! At any time, anyone could inject another virus 🦠 to the air, a new strain! It is becoming the war of the future, the biologic enemy of mankind in the recent years!

I am not going to be part of politics! I am not a hypocrite and I refused to be part of bureaucracy! Why should I follow the shaky media or be intimidated by the others! I am a man of my own and I kneel to my Lord Jesus my Savior and my God: the Armor of faith and my Shield!

So I am not taking my facemask down! I will continue to wear my facemask for now and then!

It is up to you to join me but I already made my mind! My facemask is my style and my part of my fashionable daily dress!!

Ramsis Ghaly

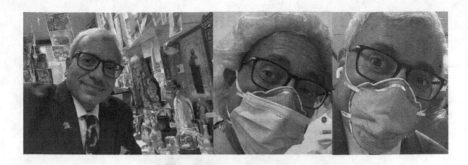

FL. Wearing my mask for sure !!

FA. Agree with you 💯 Dr Ghaly, I love my colorful masks 😊

CG. Why would you want to hide behind a mask? We can't see your good looks and great smile. I would never pass up a step towards normalcy. My mask is gone and I pray forever. 💜🙏

RH. We love you with your mask on.

JM. Me Too!! You're Looking Good Dr. Ghaly!!

JB. We are with you Dr. Ghaly!! We are fully vaccinated, but will continue to wear our masks!!

LW. Not for me. I NEED immunities

TJ. I TOTALLY agree! I will continue to wear my mask, I will continue to exercise my faith in God, and I will continue to use basic common sense. Obviously the virus is still very active and present, because people are still getting sick and some dying.

AP. I am fully vaccinated but will continue to wear my mask

LK. Only during surgery.....

VL. I won't remove my mask. Not until the end of the warm season. I will conduct my own empirical evidence. Too soon.

SP. You need to take the mask off and show off the good looking smile 😀.

SS. Giusto per fare. 👑

CR. My facemask is my best friend !!!!

RV. I like mine as well 😁👍😊💜

DM. like you ..mask will be a part of my daily attire

NC. So true!

RP. My mask has helped my allergies so much! I'm keeping it too.

MO. I feel they are stopping masks a little prematurely. I am undecided on whether I will continue to wear one. I can tolerate wearing masks for hours in a cold OR but not when I am out and it's 90 degrees outside.

Supreme COVID Scientists SCS a New Proposal to lead the COVID Taskforce!

Developed and Written by <u>Ramsis Ghaly</u>

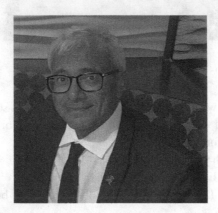

To move forward and reform the existing system if how COVID-19 was handled, let me share with you my idea to redeem it and provide the platform for future global events threatening the public health:

What about forming Supreme COVID Scientists (SCS)

Supreme COVID Scientists (SCS) must be disengaged from public media and social attachments and screened from any conflict of interest! The scientists should be left alone to do their research with no limits or restrains and be protected to find out all about COVID-19 and management not being influenced be external reasons or interrupted or redirected by various distractions!!

Perhaps, indeed, Supreme COVID Scientists (SCS) should be elected by Supreme Court Judges and must be dismissed immediately if any evidence of cheating!

If Supreme COVID Scientists (SCS) was formed from beginning December of 2019, by now one and half year later, the public should not have doubts or second thoughts with updated trustworthy abundance of data about COVID-19 and Vaccines!

And these unquestionable results will have been available, reviewed and be used to inform the public with honest information as well as be used to guide the CDC of America and UN/ WHO of the world of which direction to take and do!!

One and half years later are sufficient to produce unbiased and accurate evidence-base medicine about COVID-19 and various Vaccines supported by on-line studies available to share in public and subject to scrutinization and audit!

The COVID management and Vaccines' guidelines will be supplied with a disclaimer that the data collection is over only over 17 months duration and subject to change to reflect the incoming results of the ongoing research!

Lack of transparency and conflict of interests result in lack of confidence and distrust of the public! There are so many unanswered questions and obvious conflict of interests.

In the recent years, science is viewed as no longer pure but rather guided and supported by industry and politics and hence eroding its reputation!! It shouldn't be this way!! As Supreme Court judges elected and fo their work and duties under oath to the fullest so shall be Supreme COVID Scientists (SCS)!

Supreme COVID Scientists (SCS) is a remedy not only to ensure doing the right thing, with purity and high morals but also to earn the public trust with the undisputed data and options to chose!

Seventeen months late should be close to lift up the so called "FDA Emergency Approval no subjected to CDC Regulations" and to be subjected to interim CDC guidelines and the legal immunity be removed!

So, perhaps, the Supreme COVID Scientists (SCS) as a New Proposal to lead the COVID Taskforce, be a good trustworthy choice for handling COVID-19 and future similar events!!! Perhaps the Time is now to lift up Immunity and all COVID-19 Vaccines be Subject to CDC Regulations and the Legal Immunity to Vaccines be Removed!!

Respectfully
Ramsis Ghaly

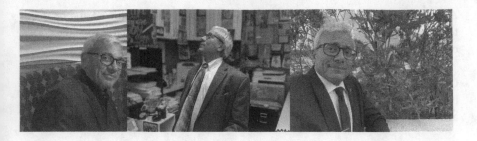

DT. Brilliant!!!!! You are Brilliant Dr. Ghaly
RH. Thank goodness for your education and truth.

Thirteen Psalms to Pray for the Ongoing Curse of COVID and Facemasks Bestowed Upon all People so that Our Savior may Lifted them up from the Face of Earth During the Holy Passion Week!!

Written by Ramsis Ghaly

Let us Pray those selected PSALMS to cast out COVID and the Face masks——

Psalm 13

FOR HOW LONG O LORD—

How long O Lord shall I keep the face mask?? How long wilt thou forget me, O Lord ? for ever? how long wilt thou hide thy face from me? [2] How long shall I take counsel of face-mask in my soul, having sorrow in my heart daily? how long shall mine COVID and the wicked (enemy) be exalted over me? [3] Consider and hear me, O Lord my God: lighten mine eyes, lest I sleep the sleep of death; [4] Lest mine COVID (COVID) say, I have prevailed against him; and those that trouble me rejoice when I am moved. [5] But I have trusted in thy mercy; my heart shall rejoice in thy salvation. [6] I will sing unto the Lord, because he hath dealt bountifully with me.

Psalm 64

Hear my voice, O God, in my prayer: preserve my life from fear of the COVID (enemy). [2] Hide me from the secret COVID and the wicked the counsel of the wicked; from the insurrection of the workers of iniquity: [3] Who whet their tongue like a sword, and bend their bows to shoot their arrows, even bitter words: [4] That they may shoot in secret at the perfect: suddenly do they shoot at him, and fear not. [5] They encourage themselves in an evil matter: they commune of laying snares privily; they say, Who shall see them? [6] They search out iniquities; they accomplish a diligent search: both the inward thought of every one of them, and the heart, is deep. [7] But God shall shoot at them with an arrow; suddenly shall they be wounded. [8] So they shall make their own tongue to fall upon themselves: all that see them shall flee away. [9] And all men shall fear, and shall declare the work of God; for they shall wisely consider of his doing. [10] The righteous shall be glad in the Lord, and shall trust in him; and all the upright in heart shall glory.

Psalm 74

O God, why hast thou cast us off for ever? why doth thine anger smoke against the sheep of thy pasture? [2] Remember thy congregation, which thou hast purchased of old; the rod of thine inheritance, which thou hast redeemed; this mount Zion, wherein thou hast dwelt. [3] Lift up thy feet unto the perpetual desolations; even all that the COVID (enemy) hath done wickedly in the sanctuary. [4] Thine COVID and the wicked (enemies) roar in the midst of thy congregations; they set up their ensigns for signs. [5] A man was famous according as he had lifted up axes upon the thick trees. [6] But now they break down the carved work thereof at once with axes and hammers. [7] They have cast fire into thy sanctuary, they have defiled by casting down the dwelling place of thy name to the ground. [8] They said in their hearts, Let us destroy them together: they have burned up all the synagogues of God in the land. [9] We see not our signs: there is no more any prophet: neither is there among us any that knoweth how long. [10] O God, how long shall the adversary reproach? shall the COVID and the wicked (enemy) blaspheme thy name for ever? [11] Why withdrawest thou thy hand, even thy right hand? pluck it out of thy bosom. [12] For God is my King of old, working salvation in the midst of the earth. [13] Thou didst divide the sea by thy strength: thou brakest the heads of the dragons in the waters. [14] Thou brakest the heads of leviathan in pieces, and gavest him to be meat to the people inhabiting the wilderness. [15] Thou didst cleave the fountain and the flood: thou driedst up mighty rivers. [16] The day is thine, the night also is thine: thou hast prepared the light and the sun. [17] Thou hast set all the borders of the earth: thou hast made summer and winter. [18] Remember this, that the COVID (enemy) hath reproached, O Lord, and that the foolish people have blasphemed thy name. [19] O deliver not the soul of thy turtledove unto the multitude of the wicked: forget not the congregation of thy poor for ever. [20] Have respect unto the covenant: for the dark places of the earth are full of the habitations of cruelty. [21] O let not the oppressed return ashamed: let the poor and needy praise thy name. [22] Arise, O God, plead thine own cause: remember how the foolish man reproacheth thee daily. [23] Forget not the voice of thine enemies: the tumult of those that rise up against thee increaseth continually. ...

Psalm 77

THE HELP IN THE WAY—-

I cried unto God with my voice, even unto God with my voice; and he gave ear unto me. [2] In the day of my trouble with COVID, I sought the Lord: my sore ran in the night, and ceased not: my soul refused to be comforted. [3] I remembered God, and was troubled: I complained, and my spirit was overwhelmed. Selah. [4] Thou holdest mine eyes waking: I am so troubled that I cannot speak. [5] I have considered the days of old, the years of ancient times. [6] I call to remembrance my song in the night: I commune with mine own heart: and my spirit made diligent search. [7] Will the Lord cast off for ever? and will he be favourable no more? [8] Is his mercy clean gone for ever? doth his promise fail for evermore? [9] Hath God forgotten to be gracious? hath he in anger shut up his tender mercies? Selah. [10] And I said, This is my infirmity: but I will remember the years of the right hand of the most High. [11] I will remember the works of the Lord: surely I will remember thy wonders of old. [12] I will meditate also of all thy work, and talk of thy doings. [13] Thy way, O God, is in the sanctuary: who is so great a God as our God? [14] Thou art the God that doest wonders: thou hast declared thy strength among the people. [15] Thou hast with thine arm redeemed thy people, the sons of Jacob and Joseph. Selah. [16] The waters saw thee, O God, the waters saw thee; they were afraid: the depths also were troubled. [17] The clouds poured out water: the skies sent out a sound: thine arrows also went abroad. [18] The voice of thy thunder was in the heaven: the lightnings lightened the world: the earth trembled and shook. [19] Thy way is in the sea, and thy path in the great waters, and thy footsteps are not known. [20] Thou leddest thy people like a flock by the hand of Moses and Aaron. ...

Psalm 88
O LORD God of my salvation, I have cried d day and night before thee: [2] Let my prayer come before thee: incline thine ear unto my cry; [3] For my soul is full of COVID troubles: and my life draweth nigh unto the grave. [4] I am counted with them that go down into the pit: I am as a man that hath no strength: [5] Free among the dead, like the slain that lie in the grave, whom thou rememberest no more: and they are cut off from thy hand. [6] Thou hast laid me in the lowest pit, in darkness, in the deeps. [7] Thy wrath lieth hard upon me, and thou hast afflicted me with all thy waves. Selah. [8] Thou hast put away mine acquaintance far from me; thou hast made me an abomination unto them: I am shut up, and I cannot come forth. [9] Mine eye mourneth by reason of affliction: Lord, I have called daily upon thee, I have stretched out my hands unto thee. [10] Wilt thou shew wonders to the dead? shall the dead arise and praise thee? Selah. [11] Shall thy lovingkindness be declared in the grave? or thy faithfulness in destruction? [12] Shall thy wonders be known in the dark? and thy righteousness in the land of forgetfulness? [13] But unto thee have I cried, O Lord ; and in the morning shall my prayer prevent thee. [14] Lord, why castest thou off my soul? why hidest thou thy face from me? [15] I am afflicted and ready to die from my youth up: while I suffer thy COVID terrors I am distracted. [16] Thy fierce wrath goeth over me; thy terrors have cut me off. [17] They came round about me daily like water; they compassed me about together. [18] Lover t and friend hast thou put far from me, and mine acquaintance into darkness. ...

Psalm 120

In my distress with COVID, I cried unto the Lord, and he heard me. [2] Deliver my soul, O Lord, from lying lips, and from a deceitful tongue. [3] What shall be given unto thee? or what shall be done unto thee, thou false tongue? [4] Sharp arrows of the mighty, with coals of juniper. [5] Woe is me, that I sojourn in Mesech, that I dwell in the tents of Kedar! [6] My soul hath long dwelt with him that hateth peace. [7] I am for peace: but when I speak, they are for war.

Psalm 121

I will lift up mine eyes unto the hills, from whence cometh my help. [2] My help cometh from the Lord, which made heaven and earth. [3] He will not suffer thy foot to be moved: he that keepeth thee will not slumber. [4] Behold, he that keepeth Israel shall neither slumber nor sleep. [5] The Lord is thy keeper: the Lord is thy shade upon thy right hand. [6] The sun shall not smite thee by day, nor the moon by night. [7] The Lord shall preserve thee from COVID and all evil: he shall preserve thy soul. [8] The Lord shall preserve thy going out and thy coming in from this time forth, and even for evermore.

Psalm 124

If it had not been the Lord who was on our side, now may Israel say; [2] If it had not been the Lord who was on our side, when COVID and the wicked rose up against us: [3] Then they had swallowed us up quick, when their wrath was kindled against us: [4] Then the waters had overwhelmed us, the stream had gone over our soul: [5] Then the proud waters had gone over our soul. [6] Blessed be the Lord, who hath not given us as a prey to their teeth. [7] Our soul is escaped as a bird out of the snare of the fowlers: the snare is broken, and we are escaped. [8] Our help is in the name of the Lord, who made heaven and earth.

Psalm 130

Out of the depths of COVID, have I cried unto thee, O Lord. [2] Lord, hear my voice: let thine ears be attentive to the voice of my supplications. [3] If thou, Lord, shouldest mark iniquities, O Lord, who shall stand? [4] But there is forgiveness with thee, that thou mayest be feared. [5] I wait for the Lord, my soul doth wait, and in his word do I hope. [6] My soul waiteth for the Lord more than they that watch for the morning: I say, more than they that watch for the morning. [7] Let Israel hope in the Lord: for with the Lord there is mercy, and with him is plenteous redemption. [8] And he shall redeem Israel from all his iniquities.

Psalm 140

Deliver me from COVID, O Lord, from the evil COVID and man: preserve me from the violent Covid and man; [2] Which imagine mischiefs in their heart;

continually are they gathered together for war. [3] They have sharpened their tongues like a serpent; adders' poison is under their lips. Selah. [4] Keep me, O Lord, from the hands of the wicked; preserve me from the COVID and violent man; who have purposed to overthrow my goings. [5] The proud have hid a snare for me, and cords; they have spread a net by the wayside; they have set gins for me. Selah. [6] I said unto the Lord, Thou art my God: hear the voice of my supplications, O Lord. [7] O God the Lord, the strength of my salvation, thou hast covered my head in the day of battle. [8] Grant not, O Lord, the desires of COVID and the wicked: further not his wicked device; lest they exalt themselves. Selah. [9] As for the head of those that compass me about, let the mischief of their own lips cover them. [10] Let burning coals fall upon them: let them be cast into the fire; into deep pits, that they rise not up again. [11] Let not an evil speaker be established in the earth: evil shall hunt the violent man to overthrow him. [12] I know that the Lord will maintain the cause of the afflicted, and the right of the poor. [13] Surely the righteous shall give thanks unto thy name: the upright shall dwell in thy presence.

Psalm 141
Lord, I cry unto thee: make haste unto me; give ear unto my voice, when I cry unto thee. [2] Let my prayer be set forth before thee as incense; and the lifting up of my hands as the evening sacrifice. [3] Set a watch, O Lord, before my mouth; keep the door of my lips. [4] Incline not my heart to any COVID or evil thing, to practise wicked works with men that work iniquity: and let me not eat of their dainties. [5] Let the righteous smite me; it shall be a kindness: and let him reprove me; it shall be an excellent oil, which shall not break my head: for yet my prayer also shall be in their calamities. [6] When their judges are overthrown in stony places, they shall hear my words; for they are sweet. [7] Our bones are scattered at the grave's mouth, as when one cutteth and cleaveth wood upon the earth. [8] But mine eyes are unto thee, O God the Lord: in thee is my trust; leave not my soul destitute. [9] Keep me from the snares which they have laid for me, and the gins of the workers of iniquity. [10] Let the wicked fall into their own nets, whilst that I withal escape.

Psalm 142
I cried unto the Lord with my voice; with my voice unto the Lord did I make my supplication. [2] I poured out my complaint about COVID before him; I shewed before him my trouble. [3] When my spirit was overwhelmed within me, then thou knewest my path. In the way wherein I walked have they privily laid a snare for me. [4] I looked on my right hand, and beheld, but there was no man that would know me: refuge failed me; no man cared for my soul. [5] I cried unto thee, O Lord: I said, Thou art my refuge and my portion in the land of the

209

living. [6] Attend unto my cry; for I am brought very low: deliver me from my persecutors; for they are stronger than I. [7] Bring my soul out of COVID prison, that I may praise thy name: the righteous shall compass me about; for thou shalt deal bountifully with me.

Psalm 143
Hear my prayer, O Lord, give ear to my supplications: in thy faithfulness answer me, and in thy righteousness. [2] And enter not into judgment with thy servant: for in thy sight shall no man living be justified. [3] For the COVID and the enemy hath persecuted my soul; he hath smitten my life down to the ground; he hath made me to dwell in darkness, as those that have been long dead. [4] Therefore is my spirit overwhelmed within me; my heart within me is desolate. [5] I remember the days of old; I meditate on all thy works; I muse on the work of thy hands. [6] I stretch forth my hands unto thee: my soul thirsteth after thee, as a thirsty land. Selah. [7] Hear me speedily, O Lord: my spirit faileth: hide not thy face from me, lest I be like unto them that go down into the pit. [8] Cause me to hear thy lovingkindness in the morning; for in thee do I trust: cause me to know the way wherein I should walk; for I lift up my soul unto thee. [9] Deliver me, O Lord, from mine COVID and enemies: I flee unto thee to hide me. [10] Teach me to do thy will; for thou art my God: thy spirit is good; lead me into the land of uprightness. [11] Quicken me, O Lord, for thy name's sake: for thy righteousness' sake bring my soul out of trouble. [12] And of thy mercy cut off mine enemies, and destroy all them that afflict my soul: for I am thy servant.

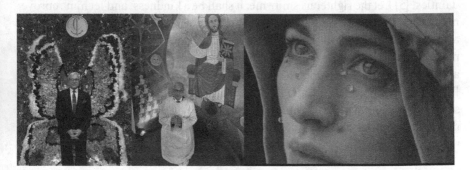

Human Life is Purely a Gift From God And Not From Man!!!

Written by Ramsis Ghaly

Human life is purely a gift from God and never from a man and only God the Almighty who has the key to life and second death!!!!

As man's dominion over the creation grows exponentially—

As man' success is claiming certification of accomplishments of so called countless mission impossible—

As man's power is conquering [obj] all enemies under the sun—-!

As man-made science and technology celebrate all the exceptional advancements—!

As man's race continues to reach out millions of miles away exploring the unlimited universe searching for the unseen—-!

As man's totality be described as unlimited and proceeds to ranks of untouched highness ruling over innumerable dynasties and islands as royalists and nobliest—-!

Be careful O man born of a woman!!! Our Lord Jesus said: "And I say unto you my friends, Be not afraid of them that kill the body, and after that have no more that they can do. [5] But I will forewarn you whom ye shall fear: Fear him, which after he hath killed hath power to cast into hell; yea, I say unto you, Fear him." Luke 12:4-5 KJV

Yet, never ever human being was, is and will be able to put a stop ◉ to death at the written predetermined time!! Furthermore, man's authority has no say and exerts no influence in the life of a man after death but God the Almighty!!

A man stands absolutely helpless before the time of death and life after death! It is no longer the man's land or man's ruling or man's home!!! Every living soul shall be taken up all alone in equity giving account for her deeds in joy or nashing with teeth. At that time the entire world shall know the Only Good Shephard and His sheep One God and one sheep!! But it is God's land, God's ruling and God's home!!

211

Man has no key for life or death but God has!! Man can never alter the clock of departure, can't call back a dead person to life again or be able to return life to a dying person to live even for few seconds longer! But only Lord Jesus and His Kingdom!

After man's departure, man will never ever rule over another fellowmen. After death, there shall be no more man-made House of Representatives, Congress, Senate, Presidents, Kings, Queens, courts, judges, teachers, headmasters, Board members, aldermen,—-nor shall it be mand-made policies, procedures, laws, guidelines, doctrine, curfews—-! Man shall never again rule over another man of have any say or criticism of one over another!!! But only Lord Jesus and His Kingdom!

At the time of death, man loses all the powers and no longer has any authorities in any human soul that departed since the beginning of ages and until the end of ages! Man is full of fantasies and high dreams of control and dominions but in reality all what man has is vanity! But only Lord Jesus and His Kingdom!

Human life is purely a gift from God and never from a man and only God the Almighty who has the key to life and second death!!!!

Revelation 1:18 "and the living One; and I was dead, and behold, I am alive forevermore, and I have the keys of death and of Hades."

John 5:21-26 "For just as the Father raises the dead and gives them life, even so the Son also gives life to whom He wishes. For not even the Father judges anyone, but He has given all judgment to the Son, so that all will honor the Son even as they honor the Father. He who does not honor the Son does not honor the Father who sent Him. read more."

1 Corinthians 15:54-57 "But when this perishable will have put on the imperishable, and this mortal will have put on immortality, then will come about the saying that is written, "Death is swallowed up in victory. O death, where is your victory? O death, where is your sting?" The sting of death is sin, and the power of sin is the law; read more."

Hebrews 2:14 "Therefore, since the children share in flesh and blood, He Himself likewise also partook of the same, that through death He might render powerless him who had the power of death, that is, the devil,-"

Revelation 20:12-14 "And I saw the dead, the great and the small, standing before the throne, and books were opened; and another book was opened, which is the book of life; and the dead were judged from the things which were written in the books, according to their deeds. And the sea gave up the dead which were in it, and death and Hades gave up the dead which were in them; and they were judged, every one of them according to their deeds. Then death and Hades were thrown into the lake of fire. This is the second death, the lake of fire."

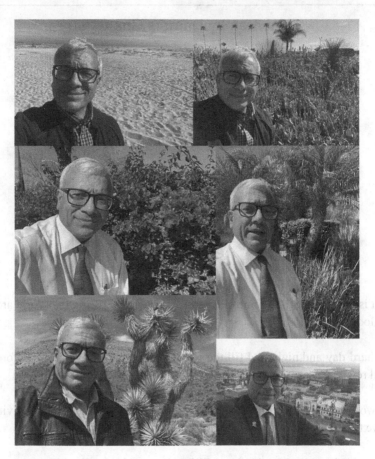

ML. My only regret working w/ you in OB/LD, OR is knowing YOU well, as a man of faith,...we we're always busy, barely had time to chat...but somehow I knew I was in "good hands" when you're "in command" though, your tone of voice was sometimes "irky nice" 😛 take care Dr. Ghaly 💚🙏

CP. Very nice. 😊

AB. Amen praise God!

CL. You Doctor are a gift from God! You help so many people. When God created you he spent special time knowing you were chosen to help others. Thank you God and thank you Dr Ghaly. 💚🙏

VG. Prelepo doktore! 🙏💜

Still a Time to Keep Working Hard filling the World around with Good Deeds!! Labor to Enter Unto Rest!

Written by Ramsis Ghaly

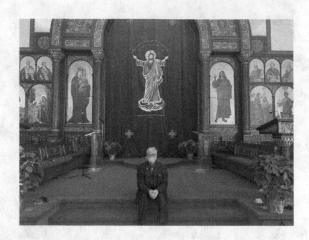

Now it is the time!! Still a Time to Keep Working Hard filling the World around with Good Deeds!!

Work hard day and night and fill the world around with good deeds before the eternal rest!

Keep working hard and filling the world around with good deeds while living to deserve the eternal comfort after death!

Be a servant keep working hard and filling the world around with good deeds to be a master!

Be a laborer keep working hard and filling the world around with good deeds to enter the Heavenly Kingdom!

Be in the field keep working hard and filling the world around with good deeds to be with the Master in His Kingdom!

Be at the streets of Jerusalem, keep working hard and filling the world around with good deeds, kneel at the gethsemane, carry the cross and be hanged on a tree at the Golgotha to resurrect in glory with Jesus at the day of the Lord!

Be in the spirit of a young child and strength of an eagle keep working hard and filling the world around with good deeds to be worthy at the Judgment Day!

No need to feel burden from working hard and filling the world around with good deeds soon the soul will be reposed forever!

Indeed, it is never enough to keep working hard and filling the world around with good deeds as what shall be coming in heaven is unspeakable and inexpressible!

Don't slow down working hard and filling the world around with good deeds before the soul shall fell unto sleep!

Why running away from working hard and filling the world around with good deeds and soon there shall be no more opportunity to do more!

Do not pause from working hard and filling the world around with good deeds as heavenly treasures and awards be awaiting!

So let all continue working hard and filling the world around with good deeds before the times of eternal relaxation and unwinding!!

Labor working hard and filling the world around with good deeds to enter to rest!

Biblical Versus

"Then said Jesus unto his disciples, If any man will come after me, let him deny himself, and take up his cross, and follow me. [25] For whosoever will save his life shall lose it: and whosoever will lose his life for my sake shall find it. [26] For what is a man profited, if he shall gain the whole world, and lose his own soul? or what shall a man give in exchange for his soul?" Matthew 16:24-26 KJV

"Again, he limiteth a certain day, saying in David, To day, after so long a time; as it is said, To day if ye will hear his voice, harden not your hearts. [11] Let us labour therefore to enter into that rest, lest any man fall after the same example of unbelief. [12] For the word of God is quick, and powerful, and sharper than any twoedged sword, piercing even to the dividing asunder of soul and spirit, and of the joints and marrow, and is a discerner of the thoughts and intents of the heart." Hebrews 4:7,11-12 KJV

Rise now is the time to keep working hard and filling the world around with good deeds as the sufferings of this present time are not worthy to be compared with the glory which shall be revealed as it is written!!

2 Corinthians 6:1-2 KJV
[1] We then, as workers together with him, beseech you also that ye receive not the grace of God in vain. [2] (For he saith, I have heard thee in a time accepted, and in the day of salvation have I succoured thee: behold, now is the accepted time; behold, now is the day of salvation.)

"Lay not up for yourselves treasures upon earth, where moth and rust doth corrupt, and where thieves break through and steal: [20] But lay up for yourselves treasures in heaven, where neither moth nor rust doth corrupt, and where thieves do not break through nor steal: [21] For where your treasure is, there will your heart be also." Matthew 6:19-21 KJV

"See then that ye walk circumspectly, not as fools, but as wise, [16] Redeeming the time, because the days are evil. [17] Wherefore be ye not unwise, but understanding what the will of the Lord is. [18] And be not drunk with wine, wherein is excess; but be filled with the Spirit;" Ephesians 5:15-18 KJV

"And I knew such a man, (whether in the body, or out of the body, I cannot tell: God knoweth;) [4] How that he was caught up into paradise, and heard unspeakable words, which it is not lawful for a man to utter. [5] Of such an one will I glory: yet of myself I will not glory, but in mine infirmities."

2 Corinthians 12:3-5 KJV
"And if children, then heirs; heirs of God, and joint-heirs with Christ; if so be that we suffer with him, that we may be also glorified together. [18] For I reckon that the sufferings of this present time are not worthy to be compared with the glory which shall be revealed in us. [19] For the earnest expectation of the creature waiteth for the manifestation of the sons of God." Romans 8:17-19 KJV

Now it is the Time!! Still a Time to Keep Working Hard filling the World around with Good Deeds!! Labor to Enter Unto Rest!!

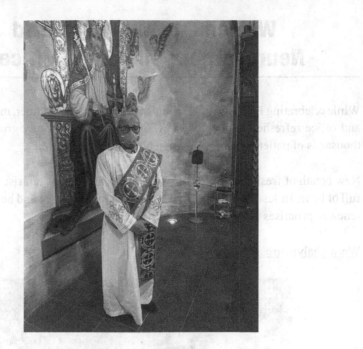

Welcome to My Post Covid Neurosurgery Clinic and Office!!

While celebrating Post-COVID Era and the beginning of summer, my entire clinic and office refreshed with New Tan Carpet in addition to my growing garden, thousands of patients thank you, gifts, blessing and stories!!!

New breath of fresh air, a smell of sweet aroma and a new sun rise with daylight full of hope, In Jesus Name we shall be blessed in His Grace and be healed in His renewed promises to His children!!

Www.ghalyneurosurgeon.com

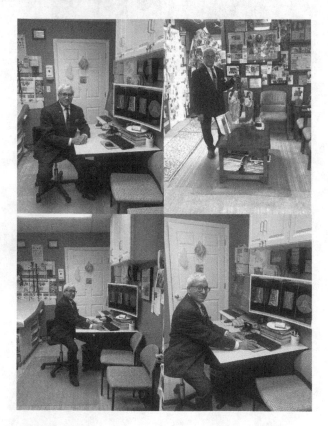

CP. Very nice. 😊
CG. Looks wonderful. I must come and see you and it one of these days. 🖤
JCB. Looks great Dr. G!!

ML. Looks great!

JC. Looks awesome, so do you Dr 🙏🙏

CB. Happy to see you without PPE

SL. ooks fantastic

NV. Great pics love the color of the walls, God Bless you 🙏

FC. Amen! God bless you! 🙏

MN. You are blessed, and we are blessed to be a patient if yours..Amen

CP. Looks great!

DM. refreshed doctor ..stayhealthy and safe

JC. Looks great Dr Ghaly!

SJ. Your clinic looks good!

Post Covid - what a nice expression

SA. Nice!

JL. I like it!! 😊 ‼️

YF. It looks great! 🖤

TW. You and your office are looking good, Dr. Ghaly. Keep soaring in your career and healing those who need you. Stay safe, my friend. 🖤🙏

KB. God bless you

EO. Office looks very nice and, you look quite dapper. Blessings.

VG. Bog Vas blagoslovio! 🙏🖤

KY. Looks great.

MN. You of all doctors deserve it Dr.Ghaly your the greatest God bless you.

CP. Looks great!

DM. refreshed doctor ..stayhealthy and safe

JC. Looks great Dr Ghaly!

SJ. Your clinic looks good!

Post Covid - what a nice expression

SA. Nice!

JL. I like it!! 😊 ‼️

YF. It looks great! 🖤

TW. You and your office are looking good, Dr. Ghaly. Keep soaring in your career and healing those who need you. Stay safe, my friend. 🖤🙏

KB. God bless you

EO. Office looks very nice and, you look quite dapper. Blessings.

VG. Bog Vas blagoslovio! 🙏🖤

KY. Looks great.

MN. You of all doctors deserve it Dr.Ghaly your the greatest God bless you.

JD. Nice

JK. BLESS is those who accept Jesus, Dr. Ghaly is the one!!! He is a preying Doctor that does for the people not what the Hospital tells him to do!!

Thank you Doc. For giving me a second chance of life threw the GRACE OF ARE LORD JESUS CHRIST.!!! You are forever in my heart & mind 😌😌 😌🙏🙏🙏

BC. Very nice!
ND. I miss visiting your office!
BK. Looking good Dr Ghaly! God bless you!
JM. Great Looking Office, Dr Ghaly 😊 Happy Day!!

Sarcasm and Funny for an Era The World Wish to Go Away and be Erased But What Remains Difficult Memories!! Here is my take about Life after Corona and the future of face masks!!

Written by Ramsis Ghaly

As the facemask nowadays is a sign of American 🇺🇸 heroism so is taking off the facemask at that time will be considered not just American 🇺🇸 heroism but patriotism!!!

We don't want to get ourselves infected again by exposing our noses and mouths in public! Then millions will die and more millions will get infected and then we get vaccinated again!! Let us keep the face masks forever!!!

I can't imagine living one more day without facemask!! Every time I forget my facemask, I feel I forget my wallet and my best half! My Face ID with facemask is my password and key to daily registrations and opening my files, websites, bank accounts, car 🚗 —-!

We all got used to muffled speech and not hearing what someone talking about! No more yelling or screams or droplets flying from the mouth!! We also got used to do staff meeting virtual from our beds 🛏 and bath tops! In fact nothing better than attending annual convention virtual from my kitchen with my pajamas!! In fact, there is hardly any traffic and not much cars outside! The homes are becoming business and need to put a suit on or dress driving the car or taking the metro train or bus. Just conduct business wireless from hone and virtual from the basement!

No way will go back to hugs or kisses or shake hands! No more opening mouth or sneezes or mouth plays. All are gross and not tolerated! Are you kidding! No one needs the bacteria and viruses of others! We will always carry hand sanitizers, sprays and air purifiers with HEPPA filters! We liked this way 6 feet apart from each other! There is no reason on earth to vine close than 6 feet. What is wrong with you people! Stay away from each other! Let us move to the deserts and countryside and build our own ranches and be away!! All we need is WIFI and digital screen!!

There is no reason for the churches to be crowded or go back to stadiums! Just watch from home under the cover in bedroom! Let us get more lazy and put on some more weights! I can't imagine people will go back to the gyms! With all the sweaty hands and reusing equipment's! No way, we like our own small gym in the basement that we never use!!

We like empty middle seats! No more tolerance to booked flights, buses or trains! They must be half capacities regardless! We love empty Restaurants and bars! We get all the attention and better service rather than be in crowded places! No one like anymore going out fur a tour! Virtual tours are as good and cheap! We love laziness and shopping on line and delivery of Amazon boxes every day! In addition, getting stimulus checks while congress, senate and house representatives getting into more arguments and disputes with no outcome! The best part is getting Supreme Court busy to decide fir then!!

In fact my kids do not recognize my face without facemask! My friends only recognize my face through my facemask!! Wives are happy seeing their husband with facemasks and Vice versa!!

O my gosh what the world will do when uncover all these rotten teeth, smelly mouth odors and cluttered lips being exposed to the public??? Imaging sitting in the plane with no facemask and next seat to you has no facemask and flight attendant 🛎 has no facemask! What about being in a room with all those people with no facemasks or convention centers and people are talking to each other with no face masks! It will not be me! No I don't think do!!! Many will get claustrophobic and chills and will run away! Many will go in strike!

In the same time, It will be shocking especially to men if women started to take off their face masks on the public places!!!

Imagine those men will go into shock and need critical care beds and urgent monoclonal antibodies to support their immune system if they spot women with exuberant make up, colorful lips, glistening white teeth, sweat mouth and fresh mouth smell!

O my gosh, CDC and Fauci have to come up with new set of guidelines for gradual easing of face masks! Those men can't handle uncovered women with exposed beauty and no longer covered with face masks!! In fact I think it should be a federal law prohibits facemask for people in order to follow the law! Remember our country is a Land of Law!!! And we must obey the law!! Peaceful protestors are allowed but must be then with no face masks!

What are we going to do with the billions of fashionable face masks, customs and designs?? Are we going to get rid of them and lose all this money?? Are you crazy?? The Wall street will crash and so is the economy!!! People will get depressed and overdosed if we remove the facemask and allow faces to be uncovered!!

You know what the president then need to implement executive order and other emergency orders to stop those aren't taking their face masks away! Furthermore, the social media google, Facebook and Twitter all of them need to suspend any organization promote facemask and spread false information against the mainstream saying facemask is good because at that time facemask will be wrong and dangerous!!

Furthermore, no one should enter any federal building with facemask. Moreover, the churches and worshipping places and businesses should not allow anyone to come with facemask otherwise they will be fined. In fact each governors will make it a state law that the facemask is prohibited and it is a felony!!

Friends, we must prepare for the next phase: faces with no facemask!! Imaging human face with no facemask will be the norm! I can just tell, it will be so many demonstrations and riots to the degree that national guards will be called to protect our statues without the face masks!!

We must learn again to see each other with our half of the face is exposed! We must teach our kids, it is okay to see lips, teeth and mouth!!! It will take time but we should be courageous to accept human faces with no masks as in the ancient days of Adam and Eve!!

Now Facebook take my post down since it is against your community guidelines and has false and misleading information!!

As the facemask nowadays is a sign of American 🇺🇸 heroism so is taking off the facemask at that time will be considered not just American 🇺🇸 heroism but patriotism!!!

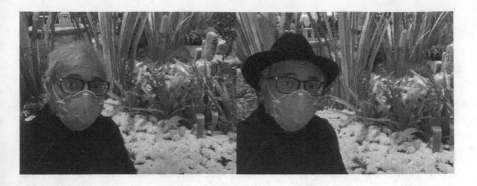

LW. I only wear one if I have to. I rarely wear on in a store or out. Never outside.

DC. Pretty funny Dr Ghaly!

CG. I can't wait until the day comes when we can throw them away. What is this nonsense about wearing two of three? We have gone a year wearing only one now we need to wear more than one? I don't think so. 😑

CR. I really appreciate your creativity in making your point. Brilliant 🙂!

RH. Gods words you share.

JM. AGREE!!

BL. I long for the days that we can share hugs, handshakes, kisses, card games, shared close space, etc.

BL. So do I! Hopefully soon "Away with the masks!"

2017 Neurosurgery/Spine Convention
These Days are gone and aren't coming back!
These days are in the memoir's archives!
Face to face and so much close and hands on freedoms are on the shelves!

Back then just 2 years ago, it was never ever accepted Zoom in or Team in or FaceTime or ——!

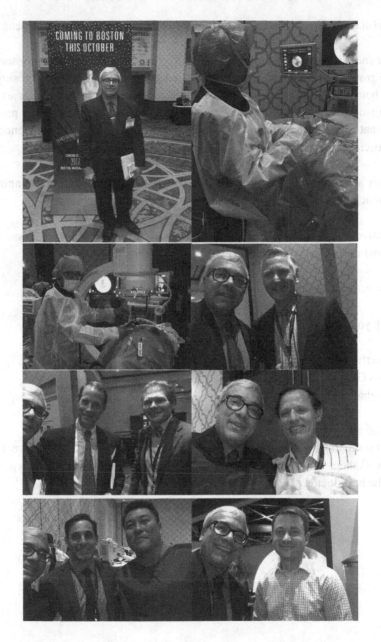

2017 Neurosurgery/Spine Convention

What a great honor to be part of every major convention, to know about each new inventions, ideas, discoveries, discuss hard cases, and grow in knowledge and skills -----: Lectures, workshop, brainstorms, debates, hands on cadaver laboratory, and case discussions every year since 1986 till present.

I cherish every time, I get the opportunity to attend and be actively present.

Never enough learning and teaching while meeting the colleagues in neurosurgery as we grow together over 30 years in the field. Each of them a legend Neurosurgeon back home---we grow together year after year and felt late our successes in a harsh world we live in with so much obstacles separating us from our patients and what we do best and enjoy every part of it: neurosurgery/ Neuroscience and Neuroscience patients.

It is my scientific neurosurgery family nationwide and worldwide. I cannot tell how much I am happy to look forward to meet each of them---

Extensive program with attendee from all over from 630 Am to 630pm. Very worthwhile and enjoyable. Appreciative to be among them all.

All is for my patients to bring and to give----

Thank you all

Respectfully
Ramsis Ghaly
www.ghalyneurosurgreon.com

JD. You are the best Dr. Ghaly!
CG. It is sad those days are gone but new ones will come soon. More conventions, workshops, ideas and all the things you miss will happen again. Keep being the best doctor. 🖤🙏

Reform Ourselves Before Asking to Reform Our System! Reform Interior Before Reforming the Exterior!

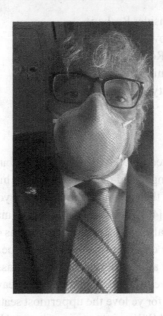

The mighty reform is that reform within the human soul before reforming the external system!

Reform inward before reforming outward!
Reform Interior before demanding reform Exterior!
Reform oneself is much difficult than reforming the system!
In fact, reforming the system comes after reforming ourselves!
Indeed reform the human soul results in reforming the system automatically!
There is no system reform without reforming ourselves!
We shall be asked about ourselves and not about the system!
Reforming the system and ignoring within the self is deemed to fail!

There is absolute no foundation in reforming the system and not reforming our human being!

How much easy to point to the system change and not to point to ourselves within!

Reform a system alone has no leg to stand before the Truth!

So what is Reform???

It is the sincere look within the self through the Eyes of Conscious Divine and open the books to re-examine the truth and depth to cleanse the inward through many ways including:

Time out. Regroup. Reconsider Reshape
Redesign. Refashion Renovate Rebuild
Reconstruct Reorganize. Remodel Remold
Rectify. Refine Revolutionize Rejuvenate
Revamp Redo Revise Restyle Transform

And———-

++Our Lord Jesus criticized severely the people who build the system and never reformed themselves saying: "And the Lord said unto him, Now do ye Pharisees make clean the outside of the cup and the platter; but your inward part is full of ravening and wickedness. [40] Ye fools, did not he that made that which is without make that which is within also? [41] But rather give alms of such things as ye have; and, behold, all things are clean unto you. [42] But woe unto you, Pharisees! for ye tithe mint and rue and all manner of herbs, and pass over judgment and the love of God: these ought ye to have done, and not to leave the other undone. [43] Woe unto you, Pharisees! for ye love the uppermost seats in the synagogues, and greetings in the markets. [44] Woe unto you, scribes and Pharisees, hypocrites! for ye are as graves which appear not, and the men that walk over them are not aware of them. [46] And he said, Woe unto you also, ye lawyers! for ye lade men with burdens grievous to be borne, and ye yourselves touch not the burdens with one of your fingers. [47] Woe unto you! for ye build the sepulchres of the prophets, and your fathers killed them. [48] Truly ye bear witness that ye allow the deeds of your fathers: for they indeed killed them, and ye build their sepulchres. [49] Therefore also said the wisdom of God, I will send them prophets and apostles, and some of them they shall slay and persecute: [50] That the blood of all the prophets, which was shed from the foundation of the world, may be required of this generation; [51] From the blood of Abel unto the blood of Zacharias, which perished between the altar and the temple: verily I say unto you, It shall be required of this generation. [52] Woe unto you, lawyers! for ye have taken away the key of knowledge: ye entered not in yourselves, and them that were entering in ye hindered." Luke 11:39-44,46-52 KJV

++Let us transform ourselves before getting critical to the outside system:

And we all, who with unveiled faces contemplate the Lord's glory, are being transformed into his image with ever-increasing glory, which comes from the Lord, who is the Spirit. 2 Corinthians 3:18 | NIV

Do not conform to the pattern of this world, but be transformed by the renewing of your mind. Then you will be able to test and approve what God's will is—his good, pleasing and perfect will. Romans 12:2 | NIV

May the Lord direct your hearts into God's love and Christ's perseverance. 2 Thessalonians 3:5 | NIV

But the fruit of the Spirit is love, joy, peace, forbearance, kindness, goodness, faithfulness, gentleness and self-control. Against such things there is no law. Galatians 5:22-23 | NIV

I appeal to you, brothers and sisters, in the name of our Lord Jesus Christ, that all of you agree with one another in what you say and that there be no divisions among you, but that you be perfectly united in mind and thought. 1 Corinthians 1:10 | NIV

Put to death, therefore, whatever belongs to your earthly nature: sexual immorality, impurity, lust, evil desires and greed, which is idolatry. Colossians 3:5 | NIV

"But whoever drinks the water I give them will never thirst. Indeed, the water I give them will become in them a spring of water welling up to eternal life." John 4:14 | NIV

Rend your heart and not your garments.

Return to the Lord your God, for he is gracious and compassionate, slow to anger and abounding in love, and he relents from sending calamity. Joel 2:13 | NIV

Repent, then, and turn to God, so that your sins may be wiped out, that times of refreshing may come from the Lord. Acts 3:19 | NIV

From that time on Jesus began to preach, "Repent, for the kingdom of heaven has come near." Matthew 4:17 | NIV

You see, at just the right time, when we were still powerless, Christ died for the ungodly. Romans 5:6 NIV

Peter replied, "Repent and be baptized, every one of you, in the name of Jesus Christ for the forgiveness of your sins. And you will receive the gift of the Holy Spirit." Acts 2:38 | NIV

Do not lie to each other, since you have taken off your old self with its practices and have put on the new self, which is being renewed in knowledge in the image of its Creator. Colossians 3:9-10

++Let us Examine Ourselves

Lamentations 3:40. Let us examine and probe our ways, And let us return to the Lord.

Ezekiel 18:27-28. Again, when a wicked man turns away from his wickedness which he has committed and practices justice and righteousness, he will save his life. Because he considered and turned away from all his transgressions which he had committed, he shall surely live; he shall not die.

Haggai 1:5-7. Now therefore, thus says the Lord of hosts, "Consider your ways! You have sown much, but harvest little; you eat, but there is not enough to be satisfied; you drink, but there is not enough to become drunk; you put on clothing, but no one is warm enough; and he who earns, earns wages to put into a purse with holes." Thus says the Lord of hosts, "Consider your ways!

Luke 15:17-24. But when he came to his senses, he said, 'How many of my father's hired men have more than enough bread, but I am dying here with hunger! I will get up and go to my father, and will say to him, "Father, I have sinned against heaven, and in your sight; I am no longer worthy to be called your son; make me as one of your hired men."'read more.

1 Corinthians 11:27-31. Therefore whoever eats the bread or drinks the cup of the Lord in an unworthy manner, shall be guilty of the body and the blood of the Lord. But a man must examine himself, and in so doing he is to eat of the bread and drink of the cup. For he who eats and drinks, eats and drinks judgment to himself if he does not judge the body rightly

Job 13:23. How many are my iniquities and sins?
Make known to me my rebellion and my sin.

Psalm 4:4. Tremble, and do not sin;
Meditate in your heart upon your bed, and be still. Selah.

Psalm 32:3-5. When I kept silent about my sin, my body wasted away. Through my groaning all day long. For day and night Your hand was heavy upon me; My vitality was drained away as with the fever heat of summer. Selah. I acknowledged my sin to You, And my iniquity I did not hide;

I said, "I will confess my transgressions to the Lord"; And You forgave the guilt of my sin. Selah.

Psalm 77:6. I will remember my song in the night;
I will meditate with my heart, And my spirit ponders:

Psalm 119:59. I considered my ways And turned my feet to Your testimonies.

Jeremiah 31:19. For after I turned back, I repented;
And after I was instructed, I smote on my thigh;
I was ashamed and also humiliated Because I bore the reproach of my youth.

++Therefore, Reform Ourselves Before Asking to Reform Our System! Reform Interior Before Reforming the Exterior!

Amen

God bless you Dr. You are loved by so many people have a restful evening.

BCD. When I see human's, I do not see color, I see Souls. Each has a history, a story of life. Try to be the best Human you can and always treat others the way you want to be treated.

JB. Hope you are ok doctor, I know it is hard for you right now but you love Jesus and he will take care of you so you can take care of your patients.
God protect you and watch over you always. 💜

KJ. YOU ARE THE DOCTOR OF CHOSEN LIFE! YOU ARE THE ANGEL OF PROMISE AND TRUE PROSPERITY!

DM. you are always full of wisdom to share people

ET. I'm going to send you some barrettes!! 😷

CG. What I see is not America. I hope that God in His infinite mercy will help us overcome the evil which we know has been growing in plain sight for too many years. 💜🙏

RC. We need to reform our way think and act quickly. Good bless you and all of us

LM. What a wonderful piece of thought from a good soul and heart. I loved reading it as it brought me to a right attitude about life and spirituality. God continue to bless you with compassion and and kindness to others.

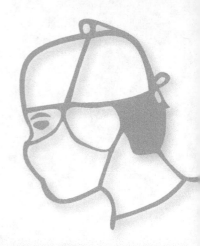

SECTION 4

Inspiring Stories Of COVID Survival

A True Story and Real Miracle of our Lord Jesus Of Two COVID Survival: They weren't sisters but they were together in the same hospital dying from COVID-19

Written by Ramsis Ghaly

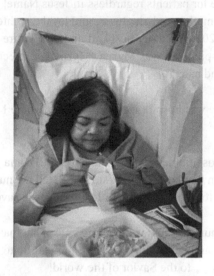

The journey began unexpectedly on November 2020! They were never sick and weren't sisters but they were together in the same hospital 🏥 dying from COVID-19.

There were two nurses fell victims of COVID-19 in the same time! They weren't sisters and they didn't know each other! What was strange was that both were from the same country of origin the Philippine!

One named Myrna and the other named Violet and they were facing each other in the critical care unit each in a private and separate sealed room with two glass doors well ventilated with negative pressure! One was in critical care bed 19 and the other in critical care bed 11!

Violet, a nursing home nurse from the Philippine originally worked all her life to care for the sick. she was a day ahead of Myrna and her COVID condition required immediate attention since her oxygenation was deteriorating so rapidly!

I was called to intubate violet! There was no time to wait! She couldn't maintain oxygenation overnight and was drifted down so low even in high oxygen flow fighting for her life to survive!

I knew Myrna for thirty years, we used to work together hand by hand and step by step along the way saving lives day and night serving the Chicagoans and indigents of the metropolitan of Chicago!

Myrna was just retired two years ago and I didn't see her since then! She believed in my mission to care for patients regardless in Jesus Name! Hardworking nurse Myrna was, a loving mother and great wife and loyal daughter! Her daughter got sick of COVID 11/3/2020, then her husband and then entire family got sick and the only one was hospitalized was Myrna. Myrna got infected while caring for her husband and grand baby!

I didn't know that she was hospitalized and she was where I was taking hospital calls!

Myrna in her early hospital days before she drifted to coma got to know that Dr Ghaly was working in that hospital! She started to tell the nursing staff all about the years of working together and how in Jesus name we saved so many lives!

Myrna told so many nurses whom were taking care of her that Dr Ghaly is blessed by the Lord of Glory and he won't permit any human life to slip by because this was his daily prayers 🙏 to the Savior of the world!

As soon as her nurse send me a message, I went directly to her room! I stopped by and she immediately screamed and held my hand saying: "Please pray for me, I don't want to die! My family are sick and they need me by all means! They aren't allowing any visitors and all I do I pray, cry and FaceTime them all the time! Look Dr Ghaly I have a a gold chain with our Virgin Mary, the Mother of Lord Jesus! Please don't leave me and keep watching over me!"

Then Myrna screamed calling the names of her personal saints St Anthony, Saint Joseph and our lady of Manaooag and called upon her Savior "O God save me" She Remember her mother kneeled before our Lady back (60) sixty years and cured her brother after all doctors gave up in her brother illness! Myrna lived Pangasinan providence in the Philippine by the ocean 🌊 and survived of many Typhons! So every year her mother would go to visit our lady and took her daughter Our Lady. As Myrna was kidding the death she said: "If I survive I will take my son and daughter to visit you Our Lady of Manaooag!

236

I cried in tears as my heart 💜 moved and pumped heavy blood 💧 ran unto the floor of the hospital bed! I said Myrna: "We love you and will continue to pray together! You will be okay. Lord Jesus can conquer COVID-19 and much more"

Whenever, I came to my on call days, I visited Myrna from the glass door and waived hello and strengthen her faith checking in her well-being thanking the hardworking nurses caring for her! Sometimes she was awake and other times laying prone awake and suffering struggling with breathing!

Day in and day out, Myrna illness was getting worse and worse and the threat in her life was becoming imminent and real! It was so much scary for me every time I come to hospital 🏥 afraid of the bad imminent news!

Each time when I saw her from the glass door, I told the nurses all about her and how she sacrificed her life for patients and recently to her family. In fact the reason she got COVID-19 was because she contracted from her own family sickness of COVID-19 while she was caring for her own! The days she was supposed to be retiring and relaxing from the heavy years of service became the days of suffering and her life was about to be taken away from COVID-19!

A week passed by and the breathing was getting difficult and her oxygen saturations were dropping to the 80's instead of 90's and 100's. From the glass door I look at her laying prone in her stomach! I cried in silence praying: "Lord Jesus as You are taking her to through this journey, please bring her back alive in thy Name O Lord of mercy and Grace" I left the critical care unit looking at the ground while passing by the nursing station! They knew my heartfelt grieving, aches and sadness!!

Many have shared with my soul the heartfelt sadness, sorrows and tears! We prayed and lightened so many candles and initiated chains of prayers all over the country of America 🇺🇸 she loved and the Philippine where she was born!

It was an evening that I was on call and I received emergency 🔔 call to come and intubate bed 19 in ICU with COVID-19. I said: "Is this our nurse Myrna?" The reply with sorrows was: "Yes she is"

I ran, put my PPE and PAPR, gowned and gloved 🧤 and got my intubating equipment and medications and rescue devices! I cried to my Lord: "O Lord Jesus please use me to save her soul! She is Your child forever. Keep the promise and keep her life, in thy name, Amen 🙏"

I entered her room, she was gasping for air, can't sleep, agitated, combative, fighting for more air and the high flow oxygen of sixty liters per minute wasn't enough! She kept turning and turning, with periods of on and off sleep and confusion. Her face, skin and lips were looking blue and her color was no longer bright and red but rather gray and dreadful!

"O Myrna, I am ready to put the tube and connect your lungs to the ventilator to help you out, give you rest and you don't have to struggle with breathing like that" She looked at me saying: "No Dr Ghaly, please don't intubate me! I will die if you put that tube in me! I am okay! Give me one more day! I have been in days with high flow oxygen! Give me an inhaler this is just another asthma attack! Let me breath some racemic epinephrine and I will be okay!"

Minutes went by and new minutes were passing by and she was getting worse and worse before our eyes. She screamed saying; "I need to talk to my son before you intubate me Dr Ghaly! Take care of me Dr Ghaly! Watch over me! Don't take the icon of my Mother Virgin Mary chain away from me keep it to my chest all the time! She is my saint!"

She Faced Time the son and exchanged few words in tears: "I am going to be intubated. I love you ❤—". She suddenly stopped! I tried to talk to her son but she immediately turned blue. I moved fast administered the medications and in seconds I put the endotracheal tube in place. Deep in the throat all looked gray and dead, as if, the virus has eaten much of her flesh!! The oxygen saturation went rapidly to the 30's". We started to ventilate her more and more pouring more oxygen in her body to revive before she goes to the grave and we gave epinephrine so that her heart won't stop!

I put an arterial line to keep track of her blood pressure and to get blood samples instead of keep sticking her for blood. Her color started to turn bright red and oxygen saturation raised up to the 90's! We all smiled and took a deep breath and a sigh of relief. I looked at her and up to heaven and said in private: "Lord Jesus thank you 🙏 for allowing me to be the chosen person to intubate her and see Your hands and made it happen while I was on call. Thank you 🙏 for giving her another lease in life"

Since then she drifted into deep coma and all her organs were shut down. She required daily kidney dialysis and high PEEP to push the air and oxygen under high pressure since her oxygenation was getting worse and worse!

Her roommate, the home health nurse next door, Violet was recovering fast on the other hand. We all continued to pray for both nurses! But more and more for the sicker Mila!

One day, I visited both Violet and Myrna. Myrna was quiet like a little baby sleeping but Violet wasn't. I did my rounds and left the unit. Violet decided with all her force to pull the tube out of her throat with her hand as soon as the nurse left the room. I was called to come back quickly to reintubate Violet! Many were angry why did she pulled the tube out. Yet as if she was in a deep sleep and drifted in a dream that she was already recovered and no more need for the tube. We all stood outside waiting for her to get worse with the oxygenation and to move forward with the intubation. But to our surprise, she was correct. It was her time to be in her own and since then she recovered completely walking out of the hospital 🏃 praising God, the Lord of hosts!

But Myrna was doing worse and her color became gray and deadly with No brightness or redness anymore!! Whenever I was on call, I stood by the glass door in tears crying to our Lord with heart full of sorrows and eyes running out of tears! In silence I pled to my Savior: "Please Lord keep the promise in thy hands she is and in thy name is our faith, Amen 🙏"

She had touched all the hearts of nurses and her previous coworkers kept asking about her progress and kept praying for her. Yet they couldn't help it but let the tears run like rivers from their eyes and grieving in her suffering!

Day after day and week after week, the prognosis was grim and no chance of living! The glimpse of life was no more! The daily conversation was about letting her go and sign the orders of "DNR" "Don't Resuscitate", pull the plug 🔌. Back and forth of "Yes" and "No" and hours and hours of uncertainties. What is the right thing to do? What should we do? We don't want to lose our mother? She is everything for us!!

The more push to withdraw life support, the more strength the family gained to say "N0" and "Do Everything for our mother Myrna"

The palliative care arrived and the family refused to withdraw life support. One day "DNR" on and another day "DNR" off! Every day, by the phone they are waiting for the bad news of the MIla life has ended. There was no sign of recovery!

Everyday update was the same and the family were told: "There is almost no chance for her to live and if she lives, she will have no quality at all! Look at her!

She is in a deep coma, not responding at all, she lost 100 pounds, she is only a skin over bones, and all her organs are shut"

I stood with the family and kept praying 🙏 of my private prayers with my Beloved: "Keep the promise in thy Name".

Yet I kept the faith and visited her from the glass door, I waived hello and I prayed while my eyes teared and my heart ached!!! she was lying in bed in coma with no response!

However, whenever I looked at Myrna, I saw life beyond the dead flesh! Initially she was ballooned and swollen from all kind of fluids and pressors to maintain her blood pressure and perfusion to the brain and her organs. Then gradually, she lost much weight as her body dried and diuresed much of the accumulated fluids!

Her face was rounded and she looked at peace! Even in her worst days of COVID-19, she looked as an innocent child face and angels all around her!

To tell you the truth, I was at peace knowing, there is life returning back to that body that once was eaten by the evil virus 🦠! One of her previous worker and former nurse and her best friend told me while she was crying: "I prayed day and night and I heard a voice from heaven: Why are you crying I didn't take her. She still alive and she will live"

While her organs were shut yet her heart was strong and recovered without any more pressors. As her lungs began to recover and oxygenation raised up to the 90's without any oxygen supplements needed but room air!

The blood counts were getting so abnormal and her immunity got to be so low. Her legs and feet turned blue and the overall perfusion wasn't sufficient. The family optimism received as not realistic and the hospital exhausted all the doors to convince the family to let her go. It has been fifty days in the hospital and close to two months in critical care in deep coma with failing organs!!

Yet the medical team, had no choice but to keep supporting her body to the last breath! A stomach tube placed direct in her stomach to feed her since she couldn't eat and a tracheostomy tube was placed directly to her throat since she couldn't breathe in her own or protect her breathing because she was still in deep coma!

"No matter what, keep doing everything! We aren't withdrawing any life support or placing her in "DNR" Give her all what she needs to fight COVID-19 and she will wake up one day! We are sure and we have faith" These were the constant words from her entire family and her friends and previous coworkers"

More and more family conference meetings and serious discussions from her medical team that the Brain 🧠 MRI showed damages and she would never recover to quality life at all.

But for the family and myself: "It isn't over until it is over and over no one knows about the long term of life and the brain but God the Lord!

Based in the determination of the family and the persistence of her support! The Medical 🏥 team made arrangements to be transferred to "long term nursing home facility with ventilator care"

In the last day prior to discharge Myrna, my heart was felt with joy that she made it all the way through the most difficult time and through the journey, God kept her life even in the eleventh hours and days of death.

I stood by the glass door in tears crying to our Lord with heart full of sorrows and eyes running out of tears! In silence I pled to my Savior: "Please Lord keep the promise in thy hands she is and in thy name us our faith, Amen 🙏"

She moved to the nursing home facility and the family started to visit her and stimulate her! They saw life in her eyes and they talked to her as if she was hearing them and seeing them. They felt her listening to them and recognizing their voices! They became more encouraged knowing a living soul underneath the skin about to burst out of the three month shell 🐚!

Gradually day by day, the days and hours of prayers and hardworking of the medical team and determination of her family and coworkers to keep her alive touched the Divine Heart and went up to Heaven!

Myrna started to Wake up and began to move her lips. She started to open her eyes and made gestures to the family as if she knew who they were and she was coming out of the three months of coma. The entire room converted from sadness and sorrows and tears to joy and laugh as in the time of Lazarus risen from the death!

Days later the ventilator was weaned off and she was breathing in her own in room air. The tracheostomy was decanulated and removed and so was the stomach tube. There wasn't any need to both of them since she was awake, eating, drinking and talking!

241

O my gosh, she remembered so many discussion and words during the illness care journey while she was in deep coma as if she was dead outside but inward was alive! Myrna is currently only few days away from coming home 🐿 sweet home 🏠 and with open arms to the coming days of more rehabilitation and reconditioning! Myrna is back to her own self and well-being!!

I informed her medical team, nurses, doctors and respiratory therapists. They were so joyful and started to cry when I saw them her pictures and videos. They all remembered her very well. Although they were surprised, yet they entrusted the Lord. The recovery of Myrna indeed renewed their faith and revived their cause! It made the days to take care of her worthwhile! It was important for me to show the results of their hardworking day and night. Despite she was in deep come and every day looked the same with no immediate feedback for Hope, yet patience and perseverance paid back in full! The entire staff were thankful and praising our Lord for the progress she had made. Soon she will go to visit the hospital and her medical team looking at the beds where she was laid and the walls she stared at! It shall bring joy with tears, memories of fears, hope for that time of despair and exaltation to the new lease in life rising from the hospital bed near death to resurrection among the family and friends! She was once a nurse caring for such patients and she became that patient for nurses!

Myrna and Violet stories brought hope to humanity in the time of the darkness and despair. It renewed faith in so many souls and the living of sickness. It made every knee bow to pray to the Lord of hosts!

It indeed brought love, admiration and inspiration to our medical profession! Never lose hope and never be fast to pull the plug 🔌!

My Lord Jesus is my Love! He has never left my sight and He is always so kind and merciful! I am not articulate as many of you but simple in my words and limited in my vocabulary! I wish I could utter all the most prolific words to describe my Lord Jesus. But He is that One that raised Lazarus from death while others were laughing since He was already buried for four days. Indeed, My Lord Jesus was never affected by the laughs and lack of faith through the illness journey of Myrna!

"Jesus said unto her, I am the resurrection, and the life: he that believeth in me, though he were dead, yet shall he live: [26] And whosoever liveth and believeth in me shall never die. Believest thou this?" John 11:25-26 KJV

Until today I remembered my words that I revealed to no one but Him: "I stood by the glass door in tears crying to our Lord with heart full of sorrows and eyes

242

running out of tears! In silence I pled to my Savior: "Please Lord keep the promise in thy hands she is and in thy name us our faith, Amen 🙏"

My Beloved said: "And he said, The things which are impossible with men are possible with God." Luke 18:27 KJV

Thank you Lord Jesus! Welcome Mila to life living among us! Go return back to thy family! Thank you 🙏 for your years of service! Lord Jesus have never ever forgotten you even in the darkest days of grim hope and deep gloominess.

The story of Myrna and Violet should comfort all of us. It is a story of faith, determination and perseverance.

O world! Be joyful Lord Jesus conquered the darkness of COVID19 and put an end to the pandemic! Spread the good news and the hope! Lightened your candles and strengthen your faith in our Lord Jesus and encourage the sick and support the weak! Indeed Lord Jesus is here and COVID-19 is casted out in a major defeat! Say Amen to Lord Jesus and Welcome our beloved Mila fully recovered from COVID-19

Psalm 16 KJV

[1] Preserve me, O God: for in thee do I put my trust. [2] O my soul, thou hast said unto the Lord, Thou art my Lord: my goodness extendeth not to thee; [3] But to the saints that are in the earth, and to the excellent, in whom is all my delight. [4] Their sorrows shall be multiplied that hasten after another god: their drink offerings of blood will I not offer, nor take up their names into my lips. [5] The Lord is the portion of mine inheritance and of my cup: thou maintainest my lot. [6] The lines are fallen unto me in pleasant places ; yea, I have a goodly heritage. [7] I will bless the Lord, who hath given me counsel: my reins also instruct me in the night seasons. [8] I have set the Lord always before me: because he is at my right hand, I shall not be moved. [9] Therefore my heart is glad, and my glory rejoiceth: my flesh also shall rest in hope. [10] For thou wilt not leave my soul in hell; neither wilt thou suffer thine Holy One to see corruption. [11] Thou wilt shew me the path of life: in thy presence is fulness of joy; at thy right hand there are pleasures for evermore.

Psalm 67 KJV

[1] God be merciful unto us, and bless us; and cause his face to shine upon us; Selah. [2] That thy way may be known upon earth, thy saving health among all nations. [3] Let the people praise thee, O God; let all the people praise thee. [4] O let the nations be glad and sing for joy: for thou shalt judge the people righteously,

and govern the nations upon earth. Selah. [5] Let the people praise thee, O God; let all the people praise thee. [6] Then shall the earth yield her increase; and God, even our own God, shall bless us. [7] God shall bless us; and all the ends of the earth shall fear him.

Psalm 22:2-25 KJV

[2] O my God, I cry in the daytime, but thou hearest not; and in the night season, and am not silent. [3] But thou art holy, O thou that inhabitest the praises of Israel. [4] Our fathers trusted in thee: they trusted, and thou didst deliver them. [5] They cried unto thee, and were delivered: they trusted in thee, and were not confounded. [6] But I am a worm, and no man; a reproach of men, and despised of the people. [7] All they that see me laugh me to scorn: they shoot out the lip, they shake the head, saying, [8] He trusted on the Lord that he would deliver him: let him deliver him, seeing he delighted in him. [9] But thou art he that took me out of the womb: thou didst make me hope when I was upon my mother's breasts. [10] I was cast upon thee from the womb: thou art my God from my mother's belly. [11] Be not far from me; for trouble is near; for there is none to help. [12] Many bulls have compassed me: strong bulls of Bashan have beset me round. [13] They gaped upon me with their mouths, as a ravening and a roaring lion. [14] I am poured out like water, and all my bones are out of joint: my heart is like wax; it is melted in the midst of my bowels. [15] My strength is dried up like a potsherd; and my tongue cleaveth to my jaws; and thou hast brought me into the dust of death. [16] For dogs have compassed me: the assembly of the wicked have inclosed me: they pierced my hands and my feet. [17] I may tell all my bones: they look and stare upon me. [18] They part my garments among them, and cast lots upon my vesture. [19] But be not thou far from me, O Lord: O my strength, haste thee to help me. [20] Deliver my soul from the sword; my darling from the power of the dog. [21] Save me from the lion's mouth: for thou hast heard me from the horns of the unicorns. [22] I will declare thy name unto my brethren: in the midst of the congregation will I praise thee. [23] Ye that fear the Lord, praise him; all ye the seed of Jacob, glorify him; and fear him, all ye the seed of Israel. [24] For he hath not despised nor abhorred the affliction of the afflicted; neither hath he hid his face from him; but when he cried unto him, he heard. [25] My praise shall be of thee in the great congregation: I will pay my vows before them that fear him.

Ramsis F Ghaly, MD
Clinical Professor of Neurosurgery and Anesthesiology
www.ghalyneurosurgeon.com

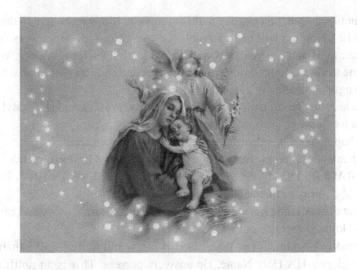

TM. ... A beautiful account of another miracle of God right before our eyes! Thank you Dr. Ghaly for taking care of her, for praying with us & for being an instrument of Faith! May God bless you more & the likes of you who bring God's words to bedside & share them with your patients & their families as well. 💜

CG. Perfect example of the power of prayer and you. This tore at my heart and so thankful they both survived. Bless you! 💜🙏

CR. This story made me cry. Your faith in Jesus and His miracles increases my faith in trusting Him more. Bless you for being His vehicle of grace and healing.

AE. Beautifully written true story. Dr. Ghaly you are a true believer and I am sure you did your prayers before you intubated her and God heard your prayers and kept her alive. Thanks a million for your support and prayers. Our hearts are filled with joy.

NA. Amen 🙏👐💜

JV. Amen 🙏🙏🙏💜💜💜💜

MD. Amen we pray. 🙏🙏🙏💜💜💜

KD. Amen, such purpose for Mila's life and for yours Dr. Ghaly

TD. Amen 🙏

NE. I love! God is good, always been going no matter the situation. Thank you Jesus for the miracle! God will continue to bless, and use you Dr. Ghaly!

ML. I deeply believe our faith in GOD & trust in our good doctors, like you Dr. Ghaly is awe inspiring, thank you for the many years & life saving efforts I have witnessed while working w/ you in OB/OR

LR. In one of the most widely known scriptures, Matthew 17:20, Jesus said, "Because you have so little faith. Truly I tell you, if you have faith like a grain of mustard seed, you can say to this mountain, Move from here to there, and it will '. Nothing will be impossible for you." Through our prayers God can speak to us and use you Dr. Ghaly to work miracles for His glory. We must come to God Completely surrender with expectancy as we see total healing, strength and recovery again for His glory.

BL. You are truly God's child and ambassador. You are so loved Dr Ghaly! Thank you for sharing! ⚒⚒⚒ Blessings.💜💜💜

NE. So happy to see my dear friend recovering, glory to God!

DLL. Thank you Dr Ghaly for sharing this ... true this is a living miracle. ⚒⚒⚒ MIRACLES DO HAPPEN IF YOU TRULY BELIEVE IN HIM.. P-U-S-H 😋😋😋 pray until something happens.

KO. What a remarkable story. Faith, prayers and extraordinary love and care, only God knows when it's our time. 💜⚒⚒

MC: Thank you so much Dr Ghaly! God is Great and Merciful. We thank Him and glorify His Holy Name, He answers prayers. This is an uplifting and humbling story of faith and persévérance!

KO. What a remarkable story. Faith, prayers and extraordinary love and care, only God knows when it's our time 💜⚒⚒

ME. Thank you so much Dr Ghaly! God is Great and Merciful. We thank Him and glorify His Holy Name, He answers prayers. This is an uplifting and humbling story of faith and perseverance!

CP. Thank you Lord Jesus Christ for bringing back Myrna to us ⚒ and Dr Ghaly as an instrument that made it possible. 💜

DL. This is a true story, my former coworker (labor and delivery) and the best anesthesiologist Dr. Ghaly..

BL. I have the EXTREME privilege of knowing Dr Ghaly; he is the most amazing (and that's a huge understatement) person I have ever met!!! He has a long list of credentials, awards, accomplishments, accolades, etc and yet treats everyone as a dear friend.

He sends posts on a regular basis and they are always a faith filled lesson.

Pm. What am amazing miracle. So glad to see Myrna active and alive. Don't even look like she has been sick and in ICU for 3 months. Praise God for Dr. Ghaly, you are such a kind soul and a prayer warrior and ambassador for our Lord Jesus, May God bless you and continue to use both of you.

Al. True A REAL miracle of Our Lord Jesus. In Jesus name we PRAY, Thy Will be done. Dr. Ghaly you are a great instrument in the field of medicine & with the Love & faith in all you do. God bless. ⚒

Mg. Truly a miracle. So glad to see Ms. Macaso healing well and coming back from the jaws of death. Thank God. 💙🙏

Gr. God is really good and Miracles do happen. Thank you Dr. Ghaly for taking care of Myrna and for this amazing story. I am so happy Myrna is back. Glory to God.

Cn. God is good, all the time. 🙏

Fm. MIRACLES INDEED HAPPEN AMEN

sa. You are a true witness for Christ Dr. Ghaly who present a testimony about the truth that we have experienced and heard. God's word is a seed once it planted it will grow and develop into the fruit the Lord intends it to become. God works in your life according to His purpose. God sent you for Myrna, and her family. Thank you Dr. Ghaly God is great, worthy to be praise. 🙏 May God continue to bless you abundantly.

FM. MIRACLES INDEED HAPPEN AMEN

JR. God is good all the time! 🙏

BR. Yes... It was a very good description of a full recovery journey Covid patient in the hands of Health doctors, nurses and health workers...we salute you for your great mission in humanity.. Amen

DR. So happy to see u God bless u always

AN. God is Good all the time. and miracle do happen everyday. We're happy to see you recovered Manang. 🙏😊

AP. Oh but God

NR. GOD IS GOOD ALL THE TIME...

GC. Praise the Lord! With faith in God Almighty all things are possible.

JB. "Miracles happen to those who believe."
If you believe in something with all your heart and mind, you bring it back to life. God is so good all the time! 🙏🙏🙏 Feel better soon Ate Myrna 💜

DR. So happy to see u God bless u always

AN. God is Good all the time. and miracle do happen everyday. We're happy to see you recovered Manang. 🙏😊

Praise the Lord! With faith in God Almighty all things are possible.

NA. God Bless Dr. Ghaly for all the things that you do and most importantly your prayers - and to all those who cared and prayed for Myrna 🙏 She is a dear friend and a nursing school classmate. God is good, He answers those who believe and have faith in Him 🙏🙏🙏

LC. Dr.Ghaly + prayer is the best medicine, you are a wonderful doctor, thank you for sharing 🙏🙏🙏

NS. Jesus is our great healer, He knows our hearts and minds. When we surrender everything to Him, our prayers will be answered as long as we ask His forgiveness. He will make us living witness of how good He is to those who have faith. While we are still strong, we have mission to do. Amen

AL. A very touching true to life story a Filipino American nurse who was infected by Covid and was in coma for 3months and with faith prayers and support from her Dr. Ghaly family co workers n friends miracle happens..

Let's us pray for all those who are sick and never give up hope...Amen — with Chicago Illinois.

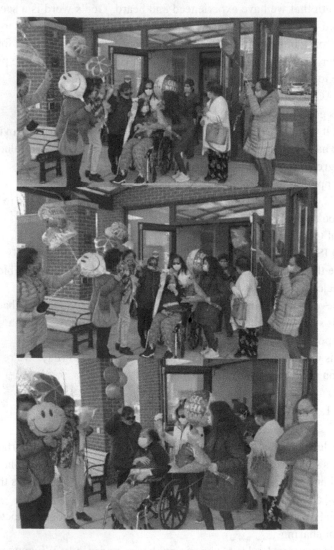

Praise our Lord four months after COVID coma and ICU on ventilator since November today going home. Today is the day to return to her hone and God blessed her with new lease in life to return to her family. Much blessing and more and more strength in recovery. We pray to all those on ventilators and in coma to recover in Jesus Name. Amen. 🙏

MM. After 3 months and 23 days... I can share the wonderful news.... MY MOM IS COMING HOME TODAY!!!

For those of you that didn't know, our mom had Covid back in November and these past few months have been the most challenging, the most anxious, the most heartbreaking, and the most depressing time of our lives. We spent all of the holidays without her, awhile she was in the ICU. Our days and nights seemed so long, and everyday our anxiety was through the roof. Every time our phones rang, we tensed up as we received updates after updates on our mom hoping for good news and improvements.

Then on Dec. 22nd, we were given the opportunity to see our mom because things weren't looking good. So there we were, standing behind a glass window looking at our mom, as she laid there intubated and on a ventilator. It's a pained image we will never forget and hope to never see again... We were then given our "options" of what we wanted to do with our mom. We were so lost, so scared.. seeing our mom suffering and enduring all the complications that stemmed from Covid... the pain was just unbearable. We spoke to our aunts, my mom's sisters, and they helped and convinced us that mom was too sedated to feel any pain, to not pull the plug and don't give up hope. When we spoke to the NP of Palliative Care and told him we've decided to continue her care and "to go all the way," his response was "ok, but I'm just letting you know, she is dying..." Those lasting words were engraved in our minds as we left the hospital speechless...

We continued to pray every day and hope for a miracle. A week or so after New Year's, the doctors called and wanted to talk about placing a trachea in and removing the tubes because mom has been sedated for about 8 weeks, they were worried if any brain damage occurred. She was approved for a tracheostomy and the procedure was successful. She then had a trachea placed in with the ventilator still attached, helping mom breath. The plan was to slowly ween her off sedation, so she can wake up and open her eyes.

We transferred her to Holy Family in Des Plaines where they specialize in ventilator weaning. Within a few days of being there, she finally opened up her eyes for the first time after 2 months! God heard our prayers. He restored our faith, gave us hope, and gave us our biggest blessing... a miracle. She was given a month at Holy Family to recover and show any improvements. By the end of the month, she was talking and she was no longer using her trachea and she was off the ventilator, but still needing help to breath with oxygen tanks. Our mom is truly a fighter! 🙏

After the month stay, she moved to a rehab facility where she received physical, occupational, and speech therapy. She's learning to walk again, regaining her strength all over, and happy to be eating all her favorite foods again. She was in rehab for only 3 weeks, but she'll continue with a day rehab program 3 hrs each day, 3 times a week for as long as she needs. Covid really did a number on her lungs and on her short term memory, but she persevered and will continue to persevere! My mom is the definition of a warrior. 💪

I share her story in hopes that people understand and see that Covid is still very much out there in our world. So please take the necessary precautions, and make smart choices!

And a quick thank you and appreciation to all the front liners putting your lives at risk to save all those who are at risk. And a huge thank you Dr. Ramsis Ghaly for saving my mom and always checking on her at Masonic. 🙏

Lastly, on behalf of my mom, dad, brother, and I.. we continue to thank all of our family and friends, near and far, for the outpour of support and prayers for our mom and for us. THANK YOU! ❤️🙏

Joint retirement party and thanksgiving Drury Lane. Though, I retired last December 20, 2020 I was thrilled and humbled that you guys planned such a sensational party in our honor. My thanks and deep appreciation for the kindness of everyone who attended and especially to ate Cristina Baculod Lacsamana, Toni Margarico Moraga, Amelia Molina-lucena, Nwanyieze Ezeikpe, Patricia Mendoza who made every detail of the party so perfect. Thank you so much. ❤️ ❤️❤️ Cook County retirees celebrants Aloysius Edakara, Glynes Roferos, Sylva Cariaga Agustin, and thanksgiving for, Sincy Vargheese.

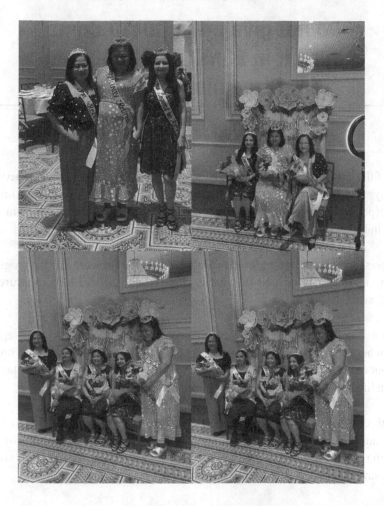

MM. Was so touched that you included us, Sincy & me to your retirement party, can't help not to cry upon seeing everyone, still have long recovery ahead. God is Good, thanks to the prayers of my family, relatives, friends,& medical team, Thanks again Cristy & your organizing team, Congratulations again to the three retirees Sheeba, Sylva, Glynes, welcome to our club, let's get together again July 31, God Bless us all.

Do not give up in COVID Coma even if in ECMO and intubated for three months in ICU!!

Written by Ramsis Ghaly

I am fully aware of three COVID patients were intubated and in coma between 55 days and three months unresponsive, not moving, not talking, lying in bed, not responding and connected to machines and full support and two of them were even in ECMO artificial lung and finally are recovering!

The pressure was high in the family to let them go and they were told the prognosis of any quality was nil and the family resisted and opposed all measures to withdrawal!

I was asked about my advice in two and my advice the same as 40 years ago: "I do not believe in human life withdrawal! Man has so many ways to take a human life but only one way to keep a life which is through God the Lord. Do let God take a life and not a man"

The three are recovering slowly but surely! They have to be rehabilitated, build their muscles back, strength and reconditioning! Two of them remember the ongoing gloomy discussion conducted while they were in coma and people around them saying hopeless and discouraging words—-!

If your loved ones start to open their eyes and show signs of communications, they are fantastic signs of recovery. Fight for their lives, search for support, ask for help and line up the therapy and support!

Show them love 💜 and care and hope! They are indeed fought the good fight! In the same time, know that because you stood close and never give up and you didn't submit to the pressure to agree and sign to withdraw, that is the reason they are with you today! Take a pride of what you did and persevere and Cherish the priceless life even for one more day!!

I used to tell many over decades of my life, "If you give the brain enough time, the brain and nerves will recover". On my series of books "Christianity and the human brains—" series of 16 books.

So many miracles and patients recovered from coma I took care of them over the years and made remarkable recovery despite majority said no way!!

Believe in yourself and your loved ones!!

This is my stories "A Miracle Worker" Chicago tribune June 2001:
https://www.chicagotribune.com/.../ct-xpm-2001-06-10...

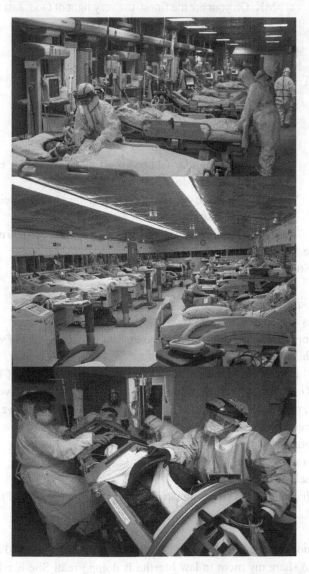

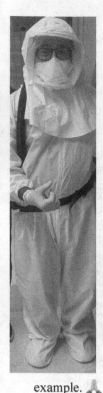

KD. Amen!

JP. Thank you for all you do Dr. Ghaly!

SS. You be are an angel. 💕

SJ. My God, please help contain this virus(s). It is heartbreaking to see these images of so many sick people and their human servants taking care of them. 🙏💜🙏

KG. Thank you!

MK. Oh your are the finest, the very light of God. Just love you Dr.

AL. Medicine & the power of prayers together 🙏, their is miracle. You are a great Doc & a believer

RC. Thank you

MA. Amen Dr. Ghaly! My brother Jorge was living proof. 🙏🙏🙏

CR. Amazing! Only God.

AB. Praise God!

MB. God bless you and protect you Doctor.

SS. Amen gloria al Dio

JB. Thank you Dr Ghaly for all that you did for my dad and continue to do for others!!

JE. Thank you, dear friend, for sharing your devoted work with us. It inspires us all.

JM. Thank you for your gift to others you are a shining example. 🙏

MH. Good Stuff! =

Prayers Inbound

VG. Bog Vas blagoslovio i čuvao!! 🙏🙏🙏

TM. Dear Lord, Bless this good man and keep him safe. He is one of your Angels on Earth. Amen. 🙏🙏🙏💜💜💜💚💚💚

JF. Beautiful words. We serve a miracle working God. May Jesus Christ be JC. Thank God you are on their side, thank you for caring for all lives. 💕😌

TJ. My God, my God - thank you for your miracles. Although we've never seen your face, we've seen what YOU can do. God's mercies are new everyday - be grateful.

LS. Thank you for sharing.

MD. A Miracle Worker

KA. I love dr ghaly. He is so passionate and cares so much for all of his patients.

NP. Amen!!!

Only God knows when our time is up... so don't give up on your loved ones. 🙏💜 So blessed to share my mom in law Martha is doing great! She is rehabilitating to gain strength to walk again 🙏👏— with Juan Contreras.

VG. Dear esteemed prof. Dr. Ramsis Ghaly. You are the only one in the world who consciously heals and respects human lives. God bless you all!! 🙏🙏🙏🖤

EP. Your message goes beyond words. It gives hope to those who have family or friends suffering from COVID or any other medical condition. This message speaks very close to my family's heart. Thank you for all you do.

CG. You are a miracle worker. You never give up where others have. God has truly blessed you with knowledge and perseverance. 🖤🙏

WK. We've had a few like that too

ME. This is so very true Dr Ghaly! Prayers and medicine working hands I hands. Thank you Doc.

VG. Amen, a 45 year old man from our town just came off life support (intubated and ECMO), for 55 days, now has started his journey in rehab!!!! Many, many prayers were and are still being said for Brian. 🖤

KB. Beautiful words. 🌹🙏🖤🙏

CG. My goodness Dr Ghaly way to represent, we are but thimble to this cup.

Sincerely, cherie

CT. You're awesome Doc, may God bless you and keep you safe. ✨🙏✨

DK. Absolutely 💯! Well said and so true. 💕

CH. You are very courageous person Dr. Ghaly! May God keep you safe! 🙏🙏🙏

VW. Thank you for sharing.

LM. You're wonderful Dr.Ghaly thank you!!! 🙏🙏🙏

DS. You are amazing inside and out Dr Ghaly. 🖤

MM. Love this. True it isn't over until God says it's over.

JP. In 1991, my son was hit by a car. He had a brain bleed, broken collar bone, ruptured spleen, and two broken legs, one a compound fracture. While in ICU, I was informed he was HIV positive. I was told" I had to consider the reality of the situation, and give them permission to let him go". Many nurses felt otherwise. They said when I spoke, read or sang to him, he responded. After a month, they removed him from his vent. Long story short, he not only recovered from all his injuries he went on to become a Christian. He did die 4yrs later at the age of 30, from complications of HIV; but he died saved and happy. Praise God for those who don't give up on their loved ones.

AP. Ain't God good

DM. Dr Ghaly is this picture in cook county? you are an awesome doctor who always give hope to people

TG. The Lord bless you and keep you. Thank you for you belief and way of thinking.

DS. You are amazing inside and out Dr Ghaly. 🖤

ES. AMNE No throw away people!!!

MM. I totally agree!!!

MW. Totally agree!

CD. God is great and my faith is immense 🖤🖤🖤🖤🖤🖤🙏🙏🙏 GV. God is great and my faith is immense 🖤🖤🖤🖤🖤🖤🙏🙏🙏 DD. You are always in our prayers cousin God is very great have faith that God in his time will give you his relief 🙏 take care of yourselves and make you really want it

KM. You are so right Dr Ghaly! God bless you! I love your faith and you are a blessing to all. Thank you. 🙏❤️

AFU. Ty Dr.God is our hope 🙏 my husband was in intubated Jan,14,21 /ICU 17 days .. he was transfer to Dignitive Oberservation Unit.less critical he spent one week and was transfer to Sub/acute Healthcare of Orange County lwas told by neurological Dr.@ Medical center ..He won't recover from 2 stroke..was undergo with tracheostomy /open his eyes twice..moving leg, jan17/21~feeding tube Jan 21/21 Dr.told me my husband won't recover due to 2 stroke /pneumonia, respiratory, diabetes and not following commands/ unresponsive..since in ICU he was moving shoulder/right hand, head, yawning, try open eyes twice..

Now in su/acute..still in coma but making lots of progress moving right hand nonstop..when video call to sing and prayer 🙏 he moves head and try to open eyes half way.. now 29 days ... since he was in hospital to sub/acute ..your prayers are needed for my miracle husband God bless!!! 🙏🙏🙏 Thank you for the beautiful and awesome encouragement of hope you have posted..You are a lifesaver and God fearing Dr....in God's timing..God is in control 🙏 I do believe and trust the LORD will heal my husband with a #miracle God bless you Dr.Ghaly Shalom!!!

JL. Check it out. Read the article on Dr. Ramsis Ghaly

JM. Simply Amazing 💙 Still Praying!!

MC. Great article. 👏

FA. Thank you Dr Ghaly... the Doctor with a heart 🤍.

SA. YOU are amazing Dr.Ghaly

AU. Amen in Jesus name

ANOTHER MIRACLE STORY
3/16/2021

What a miracle three months intubated and ICU and in ECMO and now home post COVID19. Praise our Lord Jesus.

I wonder how many lives lost by so call COVID and could have been saved!!!! And they were misinformed or weren't given the opportunity!!!

Home sweet home. Congratulations. Praise our Lord Jesus and the wife that did not give in pulling the plug or listen to advice of withdrawal of life support. Instead fought the Good fight and stood so strong in faith and loyal in love to her husband when he was sick with COVID in coma helpless!

I wonder how many lives lost by so call COVID and could have been saved!!!! And they were misinformed or weren't given the opportunity!!!

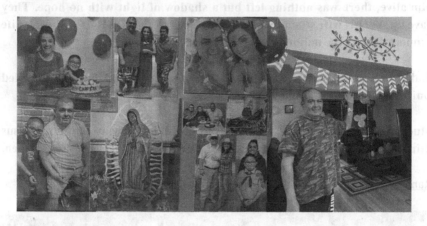

Flor De Andocutin

He kicked covid's butt!! It took him 3 months but he did it!! Thank you lord for all you do your timing is always perfect

KE. AMEN RAMSIS

AMAZING CARE

JB. Amen!!
JB. AMEN !! Welcome home.
BK. Praise God!!
EO. Praise The Lord! 🖤🖤🖤
JL. Praise God
CG. This is wonderful! Welcome home and bless you and may God keep you healthy.
AV. Praise God!! 🌊🙏
JH. Praying for continued healing blessings and strength.

July 2021
A Miracle among us!!

Four months with the worst COVID Pneumonia ever in the ventilator for three months and on artificial lung (ECMO) for two months! Salvador came to my office with sharp Mind walking in his own feet with no assistance and driving!

While Salvador was in prolonged coma, he was dying daily and listed in the death row. At the time where the medical team exhausted all means to keep him alive, there was nothing left but a shadow of light with no hope. They gave up. Yet his wife stood by him and refused to sign DNR or withdraw life support despite the majority vote to do so!

Today Salvador and his wife fought the good fight and happily married United again in a new honey moon!

Much much more blessing. Glory to our Lord Jesus. May our Lord Jesus shine more and bless you much of abundance, In Mighty Jesus Name, Amen.

Ramsis Ghaly

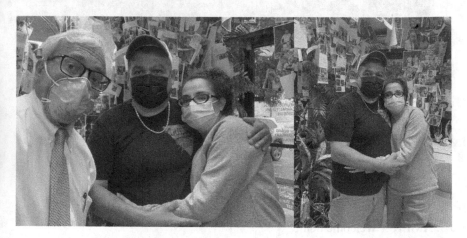

LA. Thank you Lord for the healing. 🙏

FA. Thank you for fitting us in considering i went to see you right after my surgery GOD BLESS YOU DR GHALY My husband was really impressed with all you knowledge. 🖤

MR. Thank you Lord Jesus Christ for healing. ♡ 🩹

CG. A true miracle of faith and true love! Bless them both.

SM. Dr. Ghaly, you're the best!

JU. Miracle!

AB. Praise God!

AU. 👣👣 God is good. 👣👣

DK. Praise God!! What a beautiful miracle they have received!! 🖤🙏👍

DE. A true miracle! 🙏🙏

RR. Praise the lord! 🙏

CL. Praise the Lord!!!

SD. God has a purpose for his life!! Praise to the Lord!!

CC. Miracles DO happen!

AL. God is good all the time! 🙏

JP. Praise God! 🖤🙏

GL. Que felicidad mi Rocío eres grande, tu fe lo salvó y que dios los siga bendiciendo de verdad que bonito es el amor así me encantaría pero ni modo por algo pasan las cosas un abrazote con mucho cariño y que dios los siga bendiciendo

RS. Un milagro enorme prima q dios los bendiga. 🖤

JJ. AMEN! God is HEALER! God's continued blessings to you, Salvador and your family.

AP. God is good all the time he's a plan for that young man's life

JM. AMEN

AM. Lindo final obra del Señor. 😊

DS. Great news

RH. So Thrilled for this miracle. Love is the treasure. Never take it for granite. Thank you Jesus.

AB. You're changing lives for the better always!!!

LD. raying for Salvador's continued recovery!

JG. Amen. 🙏

KD. May God continue to bless his health and their marriage. 🙏🖤

KL. Amazing

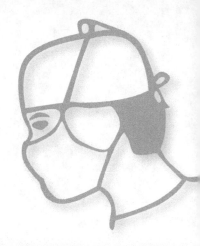

SECTION 5

Selected Patients Stories During COVID Recovery

Archangel Michael and My Patient MF. March 12, 2021

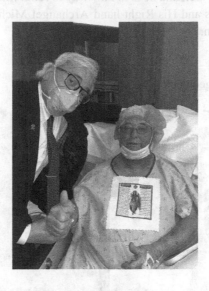

On last Friday, As I was driving early morning to do major brain surgery with deep prayers on our beloved patient, Richard, I put my hand in my suit pocket and I found a soft cloth. I took it out and it was our beloved Archangel Michael.

I became tearful and joyful since Archangel Michael is doing the surgery. The hands took the entire Timor out despite it was in a very delicate and deep place in the brain. The brain tumor is gone and will never come back.

It was so beautiful, comforting and filled the operating room and Richard hospitalization in joy. Thank you 🙏 to you Richard and your kids and sisters Eileen and Lucy and Emily. Much more blessing and your wife Arlene in heaven is watching over you!

As I talked to Richard, he said many years ago he and the church congregation established St Michael Ministry for people in grievances and suffering to provide compassion care in the church and since then he says the daily prayers: *"Saint Michael the Archangel, defend us in battle. Be our protection against the wickedness and snares of the devil; May God rebuke him, we humbly pray; And do thou, O Prince of the Heavenly Host, by the power of God, thrust into hell Satan and all evil spirits who wander through the world for the ruin of souls. Amen." A week after surgery, Richard remembered all about St Michael and now we know well heartedly St Michael is Richard Saint and St Michael never forget him and in time of need St Michael came to his Richard's surgery!*

Richard is doing very well and he is in how way to rehabilitation to get stronger. Praise our Lord Jesus and His Right hand Archangel Michael. We all pray for speed recovery. Amen. 🙏

Ramsis Ghaly
Www.ghalyneurosurgeon.com

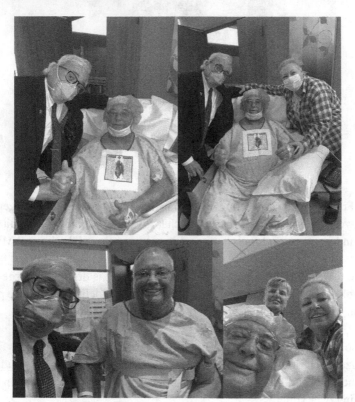

Clare, the granddaughter of my patient Richard, just send me a beautiful letter in mail. O my gosh so touching from the heart of 10 years older. I opened my mail and I read this angel words.

Richard is in his way of recovery from brain surgery.
Much blessing and thank you 🙏 Clare and Emily!!!

Ramsis Ghaly
www.ghalyneurosurgeon.com

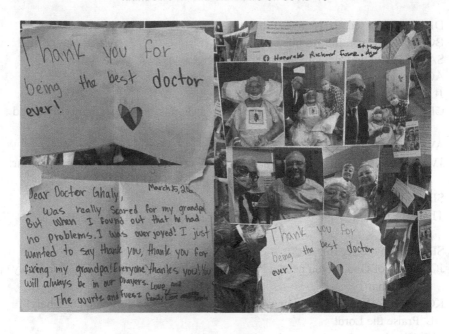

RM. God bless you Sir!

CZ. 💕🙏💕 that was so sweet !!!! God bless you & all of your patients

JB. Our prayers and thoughts are with your dad. Much love sent his way. Jo and Al Block.

VG. That's wonderful 🖤🙏🖤

CB. Clare has a way of touching people's hearts, doesn't she?!!!!

Thank you Dr Ghaly for your skill and dedication to saving people's lives. Our family loves you 🖤 Christine Fuesz - Beier

MM. That's so awesome!! Great job Claire.

BM. Sweet Clare is so adorable and caring. Give her a big hug to my flower girl. Thanksgiving to God and Dr. Ghaly for a successful surgery.

KE. Precious! 🖤

BM. How very moving the letters are, straight from the 🖤 God Bless you Dr. Ramsis Ghaly

for all you the life›s you have touched and healed. God has given you gifts and you are truly his Servant! 🖤

AH. is this your Father? Thank god for everything, I am so glad he doing good!

DC. That's awesome!

DC. So sweet!!! She has a precious heart.

CG. How precious! What a sweet and thoughtful granddaughter.

KG. So awesome!

KP. Love this! 🖤

ML. Thank God! 🖤🙏

DL. Truly blessed. Praise the Lord Jesus Christ.

BG. May God continue to bless you!!!!

SA. Beautiful and lucky to be under your care!

AG. Amen

JU. Thank you!

CE. Speedy recovery. U were and r in great hands with Dr Ghaly. May God continue to bless u Dr

AV. Praise God! Praying that he will heal quickly in Jesus name Amen! 🐦🙏

JV. Praise God! I'm glad to hear he's doing very well. Keep going with your passion and God will continue to use your healing hands 🕊️

SB. Amen!!!

Thank be to God

🙏🙏🙏🙏🙏🙏

SP. So happy to see this... 💜

JO. Hands of God, if you need a Neurosurgeon for the brain or spine, Dr Ghaly is the man.

KG: Very good and exciting news! You are such a skilled surgeon, Dr. Ghaly!

DL. Praise the Lord!

MG. Thank you for taking such good care of him.

MM. He's in my prayers f

CG. hat is so wonderful. So happy for him and his family. Bless you and him! 💜🙏

RC. Blessings for both!

BCD. Very beautiful report. Thank you

RH. Beautiful blessings and miracles. Praise God

TD. God Bless you Doctor

MP. St Michael the Archangel, pray for us.

TG. Praise God. Blessings for Boths. 🙏

MN. God Bless you Richard for a fast and safe recovery

LF. This is a great picture. So full of hope. We are so happy the surgery went well. We love and miss you. Great Picture, this one just makes me smile. We miss you all so much

DP. Blessings to you daily and all your patients!

JP. You are an amazing Christian man doctor. I'm privileged to read your posts.

ML. Wow you have multi generation fans Doc. 😙😊

PK. This is wonderful!

MM. That's right, Best Doctor ever

EF. he had a Meningioma tumor removed that was removed in full! It was large and deep. Dr. Ghaly performed a miracle through God! He is at MarianJoy

RM. God bless you Sir!

CG. How precious! What a sweet and thoughtful granddaughter.

CC. 💜🙏💜 that was so sweet !!!! God bless you & all of your patients

SA, Blessings!

266

MN. And that's the truth Dr.Ghaly is.
MN. Absolutely awesome
JF. So sweet

Richard home the weekend of Easter April 2, 2021

This is my Easter, Jesus Resurrection ftom death and return home of my patient Richard after the journey of surgery!

Home sweet home where Richard is celebrating Easter and coloring the Easter eggs with his granddaughter. What a joy and brings tears to my eyes! Hallelujah hallelujah hallelujah to the Lord and to His people! O praise our risen God Amen 🙏!

Happy Easter Jesus Risen and indeed He is Risen!

Ramsis Ghaly
Www.ghalyneurosurgeon.com

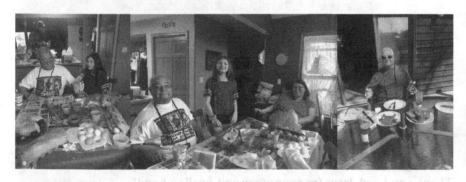

GB. Swift healing to Richard. Easter Blessings!
AB. Amen praise God
AS. Blessed Easter to you!
DL. Easter blessing to everyone.
MP. Happy Easter!
VG. Vaskršnji blagoslov svima! 🙏🙏🖤🖤
RF. Happy Easter Dr. Gahly.
MM. Happy Easter, GodBless
MR. Happy Easter doctor
SK. Happy Easter!
AH. Happy Easter to you all!
SP. Happy Easter Ramsis! 🌺🌺🌺

RM. Amen 🙏 Happy Easter Dr Ghaly! 🌞
BM. Happy Easter everyone)
JC. Happy Easter Dr! 🐰🐰💜💜

Richard loves Mimard, he went to get groceries and things to fix with his sister. Both did it. Our trip to Menards. It was uneventful. I got Richard in the car and out of the car without any casualties

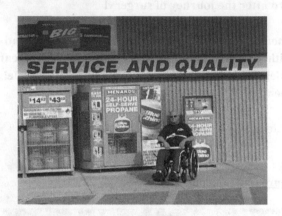

Richard and his sister Eileen came for the clinic visit today! Progressing slowly but surely. Richard is An angel living among us. He loves to shop at Menards and buy Menards Salmon in Batavia.

Richard brought me a Menards bag and a window shield blanket. He handed me a souvenir, a Ramsis Pharaoh pen from Egypt!

Thank you soo much. Bless your heart. Speed recovery. Continue to heal. Thank you Lord Jesus for your grace and healing hand!

Ramsis Ghaly

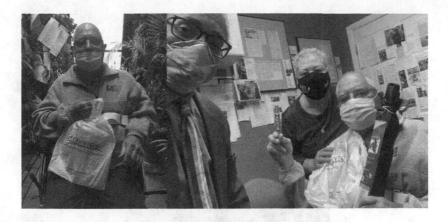

dl. You are so loved.

Every day Richard is getting better! His faith and the family faith are exceptional. His sister is by his bedside day and night. Amen to great family, positive energy and self-motivated. Only because of him and his loyal family around him that he is exceeding all expectations. They did it in their own. Great work!! Blessing to patient empowerment and strong faith in our Lord.

Thank you 🙏

Ramsis Ghaly

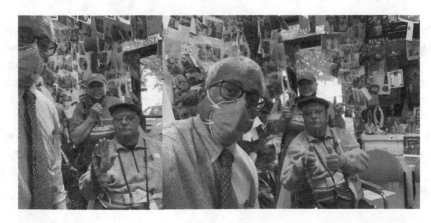

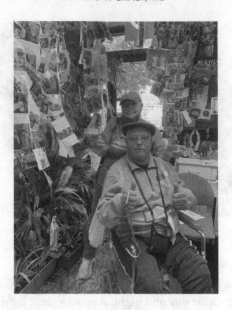

Ramsis Ghaly
May 11 at 8:39 PM ·
Shared with Only me
🔒

Look at this nan after brain surgery he is already in the basement at his own repair shop. Nothing stop his perseverance and determination.

My spectacular patient and hero brought for me his own favorite home grown plant 🌱 to planted in my office!!! So sweet!! Richard and his sister Eileen came in to the clinic visit and all sudden my clinic became a site of great celebration. Amen 🙏 to see our Lord Jesus bring healing, hope and strength. And my office garden is growing more and more by the blessed patients.

Thank you Richard and now your plant 🪴 is going to grow more and more as you heal more and more!! So proud of you, please continue to heal with speed recovery.

Ramsis Ghaly

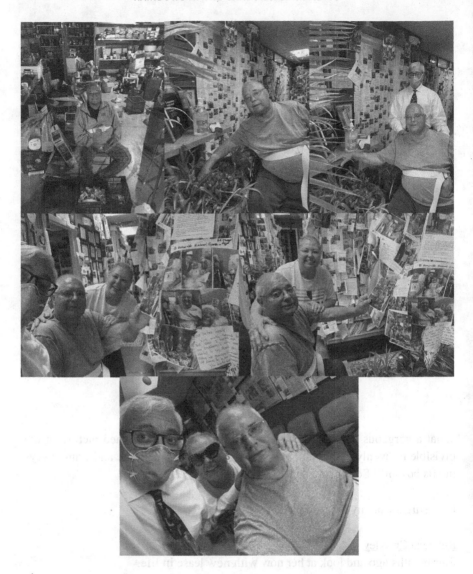

SP. To plant a garden is to believe in tomorrow. – Audrey Hepburn
So glad you're doing well. 🖤
Keep your head up, Positive thoughts 🙏

What a gorgeous touching heartfelt beautiful diamond painting of our Savior and myself in Surgery drawn by my patient RC!

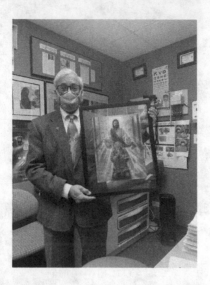

What a gorgeous touching heartfelt beautiful handmade framed picture of the invisible Heavenly Father and my Savior Jesus Christ with me and I am always in His bosom!!! So spectacular!

I did surgery on my beloved patient

Rebecca Crawley
four months ago and look at her now with new lease in life.

You have touched my heart and here is my soul praying while performing neurosurgery with my Beloved and Savior!

it's called Diamond painting. Each little piece is glued on one by one until the picture is complete. A picture this size is probably 25 to 35 hours to complete. I then seal it so none of the pieces can fall off.

Thank you Lord and God of earth and heaven for your blessing and grace and extend the healing to thy people

Thank you sooo much. Much blessing.

Ramsis Ghaly
Www.ghalyneurosurgeon.com

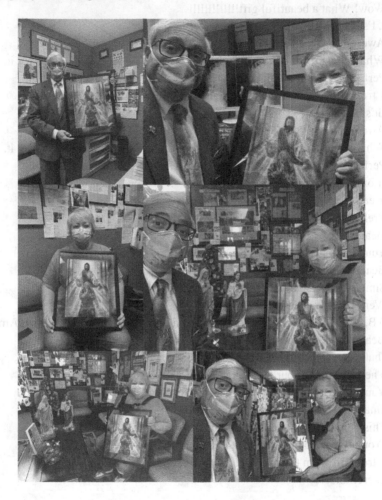

LE. How Nice, glad to see you are doing soooo well
MC. Beautiful!
TH. What a beautiful gesture.
KS. Beautiful.
DL. Wow. Very nice.
CD. Beautiful
DH. Wow. Awesome Crawls!
PK. Beautiful
LM. That is Beautiful what a special gift 💖🙏

GS. This is incredibly touching and heart warming. 🖤

SS. Glory to God to His Son Jesus and Holy Spirit Amen

GWV. This is so touching! What a wonderful gift!

JD. That is awesome Dr. Ghaly !!!

CR. Wow! What a beautiful gift!!!!!!!!!!!!!!

MSA. t's beautiful!

DC. Awesome!

CG. What a beautiful, thoughtful gift. I hope you find a special place for it.

BO. Perfect gift from one Saint to another. Love the way you framed it!

JH. A true gift from the soul and heart speechless but so deserve

MA. It's beautiful!

DC. Awesome!

CG. What a beautiful, thoughtful gift. I hope you find a special place for it.

BO. Perfect gift from one Saint to another. Love the way you framed it!

MH. Love 🐿 that picture!!

BM. Beautiful 🙏🖤🙏

VG. Prelepo, kakov poseban poklon 🙏🖤🙏

AG. Beautiful!

CC. You look amazing Becky. So glad you found him.

JM. Beautiful 🖤

JM. Simply "Gorgeous" Dr. Ghaly!!

CM. Very nice! Indeed blessed!

GV. AB. We seek the guidance, wisdom and healing virtue of our Lord. Amen

KE. Beautiful absolutely beautiful!

JD. That's awesome my friend.

DC. The Lord guides our hands and steps. 🙌✝️🙏🖤

CR. You are God's instrument of healing for sure. 🙂

JB. Amazing Dr. Ghaly, what a wonderful gift.

GS. This is incredibly touching and heart warming 🖤

MH. You are such a blessing 🙌 for giving that picture to him.

JH. A true gift from the soul and heart speechless but so

KA. Incredible! 🖤

Our special angel surprised me today in her clinic visit with another gorgeous handmade beautiful frame with Jesus our Lord holding me with His arms. Very touching sacred master piece, number two!!! it's called Diamond painting. Each little piece is glued on one by one until the picture is complete. A picture this size is probably 25 to 35 hours to complete. I then seal it so none of the pieces can fall off.

Thank you so much Rebecca Crawley. So proud of you and your perseverance and recovery. Indeed, our Lord Jesus to be praised as He had healed you and continue to overshadow your kind soul.

Thank you 🙏 and so I will be getting blessing for every surgery as you brought our Lord very close!!

Ramsis Ghaly
www.ghalyneurosurgeon.com

JM. How "Beautiful" Dr. Ghaly!!
KG. How special!!!
AS. Wow beautiful

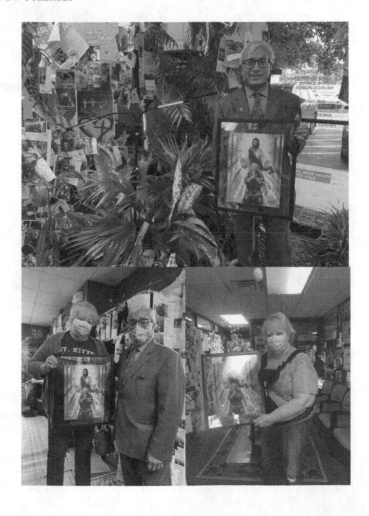

From Terry Lee Ebert Mendozza
Thinking of you with Love, as I navigate this path back to health; all because of you, my dear friend. If I don't have to go back to Mayo Clinic, then I will plan a trip to Las Vegas in early May to see Karon Kate, and hopefully you will be there, too. May God bless you always, Ramsis. I will never forget what you did for me, and no doubt, countless other people who were lost in medical quagmires. You are the Good Shepherd. Peace and love to you always. ♥♥♥

Today in my clinic a Unity of the Son to His Mother!

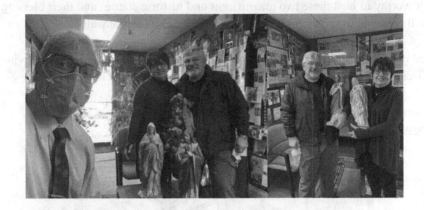

It indeed marks the Divine official end of the horrific Pandemic and peace in heaven as in earth!

Twenty years ago a wonderful patient after I removed her brain tumor, she brought me an ancient statue of Lord Jesus Sacred Heart. She dedicated her life to Service St Franciscan nuns! I cherished very much her gift and my clinic is so blessed to the degree that I put the gorgeous Sacred Heart on the top of high shelve in the middle of my clinic reception area and always was with me!

Two months ago, a wonderful mother was losing her child to a difficult disease and while she was at my clinic reception area, she spotted our Lord Jesus Sacred Heart lonely without His mother.

Immediately, her lovely spirit remembered that she has at her home, His mother, standing lonely, exactly the same height and design and almost as ancient and historic of more than a century or two.

Lynette and her husband Jim surprised me today and brought the Blessed Mother of Jesus to unit with her Son Jesus Sacred Heart. And now both are in display in the midst of my clinic United together!

After Twenty years ago, today was the day for their union. And what is really a miracle both are angelic women, despite they don't know each other and not related, yet both have the same first name, same love, same strong faith, same generosity, and same compassionate! Today both Lynettes, got to know each other by the spirit since the first Lynette now watching from heaven the unity of the Son to the Mother!

I cannot thank you 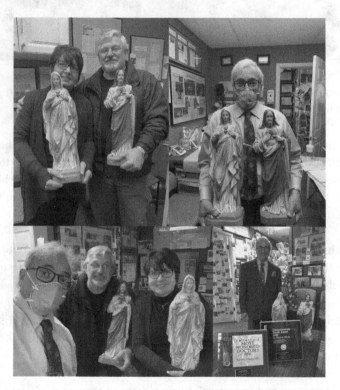 enough to both my patients and their family and love. I am not worthy to host these two magnificent and historic statues and their blessing shall continue to spread far beyond the boundaries of all the walls!

Today in my clinic a Unity of the Son to His Mother! It indeed marks the Divine official end of the horrific Pandemic and peace in heaven as in earth!

Ramsis Ghaly
www.ghalyneurosurgeon.com

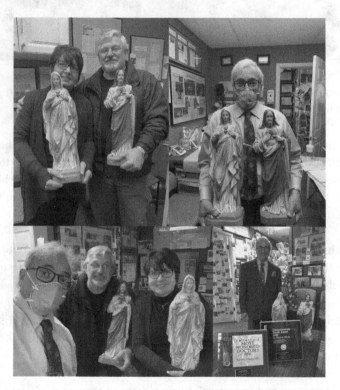

AS. Beautiful
LD. So beautiful!
AB. Beautiful
BL. The generosity of these woman reflect the well-deserved love and respect for you. The statues have a great home.
CG. The statues are beautiful. How blessed are you to be loved by so many. Congratulations on your well-deserved awards.

Words of my Patient!

My patient Deborah, last visit after I have done major Spine surgery less than a year ago. She is graduated as of today with full recovery and no pain or weakness or difficulty walking after decades of suffering!!

So Deborah said: "I am not going to see you again?"

I replied: "No but come and visit any time and remember us in your prayers and good thoughts"

Deborah replied: "I am blessed to have you as you and as neurosurgeon"

I replied: "I am so blessed to have you as you and as patient"

I love my Lord Jesus who has given me the gift to serve His children as I love His children and I am thankful with their blessing and their presence in my life!!! Thank you.

Ramsis Ghaly
Www.ghalyneurosurgeon.com

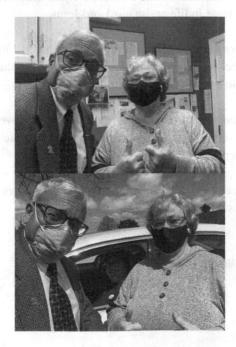

279

The Journey of Donald Sargent!

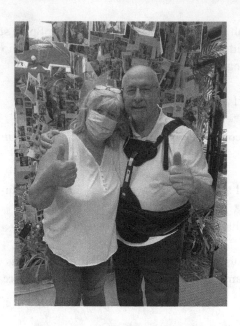

Our angel Donald and his wife Judy came today after major surgery three weeks ago. He had severe spinal stenosis and almost paralysis with severe pains All done and complete. New lease in life praise our Lord Jesus.

His daughter put horn from the marine placed in his walker!!! Patient work for the northern Illinois steel company and he was so interested in the steel in the back placed in surgery. So amazed of Donald and Judy!

Donald and Judy said "the surgery was a great journey and we fell in love again even after 37 years of marriage. We appreciate each other much more and we are together in every step"

No single pain. Never need to take pain meds. Donald us back again the normal good Donald" wife said!

Ramsis Ghaly
Www.ghalyneurosurgeon.com

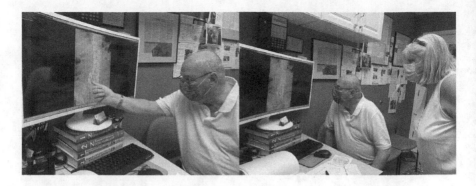

CG. Another patient who leaves your office happy and smiling. Bless him on his path to recover.

JM. Beautiful Story "Congratulations" 💕

Keep up the good recovery Don and thank you to GOD and DR <u>Ramsis Ghaly</u> for helping him walk pain free. 🙏😷

MH. Truly amazing to be out of pain & 37 yes. Together. 🖤

AU. So glad to hear he is doing well. Don and Judy are great people.

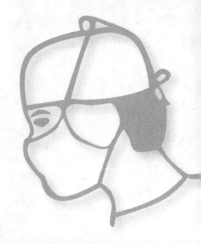

SECTION 6

Jesus Love During COVID

Jesus Love is my Thanksgivings 2020 and my Thanksgiving is Jesus Love During COVID Second Surge!

Jesus Love 🩶 is my Thanksgivings and my Thanksgiving is Jesus Love 🩶 During COVID Second Surge

Thanksgiving Poem Written by Ramsis Ghaly

Jesus Love 🩶 is my Thanksgivings and my Thanksgiving is Jesus Love 🩶

Indeed, the human soul life is worth living if in the Mighty love 🩶

Thy made an eternity out of my dust-maiden man: Thine made a purpose worth living in the Mighty Jesus love 🩶!

Jesus love 🩶 brought Merry Christmas upon the face of the Earth and salvation to the human race to return to the Heavenly kingdom!

Jesus Love 🩶 brought a heavenly New Jerusalem much much more than the very first Garden of Eden!

Jesus love brought justice and mercy together, An Incarbated God in the Flesh born in a manger to save His people and forgive their sins and be degraded from His glory and tortured and be hanged in the cross to rise again and destroy the dying of death and be the firstfruit of all things new in Him!

Jesus Love 🩶 shed blood of the God only Son for the world that He loved most to bring them to Him from the dungeon of Satan and hell of hades!

Jesus love 🩶 brought peace to earth and good will to man, True Love 🩶 to defeat hostility and aggression, rejuvenation to creation to defeat destruction and true doctrine to Hippocracy and deep rooted bureaucracy and false teaching!

Jesus love 🩶 visited man and restored back his sonship to the Heavenly Father and made him mighty, brought him to His Own and elevate him from hierley to son of God and saved the entire human race bought them with His blood to become His sheep and one sheep for One God the Almighty the Good Shephard!

"To him the porter openeth; and the sheep hear his voice: and he calleth his own sheep by name, and leadeth them out.4 And when he putteth forth his own sheep, he goeth before them, and the sheep follow him: for they know his voice.5 And a stranger will they not follow, but will flee from him: for they know not the voice of strangers.6 This parable spake Jesus unto them: but they understood not what things they were which he spake unto them.7 Then said Jesus unto them again, Verily, verily, I say unto you, I am the door of the sheep.8 All that ever came before me are thieves and robbers: but the sheep did not hear them.9 I am the door: by me if any man enter in, he shall be saved, and shall go in and out, and find pasture.10 The thief cometh not, but for to steal, and to kill, and to destroy: I am come that they might have life, and that they might have it more abundantly.11 I am the good shepherd: the good shepherd giveth his life for the sheep.12 But he that is an hireling, and not the shepherd, whose own the sheep are not, seeth the wolf coming, and leaveth the sheep, and fleeth: and the wolf catcheth them, and scattereth the sheep.13 The hireling fleeth, because he is an hireling, and careth not for the sheep.14 I am the good shepherd, and know my sheep, and am known of mine.15 As the Father knoweth me, even so know I the Father: and I lay down my life for the sheep.16 And other sheep I have, which are not of this fold: them also I must bring, and they shall hear my voice; and there shall be one fold, and one shepherd.17 Therefore doth my Father love me, because I lay down my life, that I might take it again.18 No man taketh it from me, but I lay it down of myself. I have power to lay it down, and I have power to take it again. This commandment have I received of my Father." (John 10:3-18)

Jesus love ♥ is eternal and nothing resemble it. God is Love ♥ and Live is God. Because of Jesus Love ♥, Man is no more stranger, He call men by name, they hear His voice and know His sheep, carved in Jesus Palm and no one could snatch him from His Hand set him free racing to holiness, righteousness, perfection and life eternal!

"In this was manifested the love of God toward us, because that God sent his only begotten Son into the world, that we might live through him.10 Herein is love, not that we loved God, but that he loved us, and sent his Son to be the propitiation for our sins.11 Beloved, if God so loved us, we ought also to love one another.12 No man hath seen God at any time. If we love one another, God dwelleth in us, and his love is perfected in us.13 Hereby know we that we dwell in him, and he in us, because he hath given us of his Spirit.14 And we have seen and do testify that the Father sent the Son to be the Saviour of the world.15 Whosoever shall confess that Jesus is the Son of God, God dwelleth in him, and he in God.16 And we have known and believed the love that God hath to us. God is love; and he that dwelleth in love dwelleth in God, and God in him.17 Herein is our love made perfect, that we may have boldness in the day of judgment: because as he is, so are we in this world." (1 John 4:9-17)

Jesus love 💜 reconciled the East with West and North with the South, the elect with the Gentiles an in Him mankind once again became one people as Jesus became the Second Adam!

Jesus love 💜 brought salvation to mankind and the earth, condemned darkness, brought the authorities of the world to sit in one table, globalized the world, unified the diversity and conquered the adversities, ceased the atrocities, stopped the bleeding, healed the wounds, defeated the divisions,

Jesus Love 💜 brought forgiveness to mankind, running waters to thirsty ground, bread to hunger, drink to the thirst, energy to the feeble and replaced hate with love 💜!

Jesus love 💜 replaced satanism with divinity, violence with peace, sadness with joy, death with resurrection, demotion with promotion, poverty with richness, sickness with wholeness, sins with righteousness, disobedience with obedience, darkness with light, hopeless with hope, helpless with help, loss with gain, baron with children, earth with heaven and damnation with kingdom!

Jesus love 💜 took human race from the lowly to the top, from the bottom pit to the glory, from earthly things to Spiritual things, from seen to unseen, from literal to Life, from an end to infinity, from turmoil to tranquility, from restless to deep sleep, from pains and agony to comfort, and from flooding and great waves to dry land, from drowning to shore, and from slavery to sonships and Fatherhood.

Jesus Love 💜 reconciled the educated with the illiterates, the teachers and the pupils, the children with the parents, the rich with the poor, the young with the old, the men with the women, and privileged with underprivileged!

Jesus love 💜 open the gates of heaven to all the children regardless, rescue those in trouble, refuge to the homeless, shield to the weak, mercy to the ruthless, and just to injustice. He is the King of Kings snd Lord of Lords!

Jesus love 💜 covered our sham, carried our transgression, dressed our nakedness, cleansed our dirt, and brought beauty to the human soul

Thanksgiving is all about Jesus Love 💜 in everyday of my life and always with the human soul:

The list of My Lord Jesus blessings is endless—-
While in the womb, Jesus Love 💜 breath unto my soul,
Throughout life, Jesus love gives love to my soul,
In adolescence, Jesus love 💜 matures my soul,
In days, months and years, Jesus Love 💜 gets stronger and roots deeper and deeper in my heart!
In the way, Jesus love 💜 gives wisdom to my soul,
While asleep, Jesus Love 💜 overshadow my soul,
While awake, Jesus love 💜 lead me to the green pasture,
In hunger, Jesus love 💜 feedth my soul,
In thirst, Jesus love 💜 gives drink to my soul,
In poverty, Jesus love 💜 enrich my soul,
In nakedness, Jesus love 💜 covers my soul,
In prison, Jesus Love 💜 visits my soul,
In pains, Jesus love 💜 comfort my soul,
In the freezing cold, Jesus Love 💜 warms my soul,
In the heat of the sun, Jesus love 💜 protects my soul,
In labor, Jesus love 💜 bless my soul,
In surgery, Jesus love 💜 guides my soul,
In darkness, Jesus love 💜 lightens my soul,
In tortuous road, Jesus Love 💜 carry my soul,
In tricks of Satan, Jesus love 💜 protects my soul
In wars, Jesus love 💜 rescue my soul,
In weary, Jesus love 💜 lifts my soul up,
In sorrowful, Jesus Love 💜 wipes my soul tears,
In persecution, Jesus love 💜 brings joy to my soul,
In loneliness, Jesus love 💜 accompany my soul,
In sickness, Jesus love 💜 heal my soul,
In departure, Jesus Love 💜 raises my soul up to Heaven,
In sin, Jesus love 💜 forgives my soul,
In death, Jesus love 💜 give life eternity to my soul,

O Lord Jesus, You are my Thanksgiving. To Thine I thank all the time. In the behalf of all Your creation I present You with this Poem of Thanks. Before all human race, I say Thank You

With Your son king David, I sing Psalm 138:
138 I give you thanks, O Lord, with my whole heart;
before the gods I sing your praise;
2 I bow down toward your holy temple
and give thanks to your name for your steadfast love and your faithfulness,

for you have exalted above all things
your name and your word.[a]
3 On the day I called, you answered me;
my strength of soul you increased.[b]
4 All the kings of the earth shall give you thanks, O Lord,
for they have heard the words of your mouth,
5 and they shall sing of the ways of the Lord,
for great is the glory of the Lord.
6 For though the Lord is high, he regards the lowly,
but the haughty he knows from afar.
7 Though I walk in the midst of trouble,
you preserve my life;
you stretch out your hand against the wrath of my enemies,
and your right hand delivers me.
8 The Lord will fulfill his purpose for me;
your steadfast love, O Lord, endures forever.
Do not forsake the work of your hands."
Jesus Love 🖤 is my Thanksgivings and my Thanksgiving is Jesus Love. 🖤

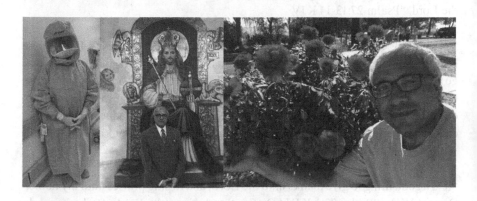

CG. Your writings always give us something to think about.. We should be
thankful for our blessings of the past year. They maybe many or few but
whatever they are we should still be thankful. Bless you! 🖤🙏

A Divine Message for Thanksgiving!

At 2020 Thanksgiving, Jesus our Lord is reaching out to each Human Soul saying:
"Wait on the Lord: be of good courage, and he shall strengthen thine heart: wait,
I say, on the Lord"

And in return, Each human soul shall lift up her heart to the Lord at Thanksgiving saying: "thou hast brought up my soul from the grave: thou hast kept me alive, that I should not go down to the pit"...

And each human soul shall say one more time: "Thou hast turned for me my mourning into dancing: thou hast put off my sackcloth, and girded me with gladness"

And every human soul shall say to the Lord Almighty: "To the end that my glory may sing praise to thee, and not be silent. O Lord my God, I will give thanks unto thee for ever"

And the entire world 🌍, At 2020 Thanksgiving, shall reply to the Lord in one voice saying: "It is a good thing to give thanks unto the Lord, and to sing praises unto thy name, O most High"

"-I had believed to see the goodness of the Lord in the land of the living. Wait on the Lord: be of good courage, and he shall strengthen thine heart: wait, I say, on the Lord. "Psalm 27:13-14 KJV

"O Lord my God, I cried unto thee, and thou hast healed me. [3] O Lord, thou hast brought up my soul from the grave: thou hast kept me alive, that I should not go down to the pit. [4] Sing unto the Lord, O ye saints of his, and give thanks at the remembrance of his holiness. [11] Thou hast turned for me my mourning into dancing: thou hast put off my sackcloth, and girded me with gladness; [12] To the end that my glory may sing praise to thee, and not be silent. O Lord my God, I will give thanks unto thee for ever. Psalm 30

"It is a good thing to give thanks unto the Lord, and to sing praises unto thy name, O most High: "Psalm 92:1 KJV "O give thanks unto the Lord ; for he is good: because his mercy endureth for ever." Psalm 118:1 KJV

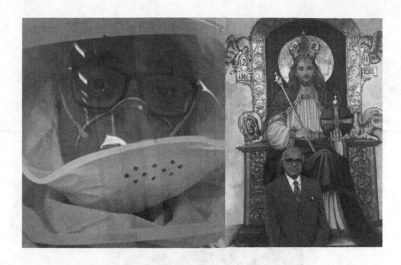

MR. our Lord Jesus Christ be with you always doctor.

Happy Valentine's Day 2021: Continue to Make a Difference! True love never be Conquered by Pandemics, Sickness and Death!

Written by Ramsis Ghaly

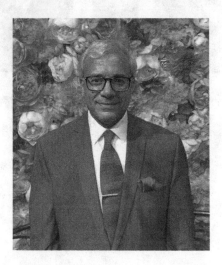

Do not let COVID pandemic and politics take the True Love 🖤 Of Valentine's away from our hearts!

In Valentine's Day commemorate those lives passed away, those in need and those in our homes, villages, schools and universities, communities, cities, states, countries, continents and all around the world!

In Valentine's Day is a day to show love 🖤, act of love 🖤, express love, spread love 🖤 and vow for more love 🖤 as we all together going through 2021!

Valentine's Day remind us with the True Love 🖤 always been Virtual and unseen!

Love 🖤 this year is more and more unconditional, non-physical but virtual!

True Love 🖤 is spiritual deep within and unseen untouched!

In Valentine's Day, let us fill the empty hearts 💜 with love and the losses with gains!

True Love does see boundaries travels thousands of miles away in the speed of the sonic wavelengths!

So what are we waiting for! Get up and write a message of Love 💜, dial the phone 📱 and utters words of love and send as much of genuine wireless Love hearts, pulses, thoughts and deeds of love!

True Love 💜 Is pure, precious and priceless!
True love 💜 never fails or be contained or obsessed!
True love 💜 never be unconquered by pandemics, sickness and death!

John 3:16 "For God so loved the world that He gave His only begotten Son, that whoever believes in Him should not perish but have everlasting life." John 15:12-13 "This is my commandment, That ye love one another, as I have loved you. [13] Greater love hath no man than this, that a man lay down his life for his friends."

My Love 💜 is but One! My Love 💜my Savior more than the love 💜 of love 💜

My Love 💜 Jesus is but One! My Love 💜 my Savior more than the love 💜 of love 💜: My Beloved is more than another beloved.

+++++
No matter how much you describe Love 💜, Love 💜 is still indescribable! No matter how much Love 💜 can be measured, love 💜 is still unmeasurable!

Love 💜 is not just a word but a Life!
Love 💜 is not just a kiss 💋 but a total embrace!
Love 💜 is not just a hug 🤗 but a heart 💜!
Love 💜 is not just a dance 💃 but doing!
Love 💜 is not just a song but a lifetime commitment!
Love 💜 is not just a gift 🎁 but a Holy Spirit!
Love 💜 is not just an experience but a sacrifice!
Love 💜 is not just a gratitude but infinite give!
Love 💜 is not just like but an absolute love!
Love 💜 is not just a moment but infinite!
Love 💜 is not a circumstance but unconditional!
Love 💜 is Eternity!
Love 💜 is God Kingdom!

Love 💜 is Life!
Love 💜 is Light!
Love 💜 is the Way!
Love 💜 is the Salvation!
Love 💜 is Destiny!
Love 💜 is the Purpose!
Love 💜 is Pure!
Love 💜 is Righteous!
Love 💜 is Unity!
Love 💜 is White like snow!
Love 💜 is the Jacob ladder between earth 🌍 and heaven!
Love 💜 is the Heart 💜💜💜 of all things!
Love 💜 is the Corner stone of all creation!
Love 💜 is the Root of all good gifts!
Love 💜 is what creation Live with!
Love 💜 is each Blood cell 🩸 running in every living soul and in each heartbeat!
Love 💜 is what every creature Breath and drink!
Love 💜 is what creation Embrace each other with!
Love 💜 is the Common Language of human race and heavenly hosts!
Love 💜 is what we live with, live for and keep us going!
Love 💜 is Sharing and what we leave behind!
Love 💜 is the Energy and the solar system!
Love 💜 is Joy, exaltation, Happiness and Secret behind laughs and smiles!
Love 💜 keep each living cell Alive!
Love 💜 is the Eye!
Love 💜 is the Center!
Love 💜 is the Engine!
Love 💜 is the Existence!
Love 💜 is the Nutrient in each living soul!
Love 💜 is Real!
Love 💜 is the Word of God and His creation made of Love 💜!

"Behold, the eye of the LORD is upon them that fear him, upon them that hope in his mercy;19 To deliver their soul from death, and to keep them alive in famine.20 Our soul waiteth for the LORD: he is our help and our shield.21 For our heart shall rejoice in him, because we have trusted in his holy name.22 Let thy mercy, O LORD, be upon us, according as we hope in thee." Psalm 33

+Love 💜 Valentine started when St Valentine 💜 gave his life for the Lord of Love Jesus in the fourth century and blessed his daughter with the pure love 💜!

294

+Love 🖤 is the Holy Trinity The Father, The Son and The Holy Spirit: Corinthians 13: 14, "The grace of the Lord Jesus Christ and the love 🖤 of God and the fellowship of the Holy Spirit be with you all."

+Love 🖤 is to love 🖤 and to love 🖤 is love 🖤 and it is all love 🖤 of love 🖤 and nothing but love 🖤!

+Divinity and humanity merged together through LOVE 🖤!

+Love 🖤 is —
Suffereth long
Sind
Envieth not
Vaunteth not itself
Not puffed up
Doth not behave itself unseemly
Seeketh not her own
Not easily provoked
Thinketh no evil
Rejoiceth not in iniquity
Rejoiceth in the truth
Beareth all things
Believeth all things
Hopeth all things
Endureth all things
"Love 🖤 never faileth:" (1 Corinthians 13:4-8)

+God himself described as all about love 🖤 God Holy Name is Love 🖤: (John 4:7-14) "Beloved, let us love one another: for love is of God; and every one that loveth is born of God, and knoweth God. 8He that loveth not knoweth not God; for God is love. 9In this was manifested the love of God toward us, because that God sent his only begotten Son into the world, that we might live through him. 10Herein is love, not that we loved God, but that he loved us, and sent his Son to be the propitiation for our sins. 11Beloved, if God so loved us, we ought also to love one another. 12No man hath seen God at any time. If we love one another, God dwelleth in us, and his love is perfected in us. 13Hereby know we that we dwell in him, and he in us, because he hath given us of his Spirit. 14And we have seen and do testify that the Father sent the Son to bethe Saviour of the world."

+LOVE 🖤 NEVER FAILETH: (1 Corinthians 13:4-8) "4Charity suffereth long, and is kind; charity envieth not; charity vaunteth not itself, is not puffed up, 5Doth not behave itself unseemly, seeketh not her own, is not easily provoked, thinketh no evil; 6Rejoiceth not in iniquity, but rejoiceth in the truth; 7Beareth all things, believeth all things, hopeth all things, endureth all things.8Charity never faileth:"

+LOVE IS THE GREATEST: (1 Corinthians 13:13) "13And now abideth faith, hope, charity, these three; but the greatest of these is charity."

++++
It is a life worth living! If you continue to make a difference! Please continue to make a difference!

It is the most Christian that human soul ever do! If you continue to make a difference! Please continue to make a difference!

It is the journey with Jesus cross to see God's Glory at the resurrection day! If you continue to make a difference! Please continue to make a difference!

It is a Nobel gain for the soul! If you continue to make a difference! Please continue to make a difference!

It is a true love to mankind! If you continue to make a difference! Please continue to make a difference!

It is the ultimate Love for God! If you continue to make a difference! Please continue to make a difference!

It is the living for one another and unconditional love one to another! If you continue to make a difference! Please continue to make a difference!

It is a service to the homeland and to mankind! If you continue to make a difference! Please continue to make a difference!

It is waters for the thirst and dry land! If you continue to make a difference! Please continue to make a difference!

It is nutrients for the weak! If you continue to make a difference! Please continue to make a difference!

It is a remedy for incapable! If you continue to make a difference! Please continue to make a difference!

It is a blossom flower in the field! If you continue to make a difference! Please continue to make a difference!

It is the hearted joy in utmost purity! If you continue to make a difference! Please continue to make a difference!

It is the sacrifice offering before the Lord! If you continue to make a difference! Please continue to make a difference!

It is the renewal of oil to lighten the lamp for others! If you continue to make a difference! Please continue to make a difference!

It is the reason for heaven to open its gates! If you continue to make a difference! Please continue to make a difference!

It is a divine purpose for the heart to beat to the last heartbeat! If you continue to make a difference! Please continue to make a difference!

It is a holy cause for the soul to breath to the last breath! If you continue to make a difference! Please continue to make a difference!

It is the morning star ⭐ to guide the new day! If you continue to make a difference! Please continue to make a difference!

It is a peace to the soul to sleep at the end of the day! If you continue to make a difference! Please continue to make a difference!

It is the being for sojourning from day to day until the end! If you continue to make a difference! Please continue to make a difference!

It is part of godly reaching out to humanity! If you continue to make a difference! Please continue to make a difference!

It is stocks added to the heavenly treasures! If you continue to make a difference! Please continue to make a difference!

It brings back hundred folds of infinite blessing! If you continue to make a difference! Please continue to make a difference!

It lives forever and carries on across generations! If you continue to make a difference! Please continue to make a difference!

It is a legacy left behind in multitudes! If you continue to make a difference! Please continue to make a difference!

It is forever a credit that never die! If you continue to make a difference! Please continue to make a difference!

It is savings that never age, never get old and never fails! If you continue to make a difference! Please continue to make a difference!

It is a duty to the fellowmen and fellow women! If you continue to make a difference! Please continue to make a difference!

It is the rescue card in the time of need! If you continue to make a difference! Please continue to make a difference!

It is considered high class and scholar greatness! If you continue to make a difference! Please continue to make a difference!

It is the absolute unselfishness of the human being! If you continue to make a difference! Please continue to make a difference!

It is the key to earn points to enter unto His kingdom! If you continue to make a difference! Please continue to make a difference!

It is written in the Book of Life! If you continue to make a difference! Please continue to make a difference!

If you continue to make a difference! It is a life worth living!

💜 Happy Valentine's Day 2021 💜: Continue to Make a Difference 💜!
💜 Happy Valentine's Day 2021 💜: Continue to Make a Difference 💜! True love 💜 never be Conquered by Pandemics, Sickness and Death!

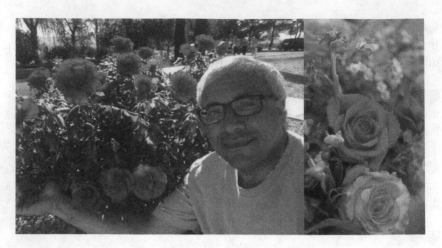

JM. Beautiful

DM. God endless love

GP. Doctor, I'm asking for a prayer request this am at 11:30. My daughter has placenta previa and seeing it's her 3rd bleed, the doctors decided a c-section at 34 weeks would be best. I am asking all my prayer warriors to hold her, the doctors and the nurses up to God for a safe and healthy delivery of my tiny grandson. God knows my heart and the love I have for Him. Thank you in advance for praying for my baby and her baby.

CB. thank you for prayers. He was born at 11:30, 5 lbs 1oz, 18 in. He is perfect. God is good .....always 🙏

RC. Happy valentine day, spreding and sending massages of love! Beutiful photos!

CB. Happy face with a happy heart. God bless Dr. Gahly.

JM. AGREE Keep The Love Always 🖤

BD. Happy valentines!!

KN. YOU are truly such a

Feb 13, 2021

No other place to spend my Valentine's Day but with my patients and Residents in duty and on call to help, save and heal! It us my honor and privilege to serve the on call residents with free hot meal 🍽 during the call.

Happy Valentine's Day
Ramsis Ghaly

300

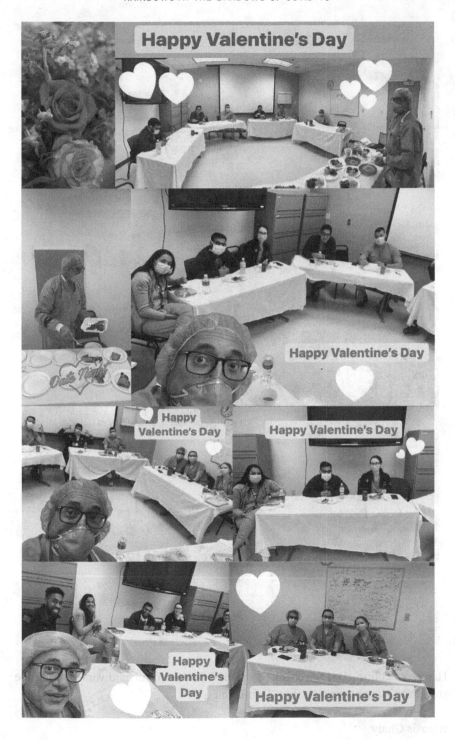

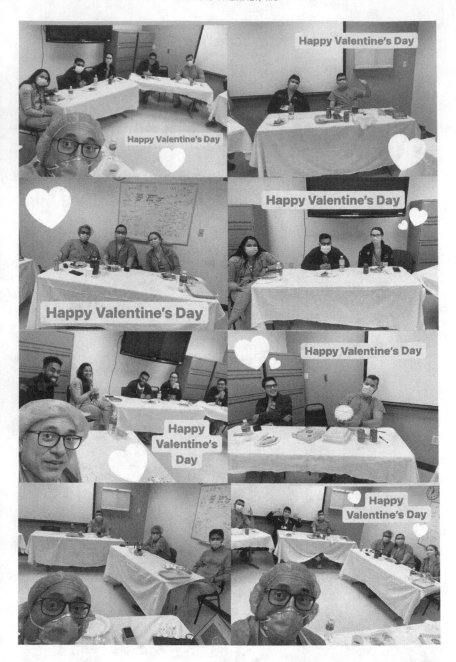

Happy Valentine's Day to you all. Snapchat with the on call hardworking frontline staff. You all are our valentines. Thank you 🙏

Ramsis Ghaly

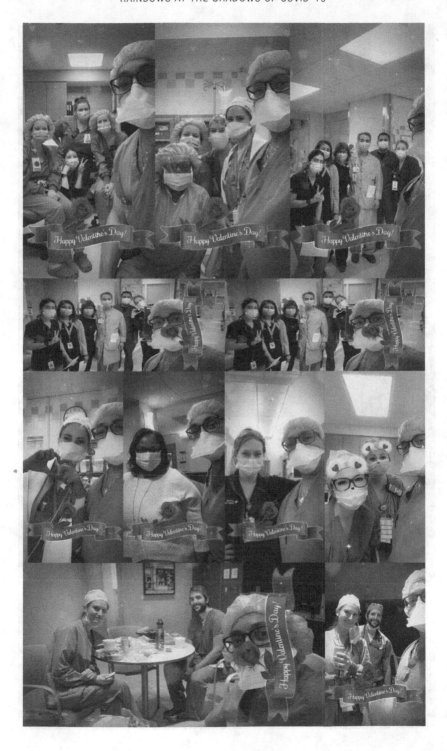

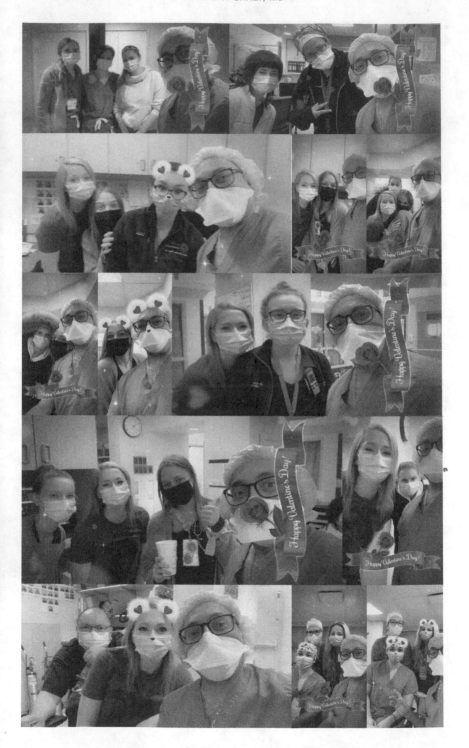

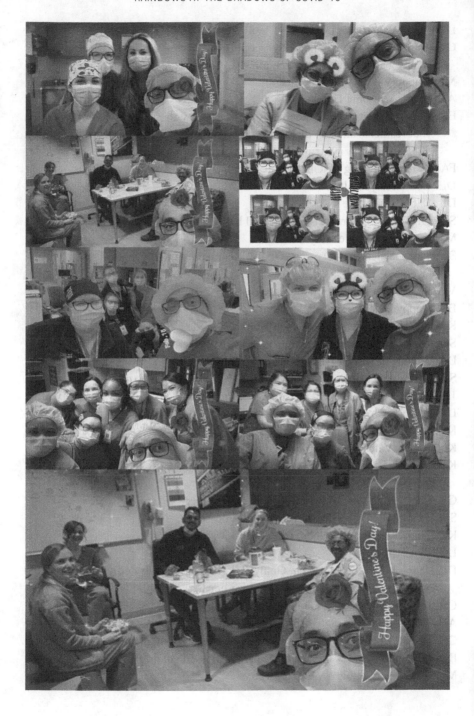

ID. Happy Valentine's Day Ghaly! You're a true saint! 🖤🖤🖤

CG. Happy you're surrounded by people who care for you and you for them. Happy Valentines' Day to you all! 😊

MS. Happy Valentine's day Dr.G

AU. That's awesome Dr.Ghaly 👏

ED. Happy Valentines Day good Doctor. How very thoughtful of you to be with your residents and buy them a free dinner. God Bless You Doctor. Thank you for sharing your amazing life with us 🙏🙏

FA. You are amazing Dr Ghaly .. the doctor with a heart of 🖤

DL. God bless you all.

DL. Happy Valentine's Day.

SM. Dr Ghaly, you are so awesome and beyond amazing!

MH. Happy Valentines Day Dr.

SJ. Happy Valentines Day Dr. Ghaly, Residents, and patients. I wish you all love 🖤

VG. Srecan dan zaljubljenih doktore!!!

BK. Happy Valentine's Day, Dr Ghaly!!

KM. 💕 Happy Valentine's Day 💕

SK. This is so amazing! You are a wonderful person and Dr!

DA. So nice of you Dr! Happy Valentine's Day! 💕

SK. Happy Valentines Day Doctor Ghaly 💕💕

JP. Happy Valentines Day Doctor. When I grow up, I want to be just like you.

LT. God bless you always

KE. Sending love 🖤

KG. Happy Valentines Day Dr Ghaly! Sending lots of love 🖤

KE. Love this 🖤 Happy Valentine's Day Dr. Ghaly. Continue doing ur amazing work

GS. Happy Valentines day Many blessings brother

SS. Happy Valentine's day to you and all your crew

KC. Thank you for all you do, Dr. Ghaly 🖤

LG. I love this 🖤

DP. Happy Valentine's Day, Dr. Ghaly. Thank you for your dedication today and every day! The world is a better place because of you!!!

CB. Happy Valentine Dr. Ghaly!

AB. 🖤🖤🖤🖤 Stay Safe, Brother!

CE. Happy Valentine's Day to a wonderful man and doctor! 💕

DM. The man with the biggest heart happy blessed valentine

MCP. Best. Attending. EVER!!!!!! 😺

I A ou guys look great! Happy Valentine's Day to you all from Egypt and Thank you for the work you do in the Covid battle and health care for all. God Bless you all!

Kc. Happy Valentines Day Dr. Ghaly!

Happy Valentine's Day to the broken-hearted

In Valentine's Day we can't forget those with broken-hearted: much love 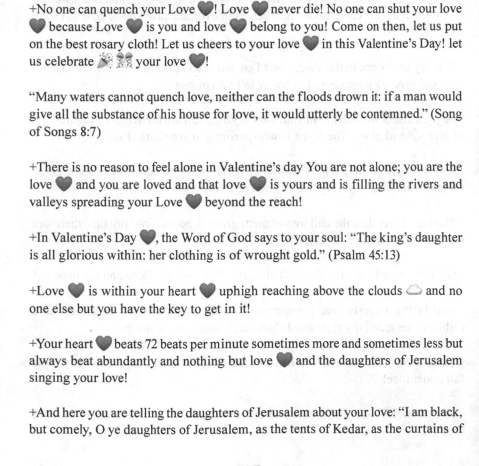 to you!

+In Valentine's Day 🖤, Indeed, Love 🖤 is within you and you are loved. You are full of love 🖤! Your candle standing and lightens 🕯 the entire universe and with your life around you is full of grace!

+No one can quench your Love 🖤! Love 🖤 never die! No one can shut your love 🖤 because Love 🖤 is you and love 🖤 belong to you! Come on then, let us put on the best rosary cloth! Let us cheers to your love 🖤 in this Valentine's Day! let us celebrate 🎉 🎊 your love 🖤!

"Many waters cannot quench love, neither can the floods drown it: if a man would give all the substance of his house for love, it would utterly be contemned." (Song of Songs 8:7)

+There is no reason to feel alone in Valentine's day You are not alone; you are the love 🖤 and you are loved and that love 🖤 is yours and is filling the rivers and valleys spreading your Love 🖤 beyond the reach!

+In Valentine's Day 🖤, the Word of God says to your soul: "The king's daughter is all glorious within: her clothing is of wrought gold." (Psalm 45:13)

+Love 🖤 is within your heart 🖤 uphigh reaching above the clouds ☁ and no one else but you have the key to get in it!

+Your heart 🖤 beats 72 beats per minute sometimes more and sometimes less but always beat abundantly and nothing but love 🖤 and the daughters of Jerusalem singing your love!

+And here you are telling the daughters of Jerusalem about your love: "I am black, but comely, O ye daughters of Jerusalem, as the tents of Kedar, as the curtains of

Solomon.6 Look not upon me, because I am black, because the sun hath looked upon me: my mother's children were angry with me; they made me the keeper of the vineyards; but mine own vineyard have I not kept.7 Tell me, O thou whom my soul loveth, where thou feedest, where thou makest thy flock to rest at noon: for why should I be as one that turneth aside by the flocks of thy companions?" (Song of Songs 1:5-7)

+Within your heart ♥ is two small rooms and one Master room and one living room. Your love ♥ is always circulating nonstop through these chambers connecting them valves open and close upon your demand pumping Love ♥ throughout your blood stream back and forth day and night 24/7 360 with immeasurable love ♥. This is who you are full of love ♥ and your love ♥ never stop filling many hearts ♥ and many more spreading to whoever comes close to you. Bless you more and more in Valentine's Day!

+Your vineyard, which is yours, is before you; thou, O Solomon, must have a thousand, and those that keep the fruit thereof two hundred. Thou that dwellest in the gardens, the companions hearken to thy voice: cause you to hear it. (Song of Songs 8:12-13)

+St Mary was alone in the Valentine's Day while sojourning with you and me but her Son' love ♥ have never left her or left you or me!

The psalmist is whispering in your ears saying: You are the King's daughter full of love ♥ and glory: The Spirit is whispering g in your ears (Psalm 45)

+Your heart is inditing a good matter: I speak of the things which I have made touching the king: my tongue is the pen of a ready writer!

+Thou art fairer than the children of men: grace is poured into thy lips: therefore God hath blessed thee for ever!

+Gird thy sword upon thy thigh, O most mighty, with thy glory and thy majesty!

+And in thy majesty ride prosperously because of truth and meekness and righteousness; and thy right hand shall teach thee terrible things!

+Thine arrows are sharp in the heart of the king's enemies; whereby the people fall under thee!

+Thy throne, O God, is for ever and ever: the sceptre of thy kingdom is a right sceptre!

+Thou lovest righteousness, and hatest wickedness: therefore God, thy God, hath anointed thee with the oil of gladness above thy fellows!

+All thy garments smell of myrrh, and aloes, and cassia, out of the ivory palaces, whereby they have made thee glad!

+You are the Kings' daughters and were among thy honourable women: upon thy right hand did stand the queen in gold of Ophir!

+Hearken, O daughter, and consider, and incline thine ear; forget also thine own people, and thy father's house!

+So shall the king greatly desire thy beauty: for he is thy Lord; and worship thou him!

+And the daughter of Tyre shall be there with a gift; even the rich among the people shall intreat thy favour!

+The king's daughter is all glorious within: her clothing is of wrought gold!

+You shall be brought unto the king in raiment of needlework: the virgins her companions that follow her shall be brought unto thee!

+With gladness and rejoicing shall they be brought: they shall enter into the king's palace!

+Instead of thy fathers shall be thy children, whom thou mayest make princes in all the earth!

+I will make thy name to be remembered in all generations: therefore shall the people praise thee for ever and ever! Psalm 45

Psalm 96
"1 O sing unto the LORD a new song: sing unto the LORD, all the earth.2 Sing unto the LORD, bless his name; shew forth his salvation from day to day.3 Declare his glory among the heathen, his wonders among all people.4 For the LORD is great, and greatly to be praised: he is to be feared above all gods.5 For all the gods of the nations are idols: but the LORD made the heavens.6 Honour and majesty are before him: strength and beauty are in his sanctuary.7 Give unto the LORD, O ye kindreds of the people, give unto the LORD glory and strength.8 Give unto the LORD the glory due unto his name: bring an offering, and come into his courts.9 O worship the LORD in the beauty of holiness: fear before him, all the

earth.10 Say among the heathen that the LORD reigneth: the world also shall be established that it shall not be moved: he shall judge the people righteously.11 Let the heavens rejoice, and let the earth be glad; let the sea roar, and the fulness thereof.12 Let the field be joyful, and all that is therein: then shall all the trees of the wood rejoice13 Before the LORD: for he cometh, for he cometh to judge the earth: he shall judge the world with righteousness, and the people with his truth."

In Valentine's Day 💜, Indeed, Love 💜 is within you and you are loved. You are full of love 💜! Your candle standing and lightens 💡 the entire universe and with your life around you is full of grace!

love
Ramsis Ghaly

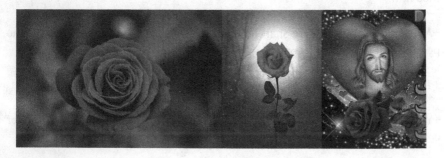

CG. This is LOVEly. This is true today and always will be. Bless you! 🙏💜
SB. Dr Ghaly

Thank you for all you do and your beautiful posts! I've been following you for a while and I'm so impressed that a doctor takes the time to reach out to people on social media! I can't wait to meet you as I have Chiari Malformation & a messed up neck! CCI, DDD, Cervical bone spurs and possible syrinx! Once this snow and cold settle down, I'll be making an appointment!

Thank you for all you do!
God Bless you

Early Happy Valentine Day During COVID 2/1/2021

Early Happy Valentine's Day with our On Call Residents wearing Face masks 😷! Our Residents and medical profession during COVID-19 is about Love, sacrifice and heroism! Thank you. 🙏

Ramsis Ghaly

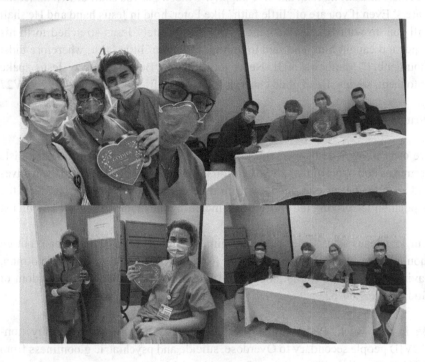

JG. God Bless you all! 🙏❤️

RH. You are all appreciated, prayed for and loved. Thank you

CG. Thank you all and may God Bless you all! ❤️🙏

FA. God bless you and your team Dr. Ghaly! 🖤

DM. happy hearts day doctors

MH. Happy Early Valentines Day! Too all of you who worked so hard to make us all well.

CCC. Spreading the word and the love...

ML. Good deal 🌷😄

Please do your part! Please spread Love 🖤, Hope, Reassurance and Peace all over and check in your neighbors and reach out to the despairs and all those in need! Please don't let them take their own lives because of daily gloomy news affecting only 0.03% of population. We all have legal responsibility to rescue them since the society is becoming insensitive and wrongful!!! Let us vow we still have each other even if all the governments failed their people! The world is still a great peaceful and prosperous healthy place to live and multiply and be fruitful!

Be smart and strong faith and live happily. Otherwise, you shall drown under the waters! Even if you are of "little faith" like Peter, hold in Jesus hand and He shall pull you up with His Divine hand: "And immediately Jesus stretched forth his hand, and caught him, and said unto him, O thou of little faith, wherefore didst thou doubt?" Matthews 14:31. Never loose hope: "But straightway Jesus spake unto them, saying, Be of good cheer; it is I; be not afraid." Matthew 14:27 KJV27

Written by Ramsis Ghaly

We can't allow it to happen and take our lives away because of the capitalists around us and opportunistic!!! So heartbreaking a family of four killed themselves and are gone because of the daily grim fake news addressing only 0,03% of the population terrorizing the entire world including the majority healthy among us!

Our lord Jesus said: "Jesus said unto him, Let the dead bury their dead: but go thou and preach the kingdom of God. [62] And Jesus said unto him, No man, having put his hand to the plough, and looking back, is fit for the kingdom of God." Luke 9:60-62

Be in the watch, PREVENTABLE deaths are sweeping into healthy non-COVID people secondary to Overdose, suicide and psychiatric gloominess from COVID-19 daily news, social curfew and hardships!!!

The world is still a great peaceful and prosperous healthy place to live and multiply and be fruitful! Please spread love 🖤 and hope and peace all over and check in your neighbors and reach out to the despairs!!!

Please don't let the opportunistic capitalists self-conflicted egocentric make you desperate and convince you to take away your life and your loved ones!

Please don't let these rumors enter your home or your household! Please don't listen to inhuman evilness of media and darkness of daily news sweep in the life of the 99.97% of the people! Always remember, the world is still a great peaceful and prosperous healthy place to live and multiply and be fruitful

Please be in peace, thankful in good cheer and strong faith in true Love 💜 one to another!

Why those are looking at the little sip at the bottom of a cup ignoring the entire cup full of honey and passion fruit!!

Let us be thankful to our Lord for the 99.97% living of all people! Our Savior is in control Colossians 3:15-17 KJV 15] And let the peace of God rule in your hearts, to the which also ye are called in one body; and be ye thankful. [16] Let the word of Christ dwell in you richly in all wisdom; teaching and admonishing one another in psalms and hymns and spiritual songs, singing with grace in your hearts to the Lord. [17] And whatsoever ye do in word or deed, do all in the name of the Lord Jesus, giving thanks to God and the Father by him. Psalm 107:1,8-9 KJV 1] O give thanks unto the Lord, for he is good: for his mercy endureth for ever. [8] Oh that men would praise the Lord for his goodness, and for his wonderful works to the children of men! [9] For he satisfieth the longing soul, and filleth the hungry soul with goodness.

Let us praise our Savior for His abundance of grace and plentiful of blessing worldwide saving 99.97% of all people! Jesus is in Control: Psalm 150:1-6 KJV 1] Praise ye the Lord. Praise God in his sanctuary: praise him in the firmament of his power. [2] Praise him for his mighty acts: praise him according to his excellent greatness. [3] Praise him with the sound of the trumpet: praise him with the psaltery and harp. [4] Praise him with the timbrel and dance: praise him with stringed instruments and organs. [5] Praise him upon the loud cymbals: praise him upon the high sounding cymbals. [6] Let every thing that hath breath praise the Lord. Praise ye the Lord.

I thought I may be missing something as I went through facts and statistics!!! I looked from my windows may be the cause of ongoing emergency 🔥 are the falling billions of rockets and explosive bombs bombarding every corner upon the face of earth but I couldn't see any!! I searched more and more and I continue to see God Grace and blessing in abundance! I thought may be Ramsis and Moses time came back with the pestilences! But o my gosh nothing like those days!!!

The world 🌍 is still a good healthy and safe place to live! God is still with us shining the sun w at day time and the moon 🌑 at nighttime, the millions of stars ⭐ covering the sky 🌑, the fresh air flowing around the planet 🌍, the ground

313

is giving plentiful of grass trees 🌱🌲 and fruits 🥭🍎🍏, the creeping animals in the fields, the birds 🦅 and towels are flying high and the whales 🐋 and fish 🐟🐠 are filling the seas and oceans and the waters erupting in the wills for the billions and billions of the living to drink!!! What is wrong of this world! God is in control and why call it crises when there isn't one since our Heavenly Father is alive and working!! Let us be thankful and give thanksgiving and joyful in the Lord!

Let us follow Jesus and let the dead bury their dead as it is written: "And he said unto another, Follow me. But he said, Lord, suffer me first to go and bury my father. [60] Jesus said unto him, Let the dead bury their dead: but go thou and preach the kingdom of God. [61] And another also said, Lord, I will follow thee; but let me first go bid them farewell, which are at home at my house. [62] And Jesus said unto him, No man, having put his hand to the plough, and looking back, is fit for the kingdom of God." Luke 9:59-62 KJV

Our Lord is with us who can be against us! COVID and rumors of pandemics and fears and terrors of pestilences shall never take over our lives and take our hears away from the love and prosperity of living day and night with our living Savior forever and ever more as it is written: "What shall we then say to these things? If God be for us, who can be against us? [32] He that spared not his own Son, but delivered him up for us all, how shall he not with him also freely give us all things? [35] Who shall separate us from the love of Christ? shall tribulation, or distress, or persecution, or famine, or nakedness, or peril, or sword? [36] As it is written, For thy sake we are killed all the day long; we are accounted as sheep for the slaughter. [37] Nay, in all these things we are more than conquerors through him that loved us. [38] For I am persuaded, that neither death, nor life, nor angels, nor principalities, nor powers, nor things present, nor things to come, [39] Nor height, nor depth, nor any other creature, shall be able to separate us from the love of God, which is in Christ Jesus our Lord." Romans 8:31-32,35-39 KJV

Be in good comfort knowing billions of people are healthy living and not touched by so called COVID!

Be of good cheer, the world 🌍 is our Savior land and a beautiful place to live! Don't live in fear! Don't let the days go by in hide: "Be strong and of a good courage, fear not, nor be afraid of them: for the Lord thy God, he it is that doth go with thee; he will not fail thee, nor forsake thee." Deuteronomy 31:6 KJV

"Cast your burden on the Lord, and He shall sustain you; He shall never permit the righteous to be moved" (Psalms 55:22)

Be in peace and give thanksgiving to the Lord in Jesus name! He is alive and our Savior and our Father! "Peace I leave with you, my peace I give unto you: not as the world giveth, give I unto you. Let not your heart be troubled, neither let it be afraid." John 14:27

Numbers 6:24-26 NKJV "The LORD bless you and keep you; The LORD make His face shine upon you, And be gracious to you; The LORD lift up His countenance upon you, And give you peace."

Emergency 🚨 and isn't Emergency! The world 🌍 is still a good healthy and safe place to live and God in Control!

Written by Ramsis Ghaly

"Be anxious for nothing, but in everything by prayer and supplication, with (B) thanksgiving, let your requests be made known to God; 7 and (C)the peace of God, which surpasses all understanding, will guard your hearts and minds through Christ Jesus." Philippians 4:6-8

https://apple.news/APVIu00ndQdGCzrX6ydffpA
https://www.cdc.gov/.../p1218-overdose-deaths-covid-19.html
https://www.centerpointehospital.com/u-s-life-expectancy.../

Please spread love and hope and peace all over and check in your neighbors and reach out to the despairs!!! The world is still a great peaceful and prosperous healthy place to live and multiply and be fruitful!

Please do your part! Please spread Love 💜, Hope, Reassurance and Peace all over and check in your neighbors and reach out to the despairs and all those in need! Please don't let them take their own lives because of daily gloomy news affecting only 0.03% of population. We all have legal responsibility to rescue them since the society is becoming insensitive and wrongful!!!

Be smart and strong faith and live otherwise you shall drown under the waters! Even if you of little faith hold in Jesus hand and He shall pull you up with His Divine hand: "And immediately Jesus stretched forth his hand, and caught him, and said unto him, O thou of little faith, wherefore didst thou doubt?" Matthews 14:31. Never lose hope: "But straightway Jesus spoke unto them, saying, Be of good cheer; it is I; be not afraid." Matthew 14:27 KJV27

Let us vow we still have each other even if all the governments failed their people! We can't allow ourselves and Neighbors to take their lives because of the acts of the evilness around us! Lord Jesus and the Savior of the World is in control!

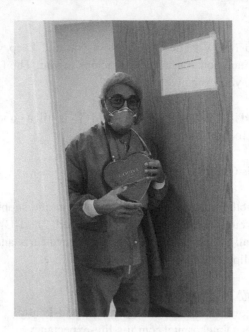

KO. Beautiful heart felt prayer, Dr Ghaly, may God bless you always Ps love is sharing those Godiva chocolates. 😄

CC. Nice Dr Ghaly truth and good advice!

MB. God bless and protect you Doctor. 🙏🤍🤍

SJ. I always knew your heart was big and sweet

LR. Great advise! I saved your post to read over and over. Definitely it lifted my spirit in this crazy world! 🙏😊

MS. Where is my box of chocolates. 😊

AB. Amen! Praise God! Thank you for your encouraging words!

CG. You are so caring and yes we must have faith in God and humanity. Let's us pray that we recognize when our neighbor, friend, or family member is depressed and needs help. May God continue to protect you. 🖤🙏

America the Country We Love!

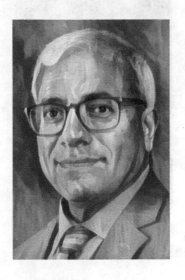

America 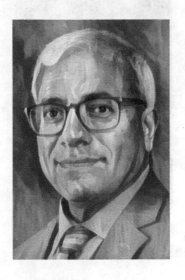 the Country we Love 💜!
America 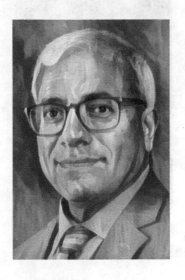 the Country we Proud!
America 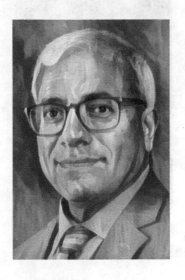 the Country we Care 💜!
America 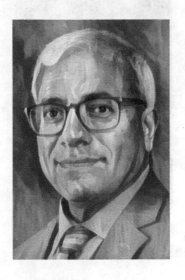 the Country worth Fighting for!
America 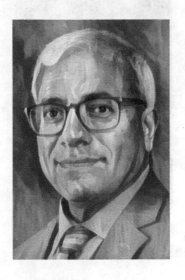 the Country we Pray for!
America 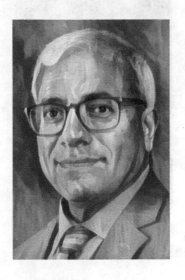 the Country we Die for!
America 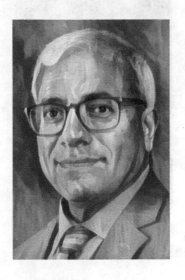 the Country we Defend!
America 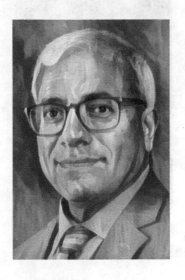 the Country we Lay our lives for!
America 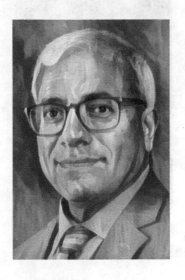 the Country we Respect most!
America 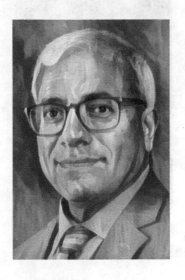 the Country we Give abundantly!
America 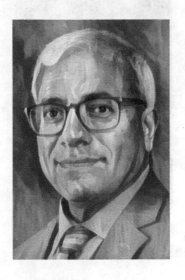 the Country we Suffer for!
America 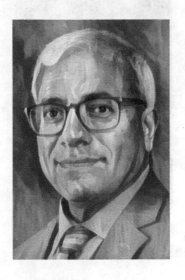 the Country we Sacrifice for!
America 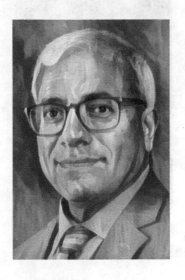 the Country we Race for!
America 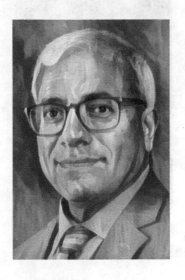 the Country we Add more!
America 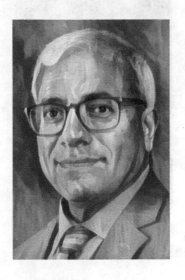 the Country we Sing for!
America 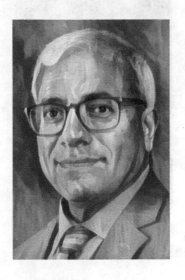 the country we Believe in!
America 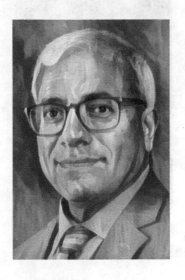 the Country our Home!
America 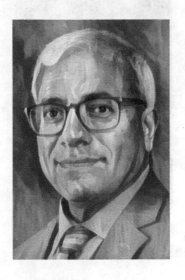 the Country our Refuge!
America 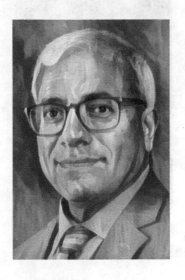 the Country our Future!

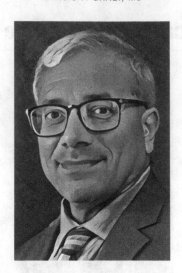

AS. God bless America
CG. Bless our country 🇺🇸
BS. 🤍🤍🤍🙏🇺🇸
TM/ Beautiful 🤍
JC. Awesome! 🇺🇸

In COVID 19 To Whom Shall my Little Soul Go to But You My Lord?

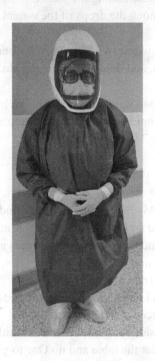

During the threats of second and third and fourth waves of COVID-19, and resistant strains with so much confusion, uprise and unrest demonstrations and unsettling election, I reflect on the Biblical Verse spoken by Peter Simon: "Then said Jesus unto the twelve, Will ye also go away? [68] Then Simon Peter answered him, Lord, to whom shall we go? thou hast the words of eternal life. [69] And we believe and are sure that thou art that Christ, the Son of the living God." John 6:67-69 KJV And Dedicated to Psalm 22

My Little Soul is So Little:

I am dust and Whom shall form my being but the Lord God!

I am nothing and Whom shall create my soul out of nothing but You the Creator of the universe!

My little soul is tiny and foreign and Whom shall make her a child but You our Heavenly Father the loving of mankind!

My little soul visited the holy mountains of the Lord, I found myself the little and the least!

My little soul is unaccountable among the sands
My little soul is so little among the drops of the waters by the seas!

Among the giants, I am the worm swirling over the stones! "But I am a worm, and no man; a reproach of men, and despised of the people." Psalm 22:6 KJV

My little soul just a smoke in nose sinned of all! "Which say, Stand by thyself, come not near to me; for I am holier than thou. These are a smoke in my nose, a fire that burneth all the day." Isaiah 65:5 KJV

Among the warriors, I was the weakest in the scale!

My little soul is voiceless! My little soul is weeping and no one to wipe her tears!
My little soul is hungry and no One with heavenly Manna!
My little soul is thirst and no One with Living waters around!
My little soul is naked and no One to cover her!
My little soul is striving no one to reach out!
My little soul is bruised and no one to soak her wounds!
My little soul is a bruised reed and no one to support!
My little soul standing outside and no One to let her in!
My little soul is sitting under the table and no One to give her food!
My little soul is in the dungeon pit and no One to raise her up to sit in the King's table!
My little soul is reproached and despised and One to go to!
My little soul is persecuted day and night and no One to deliver her!
My little soul is in the prison and One to visit!
My little soul is all alone and One to accompany her!
My little soul withered away and no One to nourish her!
My little soul is dry and no One to tender her!
My little soul is illiterate and no One to educate her!
My little soul is ignorant and One to teach her!
My little soul is indolent and One energize her!
My little soul is aging and no One to rejuvenate her!
My little soul is by dry ground and One to move her to a good ground!
My little soul is of no foundation and no One to be her rock!
My little soul is a small branch and no One to re-attach her to the Vine!
My little soul is an orphan and no One to adopt her!
My little soul is lost and no One to find her!
My little soul went astray and no One to bring her home!

My little soul is facing the great waves and no One to bring her to the shore!
My little soul is a smoking flax about to quench and no one to rescue her!
My little soul is defeated and no Conquer to defend!
My little soul is sick and no One to heal her!
My little soul is foolish and One to make wise!
My little soul is poor and no One to make her rich!
My little soul is drowning and no One is rescuing her!
My little soul is broken and no One to treat her!
My little soul is in the midst of darkness and no One to bring her to light!
My little soul is dying and no One to give her life!
My little soul is buried in sins and One forgive her sins!
My little soul is deemed to die and no One to save her!
My little soul is sinned much and no One to pay her dues!
My little soul condemned to die forever and One to die for her!
My little soul is thrown unto eternal damnation and hell and no One redeem her!

"Behold my servant, whom I have chosen; my beloved, in whom my soul is well pleased: I will put my spirit upon him, and he shall shew judgment to the Gentiles. [19] He shall not strive, nor cry; neither shall any man hear his voice in the streets. [20] A bruised reed shall he not break, and smoking flax shall he not quench, till he send forth judgment unto victory." Matthew 12:18-20 KJV

I looked up to heaven and cried: "O Lord I failed by all the measures and I have no legs to stand on, or mouth to speak, or eyes to sea or ears to hear or knees to kneel or belly to swallow or tongue to praise"

To Whom Shall my Little Soul Go to But You My Lord?

To Whom shall my little soul go to lift my soul up but You O Lord Jesus?
To Whom shall my little soul seek to rescue me but You my Lord God?
To Whom Shall my little soul journey to but You my Creator?
To Whom shall my little soul confess to but You O God of forgiveness?
To Whom shall my little soul follow but You my Master?
To Whom shall my little soul walk to but You the Living Tree!
To Whom shall my little soul wander but with You the Good Shephard?
To Whom shall my little soul take the race but You Lord of Glory?
To Whom shall my little soul dine with but with You at the Heavenly Dining Table!?
To Whom shall my little soul speak to but You my Divine Sacred Heart?
To Whom shall my little soul listen to but You my Master?
To Whom shall my little soul open the eyes to but to King of Kings Eternal God Creator of all things seen and unseen?

To Whom shall my little soul touch but You the Lord of Miracles?
To Whom shall my little soul stand before but You my Most High?
To Whom shall my little soul kneel before but You God the Lord?
To Whom shall my little soul worship but You God of Israeli Heaven and earth kneel before You?

To Whom shall my little soul praise to but Lord Lord Lord of Glory?
To Whom my little soul shall be proud but You Awesome God full of wonders the Wonderful God!

To Whom shall my little soul pray to hear the cries of my soul but to You Lord of Lords?

To Whom shall my little soul fast to but You Lord of the Lent forty days and forty nights?

To Whom shall my little soul cry to but to You God of Mercy?
To Whom my soul shall seek for strength but You King of Kings?
To Whom my soul little shall be healed but You the True Healer?

To Whom shall my little soul put her burden but You God Lord the loving of mankind!
To Whom shall my little soul put her worries but You Lord God of compassion and long-suffering full of kindness!

To Whom shall my little soul receive the Blessing but You O Lord Full of Heavenly Blessing?

To Whom shall my little soul received the Grace but You O God full of Grace?
To Whom shall my little helpless soul seek help but You my Lord and Savior?

To Whom shall my little hopeless soul seek hope but God the Lord of Heaven and Earth?

To Whom shall my little soul receive the Impossible but You God of Impossible?
To Whom shall my little soul attend to be rich but You Lord of richness!
To Whom shall my little soul receive wisdom but You Lord of wisdom!
To Whom shall my little soul look for to receive wholeness but You the Most Wholly?

To Whom shall my little soul shall receive holiness but You Lord of Holiness?

To Whom shall my little soul be sanctified but with Jesus Bloodshed in the cross!
To Whom shall my little soul be cleansed but with Your Living Spirit and waters!
To Whom shall my little soul shall die for but for thy Name Jesus Christ?

To Whom shall my little soul shall Eat the Holy Body and drink the Holy Blood
of the New Testament but You God Lord of my Salvation?

To Whom shall my little soul shall be Baptized by Your Waters O the Living
Waters and the Fountains of Spring Valley?

To Whom shall my little soul be listed under to enter to thy Kingdom but thy Holy
Name, the Holy Lamb of God?

To Whom my little soul shall get strength to climb up high to the pinnacle of the
Olive Tree to sit by You but You Master of the Aptitudes?

To Whom shall my little soul seek in the mountain of temptation with Satan but
Jesus the Nazarene?

To whom shall my little teared soul follow to the garden of Gethsemane to shed
tears as drops of blood but with You Jesus Christ the Son of Man that carried my
sins to redeem my soul?

To Whom my little soul shall follow to be tried by the aggressor at the Great Hall
but with You Lord of Righteousness and Just?

To Whom my little soul shall go to from the darkness of the World but You the
True Light?

To Whom shall my little soul seek away from the afflictions and the persecution
but You the Lord of Just!

To Whom shall my soul escape to from the sword of my enemy but You the Armor
Shield of Salvation!

To Whom shall my little soul carry my cross but You Jesus the Incarnated God
in the Flesh?

To Whom my little soul shall be hanged upon a stick of wood in the Golgotha but
with You Jesus my Savior in the Cross?

To Whom shall my little soul give up the ghost but in thy Hands my Savior?
To Whom shall I bury my little flesh but with You the garden of a new sepulcher
with you my Savior, my Glory and my Majesty?

To Whom shall my little soul be comforted in the True Loving Bosom but in You
my Heavenly Father?

To Whom shall my little soul be waiting in the middle of the night at the eleventh
hour at midnight but You my Holy Bridegroom?

To Whom shall my little soul be living but You Lord of Resurrection?
To Whom my forehead name be other than You by the Blood of Jesus Christ the
Messiah and the Savior of the world?

To Whom shall I seek to write the name of my little soul other than You Eternal
God the Lord of the Book of Life?

To Whom shall I seek to enter through the gates of Heavens other than You God
of Heavens the Owner, the Creator and Keeper of all the souls?

To Whom shall my little soul ask for to receive the Key of the Kingdom other than
You and to You the Holy, Glory, Power for ever and ever Amen?

*"Then Simon Peter answered him, Lord, to whom shall we go? thou hast the
words of eternal life. [69] And we believe and are sure that thou art that Christ,
the Son of the living God." John 6:68-69 KJV*

Psalm 22:
"My God, my God, why hast thou forsaken me? why art thou so far from helping
me, and from the words of my roaring? b [2] O my God, I cry in the daytime, but
thou hearest not; and in the night season, and am not silent. [3] But thou art holy,
O thou that inhabitest the praises of Israel. [4] Our fathers trusted in thee: they
trusted, and thou didst deliver them. [5] They cried unto thee, and were delivered:
they trusted in thee, and were not confounded. [6] But I am a worm, and no man;
a reproach of men, and despised of the people. [7] All they that see me laugh me
to scorn: they shoot out the lip, they shake the head, saying, [8] He trusted on
the Lord that he would deliver him: let him deliver him, seeing he delighted in
him. [9] But thou art he that took me out of the womb: thou didst make me hope
when I was upon my mother's breasts. [10] I was cast upon thee from the womb:
thou art my God from my mother's belly. [11] Be not far from me; for trouble is
near; for there is none to help. [12] Many bulls have compassed me: strong bulls

of Bashan have beset me round. [13] They gaped upon me with their mouths, as a ravening and a roaring lion. [14] I am poured out like water, and all my bones are out of joint: my heart is like wax; it is melted in the midst of my bowels. [15] My strength is dried up like a potsherd; and my tongue cleaveth to my jaws; and thou hast brought me into the dust of death. [16] For dogs have compassed me: the assembly of the wicked have inclosed me: they pierced my hands and my feet. [17] I may tell all my bones: they look and stare upon me. [18] They part my garments among them, and cast lots upon my vesture. [19] But be not thou far from me, O Lord: O my strength, haste thee to help me. [20] Deliver my soul from the sword; my darling from the power of the dog. [21] Save me from the lion's mouth: for thou hast heard me from the horns of the unicorns. [22] I will declare thy name unto my brethren: in the midst of the congregation will I praise thee. [23] Ye that fear the Lord, praise him; all ye the seed of Jacob, glorify him; and fear him, all ye the seed of Israel. [24] For he hath not despised nor abhorred the affliction of the afflicted; neither hath he hid his face from him; but when he cried unto him, he heard. [25] My praise shall be of thee in the great congregation: I will pay my vows before them that fear him. [26] The meek shall eat and be satisfied: they shall praise the Lord that seek him: your heart shall live for ever. [27] All the ends of the world shall remember and turn unto the Lord: and all the kindreds of the nations shall worship before thee. [28] For the kingdom is the Lord's: and he is the governor among the nations. [29] All they that be fat upon earth shall eat and worship: all they that go down to the dust shall bow before him: and none can keep alive his own soul. [30] A seed shall serve him; it shall be accounted to the Lord for a generation. [31] They shall come, and shall declare his righteousness unto a people that shall be born, that he hath done this. ..."

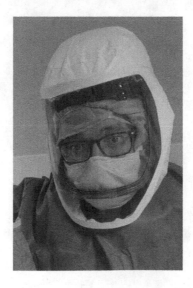

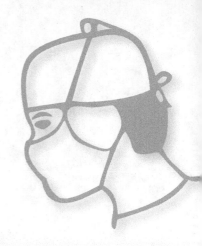

SECTION 7

CHRISTMAS DURING COVID DECLINE

Christmas During COVID Unfolding

O America 🇺🇸 Rise up at the Dawn with my soul! let us all Vote for Jesus and let us Elect Baby Jesus!! Joy on Earth 🌍! O Christmas 🌲 Tree 🌳🌲🌳!

Written by Ramsis Ghaly

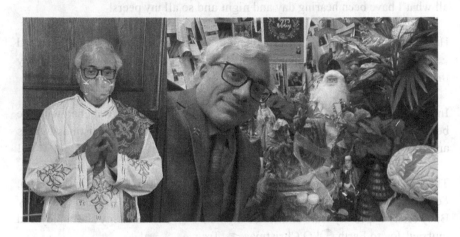

O America Rise Up at the Dawn with my soul! let us all Vote for Jesus and let us Elect Baby Jesus!! Joy to Earth 🌍! O Christmas 🌲 Tree 🌳🌲🌳!
Written by Ramsis Ghaly

O America! My heart is torn! I just heard the news from the earthly scientists that the next 6-12 weeks will be the darkest days of the entire 2020! But I just heard from my Baby Jesus: He is coming from far away descending down among the heavenly crowds flying above the white clouds ☁️☁️ running with His white horse 🐴🐎 to save His creation and protect His children from all the satanic darkness around with the voices of demons threatening our souls!

O Lord for how long??? For how long O my Lord my soul be hiding in the nitches under the ground running away fearing for my life stepped upon by the social media and news 📰🗞️📰! O my torn soul, 2020 almost over and it shouldn't be counted! All what I have been doing, I was just hiding behind a mask and covered by a gown speechless buried in Chaos under the mud and grew nothing thus far producing no fruits suited for 2020!

O America! Hear the News! Christmas 🌲 is coming early this year! I believe that the best of 2020 yet to come as we celebrate the arrival of Baby Jesus! O America 🏴 Rise Up at the Dawn with my soul! let us all Vote for Jesus and let us Elect Baby Jesus!! Joy to Earth 🌍! O Christmas 🌲 Tree 🌳🌲🌳!

I had enough and so is my soul! I prayed in tears to my Savior! O Lord why should it be this way! My soul is trapped in a cage and many are screaming at me yelling it is my end! The terrors of Chinese Coronavirus are close to take my life away is all what I have been hearing day and night and so all my peers!

Human life is short and much valuable than to surrender to fears!! So much sad 😢 news floating around! In fact, so much goodness are being shoveled away by the darkness leaving us with broken hearts 💔 and tearing 😭 eyes 👀!

In one of those gloomy nights, I couldn't sleep 💤 and I was awakened with the beautiful Christmas songs! I enjoyed very much hearing the Christmas hymns and Baby Jesus Hallelujah songs! Joy to Earth 🌍! O Christmas 🌲 Tree 🌳🌲🌳!

Through that night I gathered all my Christmas decorations! Early on at that dawn, I drove in the darkness through Chicago streets to reach my office and clinic! My Baby Jesus wiped my tears and elated my heart 💜 and lifted my soul in joy and murray! Joy to Earth 🌍! O Christmas 🌲 Tree 🌳🌲🌳!

By the time I completed the beautiful Christmas decoration, my first patient came! The Christmas songs were on and so was the good news! No more sad news my soul! Sing all the praises to Baby Jesus! Sing with the heavenly hosts and cast away all the social media and the news! I have voted for Jesus and I have Elected Baby Jesus! O America Rise Up at the Dawn with my soul! let us all Vote for Jesus and let us Elect Baby Jesus!! Joy to Earth 🌍! O Christmas 🌲 Tree 🌳🌲🌳!

As soon as I arrived, I put my Christmas 🌲 decorations saying: O America Hear the News! Christmas is coming early this year! I believe that the best of 2020 yet to come as we celebrate the arrival of Baby Jesus! O America 🏴 Rise Up at the Dawn with my soul! let us all Vote for Jesus and let us Elect Baby Jesus!! Joy to Earth 🌍! O Christmas 🌲 Tree 🌳🌲🌳!

O America! No more sad 😢 news! No more politics! No more fears! No more terrors! O America Hear the News! Christmas 🌲 is coming early this year! I believe that the best of 2020 yet to come as we celebrate the arrival of Baby Jesus! O America 🏴 Rise Up at the Dawn with my soul! let us all Vote for Jesus and let us Elect Baby Jesus!! Joy to Earth 🌍! O Christmas 🌲 Tree 🌳🌲🌳!

Be awaken O human soul! The child of Bethlehem has arrived and His salvation is perfect and eternal! No more tears or cries! No more fears! O human soul, your God has come down to visit with you and protect you from Satan and his demons and rumors of darkness! Baby Jesus shall live forever and ever more with you and shall never cut your life short. Instead, when your time comes, He shall take you up to heaven in His glory! In Jesus so I shall end! Joy to Earth 🌏! O Christmas 🌲 Tree 🌳🌲🌳!

O America Hear the News! Christmas is coming early this year! I believe that the best of 2020 yet to come as we celebrate the arrival of Baby Jesus! O America Rise Up at the Dawn with my soul! let us all Vote for Jesus and let us Elect Baby Jesus!! Joy to Earth 🌏! O Christmas 🌲 Tree 🌳🌲🌳!

As soon as I arrived my clinic, I put my Christmas 🌲 decorations saying: O America Hear the News! Christmas 🌲 is coming early this year! I believe that the best of 2020 yet to come as we celebrate the arrival of Baby Jesus! O America 🇺🇸 Rise Up at the Dawn with my soul! let us all Vote for Jesus and let us Elect Baby Jesus!! Joy to Earth 🌏! O Christmas 🌲 Tree 🌳🌲🌳!

O my soul, your True King 👑 is coming soon, *His name JESUS. He shall be great, and shall be called the Son of the Highest: and the Lord God shall give unto him the throne of his father David: And he shall reign over the house of Jacob for ever; and of his kingdom there shall be no end.—-For with God nothing shall be impossible." Luke 1:31-33,37 KJV*

As all the distressed souls from the 2020 COVID and darkness joining St Mary praise to the Heavenly King Jesus waiting for His arrival voting for Him Jesus and only Jesus, electing Him Christ and only Christ rescuing his people from suffering saving the world 🌏 from the immenient death redeeming their sins and regaining life eternity up in heaven where no more viruses, sickness and death: *"And Mary said, My soul doth magnify the Lord, [47] And my spirit hath rejoiced in God my Saviour. [48] For he hath regarded the low estate of his handmaiden: for, behold, from henceforth all generations shall call me blessed. [49] For he that is mighty hath done to me great things; and holy is his name. [50] And his mercy is on them that fear him from generation to generation. [51] He hath shewed strength with his arm; he hath scattered the proud in the imagination of their hearts. [52] He hath put down the mighty from their seats, and exalted them of low degree. [53] He hath filled the hungry with good things; and the rich he hath sent empty away. [54] He hath holpen his servant Israel, in remembrance of his mercy; [55] As he spake to our fathers, to Abraham, and to his seed for ever." Luke 1:46-55 KJV*

331

Let us go and shop with the three wisemen to receive our Savior our Voter our Elect and our King: "And when they were come into the house, they saw the young child with Mary his mother, and fell down, and worshipped him: and when they had opened their treasures, they presented unto him gifts; gold, and frankincense, and myrrh." Matthew 2:11 KJV

And at Christmas Eve, our souls shall be rejoicing with Jesus Whom we voted for Him and Whom we elected! The world Savior is born to save His people, coming soon in the midst of the heavenly hosts and the wisemen as it is written: *"And the angel said unto them, Fear not: for, behold, I bring you good tidings of great joy, which shall be to all people. [11] For unto you is born this day in the city of David a Saviour, which is Christ the Lord. [12] And this shall be a sign unto you; Ye shall find the babe wrapped in swaddling clothes, lying in a manger. [13] And suddenly there was with the angel a multitude of the heavenly host praising God, and saying, [14] Glory to God in the highest, and on earth peace, good will toward men." Luke 2:10-14 KJV*

"Glory to God in the highest, and on earth peace, good will toward men." O America Rise Up at the Dawn with my soul! let us all Vote for Jesus and let us Elect Baby Jesus!! Joy to Earth! O Christmas 🎄 Tree 🌴🎄🌳!

Wish you all and America and the world 🌍 Merry Christmas 🎄🎁 and Happy New Year 🎆🐱🔮 🎇 2021!!! Joy to Earth! O Christmas 🎄 Tree 🌴🌲🌳!

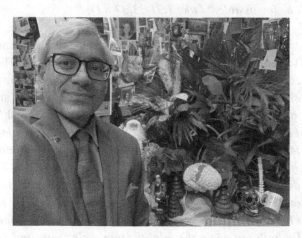

KJ. Dr. Ramis Ghaly, No demon will ever touch your soul nor mine. We see the truth and will be protected Sir. Every night before I sleep I pray for all the good people all over the World to be protected and blessed, no harm to ever come their way. A miracle happened in my life to my Son, Warren Jones. A fine bright young man age 29 was trapped in his brand new Corvette rear-ended a semi truck. His Corvette was trapped under the semi-truck, the paramedics had to cur him out. I arrived at emergency hospital as he walked out shirtless unharmed! "A true miracle Dr. Ramsis! My eyes flowing with tears of love for God protecting my Son. The other Miracle is my Daughter is Marrying a prominent Dr. and they are soon to be parents And for me, I have avoided many car accident everyday and danger that surrounds us everywhere in Las Vegas, Nevada. As you know the Demons come from everywhere and I am always protected by God, anywhere, anytime. I wish to meet you soon. I will decorate for Christmas early cuz of you! May God keep you healthy and always happy and never forget your humor!

TJ. Thank you for the inspiration Dr. . We should all try to find some happiness in the midst of this earthly chaos.

KJ. es! Rejoice!! "I believe in Miracles from the Lord Jesus- Mesiah""

We should all try to find some happiness in the midst of this earthly chaos.

MB. Amen. Be blessed, therefore safe! 🙏

CG. Your outlook brings joy to my heart. Your decorations and Christmas music will put smiles on the faces of your patients. Bless you 🖤🙏

BS. Merry Christmas to you and your family and patients. Love your writing!

KO. Ramsis, this is beautiful... it brought me and my wife to happy tears... we should all do this 🖤

FRC. I vote for Jesus and wait the arrival of Baby Jesus to elect him!

What Do You Think This Christmas 2020 Will Be Like??

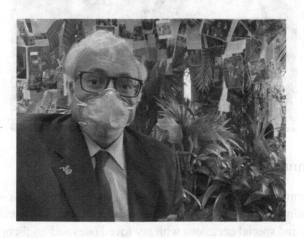

Christmas 2020

I had enough of this years and politics and media!!

I decided to play the old classic Christmas songs in my clinic to my coming patients to cheer them up with my beautiful office garden!!

I am afraid that it will be Virtual Christmas with no traditional Christmas 🎄 customs but face masks and gowns, in addition to distancing away with majority going into on line shopping and Amazon gifts???

Even the churches will be empty and so the hearts of people and minds full of worries and no much money to spend since no jobs around!!

I start to pray to Baby Jesus to brighten our coming days and make us all worthy to celebrate His birth in joy and freedom full of Indoor and outdoor songs and gathering!!! Please join my soul and let us pray!!

What do you think this Christmas will be like??

Who will tell me!!!! Open forum!!!

Ramsis Ghaly

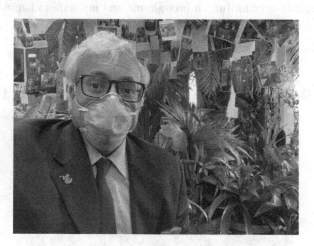

Posted Comments

IS. The government is not in charge of Thanksgiving or Christmas so we should stop waiting for them to tell us what to do. I will continue to celebrate ALL holidays and special occasions with my loved ones and go shopping at small boutiques and Ross and go to mass every Sunday no matter what! 👍👍🙏 Throw that end of the year party, Dr. Ghaly 😊 I support you!!!

LM. I believe everything will calm down after November 4th.....so pretty normal!

334

AH. I will be going to Church for sure! I am already shopping now as to beat the rush of people, I don't want my son to see any difference. I will have my family over even if we have to wear masks and eat at separate tables! God bless us all!

JC. I love Christmas and the songs, good for you, Celebrate, enjoy life. 💙💙⛪

ED. Great idea

FA. I think your patients will love Christmas 🎄 Carol's at your office Dr Ghaly

CP. I think you are very right. Merry Christmas to my favorite doctor. 😊

GH. Love this! 💜

CR. Any kind of music with power or beauty would do the same. Josh Groban, El Divo, or light, happy stuff works too. Great idea.

CP; Excellent idea, my hubby will be playing Christmas music very soon too!

BT. Christmas holidays without the Church and Christmas tradition, they will be very sad.

EA. Christmas is for family and I will be with mine the whole day laughing eating and playing games.

SA. Love Christmas Songs and Baby Jesus will see us through all this Come on 2021 🙏

CE. Yes, this year will be truly different, but with Jesus in our hearts it will all work out. We will still celebrate the holidays with our family. Bless you Dr. Ghaly!

SC. I thought of playing Christmas music, too. Sounds like a good idea to me!

NS. I love the song Mary Did You Know. Written and sung by Mark Lowry

KE. Warm and Loving

CG. Even though there will be no in person church we will still celebrate the birth of Jesus. We will be with family the way we are every Christmas. No masks will be worn. 💜🙏

JH. Great jobs we are the troopers of the hospitals!!!!

SP. Dr Ghaly, I knew there was something I liked about you other than you being an amazing surgeon. Christmas is my middle name. Lol 🎄

MA. I love music especially song of Jesus for Christmas amen

JB. I believe it will be what we make it. I will decorate as I always do. My Nativity will be on my mantel as it always is. I will have a tree in every room as I always do. I will hang my 20 stockings for my grandchildren as I always do. I love Christmas!! ‼️🎄🎄🎄🎄🎄

CS. Hopefully it will be w/ sincere repentance & rejoicing in the Lord for his faithfulness & love.

DM. Sending love 💜

DM. as head of the seniors citizen in my home town i started decorating the office with Christmas stuff to cheer the Seniors. Gift giving small token to celebrate the season .music to remind us about the birth of Jesus and above all prayers of thanksgiving. Our savior is born. MERRY CHRISTMAS....GREETING FROM THE PHILIPPINES FR KAELA AND ME..

JH Great idea finding ways to make people feel special that is my goal also

MG. If we are here and healthy we should praise god for the gift to love another day, caring for someone who needs extra care, and cherish the time we have with who ever can be with, togetherness in spirit

BF. We will be back to the simplest of times! Consider the stable and Mary and Joseph's humility and acceptance.

GG. Thinking of all the work you do! Here is my garden.. it shall be a great Christmas.

KZ. I believe I was first to hear it!!! Lol!

JJ. Families may not gather for Thanksgiving or Christmas. We must think simple and stay focused on our Savior, the Lord Jesus!

AP. Christmas is my favorite holiday but will definitely be different this year but I will be celebrating Christ birth with my family and I always start my Christmas music early.

The 2020 Virtual 🎄 Christmas 🎄! But Yet
What Christmas Calls for and Share with is
Real and Within and Never was Virtual!
Written by Ramsis Ghaly

Let us prepare for the very first The Virtual 🎄 Christmas 🎄! But yet the values and what Christmas 🎄 calling for and share were never been virtual but always have been real and within each heart, mind soul and thoughts!

The 2020 Christmas 🎄 shall be Virtual as the display of Baby Jesus birth shall be so is family and friends!

Although 2020 Christmas 🎄 is the very first Virtual Christmas but yet Baby Jesus won't! Baby Jesus is in every heart 💜 calling His Name!

Although 2020 Christmas 🎄 is the very first Virtual Christmas but yet Love 💜 won't! Love 💜 is in every heart having the birth of Baby Jesus Calling!

Let us have big screens to display brought-to-home alive family and friends gathering without being in-person!

But indeed, nothing shall stop ⬤ our generosity to one another expressed by exchanging gifts as the three wise men had done 2020 years ago to baby Jesus!

Let us begin the on-line shopping to bring joy to each home and elevate local economy in each city and state across America and globally!

Let us decorate the real non virtual Christmas Trees and make them filled with abundance of lights and variety of ornaments watered with love ♥!

Breathen let us begin today to spread the true love ♥, unity and faith all around the world!

This is because In Christmas we share -- with Baby Jesus, the truth in heart ♥ and the spirit in-action!!!

In Christmas we share --with Baby Jesus:
As Jesus Christ our Lord loved us—So we love!
As Jesus Christ our Lord gave His flesh—So we give!
As Jesus Christ our Lord sacrificed Himself—So we sacrifice!
As Jesus Christ our Lord saved us—So we save!
As Jesus Christ our Lord rescue us—-So we rescue!
As Jesus Christ our Lord taught us—So we teach!
As Jesus Christ our Lord served us— So we serve!
As Jesus Christ our Lord washed our feet— So we wash!
As Jesus Christ our Lord humbled Himself— So we humble!
As Jesus Christ our Lord forgives—So we forgive!
As Jesus Christ our Lord Faithful Servant—So we are faithful servants!
As Jesus Christ our Lord carried His Cross—So we carry our Cross!
As Jesus Christ our Lord visited us— So we visit!
As Jesus Christ our Lord prayed for us— So we pray!
As Jesus Christ our Lord fasted for us— So we fast!
As Jesus Christ our Lord fed us— So we feed!
As Jesus Christ our Lord healed the sick — So we heal!
As Jesus Christ our Lord helped us— So we help!
As Jesus Christ our Lord defend us— So we defend!
As Jesus Christ our Lord raised us from the pit— So we raise!
As Jesus Christ our Lord donated much to the poor and needy— So we donate!
As Jesus Christ our Lord supported the unfortunate and unprivileged— So we support!
As Jesus Christ our Lord covered us— So we cover!
As Jesus Christ our Lord have mercy upon us— So we have mercy!
As Jesus Christ our Lord lift us up— So we lift!
As Jesus Christ our Lord spread joy— So we spread joy!
As Jesus Christ our Lord spread hope— So we spread hope!

As Jesus Christ our Lord preached us—So we preach!
As Jesus Christ our Lord lightened our hearts—So we Lightened!
As Jesus Christ our Lord watered the dry lands—So we watered!
As Jesus Christ our Lord strengthen the weak—So we strengthen!
As Jesus Christ our Lord healed the broken bones—So we heal!
As Jesus Christ our Lord comforted us —So we comfort!
As Jesus Christ our Lord carried our burden—So we carry!
As Jesus Christ our Lord covered our nakedness—So we cover!
As Jesus Christ our Lord treat us in patience and meekness—So we treat!
As Jesus Christ our Lord the Good Shepherd—So we are His sheep among wolves!
As Jesus Christ our Lord brought us peace—So we bring!
As Jesus Christ our Lord did not judge us—So we do not judge!
As Jesus Christ our Lord calmed the winds—So we calm!
As Jesus Christ our Lord complained not—So we do not complaint!
As Jesus Christ our Lord life of longsuffering with thanksgiving—So is our life should be!
As Jesus Christ our Lord sweetness—So we are sweet!
As Jesus Christ our Lord awesome —So we are awesome!
As Jesus Christ our Lord did not deny us — So we do not deny Him!
As Jesus Christ our Lord our Heavenly Father — So we His sons and daughters follow Him and obey His Commandments!

"And the angel said unto them, Fear not: for, behold, I bring you good tidings of great joy, which shall be to all people. [11] For unto you is born this day in the city of David a Saviour, which is Christ the Lord. [12] And this shall be a sign unto you; Ye shall find the babe wrapped in swaddling clothes, lying in a manger. [13] And suddenly there was with the angel a multitude of the heavenly host praising God, and saying, [14] Glory to God in the highest, and on earth peace, good will toward men."

Luke 2:10-14 KJV
Let us all in One Spirit pray with His Son saying in One Voice:
Our Father, who art in heaven,
hallowed be thy Name,
thy kingdom come,
thy will be done,
on earth as it is in heaven.
Give us this day our daily bread.
And forgive us our trespasses,
as we forgive those
who trespass against us.

And lead us not into temptation,
but deliver us from evil.
For thine is the kingdom,
and the power, and the glory,
for ever and ever. Amen.

CG. This is something to think about! Thank you for sharing. 🖤🙏

Welcoming the Snow During COVID Second Surge!

Welcome snow to our planet 🌍 and Kiss good by to global warming!

The snow is my face mask of the day and my vaccine against Coronavirus for now!

Ramsis Ghaly

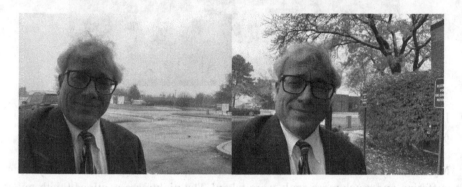

JP. Nailed it Dr Ghaly!!!! 😄
CR. I'll buy that! ❗🌨❄
CG. Stay safe and healthy doctor. I very much dislike wearing a mask but do so amongst strangers. Blessings to you. 🙏🖤
MY. ربنا هو الحافظ من كل سوء وشر وشبه شر وشكرا يا باشا حبيبي الغالي كل سنه وانت طيب
خلى بالك من نفسك والرب معك

My Meditation with my Savior for 2020 Christmas and 2021 New Year!

Written by Ramsis Ghaly

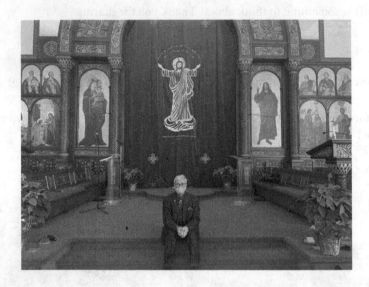

I couldn't rest my head in Christmas Eve! I didn't feel well! My heart was troubled! My eyes were teary! My heart was sad! My soul was crying! My bones were aching!

My mind drifted for a brief moment and I woke up from a nightmare of many are suffering and much more souls were taken! The nightmare continued with my early days of struggling and threats of failures and how many times!

I do not know why of such a painful dream of my previous days and nights whereas I was jobless with no food or home, living in the streets and didn't know what tomorrow should bring and times of being fired and kicked out of my dreams and refused by my own! They were very painful days when I my soul lost the loved ones I used to celebrate Christmas with! What about the days I wished to end and they didn't or the nights whereas the sun never rose!!!

O Baby Jesus: You have taken a father from the bosom of his children and love of his wife! O Baby Jesus: You have taken a mother from her kids and the love of her husband! O Baby Jesus: how many lives the Pandemic shall take for thou to stop the pandemic heal thy people! For how long O Lord the coronavirus and its family of evil viruses ▓ shall overcome thy people!

I immediately went to my little closet and cried to my Savior! In tears I spoke tonight is thy Birthday my Newborn Baby Jesus, please help my heartbroken soul and the multitudes of thy children!! Baby Jesus have mercy!

O Baby Jesus: For how long thy people be threatened by the COVID-19! O Baby Jesus, for how long we will keep a distance from each other! For how long thy people cover their faces with facemasks all the time! For how long thy people limit their outdoor activities and enjoy the nature You have formed for them!

For how long O Baby Jesus, thy children will continue to live away from their normal life and enjoy the gift of life You have granted thy soul! For how long O Baby Jesus, thy people run away and hide day and night! For how long O Baby Jesus, the curfew be imposed and social isolation!

++My soul turned to Psalm 13, and the words came out soaked in tears and trembling: "How long wilt thou forget me, O Lord Baby Jesus? forever?

How long wilt thou hide thy face from me? How long shall I take counsel in my soul, having sorrow in my heart daily?

How long shall mine enemy (COVID-19) be exalted over me?

Consider and hear me, O Lord my God: lighten mine eyes, lest I sleep the sleep of death; Lest mine enemy (COVID-19) say, I have prevailed against him; and those that trouble me rejoice when I am moved!

But I have trusted in thy mercy; my heart shall rejoice in thy salvation. I will sing unto the Lord, because he hath dealt bountifully with me! Amen ⚞ Psalm 13

++My soul became sorrowful as if I lost all my loved ones, agitated and my taste became bitter! As I fell in silence and unable to speak, the words of Psalm 22 came to my mouth. And screamed:

My God, my God, O Baby Jesus, why hast thou forsaken me? why art thou so far from helping me, and from the words of my roaring? O my God, I cry in the daytime, but thou hearest not; and in the night season, and am not silent!

But thou art holy, O thou that inhabits the praises of Israel. Our fathers trusted in thee: they trusted, and thou didst deliver them. They cried unto thee, and were delivered: they trusted in thee, and were not confounded!

O Baby Jesus, But I am a worm, and no man; a reproach of men, and despised of the people. All they that see me laugh me to scorn: they shoot out the lip, they shake the head, saying, He trusted on the Lord that he would deliver him: let him deliver him, seeing he delighted in him!

O Baby Jesus, But thou art he that took me out of the womb: thou didst make me hope when I was upon my mother's breasts. I was cast upon thee from the womb: thou art my God from my mother's belly.

O Baby Jesus, Be not far from me; for trouble is near; for there is none to help. Many bulls have compassed me: strong bulls of Bashan have beset me round. They gaped upon me with their mouths, as a ravening and a roaring lion!

O Baby Jesus, I am poured out like water, and all my bones are out of joint: my heart is like wax; it is melted in the midst of my bowels. My strength is dried up like a potsherd; and my tongue cleaveth to my jaws; and thou hast brought me into the dust of death. For dogs have compassed me: the assembly of the wicked have inclosed me: they pierced my hands and my feet. I may tell all my bones: they look and stare upon me. They part my garments among them, and cast lots upon my vesture!

O Baby Jesus, But be not thou far from me, O Lord: O my strength, haste thee to help me. Deliver my soul from the sword; my darling from the power of the dog. Save me from the lion's mouth: for thou hast heard me from the horns of the unicorns. I will declare thy name unto my brethren: in the midst of the congregation will I praise thee!

O Baby Jesus, Ye that fear the Lord, praise him; all ye the seed of Jacob, glorify him; and fear him, all ye the seed of Israel. For he hath not despised nor abhorred the affliction of the afflicted; neither hath he hid his face from him; but when he cried unto him, he heard!

My praise shall be of thee in the great congregation: I will pay my vows before them that fear him. The meek shall eat and be satisfied: they shall praise the Lord that seek him: your heart shall live for ever!

O Baby Jesus, All the ends of the world shall remember and turn unto the Lord: and all the kindreds of the nations shall worship before thee. For the kingdom is the Lord's: and he is the governor among the nations. All they that be fat upon earth shall eat and worship: all they that go down to the dust shall bow before him: and none can keep alive his own soul. A seed shall serve him; it shall be accounted

342

to the Lord for a generation. They shall come, and shall declare his righteousness unto a people that shall be born, that he hath done this! Amen 🙏 Psslm 22!

++A whirlwind came to my soul with a smile and soft breeze! I took a deep breath and I spoke these words to my soul:

The fact is I wasn't suppose to be where I am now! It was a long journey full of uncertainty and turmoil! But I couldn't believe I made it thus far and I am still standing! Thank You my Lord and Savior! Praise thy Name!

The current times are difficult! It is that time to roll back and go through our Rolodex to reflect of how my Savior was so good to me! Nowadays days aren't joyful as my ancient days! It is that day to go over my memoirs and remember how my Lord was so gracious to His people!

++ My soul was comforted much more and I became at peace as my lips to bless Baby Jesus Psalm 103:

Bless the Lord, O my soul: and all that is within me, bless his holy name!

Bless the Lord, O my soul, and forget not all his benefits: Who forgiveth all thine iniquities; who healeth all thy diseases; Who redeemeth thy life from destruction; who crowneth thee with lovingkindness and tender mercies; Who satisfieth thy mouth with good things; so that thy youth is renewed like the eagle's!

The Lord executeth righteousness and judgment for all that are oppressed. He made known his ways unto Moses, his acts unto the children of Israel!

The Lord is merciful and gracious, slow to anger, and plenteous in mercy. He will not always chide: neither will he keep his anger for ever. He hath not dealt with us after our sins; nor rewarded us according to our iniquities!

For as the heaven is high above the earth, so great is his mercy toward them that fear him. As far as the east is from the west, so far hath he removed our transgressions from us. Like as a father pitieth his children, so the Lord pitieth them that fear him!

For he knoweth our frame; he remembereth that we are dust. As for man, his days are as grass: as a flower of the field, so he flourisheth. For the wind passeth over it, and it is gone; and the place thereof shall know it no more. But the mercy of the Lord is from everlasting to everlasting upon them that fear him, and his righteousness unto children's children;!

To such as keep his covenant, and to those that remember his commandments to do them. The Lord hath prepared his throne in the heavens; and his kingdom ruleth over all!

Bless the Lord, ye his angels, that excel in strength, that do his commandments, hearkening unto the voice of his word. Bless ye the Lord, all ye his hosts; ye ministers of his, that do his pleasure. Bless the Lord, all his works in all places of his dominion: bless the Lord, O my soul! Amen 🙏 Psalm 103!

++More than Thousand years ago, a Psalm was prepared for this day, Let us open our mouth and speak the words of Psalm 77:

I cried unto God with my voice, even unto God with my voice; and he gave ear unto me,

In the day of my trouble I sought the Lord: my sore ran in the night, and ceased not: my soul refused to be comforted!

I remembered God, and was troubled: I complained, and my spirit was overwhelmed. Selah!

Thou holdest mine eyes waking: I am so troubled that I cannot speak!

I have considered the days of old, the years of ancient times!

I call to remembrance my song in the night: I commune with mine own heart: and my spirit made diligent search!

Will the Lord cast off for ever? and will he be favourable no more?

Is his mercy clean gone for ever? doth his promise fail for evermore?

Hath God forgotten to be gracious? hath he in anger shut up his tender mercies? Selah!

And I said, This is my infirmity: but I will remember the years of the right hand of the most High!

I will remember the works of the Lord: surely I will remember thy wonders of old!

I will meditate also of all thy work, and talk of thy doings!

Thy way, O God, is in the sanctuary: who is so great a God as our God?

Thou art the God that doest wonders: thou hast declared thy strength among the people!

Thou hast with thine arm redeemed thy people, the sons of Jacob and Joseph. Selah!

The waters saw thee, O God, the waters saw thee; they were afraid: the depths also were troubled!

The clouds poured out water: the skies sent out a sound: thine arrows also went abroad!

The voice of thy thunder was in the heaven: the lightnings lightened the world: the earth trembled and shook!

Thy way is in the sea, and thy path in the great waters, and thy footsteps are not known!

Thou leddest thy people like a flock by the hand of Moses and Aaron! Amen 🙏 Psalm 77!

++There is no word to express my gratitude and appreciation to all those came across my path! My life was my family at my upbringing and soon became my patients, students and residents!

My daily mission always was and us and will be: Do Your Best! Learn in Depth! Care From Your Heart! And Let God Do The Rest!

I look up to my Lord Jesus Aptitudes at the mountain of the Lord and I always pray; "Our Father which art in heaven, Hallowed be thy name. [10] Thy kingdom come. Thy will be done in earth, as it is in heaven. [11] Give us this day our daily bread. [12] And forgive us our debts, as we forgive our debtors. [13] And lead us not into temptation, but deliver us from evil: For thine is the kingdom, and the power, and the glory, for ever. Amen." Matthew 6:9-13 KJV

Living in Hope always with Christ-To Pray- To Praise- To Fast- To Serve-To Share- To Love ♥- To Give- To Heal- To Strengthen- To Lift Up- To Honor- To Renew- In the Spirit of Thanksgiving- Humility- Heartfelt ♥-Looking Up to Heaven- Racing Toward the Promise and the Unseen!

Until then: Merry Christmas 🎄 and happy new year 🥂 thank you so much. Praying for you all staying safe. Thank you all for Your kindness and wonderful heart Love and blessing.

Amen

Ramsis Ghaly

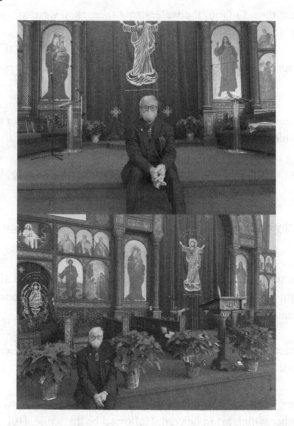

SS. Until Man heals from his wickedness.. we are put in the test of our faith... all storms that come are to clean our souls and to save humanity... believe in the lord that our faith brings us to Victory us Approaching the Lord's Throne of Love... Praying we all home in the hospitals in every place... even if we are. All separated and closed Let's all pray together with Our Savior Jesus may God forgive our

WD. Hopefully our LAST Covid Christmas 😢

CP. Very nice. 🙂

FA. Amen 🙏

AV. Amen! Thank you for these precious words! 💜🙏

MG. Angels walk amongst men!

Thy kingdom come,

Thy will be done!

On earth as it is in Heaven!

This things to shall pass!

Keep the faith,

We've got this,

Evil has not won!

🙏 Merry Christmas 🎄 and happy new year 🎊 thank you so much. Praying you staying safe. Thank you for Your kindness and wonderful heart

CR. You open your heart and faith to all of us. I can feel your pain in all of this. God has preserved you to continue to serve and heal. May you have the joy of your salvation. 🙏💜

LG. Merry Christmas, Dr. Ghaly! God bless you!

VG. Amin! Hvala na ovim divnim rečima! 💕🙏

BH. Never lose hope.

Never underestimate the power of prayer.

I wept at these words. Beautifully written.

I have hope that this too shall pass.

Stay safe!! 🙏🙏🙏💜

TG. It make me cry I'm appreciate and Thanks to God everything in my life. Love and prayers for everyone around the world 🙏💜

DL. Beautiful Dr. . Merry Christmas.

KG. We all must never lose faith and continue to pray to our Almighty God for healing. 🙏

347

Virtual 2020 Christmas and New Year

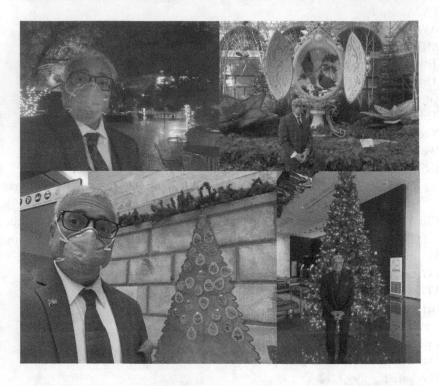

As America 🇺🇸 is awaiting post holidays COVID Surge, practicing scaled-down private Virtual 2020 Christmas 🎄 while keeping Baby Jesus within my heart and mind and thoughts dressed with 2020 stylish Christmassy suit, red tie, pocket square, cuff-links, elegant filter face mask and fashionable eye glasses/ face shield taking photos with wall images distancing away from gathering, from people and from all social events in person praying and shopping on-line saying Merry Christmas 🎁 🎄 to you all virtually through wireless technology!!!

Ramsis Ghaly
Www.ghalyneurosurgeon.com

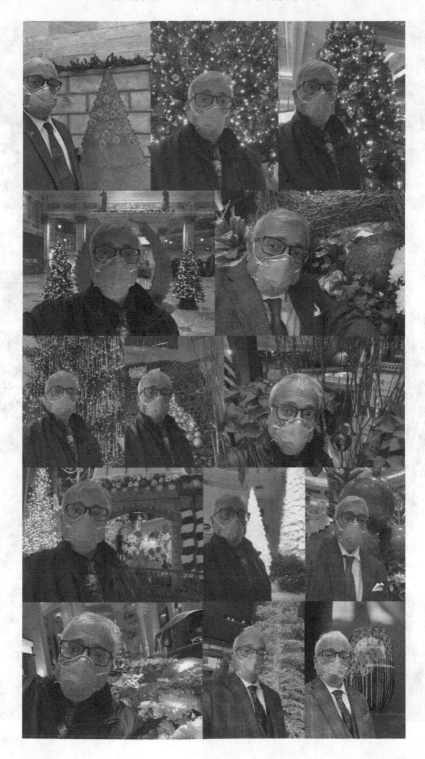

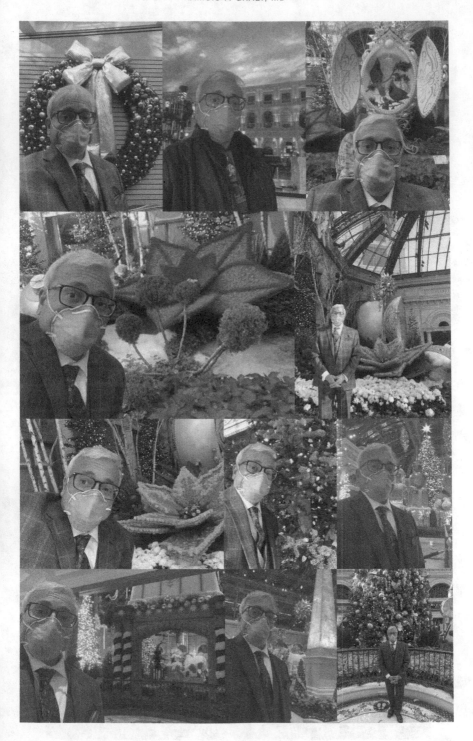

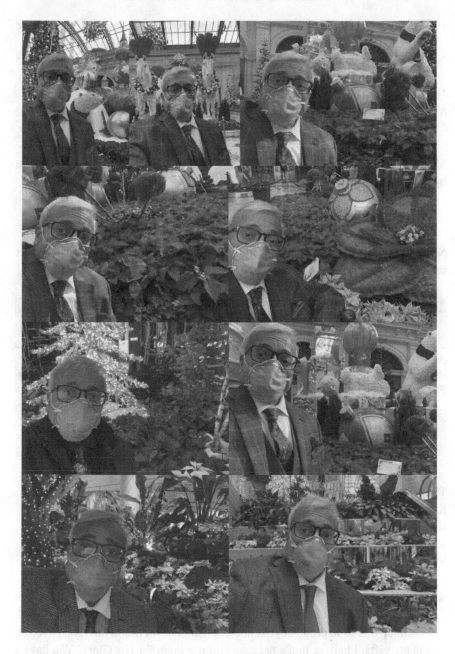

CG I hope the numbers didn't go up because of the Thanksgiving holiday. I pray that this pandemic will just disappear so we can get on with our lives. Bless you and stay safe. 🖤🙏

CP. God bless you 🙏 and take care of yourself my friend

JB. Praying so hard for the end of this. I whispered in Jesus ear last night while praying and said please end this Jesus to many people are dying.........

NE. The Lord is your strength Dr. Ghaly, God bless you for all you do! And bless everyone putting their lives on the line, the Lord is our shield and protect!

JB. Have a blessed and safe Christmas season Dr. Ghaly. 🙏 ❤️

ربنا موجود ليتمجد على صنعه يديك وارحمنا كلنا معا لان ليس لنا خلاص الابك ارحمنا كل سنه. MY.
وانت طيب ا.د.رمسيس الرب معك و يعينك وبالتوفيق والنجاح الأستاذ الدكتور الكبير رمسيس

Merry Christmas 🎄 🎁 to you all! COVID Vaccine is our special Christmas treat by the tree 🌲 🌳 🌲!

Ramsis Ghaly

No more crowd or close to each other gather in a big group as in previous years.

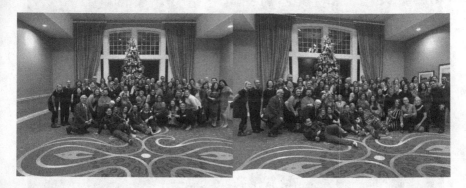

TN. Merry Christmas 💜

KO. MERRY CHRISTMAS and Happy birthday Jesus 🙏🙏 🌲

KM. Merry Christmas 🌲

SJ. A well needed read this holiday season 💜
You are such a prolific writer who never ceases to amaze me 💜

CP. Where can we buy this book and when will it be out? Thanks. ☺

KM. So proud # 17. Wow. Inspiration. I need to know which book to start from on this if it's a continuation of others preceding it. I'm not sure where to look them up at. I'm so proud of your accomplishments in life so far. God gave you many gifts. I believe that's because you use them for His Glory. You have a heart of gold & I am still wondering where sleep comes into the picture for you. Being on call, you have probably trained to sleep when your head hits the pillow. Congratulations again & keep God's light shining.

Memories of Christmas **December, 2017** ·

Some more of Christmas

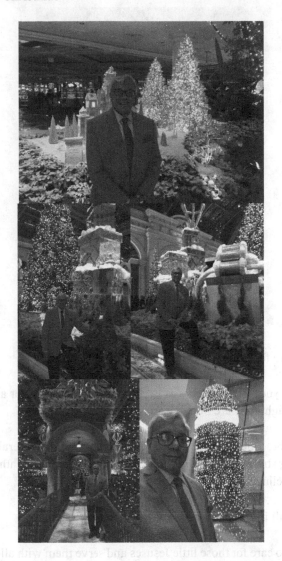

CG. Very Christmassy!

MS. Very nice, where is this place?

JV. Wonderful pictures Dr. G. Let us pray we get through this pandemic and get
   back to times like this!!

Stay safe!! 💜

My Christmas EVE PPE

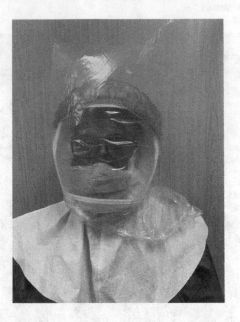

My Christmas 🌲 PPE Eve going out in a Virus Night! 🙏

Blessing to care for COVID victims in a Virus 🦠 Night!

Ready to help you! Big tgst easy as every day us getting busier and busier and many that thought they are immune are getting the Virus!

Fever, headache, flue, loss of smell and appetite, feeling miserable that never before, feeling strange and then followed by coughing and breathing difficulty and further decline!

Never ever shall I turn my back!

It is an honor to care for those little Jesuses and serve them with all my skills and from my heart!

At least I look like a nun!!!

Ramsis Ghaly

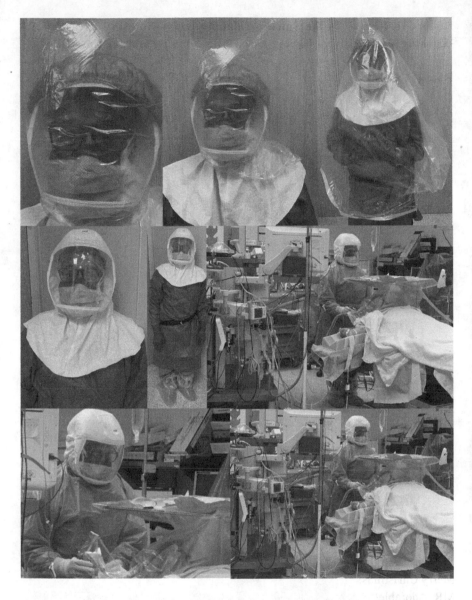

Ready to serve with my colleagues! Much virus 🦠 around! Thank you 🙏

My Christmas2019 Eve Custom!!!

In Christmas 🎄 Eve- By the Christmas Tree- In my Christmas Custom- Living in Hope always with Christ-To Pray- To Praise- To Fast- To Serve-To Share- To Love - 💜 To Give- To Heal- To Strengthen- To Lift Up- To

Honor- To Renew- In the Spirit of Thanksgiving- Humility- Heartfelt -Looking Up to Heaven- Racing Toward the Promise and the Unseen!

Ramsis Ghaly

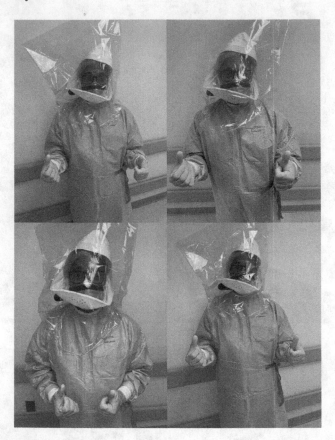

JM. Looking Good Dr. Ghaly

PL. This should "cover" many needs! 😁 Merry Christmas!

MR. Adorable!

BM. Stay safe and healthy, and God Bless you Always!

JC. Is any body in there 😀 Merry Christmas Dr 🎄🎄🎄🙏

AC. Merry Christmas Dr. Ghaly 🎄🎄😀

DM. sta clauus now in blue

SN. Merry Christmas Dr.Ghaly! 🙏✨

CP. Merry Christmas Dr.Gahly! May you receive the blessings of the Infant Jesus. God bless you.

CJ. Merry Christmas, stay safe, and bless you! 💙👍🎄

PR. A good Christmas to you my friend, much love and may 2021 be good for you.
SJ. Creative
GK. Stay safe, God bless you Doctor.
CP. Be safe! God bless you always 🙏
PV. Merry Christmas!
VG. Srecan Božic dr.Bog vas blagoslovio! 🎄🎄🎄🙏
ZC. Wishing you peace and joy throughout the season Dr.Ghally. 🎄
🌸💐🌐⚪

AH. Merry Christmas !!
TS. Merry Christmas 🎄
SI. Have a very Merry Christmas 🎄 Dr. Ghaly
LY. Merry Christmas Dr. Ghaly!
JJ. Merry Christmas!!!

May God bless you and protect you greatly. You are a great man of faith. An example to all.

GR. Merry Christmas
CT. Godspeed and God bless you my Friend, be well, Merry Christmas 🎁
KO. Merry Christmas Dr Ghaly, Lord keep you safe and healthy
God Bless you
RH. Merry Christmas to the doctor that keeps on giving. Love to you doctor
AM. I hope you have some air flowing under there Dr. AG. 🙏 merry Christmas 😷😷🎄
BH. Merry Christmas Dear Ramsis. May your holidays be filled with love, peace, hope and some semblance of normalcy. Rest and God Bless you sweet man! 🙏🖤🙏

Now, about that outfit...stay safe at all cost!

SL. Merry Christmas 🎄

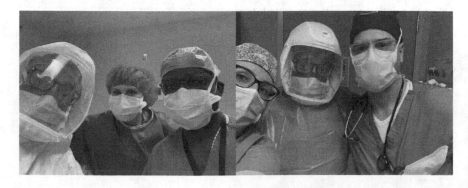

Mj. Lucky to serve with you all 🖤
Cj. Stay safe 👏
Cg. Bless you all and stay safe!
Kj. Stay safe and thank you for all that you do!

#Thanks
HEALTH
HEROES

Mg. Prayers
Kc. Looking good, Dr. Ghaly
Kn. 😊😊🙏🙏
Yf. Stay safe 🙏
Js. That looks dangerous
BK. h my goodness! How can you breathe??? 😅
ML. Stay safe DR. Ramsis Ghaly
MB. Our Lord Jesus Christ protect you 🤍🙏
SA. Stay safe and healthy
SS. Stay safe!!!
MN. Dr. Ghaly you are in my thoughts and prayers God Bless you
MR. Merry Christmas Dr. Ghaly!
KN. Merry Christmas Dr Ghaly
Thank you for your dedicated contributions
🤎🤎🤎🤎
TG. Wish you a Merry Christmas full of peace, joy and happiness. Blessings .. 🙏🙏
KW. Merry Christmas!
VG. Merry Christmas, Doctor Ghaly!
TN. Merry Christmas 🤍
KO. MERRY CHRISTMAS and Happy birthday Jesus 🙏🙏 🎄
KM. Merry Christmas 🎄
RN. Merry Christmas Dr.Ghaly, blessings 🤎🤎🙏🙏
VG. Merry Christmas Dr Ghaly!!Blessings 🙏🤍
CG. Wishing you a Merry Christmas that is full of peace, joy and happiness. 🎄🤍🙏
SK. Merry Christmas! 🎄
PH. A very distinguished looking man you are. Merry Christmas
YA. Merry Christmas 🎄💕

358

ET. MERRY CHRISTMAS to you as well! 🎄🙏
AL. That's a beautiful Christmas present (vaccine) to all. Merry Christmas
NM. Merry Christmas 🖤
CP. Merry Christmas and a Happy New Year. Very nice pictures. ☺
JF. Merry Christmas

Perhaps, it is wonderful to start the week with this song as we continue our journey with COVID second Wave Surge.

Let us sing to Our Bethlehem Baby of Light 🕯, Peace and Healing Who shall save us from all Evil including COVID! Amen 🙏

No more close together as previous years

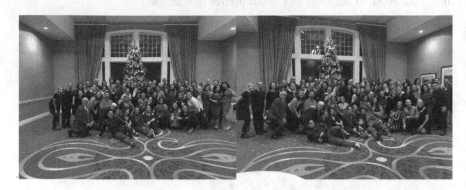

My Hospital On Call Christmas Uniform Isn't lighting Up For Sure!!!

My Christmas 🎄 Uniform, my calls aren't lighting up for sure!!!

COVID all over and many are getting sick and infected!

Whenever I turn my head, many people are getting infected and many said they followed the CDC COVID Dr Fauci guidelines and still got the Coronavirus!!

It almost feels like COVID is surrounding us all over the place including in our air, in our food, in our bags and in our homes nowadays!

"But as for me, I shall sing of Your strength; Yes, I shall joyfully sing of Your lovingkindness in the morning, For You have been my stronghold And a refuge in the day of my distress." Psalm 59:16

You all be safe!!

Ramsis Ghaly

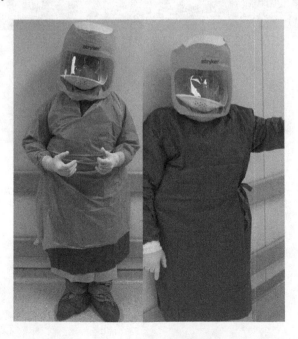

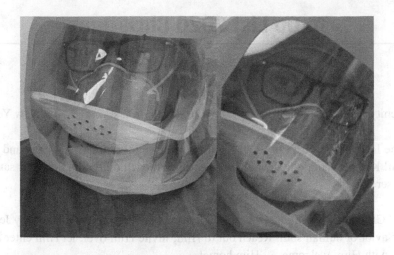

JD. Please take care of yourself Dr. Ghaly and God Bless You !!!

CR. Sending hugs and prayers to you Dr. Ghaly

Stay safe and healthy and strong 🖤🖤🙏🙏

DI. God bless you

MF. Militar bendiciones! 🙏🙏🙏

DM. God bless and protect you

ML. Our St. Ramsis Ghaly! Stay safe. 🙏🙏

CG. Blessings to you and all you do to help those in dire need. Take care. 🙏

AL. We need this outfit when we go out

TG. God Bless and Protect you! Stay safe.

JP. God bless you doctor. You are the hands and feet of Jesus to so many. Remember to be kind and minister to your own needs also. You can't pour from an empty vessel.

MY. ربنا يرحمنا ويرفع عنا ذلك الوباء العالمي وارحم صنعه يديك CP. God bless you 🙏 and take care of yourself my friend

JB. Praying so hard for the end of this. I whispered in Jesus ear last night while praying and said please end this Jesus to many people are dying.........

To Do List 2020 Christmas

Written by Ramsis Ghaly

Serenity, Solitude and Selff-Control for 2020 Christmas 🌲 and 2021 New Year!

Some Ideas for Christmas 2020! Should You have more ideas go ahead and list them! Keep sharing it is the only way to support each other and keep our sanity and serenity!!

2020 Christmas is solitude private quality tine between your soul and Bay Jesus the Savior of human soul! Reach out to Him, invite Him over, let Him enter and dine with Him, welcome 🛐 Him home!

You aren't alone and we all with you in thoughts, hearts and spirit!

Read and reflect in deep thoughts in the Holy Bible and listen and hear the words of promise, love, rejuvenation, comfort, hope and faith in Jesus Name for life on earth and life to come!

Dress up as if you going to a Christmas party!
Be in your house! Visit each room and spend special time and reflect!
Sit by the Christmas tree 🌲 by the fire wood 🪵!
Listen to Christmas music!
Sing and pray loudly and not shy!

Pray to Baby Jesus by your closet! Have a special time with our Savior, Beloved, Rescuer and Redeemer of mankind and Creator, Protector and True Healer of our human race since the establishment of the world to the End of Days!

Remember the birth of Jesus in a very harsh time among the dinners, the rulers in the midst of animals in a strange land!

Be very thankful and feel blessed and special!

Cook the best meal and prepare the best desert, bake Christmas cookies and hand the best ever Christmas tree!

Prepare meals and cookies for others! Write Christmas cards and inspiring notes to known and unknown as Good Samaritans do!

Call and zoom in wish many merry Christmas 🎁🎄 spread love, hope, optimism, laugh and joy to many you know and you don't know!

Reach out and send as much as your budget allows!
Write your diary! Gym and exercise at home!
Spend quality time with your romance and Play with your kids!
Treat yourself well and generous to others!
Go over your good times childhood and honeymoon! Tell stories —!

Decor your car, desk, office, bedroom, living room, bathroom, basement, home, house, condo, unit and RUV mobile home!

Put on Christmas decorations and display the best ever colorful ornaments!
Reflect and meditate and write songs and poets!
Explore the unknown and Read about what is new!
Play music and learn new hymns!
Do arts and learn to paint 🎨!

Try in-door new and safe entertainment such as virtual golfing, virtual plays cards and games, virtual chessboard!

Play with your pets, feed the birds 🐦 and work in the yard!
Raise dogs, cats, chicken, lamb, cattle and horses!
Plan to own a yard, an outdoor little pool, garden, ranch,—-!
Take frequent breaks and fo not keep starting at digital screens 📺📺!
Pray for eradication of COVID-19 Pandemic!
Begin write up the New Year Resolutions wishes, hopes, regrets, to do and not to do!!
Remember old good days!
Remember those lost loved ones and in need and sick, in jail, poor—etc!
Live in memories of previous Christmas!
Open old gifts and look at old albums!
Work out few hours a day!
Garden and water the plants 🪴!
Execute your manual labor hobbies!
Read books! Review novels you have read and enjoyed!
Drive alone around!
Run away to the beach, mountains and deserts if you live close by!
Keep house with effective high powered ventilations windows open!!
Learn new recipes of cooking!
Send Christmas wishes!
Call as many old and new buddies!

Be hopeful and optimistic!
No church!
No visitors! Take a break from the news, vaccines and politics!
Do not kiss or hug any strangers!
Do not you dare come close to anybody maintain 6 feet distance!
Keep your mask and eye shield if you are by someone other than your household!
Spray your house with antivirus!
No in house drinking!
No tears or cries!
Don't get upset!
No bad words or curses!
Don't blow up!
Do not jump or do something risky or stupid!
Do not be alone keep yourself busy!
No yelling or screaming!
No smoking 🚬 and no fireworks! 🧨
No fighting or arguments!
Do not spend time in the past or regrets!
Do not sleep beyond your normal hours!
Do not spend unusual time in the couch!
Do not gain weight or eat unhealthy!
Do not be lazy but active and keep yourself busy and your mind active!
Stay away from bad habits, illegal activities and wipe out side affairs!
Do not keep looking at the mirrors!
Hang up in any one make you depressed!
Open up, talk about it, don't keep it in your heart, share, laugh, smile 😊!
Don't expect much!
Cook for yourself only!
Shop on line!
Visit each room!
Look ftom the windows!
Okay to talk to yourself and yo the walls!
Take frequent breaks between tasks!
Make sure you clean up!
Take four showers!
Keep washing your hands!
Keep watching TV, movies, documentaries—!
Keep looking for messages in your phones!
Keep texting!
Zoom in only to your loved ones!
Go ahead and buy for yourself and others gifts and send them via mail!
Study in line!

And how you feel draw in a diagram and see what else you can do to make you feel better giving the circumstances!

Please share and add more ideas!!
If you are doing something different please share
Stay in touch and let us support each other digitally and wireless!!

Merry Christmas 🎁 🎄 and Happy New Year 📷🔮🎊 2021!

Ramsis Ghaly

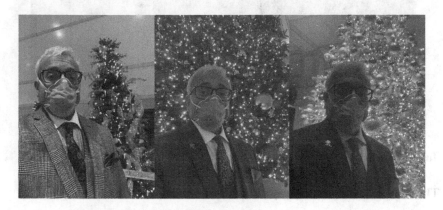

Lm. I going to run my Arabian horse in the desert.
Ko. Great plan, you're so inspirational Dr Ghaly, and you certainly speed joy unto others. 🎄
Cg. Great ideas many of which I do. I have another one to add which is feed the birds. Also contact people who live alone and try to do something to make their day a little brighter.
Hw. Bake cookies for shut ins, write in my gratitude journal, write a note of encouragement to our pastor! 🎄

Dm or these beautiful ideas and have a WONDERFIL CHRISTMAS...Greetings from the Philippines

VG, o you and your family, I wish you a happy Christmas holiday and a happy 2021 with health for all of us. And may God our Creator continue to guide our paths in this life here on earth and all eternity in heavenly villas. 🙏🙏❤️❤️❤️

Thank you 🙏 to my wonderful patient

365

CG. a beautiful Christmas music nativity scene snow globe music box. Thank you so much merry Christmas much blessing!!

HW. Bake cookies for shut ins, write in my gratitude journal, write a note of encouragement to our pastor!

Ramsis Ghaly

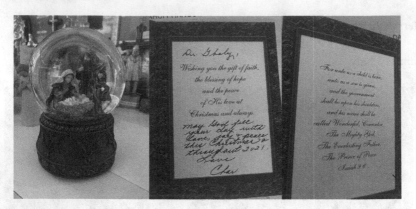

Just beautiful!! 🖤

The wonderful man Jerry my patient after brief procedure.

Many blessing merry Christmas 🎄 and happy new year and congratulations

Ramsis ghaly
Ghalyneurosurgeon.com

My Christmas life Ruby and her husband Don. Before surgery in October she was 24/7 horrific pain and couldn't walk at all. Her husband was suffering with her daily as well over at least 6 months. Look at her now and look at them both! Praise our Lord!

Before her surgery, her husband did not talk much except one tine and said: I trust you and our Lord!

With no hesitation and strong faith, Ruby underwent a very long spine surgery. Their faith stayed strong and now, Ruby has A new lease in life and now both of them to continue their love journey and happiness. Thank you Baby Jesus.

Ramsis Ghaly
www.ghalyneurosurgeon.com

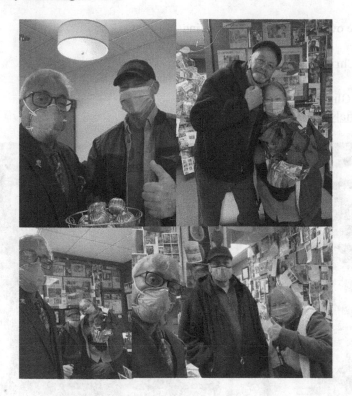

AV. Praise God! 🐶🙏

KO. That's a blessing for them, thank God, he sent you a fantastic surgeon 😊

MA. Awesome!!! Strong faith, prayers, & a great doctor!

DM. God bless your hands to heal many

CB. You are God's instrument. God bless you.

JP. Faith in God, a supportive husband and a gifted by God surgeon; The trifecta!

BM. Praise God!

CR. Praise the Lord and thanks to you!!!!

CG. So happy to hear she is doing so well. She has the best! 🖤🙏

Look at our angel

Rebecca Crawley

only 3 weeks after major surgery doing terrific, she put her own gorgeous Christmas Tree and so ready for the best Christmas without pain and new year with great inspiration! She is already planning big for 2021 and no one can stop her!

How grateful I am for my Lord you let me serve and heal with His hand. Amen our Lord Jesus our Savior and Healer. Amen!

Speed re over your angel. Keep healing

Merry Christmas 🎄 and Happy New Year

Ramsis Ghaly
Www.ghalyneurosurgeon.com

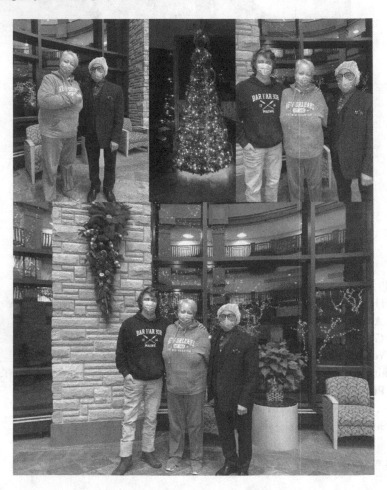

CG. How wonderful for her. What a beautiful tree. Wishes for a quick recovery. AV. Thank you Dr Ghaly! 💜🙏

Lavender Color in Christmas!

O my Lord, I received a huge compliment from a stranger. She stopped me and said: "I love your suit. You know that the Lavender Color is for Royalty" I replied: "I didn't know but now I know. Thank you. Merry Christmas 🎄"

I immediately googled and this what I found: "This shade is highly associated with elegance and grace. It has a close relation to the symbol of beauty and femininity as well. Recognized as a grown pink, lavender universally sends out a sense of delicacy, nostalgic, and romantic atmosphere."

"Lavender, a lighter version of purple, is an unconventional color with a slightly feminine touch, symbolizing gracefulness, elegance, calmness, creativity, vitality, optimism and youthfulness."

"The ancient Hebrews ascribed holiness to lavender, using it as a key component of ritual anointing oil, a fact attested to in the biblical Song of Solomon. Ancient Romans valued it so much that a pound of the plant sold for as much as a farmer's entire monthly wages."

https://www.colorpsychology.org/lavender/
https://en.m.wikipedia.org/wiki/Lavender_(color)

Ramsis Ghaly

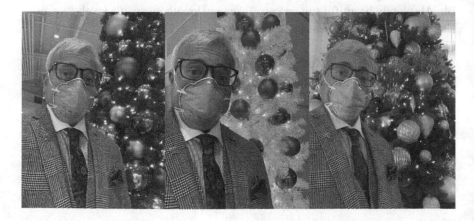

Gh. Sharing with my brother. He didn't want the lavender Ralph Lauren, cashmere sweater I was buying for him. I did my wedding in lavender years ago! Even had lavender water fountain in the cake.

Av. Great! 💜🙏

Jc. Looking very dapper - merry Christmas to you

Bm. You look very handsome. Purple and lavender are my favorite colors 💜

Jp. Looking good in that suit Doctor.

Kw. The impeccably dressed Dr Ghaly! Whether it's scrubs or designer suits, he's the man!

Cg. I think you found your color. In Europe you see alot of men wearing lavender or pink shades. It looks very attractive. 💜🙏

Al. Very festive, great looking. Have a Merry Christmas doc. Good example for wearing masks 🌲👍✌️👌

Cg. Divno! 💜🙏

Ac. Lovely... also aligned with the Advent season. 🌲💜

Tr. You are Royalty!!

Sj. Our royal doctor, Dr. Ghaly. 💜 I think all the descriptions apply

Gs. Many blessings brother

Ma. Suits you to a "T!" then! 😊👏

As. Beautiful 🎅🌲🙏

Jm. "Fabulous" What A Wonderful Compliment............handsome 💜

ml. You are such a sharp dressed man. I love your sense of style.

Rc. I love that color and all matices. You look veey nice!

Ab. Very dapper, Brother!!

Kg. Wow!!! Hit the nail on the head. 😊 Very flattering!

Bh. Absolutely beautiful suit on you. Takes my breath away. It's lovely. Have a blessed holiday season dear Dr. Ghaly!

Fl. Looks great

Pf. You ware it well my beautiful friend 💜🙏

Cl Forget the suit... even though you're a well dressed man. The fact you always smelled good was a thing for my mom!

Mp. Did you get her number? 😊

Tg. I love Lavender color you look great. Have a Blessed holiday season dear Ramsis Ghaly

It Is Sunday Let Us Be Ready to Serve Our Savior Jesus as We Approaching His Birth!

I and many don't run away from COVID patients neither we stay 6 feet apart nor turning our back to COVID Victims! They are my people, my flesh, bones and blood! But instead in courage, good faith and love as our Lord taught us, we run to serve face-to-face fearless living in His promise believing in Him unceasing!!

O my dear soul Sunday for God as God is the Lord of Sunday! Let us serve our Lord Jesus and His children according g to His calling!!

As my Master said: "And he said unto them, The sabbath was made for man, and not man for the sabbath: [28] Therefore the Son of man is Lord also of the sabbath." Mark 2:27-28 KJV

Jesus our Savior came to heal and save and He continue to do so through this horrific pandemic and man-paranoia! As He healed and saved the publican of little statue Zaccheus in the past so today, tomorrow and to the end of the world: And Jesus said unto him, This day is salvation come to this house, for so much as he also is a son of Abraham. [10] For the Son of man is come to seek and to save that which was lost.

St Paul words are: "I therefore, the prisoner of the Lord, beseech you that ye walk worthy of the vocation wherewith ye are called, [2] With all lowliness and meekness, with longsuffering, forbearing one another in love; [3] Endeavouring to keep the unity of the Spirit in the bond of peace. [4] There is one body, and one Spirit, even as ye are called in one hope of your calling; [5] One Lord, one faith, one baptism, [6] One God and Father of all, who is above all, and through all, and in you all. [7] But unto every one of us is given grace according to the measure of the gift of Christ." Ephesians 4:1-7 KJV

Ramsis Ghaly

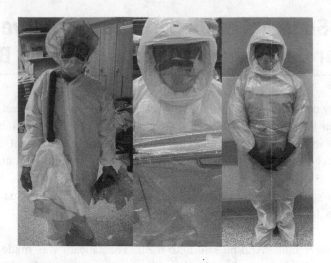

SS. 🍀🍀💜😄💜🍀 Amen
JC. Merry Christmas, Dr. Ghaly. Miss seeing you!
RN. Sending blessings Dr. Ghaly. 💜🙏🙏
ML. Many Blessings Dr. Ramsis Ghaly
🙏😊💜

The 2020 Christmas Trees are lonely This Year

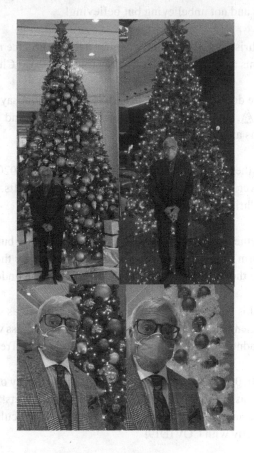

The 2020 Christmas Trees 🎄🎄🎄 are lonely This Year!! Please Don't let it Be!!! A Poem Dedicated to you all and to your children and grand great children!

The 2020 Christmas Trees 🎄🎄🎄 are lonely this year! Please don't let it be that way! The streets are dark and surrounding is gloomy! Let us spread love ♥ and help me to bring life back! The Christmas 🎄 is near and Baby Jesus newborn day is almost here! Let us receive Him in joy and be ready for His coming! Let not COVID-19 disrupt His Birthday or take our feast away! Jesus the Lord is God of the living and not of the dead! Let the pandemic have no control on us the believers and faithful servants! Jesus is our King and Lord! He is our True Healer and protector!

Let us lighten the streets and turn the lights by our cities and the Christmas hymns at our homes! Let us go out joyful obedient to the restriction but believing in the birth of our Lord Jesus and what Christmas 🎄 all about! Not in fear but in courage, not in despair but in hope, not in weakness but strength, not in sickness but in wholeness and not unbelieving but believing!

Find the 2020 Christmas 🎄 tree and give her a kiss with face mask on and hug her with your arms and tell her! "Merry Christmas thy 2020 Christmas Tree"

O my soul, please don't pass a 2020 Christmas Tree without saying: "Hello 2020 Christmas Tree 🎄, give me a kiss with my face mask on and I will give you a hug with my arms all around thee"

It is freezing out there! It is snowing out there! Enrich each 2020 Christmas Tree out there and cover her with your warmth and fill it with gifts 🎁! Please don't let any of 2020 Christmas Tree naked or abandoned!

Let us go all together distancing away 6 feet apart physically but tight spiritually and mutually warm in love 😍🥰😘 and kisses! Let us buy the ornaments, put the Star ☆ from the East on the top and the nativity scene under the tree!

Let us get busy this year, go out in joy and sing the Christmas songs! The songs sound pleasant when you sing from under the mask! Let us dress with bright colors and leave your sadness at the bottom of the 2020 Christmas Tree 🎄!

Let us feed the 2020 Christmas Tree 🎄 and let it not to be dry or malnourished!! The 2020 Christmas Tree loves ♥ water and liveth in the sweets! Let us pay a visit and light a candle and say a prayer for all people and in particular those suffered directly or indirectly with COVID19!

But let us keep the 2020 Christmas Tree 🎄 clean and neat! Let us spray it with antivirus spray and wash our hands and don't stop the breeze and let the leaves wave 👋 hellos!

Let us fear not, the 2020 Christmas shall bring much of good tidings of great joy to all people as it is written: "And the angel said unto them, Fear not: for, behold, I bring you good tidings of great joy, which shall be to all people. [11] For unto you is born this day in the city of David a Saviour, which is Christ the Lord." Luke 2:10-11 KJV

It is that time of the year, let us go shopping with the three wisemen the country shepherds watchmen at night and search for the gifts to bring and place them under the tree 🎄! Under the 2020 Christmas Tree 🎄 shall be the treasures we bring with our hearts for Baby Jesus Birthday 2020 Christmas!

I wonder who will join the shepherds to present the 2020 Christmas 🎄 gifts the gold, frankincense and myrrh, to our Newborn Savior by the manager at Bethlehem under the Christmas Tree 🎄. It is more than ever this Christmas: "And when they were come into the house, they saw the young child with Mary his mother, and fell down, and worshipped him: and when they had opened their treasures, they presented unto him gifts; gold, and frankincense, and myrrh." Matthew 2:11 KJV

Now it is the time to put on the light 💡 and thousands of bulbs 💡💡💡 and illuminate Jesus 2020 Christmas Tree 🎄! Let us praise Newborn Baby Jesus saying with the heavenly hosts: "Glory to God in the highest, and on earth peace, good will toward men." Luke 2:14 KJV You might be surprised! Baby Jesus might be under that 2020 Christmas Tree 🎄🎄🎄!

The 2020 Christmas Tree! 🎄🎄🎄

Ramsis Ghaly

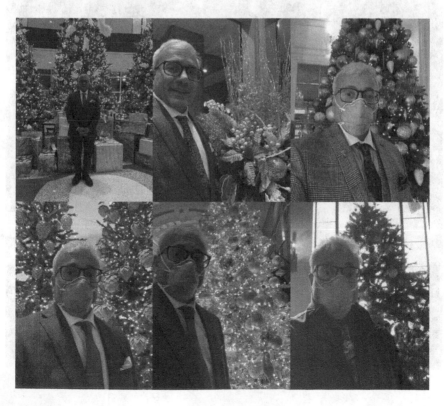

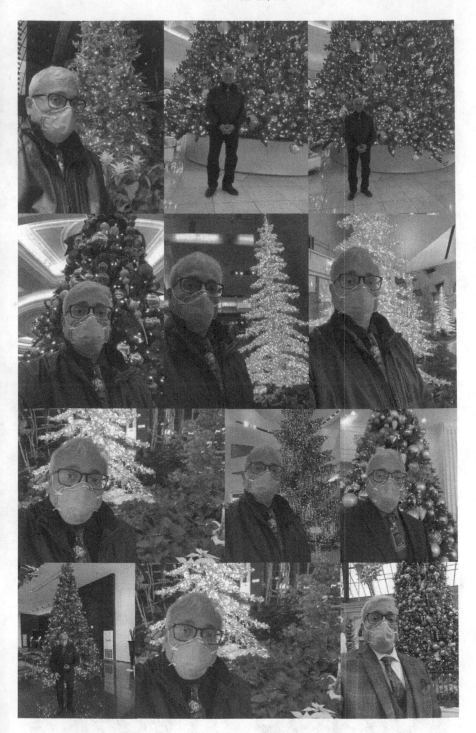

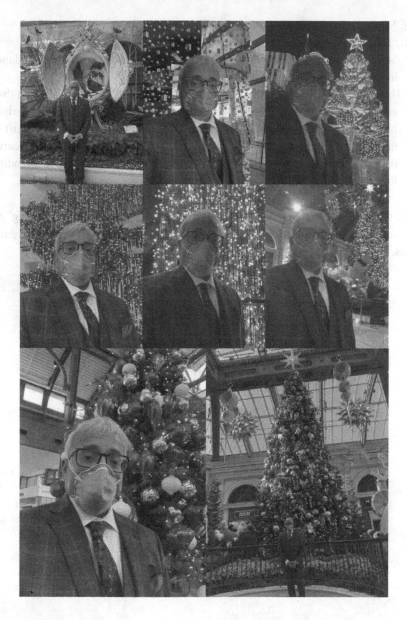

JE. Beautiful!!!! Thank you!

PP. Happy Holidays Doc!

ML. Beautiful poem Dr. Ghaly.

KG. LOVE this Dr. Ghaly 🖤. Thank you for bringing a bright smile to my face. 😃🌲🌲🌲

CG. This delightful! Thank you for bringing a little cheer into our lives. 🖤🙏🌲

RC. It is a beauty, my mother loves to put the Christmas tree

KE. M*Christmas Ramsis*

JM. "Fabulous" Photos of you and the "Christmas Trees" 💕

NP. Merry Christmas Doc! May God continue to Bless you with an Abundance in all you do 🙏

JP. Thank you fellow journeyman on our road to home. This year, more so than any other year, I have intentionally switched my focus on the One who's birthday we are celebrating. The greatest gift I can give Him, is the gift of myself serving others. When it is safe to do so, my quest will be to search the possibilities. Thank you for your inspirational posts and your unending love of all God's children. 💜

Take the time to read this post. I accidentally found this man while "snooping" on someone's posts I'm not friends with. He is the hands and feet of Jesus on a daily basis. If you like this post, like his page.

In Christmas Eve Mass in the Streets Respecting Distancing Away and Socially Protected!

Ramsis Ghaly

Look how wonderful those faithful servants are reaching out to Lord Jesus in the streets in His Christmas!!

https://www.facebook.com/100002904253741/posts/2620725801367536/?d=n

Go outside in the streets put your mask and distance away and kneel and outcry to Baby Jesus to have Mercy and to lift up the Pandemic!

Priests, Pastors, Ministers, Popes, Bishops, Deacons and Congregations go out in the streets in the open in humility and sorrowful hearts and outcry to Baby Jesus to lift up the wrath of God!

Let us get out of our hidden closets, homes, cars and fields and go out on the streets in unity join those souls in one voice lifting up our hearts and raiding our hands and looking up heaven to Our Savior!!

Let us repent and cast out evils among us especially those pedophiles committed hundreds of years of extreme sin to the little children, the angels of God on earth 🌍 The earth is cursed because of them!

Let us go out in the streets and join the prodigal son and those worshippers throughout the world 🌍!! We have sinned O Lord, have mercy on us! Let us listen to the words of Jeremiah outcry: Jeremiah 3:25 Let us lie down in our shame, and let our humiliation cover us; for we have sinned against the Lord our God, we and our fathers, from our youth even to this day. And we have not obeyed the voice of the Lord our God."

Luke 15:18 I will get up and go to my father, and will say to him, "Father, I have sinned against heaven, and in your sight; Luke 15:21 And the son said to him, 'Father, I have sinned against heaven and in your sight; I am no longer worthy to be called your son.'

379

Nehemiah 1:6 let Your ear now be attentive and Your eyes open to hear the prayer of Your servant which I am praying before You now, day and night, on behalf of the sons of Israel Your servants, confessing the sins of the sons of Israel which we have sinned against You; I and my father's house have sinned.

Psalm 106:6 We have sinned like our fathers,
We have committed iniquity; we have behaved wickedly.

Daniel 9:5 we have sinned, committed iniquity, acted wickedly and rebelled, even turning aside from Your commandments and ordinances.

Lamentations 5:16 The crown has fallen from our head; Woe to us, for we have sinned!

Psalm 41:4 As for me, I said, "O Lord, be gracious to me; Heal my soul, for I have sinned against You."

Daniel 9:11 Indeed all Israel has transgressed Your law and turned aside, not obeying Your voice; so the curse has been poured out on us, along with the oath which is written in the law of Moses the servant of God, for we have sinned against Him.

Daniel 9:15 And now, O Lord our God, who have brought Your people out of the land of Egypt with a mighty hand and have made a name for Yourself, as it is this day—we have sinned, we have been wicked.

Numbers 21:7 So the people came to Moses and said, "We have sinned, because we have spoken against the Lord and you; intercede with the Lord, that He may remove the serpents from us." And Moses interceded for the people.

Deuteronomy 1:41 Then you said to me, 'We have sinned against the Lord; we will indeed go up and fight, just as the Lord our God commanded us.' And every man of you girded on his weapons of war, and regarded it as easy to go up into the hill country.

Judges 10:10 Then the sons of Israel cried out to the Lord, saying, "We have sinned against You, for indeed, we have forsaken our God and served the Baals."

Judges 10:15 The sons of Israel said to the Lord, "We have sinned, do to us whatever seems good to You; only please deliver us this day."

1 Samuel 7:6 They gathered to Mizpah, and drew water and poured it out before the Lord, and fasted on that day and said there, "We have sinned against the Lord." And Samuel judged the sons of Israel at Mizpah.

1 Samuel 12:10 They cried out to the Lord and said, 'We have sinned because we have forsaken the Lord and have served the Baals and the Ashtaroth; but now deliver us from the hands of our enemies, and we will serve You.'

Jeremiah 14:7 Although our iniquities testify against us, O Lord, act for Your name's sake!

Truly our apostasies have been many,

We have sinned against You.

Jeremiah 14:20 We know our wickedness, O Lord,
The iniquity of our fathers, for we have sinned against You.

Daniel 9: Open shame belongs to us, O Lord, to our kings, our princes and our fathers, because we have sinned against You.

Lamentations 3:42 We have transgressed and rebelled, You have not pardoned.

1 Kings 8:47 if they take thought in the land where they have been taken captive, and repent and make supplication to You in the land of those who have taken them captive, saying, 'We have sinned and have committed iniquity, we have acted wickedly';

Genesis 20:9 Then Abimelech called Abraham and said to him, "What have you done to us? And how have I sinned against you, that you have brought on me and on my kingdom a great sin? You have done to me things that ought not to be done."

1 Kings 1:21 Otherwise it will come about, as soon as my lord the king sleeps with his fathers, that I and my son Solomon will be considered offenders."

2 Kings 7:9 Then they said to one another, "We are not doing right. This day is a day of good news, but we are keeping silent; if we wait until morning light, punishment will overtake us. Now therefore come, let us go and tell the king's household."

Joshua 7:20 So Achan answered Joshua and said, "Truly, I have sinned against the Lord, the God of Israel, and this is what I did:

Numbers 22:34 Balaam said to the angel of the Lord, "I have sinned, for I did not know that you were standing in the way against me. Now then, if it is displeasing to you, I will turn back."

2 Samuel 12:13 Then David said to Nathan, "I have sinned against the Lord." And Nathan said to David, "The Lord also has taken away your sin; you shall not die.

2 Samuel 24:10 Now David's heart troubled him after he had numbered the people. So David said to the Lord, "I have sinned greatly in what I have done. But now, O Lord, please take away the iniquity of Your servant, for I have acted very foolishly."

2 Kings 18:14 Then Hezekiah king of Judah sent to the king of Assyria at Lachish, saying, "I have done wrong. Withdraw from me; whatever you impose on me I will bear." So the king of Assyria required of Hezekiah king of Judah three hundred talents of silver and thirty talents of gold.

Job 7:20 Have I sinned? What have I done to You,

O watcher of men? Why have You set me as Your target, So that I am a burden to myself?

Matthew 27:4 saying, "I have sinned by betraying innocent blood." But they said, "What is that to us? See to that yourself!"

Exodus 9:27 Then Pharaoh sent for Moses and Aaron, and said to them, "I have sinned this time; the Lord is the righteous one, and I and my people are the wicked ones.

Exodus 10:16 Then Pharaoh hurriedly called for Moses and Aaron, and he said, "I have sinned against the Lord your God and against you.

1 Samuel 15:24 Then Saul said to Samuel, "I have sinned; I have indeed transgressed the command of the Lord and your words, because I feared the people and listened to their voice.

1 Samuel 15:3 Then he said, "I have sinned; but please honor me now before the elders of my people and before Israel, and go back with me, that I may worship the Lord your God."

1 Samuel 26:21 Then Saul said, "I have sinned. Return, my son David, for I will not harm you again because my life was precious in your sight this day. Behold, I have played the fool and have committed a serious error."

2 Samuel 19:20 For your servant knows that I have sinned; therefore behold, I have come today, the first of all the house of Joseph to go down to meet my lord the king."

Job 33:27 He will sing to men and say,
'I have sinned and perverted what is right,
And it is not proper for me.

Cr. Lord hear the cries of your children!

Merry Christmas and happy new year!

Praying for you all staying safe. Thank you for Your kindness and wonderful heart Love and Blessing!

Early morning joining the worshippers worldwide in the Church of our Lord and Savior listening to the heavenly hosts "Glory to God in the highest, and on earth peace, good will toward men." Luke 2:14

Going to the manger of our Savior incarnated Son God in the flesh praising Him and praying 🙏 with the three countrymen offering gold, and frankincense, and myrrh.

"For unto you is born this day in the city of David a Saviour, which is Christ the Lord. [12] And this shall be a sign unto you; Ye shall find the babe wrapped in swaddling clothes, lying in a manger. [13] And suddenly there was with the angel a multitude of the heavenly host praising God, and saying, [14] Glory to God in the highest, and on earth peace, good will toward men." Luke 2:11-13

"And when they were come into the house, they saw the young child with Mary his mother, and fell down, and worshipped him: and when they had opened their treasures, they presented unto him gifts; gold, and frankincense, and myrrh." Matthew 2:11 KJV

And in Joy uttering psalm 100: Make a joyful noise unto the Lord, all ye lands. [2] Serve the Lord with gladness: come before his presence with singing. [3] Know ye that the Lord he is God: it is he that hath made us, and not we ourselves; we are his people, and the sheep of his pasture. [4] Enter into his gates with thanksgiving, and into his courts with praise: be thankful unto him, and bless his name. [5] For the Lord is good; his mercy is everlasting; and his truth endureth to all generations. Psalm 100

[OBJ] Merry Christmas 🎄 and happy new year to you all!

Praying for you all staying safe!

Thank you for Your kindness and wonderful hearts 💜! Love and Blessing

Ramsis Ghaly

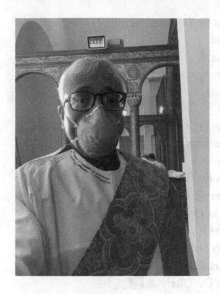

HC. Merry Christmas

AS. Merry Christmas

VG. Merry Christmas Dr Ghaly 🎄🎄

PV. Merry Christmas Dr Ghaly

JB. Amen and Merry Christmas and a Happy, Healthy New Year Dr. Ghaly! 🙏💜

RS. ميلاد مجيد و كل عام وانت بالف خير

VS. Merry Christmas 🎁🎄

BM. Merry Christmas and God Bless you always!

AB. Merry Christmas, Brother!

LP. Merry Christmas to you and your family!

DS. Merry Christmas

JP. Merry Christmas

NP. Happy Birthday Jesus 💜 Today is a day to rejoice for the King was born, glory to God 🙌 Merry Christmas Sweetheart 🎄 May you and your Beautiful Family enjoy this blessed day 🙏💜

BS. Merry Christmas!

DZ. MR. Wish you a blessed merry Christmas doctor and God bless you

JC. Merry Christmas Dr.Ghaly 🎄✨🎁🎄

CP. Merry Christmas & Happy New Year. 😊

JC. VV. Merry Christmas

DE. Merry Christmas 🎄

RN. Merry Christmas Dr. Ghaly many blessings to you 💜💜

AG. Merry Christmas Dr RW. Merry Christmas and Happy New Year!

IM. Merry Christmas 🎁🎄

DS. Merry Christmas! Dr. Ghaly..Be safe! Be Blessed 🤍🎄💜🙏

385

PR. Merry Christmas to YOU and family.
DC. Merry Christmas
DT. Merry Christmas 🎄
DS. Merry Christmas brother. 😊😊
MW. Merry Christmas
AL. Feliz navidad 🎄
AS. Merry Christmas Dr. G
SH. Merry Christmas!! 🖤
SK. Merry Christmas!! 🎄
DI. Merry Christmas Dr Ghaly!
AR. Merry Christmas dr. Ghaly!
MA. Merry Christmas Dr.
AA. Merry Christmas Ramsis, many blessings.
CC. Merry Christmas Dr. Ghaly
NH. Merry Christmas & Happy New year
SP. Merry Christmas Dr. Ghaly 🎄🖼️🙏
WP. Same to you, Dr. Ghaly 🎄
SS. Merry Christmas
CP. Merry Christmas Dr. Ghaly. God bless. 🖤🙏🎄
KG. Merry Christmas Dr. Ghaly 🎄. God bless you 🙏
PP. Merry Christmas Dr. Ghaly!
RW. Merry Christmas Dr. Ghaly! It's a perfect Christmas because Hunter is doing great thanks to you! God bless you
PP. Merry Christmas 🎄
RM. Merry Christmas Dr Ghaly 🎄 Have a wonderful day 💐
VW. Merry Christmas 🎁
MB. Merry Christmas 🎄
TA. merry Christmas 🎄🎁
LS. Merry Christmas. 🎄
NE. Merry Christmas 🎄🎁
SN. Merry Christmas Dr.Ghaly. ✨🙏🖤
CS. Merry Christmas
JS. Merry Christmas 🎄
RB. Merry Christmas
EB. Merry Christmas 🎁✨
TM. Merry Christmas 🎁🖤🙏
KC. Merry Christmas, Dr. Ghaly!
BP. Merry Christmas doc!
Hope the New Year grants your every wish! 🖤
HM. Merry Christmas Dr. Ghaly!
MC. Feliz Navidad Dr.Ghaly y familia!!
AP. GC/. erry Christmas! Peace and Joy to you always!!

RP. Merry Christmas doctor and God bless you 🤗😊🎄🙏

SH. Merry Christmas 🎄🥂

KO. Merry Christmas 🎄🎁

HW. God bless you, merry Christmas 🖤

BL. I will be praying for you as well, Dr Ghaly. Have a blessed new year.

LS. Merry Christmas 🎄

MP. Feliz Navidad, Dios lo bendiga Doctor.

EH. Merry Christmas

JP. Merry Christmas

GK. ميلاد مجيد، لقد ولد مخلصنا يسوع المسيح.

CP. Be safe! God bless you always 🙏

PV. Merry Christmas!

VG. Srecan Božic dr.Bog vas blagoslovio! 🎄🎄🎄🙏

ZC. Wishing you peace and joy throughout the season Dr.Ghally. 🎄
🌹🌷🌐🌞

AH. Merry Christmas !!

TS. Merry Christmas 🎄

SI. Have a very Merry Christmas 🎄 Dr. Ghaly

LY. Merry Christmas Dr. Ghaly!

JJ. Merry Christmas!!!

May God bless you and protect you greatly. You are a great man of faith. An example to all.

JR. Merry Christmas

CT. Godspeed and God bless you my Friend, be well, Merry Christmas 🎁

KO. Merry Christmas Dr Ghaly, Lord keep you safe and healthy

RH. God Bless you Merry Christmas to the doctor that keeps on giving. Love to you doctor

AM. I hope you have some air flowing under there Dr.

AS. 🙏 merry Christmas 🍪🎂🎄

BH. Merry Christmas Dear Ramsis. May your holidays be filled with love, peace, hope and some semblance of nornalcy. Rest and God Bless you sweet man! 🖤🙏🖤

Now, about that outfit...stay safe at all cost!

SL. Merry Christmas 🎄🎁

YA. Merry Christmas 🎄🎁

JC. Merry Chrtistmas!

BM. Merry Christmas Dr. Ghaly.

KG. Merry Christmas 2020. God Bless you

Stay safe

Stay well…

RF. Merry Christmas

SA. Merry Christmas! Christ is the reason for this season. Gods blessings

NV. Merry Christmas 🌲 Doctor Ghaly, God Bless you and stay safe

TF. Merry Christmas 🌲🎁

VM. Merry Christmas bff

LW. You could have scared me......enjoy the holidays despite 🙏🙏

JS. 🎊🎁🎿🎄🌲🌲🌳 Merry Christmas & Blessed New Year 🌲🌲🎍🎊🎁🎿 🏘️⛪😇 May God Bless 🙏✝️😇, Protect, And Lead You & Your Blessed Family 👪💕👫 The Way Unto His Kingdom! 📩🏰⛪

AV. Merry Christmas

LA. Wishing you a very Blessed, Peaceful, and Merry Christmas, Dr. !! Praying for a hedge of God's protection around you as you care for and serve others. 💚🙏💜

AG. same to you Dr. Ghaly. Wishing you healthy happiness love and lots more

In the Post-Christmas Day I am for another day in the Service!

But thanks God COVID Chicago cases are slowing down, But Not because of the Vaccine! Hope it last forever!!

Nonetheless, there is still a threat of new strains moving from CA, UK, Japan and France!

https://www.latimes.com/.../l-a-county-is-probing-whether...
https://apple.news/AzABWLHZvRmyTK2WSrBF7ZQ

Let us pray!

Ramsis Ghaly

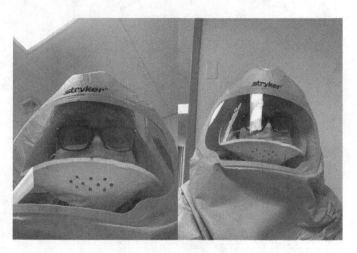

JB. Stay safe and healthy! 🖤🙏
DE. 🙏🙏🙏
CD. Merry Christmas and Happy New Year!
CP. Stay safe 🖤🙏
CP. Happy New Year. ☺
VG. 🙏🙏🙏
BL. I hope you had a blessed Christmas Day. Thank you for the update on the COVID status in Chicago. 💜
CD. Merry Christmas and Happy New Year

NV. 🙏

MB. Oh Lord have Mercy! 🙏🙏🙏 Be safe Dr. Ghaly.

BCD. Thank you for your dedication Sir

ML: You are an angel Dr. Ramsis Ghaly

!❤🙏

KJ. Praying always for your health and safety. Right now my best m'y dearest best friend is on life support and is failing. He has Coronavirus and is in I.C.U. in Palm Springs, Ca.. His name is STOGE AMAROV. His Daughter Jenny just called me. PLEASE PRAY FOR HIM IN THE NAME OF GOD. AMEN, Love, Kammy Jones

Christmas 2020 by the
Mountains of the Lord!

A calling to my soul: "Rise my son and head to the mountains of the Lord where a Christmas feast of the Birthday of Jesus the Savior be for 2020. Tell the people and the inhabitants of earth. The pandemic is dispersing the children of the lord and running them away from celebrating our Savior Birth"

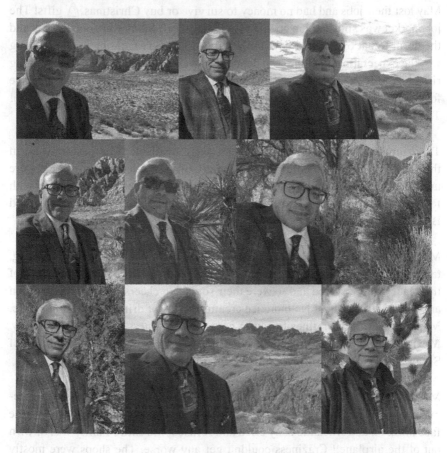

I immediately jumped took a shower washed and out my mountain Christmasy cloth, jeans 👖 with leather jacket 🧥 and Santa Claus tie **Père Noël [pɛʁ nɔ.ɛl]**), 'Papa Noël'. I packed my car with hiking 👟 materials and bottles of water!

Merry Christmas was indeed rare in 2020 as if it was the determination of Satan and his followers!!

It was early on the dawn and many sleeping in their homes. There was nothing going on outside but dark streets and signs of Don in, stay at home order and limit the outdoors social gathering!

Things happen so fast and I didn't see a need to wake up my neighbors or inform my family and friends! The mood anyhow was gloomy with no much of Christmas celebration outside and inside the homes were silent Christmas trees with sadness across the globe 🌎!

May lost their jobs and had no money to survive or buy Christmas 🎄 gifts! The job market was slim and job opening was almost nil! Many were out of work and the norm to eat one meal a day! Poverty became overwhelming and borrowing was the expectations! Famine and depression were in the way! Many were taking risks just to feed their children and support loved ones! Families might survive for few weeks with no jobs but no one could survives with months with no job! There were no much of savings or credits but majority was on debt!

The churches were closed and few seats were available. The pastors were in the hid and so were the politicians and many of the leaders and ministers were unreachable. The restaurants were shut and those were open were numbered with few seats! No more social gathering or getting together. The outing, cinemas and Bars were forbidden. The city walls were shut and the law was enforced.

Madness to say the least. I say again madness say the soul. People were walking, talking and working with face masks and further away from each other. Half of their faces were covered and so were their souls! No cheers but rather depression and hidden nightmares! No more ice creams or sips of drinks allowed in public. Many were waiting in lines trying to cover their sadness and limit the curfew. **Merry Christmas was indeed rare in 2020 as if it was the determination of Satan and his followers!!**

Many had enough and were coming out their cloths. I saw many threw their face-masks away! Can you imagine a flight attendant demand a two years old to put the face mask on and when the baby cried and refused, the entire family was thrown out of the airplane!! Craziness couldn't get any worse. The shops were mostly closed and those open were allowed to function in half and the stores must limit their customers. Yet the retails still suppose to make living to fight the imminent crash in economy!

Common sense weren't in existence as the gab was widened between reality and fake distant reality. Walking lonely and shopping 🛍 on line became the

norm as Telemedicine, Teleconferencing, Microsoft Team and video zooming. And man more were conducted through wireless and digital technology through the complex electronics and circuitries!

It is a stand of artificial technology and man made electronic minds against humanity and human brains! It is a war between man for technology or technology for man. Human independence or human subservient to artificial technology and robots!!!

Virtual reality was the actual reality and remote learning the 2020 tutoring agenda! Who knows perhaps coming soon total transformation of True Reality to Virtual Reality and Personal Existence to Virtual Existence!! God forbid man grandiosity will ever thought that he could create an electronic brain to replace a human brain ☺ created by the Almighty!!! At that time, God shall disperse man and do what He had done to man behind tower of Babylon! "And they said, Go to, let us build us a city and a tower, whose top may reach unto heaven; and let us make us a name, lest we be scattered abroad upon the face of the whole earth. [5] And the Lord came down to see the city and the tower, which the children of men builded. [6] And the Lord said, Behold, the people is one, and they have all one language; and this they begin to do: and now nothing will be restrained from them, which they have imagined to do. [7] Go to, let us go down, and there confound their language, that they may not understand one another's speech. [8] So the Lord scattered them abroad from thence upon the face of all the earth: and they left off to build the city. [9] Therefore is the name of it called Babel; because the Lord did there confound the language of all the earth: and from thence did the Lord scatter them abroad upon the face of all the earth." Genesis 11:4-9 KJV

The ambulance Sirens were heard every day and many go and few come back to their homes! The sorrows and screams were heard from faraway and the rivers of tears were sweeping from under the doors and gates!

It was heartbreaking and I couldn't take it anymore every night I went to my bed and hit my sacks I prayed to my Lord and plead for help! Life on our land was shut down. Break through humanity and winds blow in their faces and flipped daily living upside down. Much loss with no gain. Terrors, fears and unhappiness were spreading everyday with no sign of relief.

The calling was timely as the heaven heard my supplication. I didn't hesitate to leave my nest and run away to the Lord of mountains!

The mountains ⚠ are made for Christmas as Christmas also made for the mountains of the Lord. Let us go O my soul and spend the 2020 Christmas faraway from the world and it's COVID!

The winds were hard and the fresh air free of viruses 〇〇〇 was abundantly, and word of unlimited or too much wasn't enough to describe! I was certain the coronavirus virus 〇〇〇 won't dare to come close and would be crushed instantly!

O my Lord Jesus thank you ⚒ for taking my soul away from the world 📖 of madness and the craziness of the governors! The rulers of the earth had nothing to offer except house arrest and send the people away with empty hands! In fact the science 💊 💊 of human minds developed no treatment to cure and Medicine officials have nothing to administer except experimental mixtures to try!

Indeed my Lord, these tiny particles and the invisible nano viruses 〇〇〇 showed that man is nothing and his brain worth pennies without You our Heavenly Father!

Christmas at the mountains ⚠ full of serenity and tranquility away from the turmoil of the world and COVID-19!

The distraction is disturbing between the COVID-19 and election results and the pending crash in economy and who knows what else artificial intelligence and little satans are planning to do!

It is all meant to distract the children of Jesus from His Birthday! Therefore, let us go the mountains away away from the noisy world 🌍 and be with our Lord Jesus and His parents and the three wisemen!

The holy family isn't in the Inn but they will be by the manager in the mountains ⚠ of the Lord! There is no facemask required or PPE or distancing away since COVID never made it by the deserts! COVID-19 will never dare to come close to the mountains of the Lord. The fresh air is flowing and the winds are blowing and there is nothing to worry about but be at peace with the Lord be cheerful at Christmas by the mountains ⚠.

As I was walking slowly, I heard sounds of moving waters followed by a soft breeze. I walked toward the waters and I saw green trees and a small lake with little fish swimming in it. The spring waters was a good treat for my journey and was good break to witness life and living in the way to the mountains. The soil was rich in the middle of the desert. It is a gorgeous little park made possible by desert springs. The fain falling in the deserts and highlands let the rainwaters seeps unto the ground to an aquifer as the waters mix with inner rock brings heat to the spring waters and life with minerals!

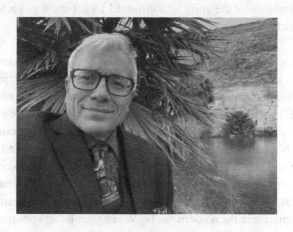

I took a little break praising my Lord fur His treat and kept driving to reach my Destiny! To my surprise, I wasn't alone. The Holy Spirit invited many souls and has put it in the hearts of many to leave the city and meet Him by the mountains at the Lord's Day in Christmas 2020. However, only the sincere worshippers shall join our journey to meet Baby Jesus by the Mountains ⛰ of the Lord!

It is the time to celebrate Christmas 🎄 by the mountains ⛰⛰ whereas neither COVID-19 nor laws of man-made restrictions!

At the mountains God the Almighty enforces neither curfews nor masks and PPE but freedom and truth without limits!

Up high the sky has no limit as the top of the mountains continues with the clouds ☁ where the earth and heaven become one and diffuse together boundless.

At the mountains ⛰⛰ the Heavenly Father rejuvenate the human soul and dress her with the wings to fly like an eagle 🦅!

At the mountains ⛰⛰ where the sand meet the snow and the sun ☀ meets the clouds ☁☁, the greenery with the yellow leaves and the dry land with the wells!

I parked my SUV 🚐 by the Base and walked my way then. Step by step singing Christmas 🎄 songs and praising the Newborn Baby Jesus with the Christmas hymns. The Spirit of the Lord overshadowed the mountains as at the times of my father Moses by the Sinai!

The air was blowing harshly and pushed me from side to side and in between the by the quiescence of the spirit of solitude! I forgot my way back and I didn't remember which direction I left my car!

I start to sing with my father David the Psalmist Psalm 95 "O come, let us sing unto the Lord: let us make a joyful noise to the rock of our salvation. [2] Let us come before his presence with thanksgiving, and make a joyful noise unto him with psalms. [3] For the Lord is a great God, and a great King above all gods. [4] In his hand are the deep places of the earth: the strength of the mountains is his also. [5] The sea is his, and he made it: and his hands formed the dry land. [6] O come, let us worship and bow down: let us kneel before the Lord our maker. [7] For he is our God; and we are the people of his pasture, and the sheep of his hand. To day if ye will hear his voice, [8] Harden not your heart, as in the provocation, and as in the day of temptation in the wilderness: [9] When your fathers tempted me, proved me, and saw my work. [10] Forty years long was I grieved with this generation, and said, It is a people that do err in their heart, and they have not known my ways: [11] Unto whom I sware in my wrath that they should not enter into my rest."

I took frequent breaks, walk much, rest little until I finally I got tired from walking as I felt it was many miles had been with these heavy boots 🥾. It was freezing cold with showers of snows. The mountain sands were covered with snow!

I reached a den deep within the rock as I ran out of energy and fatigued. It was God sent a Rest stop ⬤. I took out two wood sticks and made fire 🔥 wood 🪵 to warm up. It was a romantic night with my Lord at the mountains 🏔 faraway from the world and the noise of the cities.

There were no announcement boards or earthly proclamation or by manmade laws! It was all for the Lord and all things are His and His Name was written allover the mountains! Gorgeous and splendid to spend Christmas by the mountains 🏔 all alone. He has my soul and I have Him and nothing in between or any excuse to separate Us apart!

I sang with the psalmist psalm 121: "I will lift up mine eyes to the mountains, from whence cometh my help. [2] My help cometh from the Lord, which made heaven and earth. [3] He will not suffer thy foot to be moved: he that keepeth thee will not slumber. [4] Behold, he that keepeth Israel shall neither slumber nor sleep. [5] The Lord is thy keeper: the Lord is thy shade upon thy right hand. [6] The sun shall not smite thee by day, nor the moon by night. [7] The Lord shall preserve thee from all evil: he shall preserve thy soul. [8] The Lord shall preserve thy going out and thy coming in from this time forth, and even for evermore."

I kneeled and said my midnight prayers. It was dark deep in the den but the moon and stars lightened the mountains. My mind drifted deep in the heart of the Spirit. It was a night of meditations and reflections!

I fell unto deep sleep wandering where could I put my Christmas tree and prepare the manger to celebrate Jesus Birthday. I cried unto the Lord to show me the way!

I didn't know that the night was the night and Christmas was about to begin! By the dawn next day, I saw unimaginable manger already prepared and ready to go. There was a light 💡 emanated from within and little ❄️ by the top!

I screamed loudly calling upon the Lord of Lord: Hallelujah hallelujah hallelujah to the Lord God Glory to You and welcome to thy land. I ran as fast as I could gasping from my breath.

And suddenly, I heard with my ears the words spoken to the three wisemen 2020 years ago singing and saying: "And the angel said unto them, Fear not: for, behold, I bring you good tidings of great joy, which shall be to all people. [11] For unto you is born this day in the city of David a Saviour, which is Christ the Lord. [14] Glory to God in the highest, and on earth peace, good will toward men." Luke 2:10-11,14 KJV

It was like a dream and spiritual vision out of space. I was overwhelmed with excitement and kept telling my soul my soul bear with me for a little while. It is the birthday celebration of our Savior.

It is the visitation of my dream 💭, Baby Jesus descended from heaven laying in a manger with swaddling clothes! Praise thy Lord O my Soul praise thy Lord O my soul! "And this shall be a sign unto you; Ye shall find the babe wrapped in swaddling clothes, lying in a manger." I sang with the multitudes of heavenly host singing with them: "And suddenly there was with the angel a multitude of the heavenly host praising God, and saying, [14] Glory to God in the highest, and on earth peace, good will toward men." Luke 2:12-14 KJV

I started to smell the incense filling up the manger and I saw the three wisemen countrymen 🎁 laying by our Savior: the frankincense and the gold and myrrh. I joined them I bowed to the Child Merry Christmas 🏺🎁 my Dear Lord and Savior singing: "Thank You for coming to the world thy created and save the souls of thy children. Welcome 🙏 our Beloved the the Rose of Sharon, the Creator of all things seen and unseen. Holy Holy Holy is thy Name above all names and gods forever and ever Amen 🙏".

My soul was full of joy 😊 and warmth. It was glamorous scenery full of holiness and purity. The Christmas hymns were heard throughout the mountains 🏔️🏔️ and no one could say a word!

I talked my Lord and uttered St Peter words: "Then answered Peter, and said unto Jesus, Lord, it is good for us to be here: if thou wilt, let us make here three tabernacles; one for thee, and one for Moses, and one for Elias." Matthew 17:4 KJV

I heard the biblical words to follow: "While he yet spake, behold, a bright cloud overshadowed them: and behold a voice out of the cloud, which said, This is my beloved Son, in whom I am well pleased; hear ye him." Matthew 17:5 KJV

I immediately found myself my SUV and the voice came: "Go and spread the word of the Gospel and Christmas of Emmanuel which means God is with us" "Now all this was done, that it might be fulfilled which was spoken of the Lord by the prophet, saying, [23] Behold, a virgin shall be with child, and shall bring forth a son, and they shall call his name Emmanuel, which being interpreted is, God with us." Matthew 1:22-23 KJV

Indeed it was an experience of my life time! It was a miniature of what about to come when thy children liveth in thy tabernacle as it is written: "And I heard a great voice out of heaven saying, Behold, the tabernacle of God is with men, and he will dwell with them, and they shall be his people, and God himself shall be with them, and be their God." Revelation 21:3 KJV

"And, behold, I come quickly; and my reward is with me, to give every man according as his work shall be. [13] I am Alpha and Omega, the beginning and the end, the first and the last. [14] Blessed are they that do his commandments, that they may have right to the tree of life, and may enter in through the gates into the city. [17] And the Spirit and the bride say, Come. And let him that heareth say, Come. And let him that is athirst come. And whosoever will, let him take the water of life freely. [20] He which testifieth these things saith, Surely I come quickly. Amen. Even so, come, Lord Jesus. [21] The grace of our Lord Jesus Christ be with you all. Amen." Revelation 22:12-14,17,20-21 KJV

Amen 🙏 Come Lord Jesus Amen 🙏 Come Baby Jesus Amen 🙏 Come!

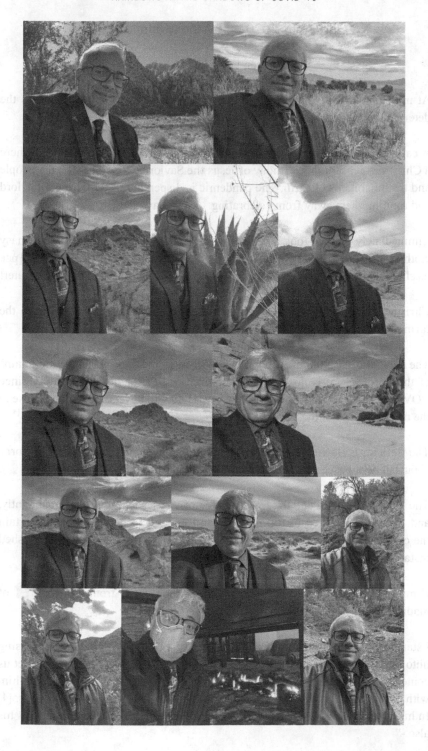

Christmas 2020 🌲 by the Mountains 🏔️!

Written by Ramsis Ghaly

At my Hometown, Merry Christmas was indeed rare in 2020 as if it was the determination of satan and his followers!!

A calling to my soul: "Rise my son and head to the mountains of the Lord where a Christmas feast of the Birthday of Jesus the Savior be for 2020. Tell the people and the inhabitants of earth. The pandemic is dispersing the children of the lord and running them away from celebrating 🐱 our Savior Birth"

I immediately jumped took a shower washed and out my mountain Christmasy cloth, jeans 👖 with a suit, a leather jacket 🧥 and Santa Claus tie Père Noël [pɛʁ nɔ.ɛl]), 'Papa Noël'. I packed my car with hiking 🥾 materials and bottles of water!

Christmas at the mountains 🏔️ full of serenity and tranquility away from the turmoil of the world and COVID-19!

The holy family isn't in the Inn but they will be by the manager in the mountains of the Lord! There is no facemask required or PPE or distancing away since COVID never made it by the deserts! COVID-19 will never dare to come close to the mountains 🏔️ of the Lord.

The fresh air is flowing and the winds are blowing and there is nothing to worry about but be at peace with the Lord be cheerful at Christmas by the mountains 🏔️.

The winds were hard and the fresh air free of viruses 🦠🦠🦠 was abundantly, and word of unlimited or too much wasn't enough to describe! I was certain the coronavirus virus 🦠🦠🦠 won't dare to come close and would be crushed instantly!

O my Lord Jesus thank you 🙏 for taking my soul away from the world 📖 of madness and the craziness!

I start to sing with my father David the Psalmist Psalm 95 "O come, let us sing unto the Lord: let us make a joyful noise to the rock of our salvation. [2] Let us come before his presence with thanksgiving, and make a joyful noise unto him with psalms. [3] For the Lord is a great God, and a great King above all gods. [4] In his hand are the deep places of the earth: the strength of the mountains is his also.-"

As I was driving slowly, I heard sounds of moving waters followed by a soft breeze. I walked toward the waters and I saw green trees and a small lake with little fish swimming in it. The spring waters was a good treat for my journey and was good break to witness life and living in the way to the mountains. The soil was rich in the middle of the desert. It is a gorgeous little park made possible by desert springs. The rain falling in the deserts and highlands let the rainwaters seeps unto the ground to an aquifer as the waters mix with inner rock brings heat to the spring waters and life with minerals!

To my surprise, I wasn't alone. The Holy Spirit has put it in the hearts of many to leave the city and meet Our Savior by the mountains at the Lord's Day in Christmas 🎄 2020. However, only the sincere worshippers shall join our journey to meet Baby Jesus by the Mountains ⛰ of the Lord!

The fresh air is flowing and the winds are blowing and there is nothing to worry about but be at peace with the Lord be cheerful at Christmas by the mountains ⛰.

It is the time to celebrate Christmas 🎄 by the mountains ⛰⛰ whereas neither COVID-19 nor laws of man-made restrictions!

At the mountains God the Almighty enforces neither curfews nor masks and PPE but freedom and truth without limits!

Up high the sky has no limit as the top of the mountains continues with the clouds ☁ where the earth and heaven become one and diffuse together boundless.

At the mountains ⛰⛰ the Heavenly Father rejuvenate the human soul and dress her with the wings to fly like an eagle 🦅!

At the mountains ⛰⛰ where the sand meet the snow and the sun ☀ meets the clouds ☁☁, the greenery with the yellow leaves and the dry land with the wells!

Gorgeous and splendid to spend Christmas by the mountains ⛰ all alone. He has my soul and I have Him and nothing in between or any excuse to separate Us apart! I sang with the psalmist psalm 121: "I will lift up mine eyes to the mountains, from whence cometh my help. [2] My help cometh from the Lord, which made heaven and earth—"

It is the visitation of my dream ☁, Baby Jesus descended from heaven laying in a manger with swaddling clothes! Praise thy Lord O my Soul praise thy Lord O my soul! "And this shall be a sign unto you; Ye shall find the babe wrapped in swaddling clothes, lying in a manger." I sang with the multitudes of heavenly host singing with them: "And suddenly there was with the angel a multitude of the heavenly host praising God, and saying, [14] Glory to God in the highest, and on earth peace, good will toward men." Luke 2:12-14 KJV

I started to smell the incense filling up the manger and I saw the three wisemen countrymen 🧳 laying by our Savior: the frankincense and the gold and myrrh. I joined them I bowed to the Child Merry Christmas 🕯️🧳 my Dear Lord and Savior singing: "Thank You for coming to the world thy created and save the souls of thy children. Welcome our Beloved the the Rose of Sharon, the Creator of all things seen and unseen. Holy Holy Holy is thy Name above all names and gods forever and ever Amen 🙏".

My soul was full of joy 😊🤩 and warmth. It was glamorous scenery full of holiness and purity. The Christmas hymns were heard throughout the mountains 🏔️🏔️ and no one could say a word!

AS. Beautiful
JO. Enjoy your vacation and spiritual retreat! God Bless your time away and may He restore your soul. Merry Christmas! 🎁🌲🌟
DC. God bless and keep you. ✝️🌲🌟
LR. I'm happy for you that you were able to get away to the mountain...and restore your soul.
DL. Peace on Earth.. Good will too you Dr. enjoy your retreat..be Blessed 🙏❤️
NV. Merry Christmas 🌲 and God Bless you 🙏 enjoy your trip 🏔️
CP. Merry Christmas, very nice pictures. ☺️
TF. God Bless and a Merry Christmas 🌲.
HD. Merry Christmas
How wonderful to get away and rejuvenate your mind, body, & spirit with the Lord 🙏❤️
KG. Merry Christmas to you, Dr. Ghaly 🌲
MS. Looking good 😌
SP. Merry Christmas Dr. May God and all of his Angels bless you and keep you safe 🙏🙏🙏
AV. Thank you Dr Ghaly for sharing these beautiful thoughts & prayers! So glad u can get some rest & refresh your body mind & soul with our Lord & Saviour Jesus! God Bless u & watch over you!! 🙏🙏
AR. Merry Christmas!
JT. No mask in all the photos

LM NEnjoy your time away from reality doc. You work hard and desire a break! Happy Holidays to you!

VA. men! 💜

CR, So glad you finally did something for yourself to bring some peace and joy back into your soul and spend this time with Jesus.

AP. Merry Christmas so glad you were able to get well deserved retreat

HH. Merry Christmas My Dr. Ramsis Ghaly and goodwill to all.!!

MR. Merry Christmas 🎄 to you and God bless you

JM. Happy Holidays 💜 Enjoy

CG. You are a master of story telling and of words. Thank you! 💜🗼

JC. Enjoy your relaxing retreat Dr. Ghaly! It looks beautiful there 🏔️☀️🌲 Merry Christmas 🦌 🎄

EM. Enjoy your time with the Lord. Have a wonderful Christmas 💜

RH. I love your tie. Very sharp dressed man. God bless you Dr. in your travels

CG. ou are a master of story telling and of words. Thank you! 💜🗼

JC. Enjoy your relaxing retreat Dr. Ghaly! It looks beautiful there 🏔️☀️🌲 Merry Christmas 🦌 🎄

EM. Enjoy your time with the Lord. Have a wonderful Christmas 💜

RH The rock behind you looks like it's ready to devour you when you weren't looking back

Rhonda Lee Burgess
I see the face of Jesus looking down at you with a pleased expression.

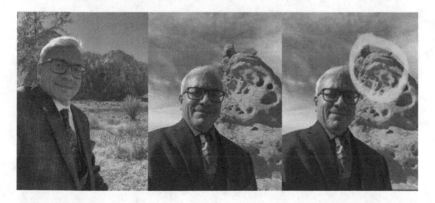

Ramsis Ghaly I pray and trust in Him all the time as you do. I dress for Him Thank you

DS. Ramsis Ghaly

I see it too 🙏🖤

RM. I see it too and it looks like his arm is touching you 🙏🙏🙏

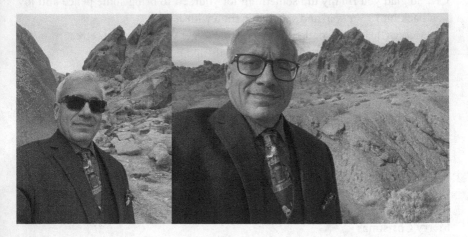

It is That Time to Cry in Sorrows and Griefs by the 2020 Christmas Tree!

Dedicated to Those in Sadness and Grieving in Christmas!

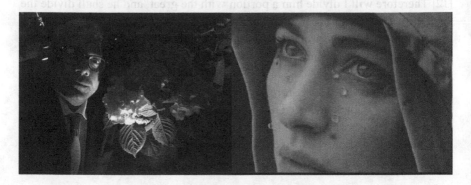

"Blessed are they that mourn: for they shall be comforted." **Matthew 5:4 KJV**

"They that sow in tears shall reap in joy. [6] He that goeth forth and weepeth, bearing precious seed, shall doubtless come again with rejoicing, bringing his sheaves with him." **Psalm 126:5-6 KJV**

It is That Time to Cry 😭 in Sorrows and Griefs by the 2020 Christmas Tree 🎄! It is okay to cry! It is my time to uncover my weakness and shed my tears 😭! There is more words remained and no more could I do but to shed my tears 😭 and cry 😭 by the Christmas Tree!

In Christmas, join me to remember Baby Jesus and all His unbelievable afflictions, sorrows, griefs and pains for our salvations since His birth until His death whom done no wrong and commit no sin. As we walk to the 2020 Christmas Tree 🎄, we carry our own sorrows and griefs and those of our loved ones and of the entire the globe 🌍. Let us shed our tears 😭 by the 2020 Christmas Tree 🎄!

"He is despised and rejected of men; a man of sorrows, and acquainted with grief: and we hid as it were our faces from him; he was despised, and we esteemed him not. [4] Surely he hath borne our griefs, and carried our sorrows: yet we did esteem him stricken, smitten of God, and afflicted. [5] But he was wounded for our transgressions, he was bruised for our iniquities: the chastisement of our peace was upon him; and with his stripes we are healed. [7] He was oppressed, and he was afflicted, yet he opened not his mouth: he is brought as a lamb to the slaughter, and as a sheep before her shearers is dumb, so he openeth not his mouth. [8] He was taken from prison and from judgment: and who shall declare his generation? for he was cut off out of the land of the living: for the transgression of my people was he stricken. [9] And he made his grave with the wicked, and with the rich in his death; because he had done no violence, neither was any deceit in his mouth. [12] Therefore will I divide him a portion with the great, and he shall divide the spoil with the strong; because he hath poured out his soul unto death: and he was numbered with the transgressors; and he bare the sin of many, and made intercession for the transgressors." Isaiah 53:3-5,7-9,12 KJV

It is That Time to Cry 😭 in Sorrows and Griefs by the 2020 Christmas Tree 🎄! I wish together with many could reach out to each of you and wipe your tears and take your sadness away! We all in loss and in each household a mourning rising up to the Lord of Lords and river of tears running through the land and much aches drilling in our bones!

****

It is That Time to Cry 😭 in Sorrows and Griefs by the 2020 Christmas Tree 🎄! It is okay to cry! It is my time to uncover my weakness and shed my tears 😭! There is more words remained and no more could I do but to shed my tears 😭 and cry 😭 by the Christmas Tree!

I sat down by River of Babylon wept when I remembered those in sadness and sorrows especially the COVID Victims: "By the rivers of Babylon, there we sat down, yea, we wept, when we remembered Zion. [2] We hanged our harps upon the willows in the midst thereof. [3] For there they that carried us away captive required of us a song; and they that wasted us required of us mirth, saying, Sing us one of the songs of Zion. [5] If I forget thee, O Jerusalem, let my right hand forget her cunning. [6] If I do not remember thee, let my tongue cleave to the roof of my mouth; if I prefer not Jerusalem above my chief joy. [7] Remember, O Lord, the children of Edom in the day of Jerusalem; who said, Rase it, rase it, even to the foundation thereof. [8] O daughter of Babylon, who art to be destroyed; happy shall he be, that rewardeth thee as thou hast served us. [9] Happy shall he be, that taketh and dasheth thy little ones against the stones." Psalm 137:1-3,5-9 KJV

It is That Time to Cry 😭 in Sorrows and Griefs by the 2020 Christmas Tree 🎄! I wish together with many could reach out to each of you and wipe your tears and take your sadness away! We all in loss and in each household a mourning rising up to the Lord of Lords and river of tears running through the land and much aches drilling in our bones!

****

It is That Time to Cry 😭 in Sorrows and Griefs by the 2020 Christmas Tree 🎄! It is okay to cry! It is my time to uncover my weakness and shed my tears 😭! There is more words remained and no more could I do but to shed my tears 😭 and cry 😭 by the Christmas Tree!

I am a grieving father full of sorrows and have not seen my only son since he attracted COVID four weeks ago! My baby, my flesh and my blood thrown in the intensive care fighting fur his life connected to machines and on life support! I am the dying father about to lose my son, I wish God take my life away and keep my son instead! O my Lord hear my out cry and be attentive to my cry!

"The eyes of the Lord are upon the righteous, and his ears are open unto their cry. [17] The righteous cry, and the Lord heareth, and delivereth them out of all their troubles. [18] The Lord is nigh unto them that are of a broken heart; and saveth such as be of a contrite spirit. [19] Many are the afflictions of the righteous: but the Lord delivereth him out of them all. [20] He keepeth all his bones: not one of them is broken. [21] Evil shall slay the wicked: and they that hate the righteous shall be desolate. [22] The Lord redeemeth the soul of his servants: and none of them that trust in him shall be desolate." Psalm 34:15,17-22 KJV

It is That Time to Cry 😭 in Sorrows and Griefs by the 2020 Christmas Tree 🎄! I wish together with many could reach out to each of you and wipe your tears and take your sadness away! We all in loss and in each household a mourning rising up to the Lord of Lords and river of tears running through the land and much aches drilling in our bones!

****

It is That Time to Cry in Sorrows and Griefs by the 2020 Christmas Tree 🎄! It is okay to cry! It is my time to uncover my weakness and shed my tears 😭! There is more words remained and no more could I do but to shed my tears 😭 and cry 😭 by the Christmas Tree!

I am a bride 👰♂ soon to be until one night my love started to cough, reluctantly I called 911 against his will and since then I am not allowed to see him or visit him! Every day I am by my phone waiting for an update and I was only told the gloomy news! My love isn't doing any better. He is laying in the critical care and can't breath. His hear has hard time beating right and the kidney is shutting down. They started him in dialysis and I was asked to let him go! O. Y God have mercy upon my soul he is my sol mate and I am about to marry the love of my life and tell him I do. Please Lord in thy name don't take him away!!

"Have mercy upon me, O Lord, for I am in trouble: mine eye is consumed with grief, yea, my soul and my belly. [10] For my life is spent with grief, and my years with sighing: my strength faileth because of mine iniquity, and my bones are consumed. [12] I am forgotten as a dead man out of mind: I am like a broken vessel. [15] My times are in thy hand: deliver me from the hand of mine enemies, and from them that persecute me." Psalm 31:9-10,12,15 KJV

It is That Time to Cry 😭 in Sorrows and Griefs by the 2020 Christmas Tree 🎄! I wish together with many could reach out to each of you and wipe your tears and take your sadness away! We all in loss and in each household a mourning rising up to the Lord of Lords and river of tears running through the land and much aches drilling in our bones!

****

It is That Time to Cry 😭 in Sorrows and Griefs by the 2020 Christmas Tree 🎄! It is okay to cry! It is my time to uncover my soul from under the clouds ☁ of the world and shed my tears 😭! There is more words remained and no more could I do but to shed my tears 😭 and cry 😭 by the 2020 Christmas Tree 🎄!

I saw a baby child crying 😭! The 6 months years old baby child 👶 was crawling soaked with tears! Mommy mommy the baby 👶 scream and scream! Mommy no more COVID-19 just took her away! Mommy was in the intensive care intubated for three weeks and the family just got the new! A mother of three and since she was transported to the hospital, no one of her family could see her! Even her funeral is being arranged virtual! For three weeks the child never saw his mommy and was never fed by mommy breast milk! The child 👶 didn't receive much love nether a hug or a kiss!

My soul in loss! I can't eat or drink! I just want to cry 😭 with the baby child! O evil COVID, why have you taken mommy away? What have you gained? O COVID you have killed an innocent mommy and left behind a baby child without mommy and a husband without a wife! The world lost a mother and now a baby child in forever grief!

It is That Time to Cry 😭 in Sorrows and Griefs by the 2020 Christmas Tree 🎄! I wish together with many could reach out to each of you and wipe your tears and take your sadness away! We all in loss and in each household a mourning rising up to the Lord of Lords and river of tears running through the land and much aches drilling in our bones!

****

It is That Time to Cry 😭 in Sorrows and Griefs by the 2020 Christmas Tree 🎄! It is okay to cry! It is my time to uncover my soul from under the clouds ☁ of the world and shed my tears 😭! There is more words remained and no more could I do but to shed my tears 😭 and cry 😭 by the 2020 Christmas Tree 🎄!

I am the Unknown got ill and lost all what I had from years of wealth! I am sick a d can't afford to get help! I am the unknown and no one around me! I lived my life in sweats and tears! I paid my dues and just got the news; I attracted COVID and I must stay in doors! I can't work and lost all my saving waiting for a check! I just lost my best friend in nursing home and my children are grown and aren't near! I am suffering and in permanent pains and getting nowhere! What remained of me is skeleton of bone and eyes shedding tears 😭!

My father Isiah described me; "In their streets they have girded themselves with sackcloth; On their housetops and in their squares Everyone is wailing, dissolved in tears." Isaiah 15:3 "Therefore I say, "Turn your eyes away from me, Let me weep bitterly, Do not try to comfort me." Isaiah 22:4

It is That Time to Cry 😭 in Sorrows and Griefs by the 2020 Christmas Tree 🎄! I wish together with many could reach out to each of you and wipe your tears and take your sadness away! We all in loss and in each household a mourning rising up to the Lord of Lords and river of tears running through the land and much aches drilling in our bones!

****

It is That Time to Cry 😭 in Sorrows and Griefs by the 2020 Christmas Tree 🎄! It is okay to cry! It is my time to uncover my weakness and shed my tears 😭! There is more words remained and no more could I do but to shed my tears 😭 and cry 😭 by the Christmas Tree!

I am deeply torn between the love ❤ to my patients and the fact that COVID is taken them one by one away from me!

Since my years in High School, my Heavenly Father invited me to shadow His steps to medicine! It was a fearful moment in the midst of my sleep! I wasn't exact of that dream or vision or fantasy from my own subconscious ambition!

Nonetheless, since that dream I haven't been the same but my soul was transferred to an engine wishing to save the sick of the world and eradicate all the illnesses from the face of earth!! 🌍 Since then I prayed to my Father to open my eyes and help me to make the correct diagnosis: to give me wisdom to guide their management and to to hold my hands throughout their surgeries and care! I showed them the way of the Lord and asked them to give our Savior the Glory as it is written: "Let your light so shine before men, that they may see your good works, and glorify your Father which is in heaven." Matthew 5:16 KJV

He continued in His promise even in the times that I didn't recognize His hands, He was always there! I remember my early careers years when I didn't know what I am doing, and He took my hands and led the way! All I did is call upon His Name! O Lord I do not know but You know! I won't ever let You go!

It is That Time to Cry 😢 in Sorrows and Griefs by the 2020 Christmas Tree 🎄! I wish together with many could reach out to each of you and wipe your tears and take your sadness away! We all in loss and in each household a mourning rising up to the Lord of Lords and river of tears running through the land and much aches drilling in our bones!

****

It is That Time to Cry 😢 in Sorrows and Griefs by the 2020 Christmas Tree 🎄! It is okay to cry! It is my time to uncover my soul from under the clouds ☁ and shed my tears! There is more words remained and no more could I do but to shed my tears 😢 and cry 😢 by the 2020 Christmas Tree 🎄!

Back in January the early days of the 2020, the voice came: "Be ready My son, the time is near and the nations must mourn" it was a nightmare I will never forget and I cried in fears and screamed to the world 🌐! But I was immediately asked to shut up and my sayings were pushed to the side.

The virus 🦠 hit hard and in no time spread fast! Many were in denial and others didn't see what I and others saw and heard what I and others heard! Many more fell victims to the virus 🦠 and only recently during the second wave surge when the virus almost affected each household! The outcry is so severe! Lamentations and weeping, many lives are taken so soon and so fast and every day bring about more and more causalities. It is Rama "In Rama was there a voice heard, lamentation, and weeping, and great mourning, Rachel weeping for her children, and would not be comforted, because they are not." Matthew 2:18 KJV

It is as in Herod time where he —slew all the children that were in Bethlehem, and in all the coasts thereof, from two years old and under, according to the time which he had diligently enquired of the wise men." Matthew 2:16 KJV

Nonetheless, I didn't surrender and I plead to my Lord: "O My Lord please save the world! Keep thy promise! Every patient is to be healed regardless of what is written to be!

Yet I had a hard talk, one to One with my Savior! I said at that night, I am thy vessel and You are my Lord; My soul is all Yours but let no one of my patient go! It is the only thing I ask of You, O Lord! One thing my Lord not to let be that one! Please Lord heal each one of them! They are thy children after all and I am the barren soul the unworthy servant!

It is That Time to Cry 😭 in Sorrows and Griefs by the 2020 Christmas Tree 🎄! I wish together with many could reach out to each of you and wipe your tears and take your sadness away! We all in loss and in each household a mourning rising up to the Lord of Lords and river of tears running through the land and much aches drilling in our bones!

****

It is That Time to Cry 😭 in Sorrows and Griefs by the 2020 Christmas Tree 🎄! It is okay to cry! It is my time to uncover my soul from under the clouds ☁ and shed my tears 😭! There is more words remained and no more could I do but to shed my tears 😭 and cry 😭 by the 2020 Christmas Tree 🎄!

After heavy day with much of corps and bodies eaten by COVID, I couldn't take it anymore! My heart was heavy, my body was shaky, my soul was trembling and I wished my day to go was now. I rushed to the mountain of the Lord in solitude and uttered with the psalmist: Be merciful unto me and my people all Lord and don't let COVID swallow thy people—-

"Be merciful unto me, O God: for COVID (man) would swallow me up; COVID (he) fighting daily oppresseth me. [2] Mine enemies COVID would daily swallow me up: for they COVID be many that fight against me, O thou most High. [4] In God I will praise his word, in God I have put my trust; I will not fear what flesh can do unto me. [9] When I cry unto thee, then shall mine enemies COVID turn back: this I know; for God is for me. [10] In God will I praise his word: in the Lord will I praise his word. [11] In God have I put my trust: I will not be afraid what COVID man can do unto me. [12] Thy vows are upon me, O God: I will render praises unto thee. [13] For thou hast delivered my soul from death: wilt not thou deliver my feet from falling, that I may walk before God in the light of the living?" Psalm 56:1-2,4,9-13 KJV

It is That Time to Cry 😭 in Sorrows and Griefs by the 2020 Christmas Tree 🎄! I wish together with many could reach out to each of you and wipe your tears and take your sadness away! We all in loss and in each household a mourning rising up to the Lord of Lords and river of tears running through the land and much aches drilling in our bones!

****

It is That Time to Cry 😭 in Sorrows and Griefs by the 2020 Christmas Tree 🎄! It is okay to cry! It is my time to uncover my soul from under the clouds ☁ of the world and shed my tears 😭! There is more words remained and no more could I do but to shed my tears 😭 and cry 😭 by the Christmas Tree 🎄!

I am deeply sad 😔 and my heart is full of sorrows, I lost 😠 some of my patient and I can't let it go! I kneeled crying to my Lord why did you take them and I received no reply! I realized is their time to wave goodbye under these circumstances! My soul is torn between the love ❤ to my patients and the fact that COVID is taken them one by one away from me!

In my loss while I am totally soaked in my tears, my Heavenly Father opened my eyes! I saw so many souls are also crying 😭 and shedding their tears for the great loss of their innumerable souls of the loved ones!! Suddenly, the angel of Lord flew and appeared before our teary eyes saying: "As it is written: "—see that ye be not troubled: for all these things must come to pass, but the end is not yet. All these are the beginning of sorrows.—And because iniquity shall abound, the love of many shall wax cold. But he that shall endure unto the end, the same shall be saved." Matthew 24:6,8,12-13 KJV

I remembered my Savior words: "Watch and pray, that ye enter not into temptation: the spirit indeed is willing, but the flesh is weak." Matthew 26:41 KJV

I remembered the last days of Jesus in agony, I dressed in sackcloths, beaten my chest and I fell down in my face as my tears became droplets of blood. I uttered my Lord Jesus Heavenly word with broken hearted spirit 💔 saying to my Beloved: "- My soul is exceeding sorrowful, even unto death: —And he went a little further, and fell on his face, and prayed, saying, O my Father, if it be possible, let this cup pass from me: nevertheless not as I will, but as thou wilt. He went away again the second time, and prayed, saying, O my Father, if this cup may not pass away from me, except I drink it, thy will be done.

I prayed: "O my Lord, please let it pass from us: nevertheless not as I will, but as thou wilt."

412

I was signaled to read Revelations chapter 21! It is okay to cry 😭 now and shed tears 😭 now! It shall guard the human soul from the second cry 😭! Only at the Heavenly Jerusalem shall everything be new and shall no more cry no more tears, no more pains and no more suffering!! God himself shall be with them, and be their God. And God shall wipe away all tears from their eyes; and there shall be no more death, neither sorrow, nor crying, neither shall there be any more pain: for the former things are passed away—-: "And I John saw the holy city, new Jerusalem, coming down from God out of heaven, prepared as a bride adorned for her husband. [3] And I heard a great voice out of heaven saying, Behold, the tabernacle of God is with men, and he will dwell with them, and they shall be his people, and God himself shall be with them, and be their God. [4] And God shall wipe away all tears from their eyes; and there shall be no more death, neither sorrow, nor crying, neither shall there be any more pain: for the former things are passed away. [5] And he that sat upon the throne said, Behold, I make all things new. And he said unto me, Write: for these words are true and faithful. [6] And he said unto me, It is done. I am Alpha and Omega, the beginning and the end. I will give unto him that is athirst of the fountain of the water of life freely. [7] He that overcometh shall inherit all things; and I will be his God, and he shall be my son." Revelation 21:2-7 KJV

It is That Time to Cry 😭 in Sorrows and Griefs by the 2020 Christmas Tree 🎄! I wish together with many could reach out to each of you and wipe your tears and take your sadness away! We all in loss and in each household a mourning rising up to the Lord of Lords and river of tears running through the land and much aches drilling in our bones!

****

Spiritual Vision by 2020 Christmas Tree 🎄

It is That Time to Cry 😭 in Sorrows and Griefs by the 2020 Christmas Tree 🎄! It is okay to cry! It is my time to uncover my soul from under the clouds ☁ of the world and shed my tears! There is more words remained and no more could I do but to shed my tears 😭 and cry 😭 by the Christmas Tree 🎄!

The Lord is attentive to those in sorrows and cried as it is written: "The eyes of the Lord are upon the righteous, and his ears are open unto their cry. [17] The righteous cry, and the Lord heareth, and delivereth them out of all their troubles. [18] The Lord is nigh unto them that are of a broken heart; and saveth such as be of a contrite spirit. [19] Many are the afflictions of the righteous: but the Lord delivereth him out of them all. [20] He keepeth all his bones: not one of them is

413

broken. [22] The Lord redeemeth the soul of his servants: and none of them that trust in him shall be desolate." Psalm 34:15,17-20,22 KJV

No matter what the world do or say, only Baby Jesus of the 2020 Christmas 🎄 can raise Lazarus from death even if the flesh was smelly and destroyed with the evil 🦠♂ COVID-19! I ran to the 2020 Christmas Tree 🎄 and watered 🌿 the tree with my unceasing river of tears 😭. I ran to Baby Jesus crying 😭 and crying and saying Martha words: "Lord, if thou hadst been here, my brother had not died." John 11:21 KJV. Baby Jesus opened His mouth: "Thy brother shall rise again." John 11:23 KJV I cried and said: "I know that he shall rise again in the resurrection at the last day." John 11:24 KJV Baby Jesus raised His arms to reach my heart and said: "Jesus said unto her, I am the resurrection, and the life: he that believeth in me, though he were dead, yet shall he live: [26] And whosoever liveth and believeth in me shall never die. Believest thou this?" John 11:25-26 KJV I worshipped and kneeled to floor saying: "She saith unto him, Yea, Lord: I believe that thou art the Christ, the Son of God, which should come into the world." John 11:27 KJV

Voice of the Lord came to me and the widow: "And when the Lord saw her, he had compassion on her, and said unto her, Weep not." Luke 7:13 KJV And we saw a Hand touched the dead: "And he came and touched the bier: and they that bare him stood still. And he said, Young man, I say unto thee, Arise. [15] And he that was dead sat up, and began to speak. And he delivered him to his mother." Luke 7:14-15 KJV

Baby Jesus whipped with me I continued to cry: "Jesus wept." O my Lord and God Your Love to Your children much much more than that of the suckling mother to her baby: "Can a woman forget her sucking child, that she should not have compassion on the son of her womb? yea, they may forget, yet will I not forget thee. [16] Behold, I have graven thee upon the palms of my hands; thy walls are continually before me." Isaiah 49:15-16 KJV

"Then said the Jews, Behold how he loved him!" John 11:35-36 KJV

The former things are come to pass and new things shall be declared says the Lord of hosts and our Heavenly Father: "A bruised reed shall he not break, and the smoking flax shall he not quench: he shall bring forth judgment unto truth. [7] To open the blind eyes, to bring out the prisoners from the prison, and them that sit in darkness out of the prison house. [8] I am the Lord: that is my name: and my glory will I not give to another, neither my praise to graven images. [9] Behold, the former things are come to pass, and new things do I declare: before they spring forth I tell you of them. [10] Sing unto the Lord a new song, and his praise from the end of the earth, ye that go down to the sea, and all that is therein; the isles, and the inhabitants thereof." Isaiah 42:3,7-10 KJV

Baby Jesus reached out with His holy hand whipped my tears and told me: My son, My daughter, My love; it is okay to cry! My heart is weeping for all my children— Hear, O heavens, and give ear, O earth: for the Lord hath spoken, I have nourished and brought up children, and they have rebelled against me. [The ox knoweth his owner, and the ass his master's crib: but Israel doth not know, my people doth not consider." Isaiah 1:2-3 KJV

Baby Jesus looked at me with His shinning Newborn eyes and said: "-and, lo, I am with you alway, even unto the end of the world. Amen."—Matthew 28:20 KJV

We all shall see Your glory soon our Savior as You spoke: "Jesus saith unto her, Said I not unto thee, that, if thou wouldest believe, thou shouldest see the glory of God?" John 11:40 KJV

It is no longer death but sleep in our Lord Jesus salvation: "But we do not want you to be uninformed, brethren, about those who are asleep, so that you will not grieve as do the rest who have no hope. For if we believe that Jesus died and rose again, even so God will bring with Him those who have fallen asleep in Jesus. For this we say to you by the word of the Lord, that we who are alive and remain until the coming of the Lord, will not precede those who have fallen asleep."1 Thessalonians 4:13-18 "And I heard a voice from heaven, saying, "Write, 'Blessed are the dead who die in the Lord from now on! "Yes," says the Spirit, "so that they may rest from their labors, for their deeds follow with them." Revelation 14:13 "Your dead will live; Their corpses will rise. You who lie in the dust, awake and shout for joy, For your dew is as the dew of the dawn, And the earth will give birth to the departed spirits."" Isaiah 26:19

Come with Me son see what shall come soon: "And I saw a new heaven and a new earth: for the first heaven and the first earth were passed away; and there was no more sea. [2] And I John saw the holy city, new Jerusalem, coming down from God out of heaven, prepared as a bride adorned for her husband. [3] And I heard a great voice out of heaven saying, Behold, the tabernacle of God is with men, and he will dwell with them, and they shall be his people, and God himself shall be with them, and be their God. [4] And God shall wipe away all tears from their eyes; and there shall be no more death, neither sorrow, nor crying, neither shall there be any more pain: for the former things are passed away. [5] And he that sat upon the throne said, Behold, I make all things new. And he said unto me, Write:

for these words are true and faithful. [6] And he said unto me, It is done. I am Alpha and Omega, the beginning and the end. I will give unto him that is athirst of the fountain of the water of life freely. [7] He that overcometh shall inherit all things; and I will be his God, and he shall be my son." Revelation 21:1-7 KJV

It is That Time to Cry in Sorrows and Griefs by the 2020 Christmas Tree! Dedicated to Those in Sadness and Grieving in Christmas!

For now and every day, please Our Heavenly Father turn our sorrows and lamentation unto joy in thy Name, the Only Name we know and was given to us Jesus Christ our Lord and Savior as it is written: "Verily, verily, I say unto you, That ye shall weep and lament, but the world shall rejoice: and ye shall be sorrowful, but your sorrow shall be turned into joy. [21] A woman when she is in travail hath sorrow, because her hour is come: but as soon as she is delivered of the child, she remembereth no more the anguish, for joy that a man is born into the world. [22] And ye now therefore have sorrow: but I will see you again, and your heart shall rejoice, and your joy no man taketh from you. [23] And in that day ye shall ask me nothing. Verily, verily, I say unto you, Whatsoever ye shall ask the Father in my name, he will give it you." Savior: John 16:20-23 KJV

Fear thou not; for I am with thee: be not dismayed; for I am thy God: I will strengthen thee; yea, I will help thee; yea, I will uphold thee with the right hand of my righteousness. Isaiah 41:10 KJV

Biblical verses of Sorrows and Cries

Revelation 21:4 - And God shall wipe away all tears from their eyes; and there shall be no more death, neither sorrow, nor crying, neither shall there be any more pain: for the former things are passed away.

John 11:35 - Jesus wept.

Isaiah 41:10 - Fear thou not; for I [am] with thee: be not dismayed; for I [am] thy God: I will strengthen thee; yea, I will help thee; yea, I will uphold thee with the right hand of my righteousness.

John 14:1-31 - Let not your heart be troubled: ye believe in God, believe also in me.

1 Corinthians 12:26 - And whether one member suffer, all the members suffer with it; or one member be honoured, all the members rejoice with it.

Psalms 56:8 - Thou tellest my wanderings: put thou my tears into thy bottle: [are they] not in thy book?

Luke 7:13 - And when the Lord saw her, he had compassion on her, and said unto her, Weep not.

John 20:11 - But Mary stood without at the sepulchre weeping: and as she wept, she stooped down, [and looked] into the sepulchre,

Ecclesiastes 3:8 - A time to love, and a time to hate; a time of war, and a time of peace.

Isaiah 53:5 - But he [was] wounded for our transgressions, [he was] bruised for our iniquities: the chastisement of our peace [was] upon him; and with his stripes we are healed.

Romans 10:9 - That if thou shalt confess with thy mouth the Lord Jesus, and shalt believe in thine heart that God hath raised him from the dead, thou shalt be saved.

Ecclesiastes 3:4 -A time to weep and a time to laugh, a time to mourn and a time to dance" (.

Psalm 30:5) "For his anger lasts only a moment, but his favor lasts a lifetime; weeping may stay for the night, but rejoicing comes in the morning" (

Psalm 34:15) "The eyes of the Lord are on the righteous, and his ears are attentive to their cry"

Luke 13:28- "There will be weeping there, and gnashing of teeth, when you see Abraham, Isaac and Jacob and all the prophets in the kingdom of God, but you yourselves thrown out"

(John 11:33, 35) "When Jesus saw her weeping, and the Jews who had come along with her also weeping, he was deeply moved in spirit and troubled … Jesus wept".

Revelation 21:4). "He will wipe every tear from their eyes. There will be no more death or mourning or crying or pain, for the old order of things has passed away"

Psalm 90:10 "Put my tears in Your bottle"

Psalm 56:8 As for the days of our life, they contain seventy years, Or if due to strength, eighty years, Yet their pride is but labor and sorrow; For soon it is gone and we fly away.

Psalm 13:1-2 How long, O Lord? Will You forget me forever? How long will You hide Your face from me?

How long shall I take counsel in my soul, Having sorrow in my heart all the day? How long will my enemy be exalted over me?

Psalm 31:9 Be gracious to me, O Lord, for I am in distress; My eye is wasted away from grief, my soul and my body also.

Jeremiah 20:18 Why did I ever come forth from the womb. To look on trouble and sorrow, So that my days have been spent in shame?

1 Peter 1:6 In this you greatly rejoice, even though now for a little while, if necessary, you have been distressed by various trials,

Matthew 26:38 Then He *said to them, "My soul is deeply grieved, to the point of death; remain here and keep watch with Me."

Philippians 2:27 For indeed he was sick to the point of death, but God had mercy on him, and not on him only but also on me, so that I would not have sorrow upon sorrow.

Isaiah 38:2-3 Then Hezekiah turned his face to the wall and prayed to the Lord, and said, "Remember now, O Lord, I beseech You, how I have walked before You in truth and with a whole heart, and have done what is good in Your sight." And Hezekiah wept bitterly.

Psalm 6:1-7 O Lord, do not rebuke me in Your anger, Nor chasten me in Your wrath. Be gracious to me, O Lord, for I am pining away; Heal me, O Lord, for my bones are dismayed. And my soul is greatly dismayed; But You, O Lord—how long?

1 Samuel 1:16 Do not consider your maidservant as a worthless woman, for I have spoken until now out of my great concern and provocation."

Acts 20:37 And they began to weep aloud and embraced Paul, and repeatedly kissed him,

Matthew 17:23 and they will kill Him, and He will be raised on the third day." And they were deeply grieved.

Luke 22:45 When He rose from prayer, He came to the disciples and found them sleeping from sorrow,

John 16:6 But because I have said these things to you, sorrow has filled your heart.

Genesis 23:2 Sarah died in Kiriath-arba (that is, Hebron) in the land of Canaan; and Abraham went in to mourn for Sarah and to weep for her.

John 20:11 But Mary was standing outside the tomb weeping; and so, as she wept, she stooped and looked into the tomb;

Genesis 50:1 Then Joseph fell on his father's face, and wept over him and kissed him.

Deuteronomy 34:8 So the sons of Israel wept for Moses in the plains of Moab thirty days; then the days of weeping and mourning for Moses came to an end.

2 Samuel 19:2 The victory that day was turned to mourning for all the people, for the people heard it said that day, "The king is grieved for his son."

Luke 7:12-14 Now as He approached the gate of the city, a dead man was being carried out, the only son of his mother, and she was a widow; and a sizeable crowd from the city was with her. When the Lord saw her, He felt compassion for her, and said to her, "Do not weep." And He came up and touched the coffin; and the bearers came to a halt. And He said, "Young man, I say to you, arise!"

Luke 8:52 Now they were all weeping and lamenting for her; but He said, "Stop weeping, for she has not died, but is asleep."

John 11:33-35 When Jesus therefore saw her weeping, and the Jews who came with her also weeping, He was deeply moved in spirit and was troubled, and said, "Where have you laid him?" They *said to Him, "Lord, come and see." Jesus wept.

Acts 8:2 Some devout men buried Stephen, and made loud lamentation over him.

Psalm 137:1 By the rivers of Babylon, There we sat down and wept, When we remembered Zion.

Isaiah 15:3 In their streets they have girded themselves with sackcloth; On their housetops and in their squares Everyone is wailing, dissolved in tears.

Isaiah 22:4 Therefore I say, "Turn your eyes away from me, Let me weep bitterly, Do not try to comfort me concerning the destruction of the daughter of my people."

Jeremiah 22:10 Do not weep for the dead or mourn for him, But weep continually for the one who goes away; For he will never return Or see his native land.

Jeremiah 48:17 "Mourn for him, all you who live around him, Even all of you who know his name; Say, 'How has the mighty scepter been broken, A staff of splendor!'

Ezekiel 21:6 As for you, son of man, groan with breaking heart and bitter grief, groan in their sight.

Ezekiel 27:30 And they will make their voice heard over you And will cry bitterly. They will cast dust on their heads, They will wallow in ashes.

Psalm 34:18 The Lord is near to the brokenhearted And saves those who are crushed in spirit.

Psalm 10:14 You have seen it, for You have beheld mischief and vexation to take it into Your hand. The unfortunate commits himself to You; You have been the helper of the orphan.

Isaiah 53:4 Surely our griefs He Himself bore, And our sorrows He carried; Yet we ourselves esteemed Him stricken, Smitten of God, and afflicted.

John 11:35 Jesus wept.

Jeremiah 31:13 "Then the virgin will rejoice in the dance, And the young men and the old, together, For I will turn their mourning into joy And will comfort them and give them joy for their sorrow.

Isaiah 35:10 And the ransomed of the Lord will return. And come with joyful shouting to Zion, With everlasting joy upon their heads. They will find gladness and joy, And sorrow and sighing will flee away.

Lamentations 3:32-33 For if He causes grief,

Then He will have compassion. According to His abundant lovingkindness. For He does not afflict willingly. Or grieve the sons of men.

John 16:20 Truly, truly, I say to you, that you will weep and lament, but the world will rejoice; you will grieve, but your grief will be turned into joy.

1 Thessalonians 4:13-14 But we do not want you to be uninformed, brethren, about those who are asleep, so that you will not grieve as do the rest who have no hope. For if we believe that Jesus died and rose again, even so God will bring with Him those who have fallen asleep in Jesus.

Revelation 21:4 and He will wipe away every tear from their eyes; and there will no longer be any death; there will no longer be any mourning, or crying, or pain; the first things have passed away."

Psalm 16:4 The sorrows of those who have bartered for another god will be multiplied; I shall not pour out their drink offerings of blood, Nor will I take their names upon my lips.

1 Samuel 2:33 Yet I will not cut off every man of yours from My altar so that your eyes will fail from weeping and your soul grieve, and all the increase of your house will die in the prime of life.

2 Corinthians 2:4-5 For out of much affliction and anguish of heart I wrote to you with many tears; not so that you would be made sorrowful, but that you might know the love which I have especially for you. But if any has caused sorrow, he has caused sorrow not to me, but in some degree—in order not to say too much—to all of you.

Genesis 34:7 Now the sons of Jacob came in from the field when they heard it; and the men were grieved, and they were very angry because he had done a disgraceful thing in Israel by lying with Jacob's daughter, for such a thing ought not to be done.

1 Samuel 20:34 Then Jonathan arose from the table in fierce anger, and did not eat food on the second day of the new moon, for he was grieved over David because his father had dishonored him.

Ezra 10:6 Then Ezra rose from before the house of God and went into the chamber of Jehohanan the son of Eliashib. Although he went there, he did not eat bread nor drink water, for he was mourning over the unfaithfulness of the exiles.

Ezekiel 9:4 The Lord said to him, "Go through the midst of the city, even through the midst of Jerusalem, and put a mark on the foreheads of the men who sigh and groan over all the abominations which are being committed in its midst."

Romans 9:2 that I have great sorrow and unceasing grief in my heart.

1 Corinthians 5:2 You have become arrogant and have not mourned instead, so that the one who had done this deed would be removed from your midst.

Matthew 5:4 "Blessed are those who mourn, for they shall be comforted.

Matthew 26:75 And Peter remembered the word which Jesus had said, "Before a rooster crows, you will deny Me three times." And he went out and wept bitterly.

2 Corinthians 7:9-11mI now rejoice, not that you were made sorrowful, but that you were made sorrowful to the point of repentance; for you were made sorrowful according to the will of God, so that you might not suffer loss in anything through us. For the sorrow that is according to the will of God produces a repentance without regret, leading to salvation, but the sorrow of the world produces death. For behold what earnestness this very thing, this godly sorrow, has produced in you: what vindication of yourselves, what indignation, what fear, what longing, what zeal, what avenging of wrong! In everything you demonstrated yourselves to be innocent in the matter.

James 4:9 Be miserable and mourn and weep; let your laughter be turned into mourning and your joy to gloom.

Lamentations 1:5 Her adversaries have become her masters, Her enemies prosper; For the Lord has caused her grief Because of the multitude of her transgressions; Her little ones have gone away As captives before the adversary.

Nehemiah 1:4 When I heard these words, I sat down and wept and mourned for days; and I was fasting and praying before the God of heaven.

Jeremiah 8:21 For the brokenness of the daughter of my people I am broken; I mourn, dismay has taken hold of me.

Jeremiah 10:19 Woe is me, because of my injury! My wound is incurable. But I said, "Truly this is a sickness, And I must bear it."

Jeremiah 13:17 But if you will not listen to it, My soul will sob in secret for such pride; And my eyes will bitterly weep And flow down with tears, Because the flock of the Lord has been taken captive.

Jeremiah 14:2 "Judah mourns And her gates languish; They sit on the ground in mourning, And the cry of Jerusalem has ascended.

Amos 5:16-17 Therefore thus says the Lord God of hosts, the Lord, "There is wailing in all the plazas, And in all the streets they say, 'Alas! Alas!' They also call the farmer to mourning And professional mourners to lamentation."And in all the vineyards there is wailing, Because I will pass through the midst of you," says the Lord.

Amos 8:10 "Then I will turn your festivals into mourning And all your songs into lamentation; And I will bring sackcloth on everyone's loins And baldness on every head. And I will make it like a time of mourning for an only son, And the end of it will be like a bitter day.

Micah 1:8 Because of this I must lament and wail, I must go barefoot and naked; I must make a lament like the jackals And a mourning like the ostriches.

Zephaniah 1:15 A day of wrath is that day, A day of trouble and distress, A day of destruction and desolation, A day of darkness and gloom, A day of clouds and thick darkness,

Zechariah 12:10 "I will pour out on the house of David and on the inhabitants of Jerusalem, the Spirit of grace and of supplication, so that they will look on Me whom they have pierced; and they will mourn for Him, as one mourns for an only son, and they will weep bitterly over Him like the bitter weeping over a firstborn.

Matthew 8:12 but the sons of the kingdom will be cast out into the outer darkness; in that place there will be weeping and gnashing of teeth."

Matthew 24:30 And then the sign of the Son of Man will appear in the sky, and then all the tribes of the earth will mourn, and they will see the Son of Man coming on the clouds of the sky with power and great glory.

Revelation 1:7 Behold, He is coming with the clouds, and every eye will see Him, even those who pierced Him; and all the tribes of the earth will mourn over Him. So it is to be. Amen.

Luke 19:41-42 When He approached Jerusalem, He saw the city and wept over it, saying, "If you had known in this day, even you, the things which make for peace! But now they have been hidden from your eyes.

Revelation 21:4 ESV He will wipe away every tear from their eyes, and death shall be no more, neither shall there be mourning, nor crying, nor pain anymore, for the former things have passed away."

Psalm 34:15 ESV The eyes of the Lord are toward the righteous and his ears toward their cry.

Psalm 34:17 ESV When the righteous cry for help, the Lord hears and delivers them out of all their troubles.

Isaiah 41:10 ESV Fear not, for I am with you; be not dismayed, for I am your God; I will strengthen you, I will help you, I will uphold you with my righteous right hand.

John 11:35 ESV / 200 helpful votes Helpful Not Helpful

Jesus wept.

Psalm 126:5-6 Those who sow in tears shall reap with shouts of joy! He who goes out weeping, bearing the seed for sowing, shall come home with shouts of joy, bringing his sheaves with him.

Hebrews 5:7 ESV In the days of his flesh, Jesus offered up prayers and supplications, with loud cries and tears, to him who was able to save him from death, and he was heard because of his reverence.

John 14:1-31 ESV "Let not your hearts be troubled. Believe in God; believe also in me. In my Father's house are many rooms. If it were not so, would I have told you that I go to prepare a place for you? And if I go and prepare a place for you, I will come again and will take you to myself, that where I am you may be also. And you know the way to where I am going." Thomas said to him, "Lord, we do not know where you are going. How can we know the way?" ...

1 Corinthians 12:26 ESV If one member suffers, all suffer together; if one member is honored, all rejoice together.

Luke 7:13 ESV And when the Lord saw her, he had compassion on her and said to her, "Do not weep."

Isaiah 38:5 ESV "Go and say to Hezekiah, Thus says the Lord, the God of David your father: I have heard your prayer; I have seen your tears. Behold, I will add fifteen years to your life.

Psalm 145:19 ESV He fulfills the desire of those who fear him; he also hears their cry and saves them.

Psalm 56:8 ESV You have kept count of my tossing's; put my tears in your bottle. Are they not in your book?

John 20:11 ESV But Mary stood weeping outside the tomb, and as she wept she stooped to look into the tomb.

Ecclesiastes 3:8 ESV A time to love, and a time to hate; a time for war, and a time for peace

Ecclesiastes 3:4 ESV / 24 helpful votes Helpful Not Helpful

A time to weep, and a time to laugh; a time to mourn, and a time to dance;..

1 Corinthians 15:51 ESV / 22 helpful votes Helpful Not Helpful

Behold! I tell you a mystery. We shall not all sleep, but we shall all be changed,

Revelation 13:8 ESV / 10 helpful votes Helpful Not Helpful

And all who dwell on earth will worship it, everyone whose name has not been written before the foundation of the world in the book of life of the Lamb who was slain.

Ephesians 2:10 ESV / 10 helpful votes Helpful Not Helpful

For we are his workmanship, created in Christ Jesus for good works, which God prepared beforehand, that we should walk in them.

Ephesians 1:20 ESV / 10 helpful votes Helpful Not Helpful

That he worked in Christ when he raised him from the dead and seated him at his right hand in the heavenly places,

Acts 20:19 ESV Serving the Lord with all humility and with tears and with trials that happened to me through the plots of the Jews;

John 11:33 ESV When Jesus saw her weeping, and the Jews who had come with her also weeping, he was deeply moved in his spirit and greatly troubled.

Proverbs 21:15 ESV When justice is done, it is a joy to the righteous but terror to evildoers.

Proverbs 8:1 ESV Does not wisdom call? Does not understanding raise her voice?

Psalm 30:5 ESV / 10 helpful votes Helpful Not Helpful

For his anger is but for a moment, and his favor is for a lifetime. Weeping may tarry for the night, but joy comes with the morning.

1 Timothy 3:1-16 ESV The saying is trustworthy: If anyone aspires to the office of overseer, he desires a noble task. Therefore an overseer must be above reproach, the husband of one wife, sober-minded, self-controlled, respectable, hospitable, able to teach, not a drunkard, not violent but gentle, not quarrelsome, not a lover of money. He must manage his own household well, with all dignity keeping his children submissive, for if someone does not know how to manage his own household, how will he care for God's church? ...

Philippians 4:6-7 ESV Do not be anxious about anything, but in everything by prayer and supplication with thanksgiving let your requests be made known to God. And the peace of God, which surpasses all understanding, will guard your hearts and your minds in Christ Jesus.

John 11:1-57 ESV Now a certain man was ill, Lazarus of Bethany, the village of Mary and her sister Martha. It was Mary who anointed the Lord with ointment and wiped his feet with her hair, whose brother Lazarus was ill. So the sisters sent to him, saying, "Lord, he whom you love is ill." But when Jesus heard it he said, "This illness does not lead to death. It is for the glory of God, so that the Son of God may be glorified through it." Now Jesus loved Martha and her sister and Lazarus. ...

Matthew 24:36 ESV "But concerning that day and hour no one knows, not even the angels of heaven, nor the Son, but the Father only.

Psalm 50:15 And call upon me in the day of trouble; I will deliver you, and you shall glorify me."

Hebrews 9:27 And just as it is appointed for man to die once, and after that comes judgment,

John 20:17 Jesus said to her, "Do not cling to me, for I have not yet ascended to the Father; but go to my brothers and say to them, 'I am ascending to my Father and your Father, to my God and your God.'"

Luke 16:19-31 ESV There was a rich man who was clothed in purple and fine linen and who feasted sumptuously every day. And at his gate was laid a poor man named Lazarus, covered with sores, who desired to be fed with what fell from the rich man's table. Moreover, even the dogs came and licked his sores. The poor man died and was carried by the angels to Abraham's side. The rich man also died and was buried, and in Hades, being in torment, he lifted up his eyes and saw Abraham far off and Lazarus at his side. ...

Luke 13:28 ESV In that place there will be weeping and gnashing of teeth, when you see Abraham and Isaac and Jacob and all the prophets in the kingdom of God but you yourselves cast out.

Matthew 25:1-46 ESV "Then the kingdom of heaven will be like ten virgins who took their lamps and went to meet the bridegroom. Five of them were foolish, and five were wise. For when the foolish took their lamps, they took no oil with them, but the wise took flasks of oil with their lamps. As the bridegroom was delayed, they all became drowsy and slept. ...

Genesis 21:17 ESV And God heard the voice of the boy, and the angel of God called to Hagar from heaven and said to her, "What troubles you, Hagar? Fear not, for God has heard the voice of the boy where he is.

Revelation 17:14 ESV They will make war on the Lamb, and the Lamb will conquer them, for he is Lord of lords and King of kings, and those with him are called and chosen and faithful."

1 Peter 1:1-25 ESV Peter, an apostle of Jesus Christ, To those who are elect exiles of the dispersion in Pontus, Galatia, Cappadocia, Asia, and Bithynia, according to the foreknowledge of God the Father, in the sanctification of the Spirit, for obedience to Jesus Christ and for sprinkling with his blood: May grace and peace be multiplied to you. Blessed be the God and Father of our Lord Jesus Christ! According to his great mercy, he has caused us to be born again to a living hope through the resurrection of Jesus Christ from the dead, to an inheritance that is imperishable, undefiled, and unfading, kept in heaven for you, who by God's power are being guarded through faith for a salvation ready to be revealed in the last time. ...

John 16:33 ESV I have said these things to you, that in me you may have peace. In the world you will have tribulation. But take heart; I have overcome the world."

Luke 19:41 ESV And when he drew near and saw the city, he wept over it,

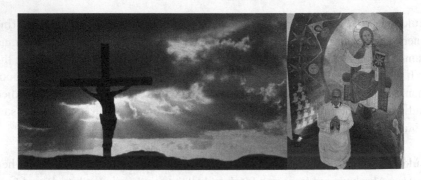

KG. I'm sure know better than most the sadness and grief surrounding Covid!!!
PP. Well said 🖤
JP. So sad for so many.

My Patient Michael Stroud passed away 12/06/2020
<u>December 6 at 9:27 AM</u> ·
🌐

COVID TOOK OUR ANGEL MIKE AWAY!

MIKE DID EVERYTHING TO STAY AWAY FROM COVID BUT COVID SOMEHOW GOT HIM!!

COVID WENT TO HIS LUNGS AND AFTER HE WENT HOME, COVID WENT TO HIS HEART AND ENDED HIS LIFE!

YOU ALL PLEASE TAKE COVID SERIOUSLY, MIKE WAS ONLY 49 YEARS OLD!

AFTER MY SURGERY LAST YEAR M, HE WAS GOLFING AND DOING GREAT UNTIL COVID.

SO SAD! COVID IS AN EVIL ENEMY TO MANKIND!

December 6, 2018 post

Repose in peace our angel; Mike. You were taken so soon. Much love and blessing to your soul and comfort to your family and friends. I was so honored and blessed to be your neurosurgeon and bro and part of your family for decades.

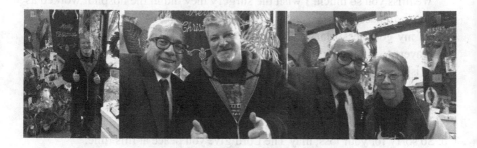

My patient ready to celebrate Christmas and New Year with no pain, back in his feet and soon ready to go back to work after a dead road full of miserable suffering.

Our Baby Jesus grant Michael a new lease in life with so much blessing

Merry Christmas and happy new year

Ramsis Ghaly

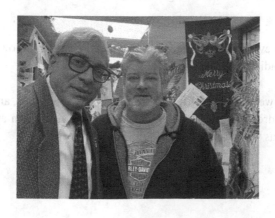

January 10, 2019 ·
Shared with Public

So proud of you Michael. You did great after surgery. You persevered and endured and now you won. Back to work and happy with no pain. Thank you Lord Jesus

Ramsis Ghaly
www.ghalyneurosurgeon.com

NC. Each day is harder to know your gone and my nephews are without a dad! We miss you so much! I wish the surgery they did in the hospital worked as yours did last year! 🖤🖤

Jw. Oh my goodness Mary and family I am so so sorry to hear this love and prayers to all of you

Lm. Wish this would end so sorry for the loss of your patient and friend sending condolences and prayers 🙏🙏🙏😞

Mp. So sorry for Mike Dr. Ghaly. May he rest in peace. And you take care of yourself as well dear friend. 🙏🙏🙏

Cb. So sorry for your loss, may The Lord give you peace at this time.

My Patient CARMEL PERINO passed away 12/14/ 2020

December 14 at 11:48 AM · What a loss! My patient I have known for almost three decades just passed away!! We are crying heavily with running tears! You were just an eagle 🦅 flying full of love 💜 always be in our hearts and homes! Rest in peace

Carmel Perino
! This year need to end soon enough enough O lord we pray!!

Carmel Perino
was the best in every aspect. She was our angel on earth and now she is joining the eternal paradise in Jesus hand in His bosom and St Mary.

Carmel served well her entire life and brought up gorgeous kids, and her children and grand children were all her life and love. They are grown and she always proud of them as we all are,

Onnie Richter
Angi and Louis. Her grand children are her testimony with her children, friends and all whoever met her.

I did her surgery years ago and became so close to them all and became part of their family. In Christmas, in thanksgiving and many many times, visits and phones. Her children are part of Me. I saw her two month ago and she was doing well.

Back then, many told her she won't recover from brain surgery and couldn't talk. Her two beautiful daughters Onni and Angi listen to no one and their love and Italian determination, Carmel lived two decades after surgery doing fantastic and got to see her grandchildren. Her own children continued to train her daily for two straight years when hospital and therapists said no hope until she regained her speech and ability to talk and converse! Never once her two daughters Angi and Onni left her sight. She loved them so much. What a strong woman was full of love. She did all by her own hands and her will took her thousands of Miles and her love 💜 filled the earth! I can't speak enough about you Carmel! You conquered the impossible during your earthly journey and now you are triumphant up high in heaven!

The death is all of a sudden, she was taken to Rush St Luke hospital and no much of information because of COVID mess! Michael was of great support to Carmel. So sorry Michael and all her friends and family members about your all loss!

Carmel your soul is in joy, you have done well and fought the good fight. We loved you so much and we will miss you much.

Onni, Angi and Louis no words that I could express our loss and deep sorrows and sadness. She was always proud of each of you and so we all are. She is in good comfort praying for us and holding our hearts always. Repose in peace Carmel with joy with the angels of our Lord Jesus, Amen 🙏 we all pray

"I have fought a good fight, I have finished my course, I have kept the faith:8 Henceforth there is laid up for me a crown of righteousness, which the Lord, the righteous judge, shall give me at that day: and not to me only, but unto all them also that love his appearing."2 Timothy 4:7-8

Ramsis Ghaly

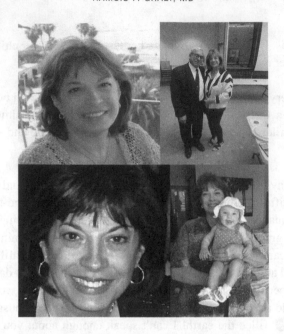

BS. I am so sorry for your loss, Dr. Ghaly

SM. Sorry for your loss Dr. Ghaly!

JM. A Beautiful Girl 🖤 Prayers For The Family 🖤

SS. I'm so sorry for your loss! All of you are in my prayers.

NW. So sorry for your loss. May the Lord comfort you and her family as you all grieve. 🙏

JM. So sorry 🥺 our Deepest Condolences and prayers

LM. My condolences to you and her family 🙏

RN. My condolences to you and to her family 🕊️✝️🙏😞

FL. Sorry it's never easy to loose friends

LP. So sad. I remember her when we were CINN

PH. I am so sorry. God has plans, but we never understand, do we.

NP. So sorry for your loss 🙏 My deepest condolences for you and her family 🙏

JB. So very sorry for your loss! May she rest in the loving arms of her heavenly Father and may God grant comfort and peace to her family and friends.

LC. SO SORRY TO HEAR THIS She is flying with the Angels now R,I,P,AND GOD BLESS

CD. Lovely lady. I met her here at Silver Cross. RIP.

ML. Such a loss. I pray for her family during this time of grief. May her spirit live on in the hearts of her family. 🙏

RP. y deepest condolences 🙏 such a beautiful woman.

RF. I am so sorry. We know God has her now and is waiting for all of us to join her in Eternal Life.

Claudia and Robert Flaws 12/15/2020 Passed away

Robert and Claudia a beautiful story to share
Years and years ago, I have been blessed with a special patient name Robert.
He was suffering so much and no one could figure out what he had. The man
continued to suffer of pains for years. His prayers heard by Baby Jesus.

I was blessed by him and his dedicated wife Claudia. Claudia stood by his bed
day and night. The children and grandchildren visited him daily. His spectacular
daughter a nurse Jean was and still is the right hand in his care.

Robert loved all about his children and grandchildren and if you want him to
forget about his pains or move his foot ask his grandchildren to tell him

Years and years later, today. I made a surprise visit. I am honored to visit them
all in their home that I visited so many years ago. Although Robert left us, yet he
is alive in his house, his wife Claudia, his children and grandchildren. They are
growing with Robert and Claudia Prayers They are angels in the house

Merry Christmas 🎁 🎄 and happy new year to you all

Ramsis Ghaly

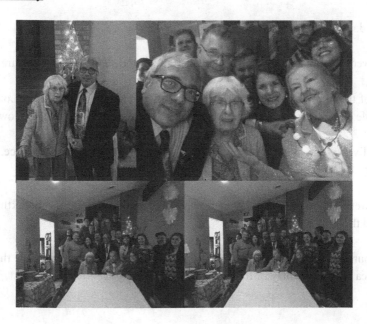

433

AF. So sad I missed meeting you! My family is so grateful for you! Happy New Year! 🖤

MF. So sorry we missed each other. It was a good time to step away and go to the cemetery to visit my Mom. Thank you for taking care of our family and for your continue support and dedication 🖤

MF. Dr. Ghaly, you truly are a kind caring man. We will never forget how you focused on our Dad's care, determined to relieve him of his pain to give him quality of life. You are a warrior angel from God. Thank you for the good fight.

KF. I am not too sure if you saw but i wanted to let you know that my Grandmother, Claudia Flaws, passed away on Tuesday. You were a good friend to her and my Grandfather and still are of this family!

Those Days are Gone!

Written by Ramsis Ghaly

Only few years, we were all together at Bagel Cafe with Sheldon Adelson, Lou Toomin and Marty Allan!

Those days are gone and they took the three giants with them!

Those days are gone and they passed away!

They were 🤩 fun and joy with so much laugh 😄 and share! Those days are gone!

Each of those three American Heroes 🧓🧓🧓, Sheldon, Marty and Lou took their life story with them and left the steps of their journeys to us to follow!

Their lives were much of true struggle from nothing to magnificence, from poverty to richness, and from baby steps to the road to fame!

They were visionaries in their own ways and they had done the breakthrough beyond the impossible!

They pursued their American dream to its fullest and in fact they made the new America 🏴 the country of the brave and the country we love!

434

And at the end of day, we all get together to share the good times and at the weekend we eat breakfast together at the bagel Cafe in casual dress and informal and tell stories and say things as it is uncoated with no fear!

Those days were fun and full of laughs! Our hearts are empty and we all are grieving for their loss!! Those days are gone! We were so fortunate to get to know each of them and to share much in one table! Indeed those days are gone!!

My soul is sorrowful! I am afraid 🙀 America won't produce such legends any longer! Those were true men started from scratch and build towers stood against status quo and never bowed down to opposition and adversities made them strong and even at their later years, they still contributed more and more and shared do much! They taught many generations!

Repose in peace Sheldon, Marty and Lou!! We pray for their families and sure they too will run with the Olympic flame 🔥 taking America to the frontier as their dads did too! Amen 🙏

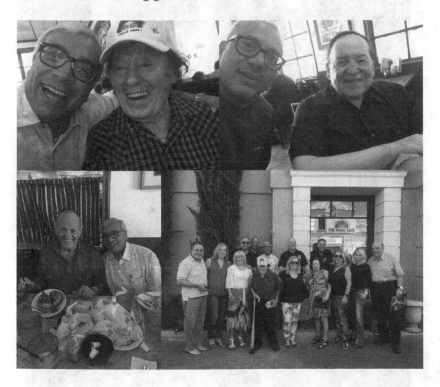

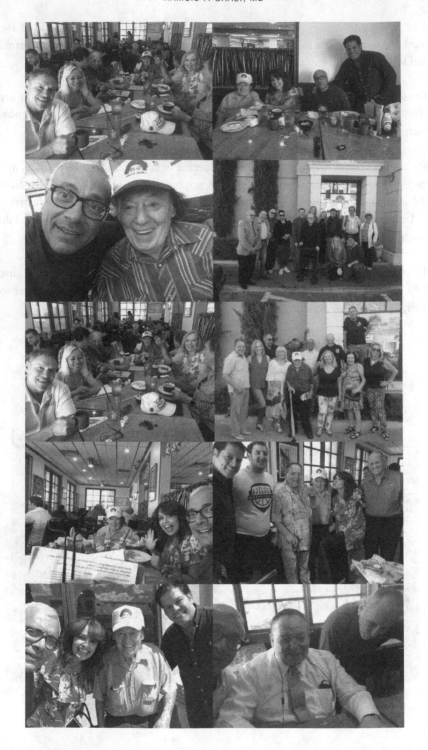

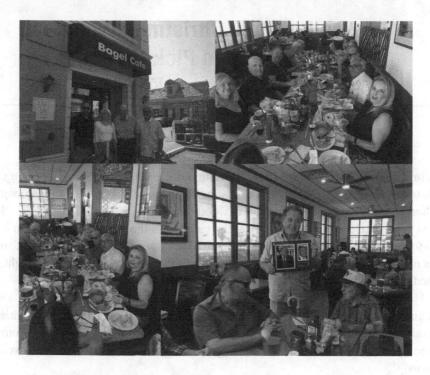

Cg. So sorry for your loss of your friend Sheldon Adelson yesterday

They all may be gone but look at all the great memories you will have forever.

Mn. i know you will remember all the good times I'm sorry to hear that Dr. Ghaly.
da. Miss my guys
Ls. 💕🙏
Lw. So much sorrow but also so many pleasant memories...
Tm. Ramsis, the loss of Sheldon, along with Marty is just too much to bear. I cry
with you. Every day I think of Marty. I only met Sheldon a few times, but he
was such a sweet man. His son-in-law looked at our home in Manalapan to
purchase, but then decided on Palm Beach. Funny how our lives intertwined
without our even knowing it. I will be in Las Vegas in February, and would
love to see you again, my friend. God bless, and keep fighting the good
fight 🩶

Roses for 2020 Christmas Would You All Join Me to Pick Up Roses for the Newborn King!!

A Poem Written by Ramsis Ghaly

Christmas 🎄 Spirit is Love, Joy, Blessing, Grace, Cheering, Sharing, Giving, Humility, and Forgiveness. My Lord is the Rose 🌷 of Sharon, the Lily among thorns, Apple Tree among the trees of wood full of love, Sweet and Awesome: "I am the rose of Sharon, and the lily of the valleys. As the lily among thorns, so is my love among the daughters. As the apple tree among the trees of the wood, so is my beloved among the sons. I sat down under his shadow with great delight, and his fruit was sweet to my taste." (Song of songs 2:1-3)

I kneeled to the Newborn King 👼 saying: "O Lord for Your Christmas 🎄 this year, instead of gold, frankincense and myrrh, I will go to the fields with Your people all together and pick up Roses 🌷 Roses 🌷 for Baby Jesus and my loved ones,

Since Roses are all about love 💜, unity, friendship, blessing, sharing, beauty, Joy, happiness, dignity and respect to all do is Christmas 🎄 the Spirit of a Truth, Love and Grace!

Love is what Christmas 🎄 all about and Love 💜 is the gift and Peace and blessing are the fruits!

Therefore, Roses are my gift, I wish you can come along with me, Together will hand the Roses to the hearts in need!

Together will hand the Roses 🌷 to the hearts in need! Who is coming with me to pick the loving red beautiful Roses 🌷 to hand them to the tender hearts 💜 of the human souls in need!

Christmas 🎄 is Eve is here! Who is joining me to harvest the white, yellow and pink Roses 🌷 for the sorrowful souls away from home!

Christmas 🎄 is at the door! Who is coming to gather the burgundy, the orange, the purple, and the lavender Roses 🌷 for the loved ones!

+++++++++
I called upon my Lord! I walked down the streets! I raised my hands and lifted my heart and asked baby Jesus: Lord this Christmas, I will go to the field with all your people, together will pick up the loving Roses 🌹 and be the gifts for You, the Newborn King. It will be all about love and not gold, frankincense and myrrh!

My Lord came down to me, sat by my side, hold my hand, smiled and freed me to go to the fields and spread the words to the ends of earth------!

I am going to pick up the loving Roses for Christmas, can you come with me? Come join me and hold the Roses 🌹 and sing to the Newborn King: "Glory to God in the highest, and on earth peace, good will toward men."

++++++=
Christmas 🎄 is love 🖤 and love 🖤 is Christmas 🎄. It is time to love 🖤, Christmas 🎄 is all about love: "For God so loved the world, that he gave his only begotten Son, that whosoever believeth in him should not perish, but have everlasting life." (John3:16)

Friends, Satan is racing to to kidnap the human souls away from the Newborn King, Jesus the Savior of the World 🌍 taking a Jesus name away from Christmas! Our world is in need of love! I choose Roses 🌹 as my gift and I wish you can come along with me!

Friends, I wish you come with me and pick up from the field the loving orange beautiful Roses 🌹 to take them to broken hearts! let us join in love, peace and faith carrying our loving Roses 🌹 in unity together with three wise men to visit the true King in the manger!

Come and join me! The field has so many beautiful Roses 🌹, call your friends, all people and all Human souls, let us turn away from all the divisions and Satan-hood deeds and in one Spirit let us sing to Our Savior: "Glory to God in the highest, and on earth peace, good will toward men."(Luke 2:14)

++++
It is the Christmas season! Who is joining me to pick the loving pink beautiful Roses gifts for the sorrowful and sick human souls?

It is the Christmas time! I am going to the field to pick the loving Yellow Roses for Christmas, would you please rise and together we bring them to all the people?

Friends, Christmas is coming soon, I wish you come with me and pick up from the field the loving orange beautiful Roses to take them to broken hearts!

Friends, this year more than ever, let us join in love, peace and faith carrying our loving Roses in unity together with three wise men to visit the true King in the manger.

Come and join me, the field has so many beautiful Roses, call your friends, all people and all Human souls, let us turn away from all the divisions and Satan-hood deeds and in one Spirit let us sing to Our Savior:

"Glory to God in the highest, and on earth peace, good will toward men."(Luke 2:14)

Two thousand and Twenty years later, the living human souls, each picked up the beautiful loving Roses -----We walked all night long---We followed the Star of the King---We met the three wisemen with their three gifts: Gold, Frankincense (an aromatic gum resin used in incense and perfumes), and Myrrh (aromatic plant resin).

(Matthew 2:10-11) "When they saw the star, they rejoiced with exceeding great joy. 11 And when they were come into the house, they saw the young child with Mary his mother, and fell down, and worshipped him: and when they had opened their treasures, they presented unto him gifts; gold, and frankincense, and myrrh."

For unto you is born this day in the city of David a Saviour, which is Christ the Lord." (Luke 2:11)

(Luke 2:13-14) "And suddenly there was with the angel a multitude of the heavenly host praising God, and saying, 14Glory to God in the highest, and on earth peace, good will toward men."

Peace, love and blessing to you all,
let us pray all together with one voice to the Everlasting One Jesus Christ, Amen
May you all and the world accept my Rose 🌷 for Christmas 🌲 2020. Amen 🙏

Ramsis Ghaly
Www.ghalyneurosurgeon.com

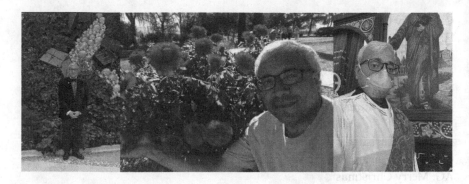

AC. Merry Christmas and happy New Year 🌲🎁🌲 Merry Christmas Dear, I believe, that beauty and faith will save the world. Thank You for Your prayers, I very appreciate. 🌷

AK. Merry Christmas, Doctor. Thank you, for all you did this year. God Bless you.

AV. Beautiful! 💚🙏

RP. Merry Christmas 🌲🎁

RM. Merry Christmas 🎄 Sir ❗ I wish a safe and Happy new year 💜

KE. Blessed Christmas

MM. Merry Christmas! 🤎

VW. Merry Christmas, Dr. Ghaly!

DS. Merry Christmas! 🎁🌲

MH. Merry Christmas 🍪

SS. Merry Christmas

ID. Merry Christmas!

RH. I love your prayers 🙏🕊️🌲✝️

AF. رمسيس المحبوب د. يا وسعادة وبخير طيب وانت سنة كل . حضرتك على سعيده اعياد .

JV. Merry Christmas Doc

MS. Merry Christmas Dr. Ghaly 🌷💚💜🌲

NE. Merry Christmas Dr. Ghaly!

YB. Merry Christmas

LN. Merry Christmas Doc!

MA. Merry Christmas and happy new year

KB. Merry Christmas.

GR. MERRY CHRISTMAS !!!

SM. Merry Christmas Doc!!

JB. Merry Christmas!!

MB. Merry Christmas and be safe Dr. Ghaly.

LH. Merry Christmas!

MY. SS. Merry Christmas

NG. Merry Christmas!

JP. DL. Yes. Happy Birthday Jesus.

CH. Merry Christmas 🎄

HM. Merry CHRISTmas 🎄

AP. Merry Christmas 🎄 !

LM. Merry Christmas 🎄 Dr. Ramsis 🎅

NW. Merry 🎄 Christmas!

SJ. Merry Christmas, Dr. Ghaly. May God's light shine brightly on you and this world. 💡🌐

LT. Merry Christmas

CG. TMN. You are looking very nice Dr.Ghaly

AG. Merry Christmas 🎁🎄

RW. Merry Christmas!

AC. Merry Christmas and happy New Year 🎄🎁🎄

Wonderful roses, I like to send You Dear Dr. Ramsis Ghaly, roses from my garden 🌷🌷🌷

Beautiful. Thank you. Merry Christmas 🎄 and happy new year 🎊 thank youso much. Praying for you staying safe. Thank you for Your kindness and wonderful heart Love and blessing. Ramsis ghaly

AC. Merry Christmas Dear Ramsis Ghaly, I believe, that beauty and faith will save the world. Thank You for Your prayers, I very appreciate. 🌷

AK. Merry Christmas, Doctor. Thank you, for all you did this year. God Bless you.

AV. Beautiful! 💐🙏

RP. Merry Christmas 🎄🎁

RM. Merry Christmas ⛄ Sir ❗ I wish a safe and Happy new year 💜

KE. Blessed Christ

MM. Merry Christmas! 🦀

CM. Merry Christmas ❄🎄❄

BC. What a nice photo!

DM. merry blessed christmas

JP. Merry Christmas Dr. Ghaly

SM. Merry Christmas 🎄

BCD. Shirt sleeves??? It's freezing in VIRGINIA

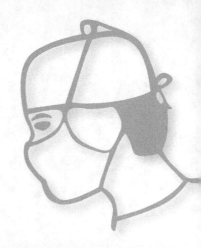

SECTION 8

Good Friday and Easter during COVID-19 Recovery

Good Friday By the Monastery faraway to comply with COVID Restriction and Resurrection Feast 2021! Easter during COVID-19 Recovery

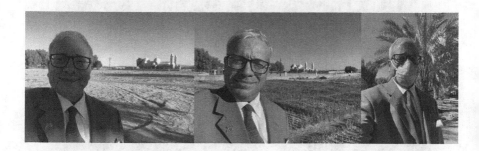

I think I made trouble today!!

I decided to sneak through the back door with my mask to enter the Egyptian Coptic Orthodox Monastery and get my Heavenly Father blessing and His mother St Mary and St Antony by the remote desert! The orthodox faith is still in lent and all fasting with no food or animal products but only living vegetable!!

It has been a year plus and no one was allowed to enter because of the COVID and I missed the holy place much!

Then as I entered, I could no longer be silent as soon we realized we missed each other very much!!

So, as soon as I was seen, many were so happy to see me as my soul was exalted to be with them once more!!

I walked and kissed the sand as I saw the farm and the fields are growing fast in the desert and blossoming greens, vegetables, fruits and domestic animals by God blessing among the silent monks of our Lord Jesus.

It was three hours in heaven and it came the time, I must leave before the dark!

The orthodox Christian faith Easter and Resurrection is in May 2, 2021. Happy Resurrection to you all. Our Lord Jesus is Risen! Indeed He is Risen!

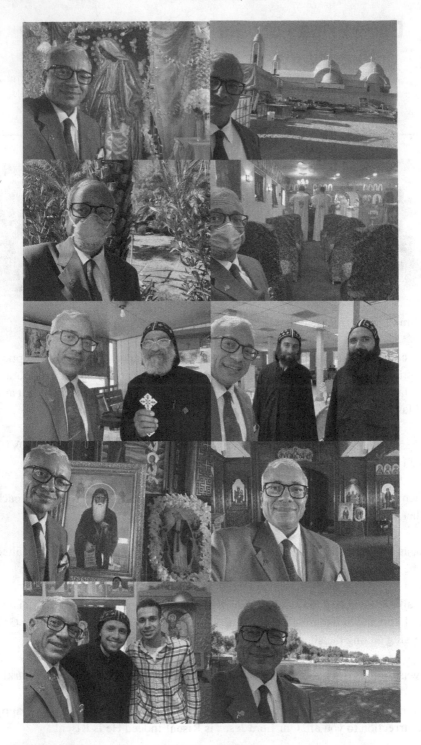

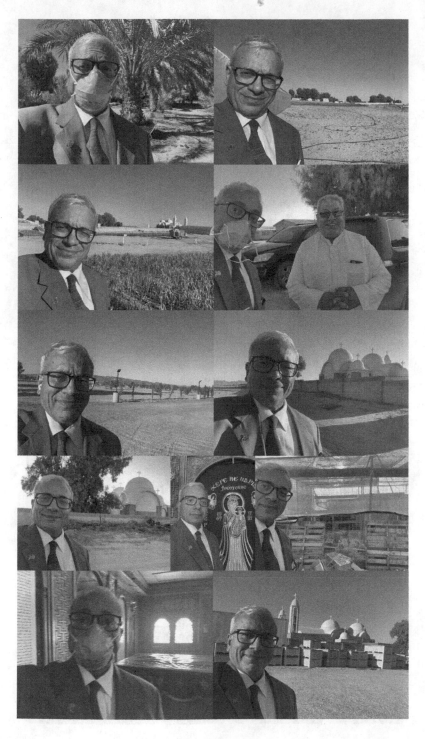

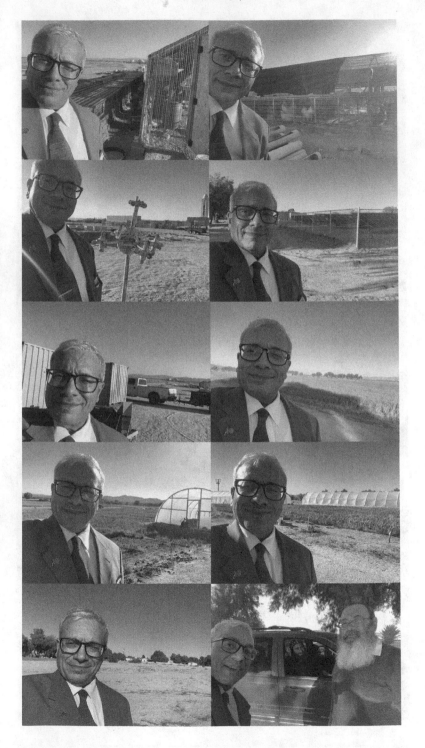

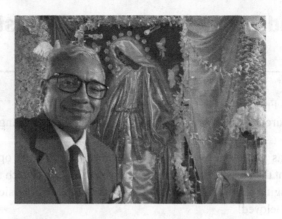

JB. We are glad you are in your happy place Dr. G. We know you love visiting the Monastery as well as the desert. Have a blessed Easter! 💜🙏

AM. Lucky Dr. Ramsis, May God bless you and all your work.

GR. God bless you

DL. So wonderful. May God continue to bless you. Happy Easter Dr. <u>Ramsis Ghaly</u>

YLJ¡Love your strong Christian faith.

VG. Srecan Uskrs, Bog Vas blagoslovio. 🙏💜

NC. Love your dedication

EB. I wish we can visit. God protect Abouna.

EM. Have a blessed Easter! Jim and I are so happy the Lord brought you into our lives. 💜

AR. Happy Easter!

CR. Blessing upon blessing. My sister is also orthodox so I understand and appreciate all of this.

RC. Is good to see tour in one of tour favorite place

SJ. Happy Resurrection and Easter to you, Dr. Ghaly.

Thank you very much for taking us on a photographic tour of your beloved Egyptian Coptic Orthodox Monastery. I absolutely loved seeing how self sustaining and beautiful it is 💜✝️💜

Many blessings to you during these holy days

MN. Nothing surprises me Dr. Ghaly you are amazing man you do what you have to pray to the Lord Jesus Christ God Bless you Dr. Ghaly with all my heart.

I know he has risen i kneel in front of a cross. In my room and pray to the Lord Happy Easter Dr. Ghaly.

Good Friday and Easter of Christian Orthodoxy April 2021

It is the Good Friday for my Orthodoxy faith and I arrived late! The cars were leaving the church parking garage and here I am a stranger coming and so tardy!

The traffic was going one way and I was walking fast in the opposite way! I couldn't look at the blessed faces whom were attending the church the entire day! They were singing all the sad rituals and sorrowful hymns classic for the Good Friday of my Beloved!

Finally I made it to the church and was almost empty! I kneeled to alter and bowed to the buried body of Jesus by Golgotha! I prayed twenty of Psalms of David before my Love Holy Body!

As I was leaving the Alter, my eyes fell on the picture of my Beloved in the Cross!! I ran to it and I kneeled before my Lord! I stared at Him and He wasn't responding!!!

My Love was lonely and the crowd already home! My heart moved as the Good Friday rituals were over and the people took the blessing home after close to one hundred of sixty right kneeling before the Cross saying Lord have merry Lord have mercy Lord Have mercy!!!

My Lord was alone and neither His heart 💜 was beating nor His lungs 🫁 were exchanging air! His Head bowed down and His eyes were shut and He no longer could open His mouth 👄 to speak!

My Beloved no longer could walk or move His arms or legs! I no longer could see Him or hear His voice again!

I screamed and He didn't answer me! I yelled and He didn't reply! I cried and He didn't respond to my grieving soul! I shed rivers of tears 😰 and He didn't look at my dying soul!

The transgressors had already murdered Him and they all ran away to their home celebrating their evilness with wine and toasts!!

My Beloved's enemies wanted Him to die and His Holy Name perish fir ever! Falsely and injustice, they surrounded Him and cut Him among His people!!

450

He was tried by the court to falsely accuse Him, tortured severely to suffer, crowned to be punished, dragged to be humiliated, hanged high to die, stabbed to bleed, murdered to die and buried in a dug tomb in the rock with large stone so that won't be seen forever anymore!

My Love just passed away! For me, He gave Himself up to the transgressors! My Love died for me! He Is and no one Like Him and no One but Him!

My God my God attend to me! My God my God why you have forsaken Me?? They gave Me vinegar and mocked Me I am poor and sorrowful They placed in low den in the shallow of death. But I rested snd I slept and I rose for the Lord helped. Lord have mercy upon me and raise me up! But You are my God! You brought me from the den and sorrows and the mud of hardship!

My Love is my Holy Lamb and Sacrifice and gave Himself Random for me and gave His Body and Blood for my Salvation!

My Love 😍 was all alone! My Savior was gone! My soul was all alone by His feet kneeling at the crucifix picture painted in oil and framed in wood!!

O daughters of Jerusalem!! Why you all left my Love by Himself alone! The crowd was no more and so His children ran away and from the fears they were locked at homes!!

Nonetheless, O daughters of Jerusalem, if you decide to come back and be with my Beloved, you shall find me by His feet! I know the show was over but believe it never fade away! My soul is living with Him all the way!

I shall keep talking to my Savior and I will keep crying shedding my tears to my Savior! I loved Him much and my Love is endless for Him! I shall live in the memories of the last three years that I got to know Him so close in the flesh! I remember when He called me as I was walking astray!

O daughters of Jerusalem, don't you all know my Beloved! I know Him well! I ate from His hands. I drank from His cup! I listened to His words and followed His steps! My soul was nourished day and night from His endless blessing and grace! In His bosom I never needed anything else! He rose the dead, healed the sick, covered the naked, taught the literate and illiterate, fed the hunger, fulfilled the thirst, strengthened the weak, defended the victims and rescued the drowned, revived the entire human race, set free the accusers, and gave eternal life to those who believe in Him!!

My Love is risen from death and my Firstfruit ever and so I shall follow: "But now is Christ risen from the dead, and become the firstfruits of them that slept. [21] For since by man came death, by man came also the resurrection of the dead. [22] For as in Adam all die, even so in Christ shall all be made alive. [23] But every man in his own order: Christ the firstfruits; afterward they that are Christ's at his coming."1 Corinthians 15:20-23 KJV

My Love to Whom is the Cherubim, Seraphim, angels, archangels, authorities, prinicipslities, all powers and dominions worship to and praising His Name: "And I beheld, and I heard the voice of many angels round about the throne and the beasts and the elders: and the number of them was ten thousand times ten thousand, and thousands of thousands; [12] Saying with a loud voice, Worthy is the Lamb that was slain to receive power, and riches, and wisdom, and strength, and honour, and glory, and blessing. [13] And every creature which is in heaven, and on the earth, and under the earth, and such as are in the sea, and all that are in them, heard I saying, Blessing, and honour, and glory, and power, be unto him that sitteth upon the throne, and unto the Lamb for ever and ever. [14] And the four beasts said, Amen. And the four and twenty elders fell down and worshipped him that liveth for ever and ever." Revelation 5:11-14 KJV

"After this I beheld, and, lo, a great multitude, which no man could number, of all nations, and kindreds, and people, and tongues, stood before the throne, and before the Lamb, clothed with white robes, and palms in their hands; [10] And cried with a loud voice, saying, Salvation to our God which sitteth upon the throne, and unto the Lamb. [11] And all the angels stood round about the throne, and about the elders and the four beasts, and fell before the throne on their faces, and worshipped God, [12] Saying, Amen: Blessing, and glory, and wisdom, and thanksgiving, and honour, and power, and might, be unto our God for ever and ever. Amen." Revelation 7:9-12 KJV

For now until, He comes again, I shall keep talking to my Beloved and Love! I shall keep praying day and night to Him and be always in the watch as He previously told me by the mountains of Olive 🜚 and while We were walking together by the trees!

My Beloved's commandments is my doctrine and my daily homework! My beloved is alive and He never die! He is with me all the time! He is dead to the transgressors but He is alive within my soul!

However, I still miss His days in the flesh! We shared much together: the walks by the wayside and by the shore and the meals of fish and the mana bread!

With deep sadness and sorrows of the passion week, O my soul, let us rejoice! Let us be glad and rejoice, and give honour to him: for the marriage of the Lamb is come, and his wife hath made herself ready.: "And after these things I heard a great voice of much people in heaven, saying, Alleluia; Salvation, and glory, and honour, and power, unto the Lord our God: [2] For true and righteous are his judgments: for he hath judged the great whore, which did corrupt the earth with her fornication, and hath avenged the blood of his servants at her hand. [3] And again they said, Alleluia. And her smoke rose up for ever and ever. [4] And the four and twenty elders and the four beasts fell down and worshipped God that sat on the throne, saying, Amen; Alleluia. [5] And a voice came out of the throne, saying, Praise our God, all ye his servants, and ye that fear him, both small and great. [6] And I heard as it were the voice of a great multitude, and as the voice of many waters, and as the voice of mighty thunderings, saying, Alleluia: for the Lord God omnipotent reigneth. [7] Let us be glad and rejoice, and give honour to him: for the marriage of the Lamb is come, and his wife hath made herself ready. [11] And I saw heaven opened, and behold a white horse; and he that sat upon him was called Faithful and True, and in righteousness he doth judge and make war. [12] His eyes were as a flame of fire, and on his head were many crowns; and he had a name written, that no man knew, but he himself. [13] And he was clothed with a vesture dipped in blood: and his name is called The Word of God. [14] And the armies which were in heaven followed him upon white horses, clothed in fine linen, white and clean. [15] And out of his mouth goeth a sharp sword, that with it he should smite the nations: and he shall rule them with a rod of iron: and he treadeth the winepress of the fierceness and wrath of Almighty God. [16] And he hath on his vesture and on his thigh a name written, KING OF KINGS, AND LORD OF LORDS." Revelation 19:1-7,11-16 KJV

O my Love, they thought You are dead but You never die! "I am Alpha and Omega, the beginning and the ending, saith the Lord, which is, and which was, and which is to come, the Almighty. [12] And I turned to see the voice that spake with me. And being turned, I saw seven golden candlesticks; [17] And when I saw him, I fell at his feet as dead. And he laid his right hand upon me, saying unto me, Fear not; I am the first and the last: [18] I am he that liveth, and was dead; and, behold, I am alive for evermore, Amen; and have the keys of hell and of death." Revelation 1:8,12,17-18 KJV

When You are coming, You shall find my soul waiting for You my Holy Bridegroom! My Savior and my love, today is Good Friday but Sunday shall be thy glory the Holy Resurrection of my Love and the day after those days, it shall be the second coming of Jesus Christ in His Glory up high in the crowds! Amen Lord Jesus Come Soon Please Come!! "And, behold, I come quickly; and my reward is with me, to give every man according as his work shall be. [13] I am Alpha and Omega, the beginning and the end, the first and the last. [14] Blessed are they that do his commandments, that they may have right to the tree of life, and may enter in through the gates into the city. [15] For without are dogs, and sorcerers, and whoremongers, and murderers, and idolaters, and whosoever loveth and maketh a lie. [16] I Jesus have sent mine angel to testify unto you these things in the churches. I am the root and the offspring of David, and the bright and morning star. [20] He which testifieth these things saith, Surely I come quickly. Amen. Even so, come, Lord Jesus." Revelation 22:12-16,20 KJV

Jesus Christ is Risen Indeed He is Risen! Happy Resurrection and happy Easter to all the Christians Orthodox worldwide and the Copts of Egypt 🇪🇬 my hometown! Amen 🙏

Happy Easter
Happy Resurrection
Ekhristos Anesti.
Alithos Anesti.
Christ is risen.
Indeed He is Risen
Albanian – Gezuar Pashket
Arabic – Fish sa'id / El Maseeh Qam (Christ has risen
Chinese – Fu huo jie kuai le
Croatian – Sretan Uskrs
Czech – Vesele Velikonoce
Danish – Glædelig Paske / God paske
Dutch – Gelukkig Paasfest / Vrolijk Pasen
English – Happy Easter
French – Joyeuses Pâques
Finnish – Hyvaa Paasiaista / Iloista paasiaista
German – Frohe Ostern
German (Swiss) – Schoni Oschtere
Greek – Kalo Pascha
Hungarian – Boldog Husveti Unnepeket
Hebrew – Chag pesach same'ach
Hindi – Subh Istar
Italian – Buona Pasqua
Indonesian – Selamat Paskah
Lithuanian – Linksmu Velyku
Latvian – Priecigas Lieldienas
Maltese – LGhid it-tajjeb

Norwegian – God paske
Polish – Szczęśliwej Wielkanocy
Portuguese – Feliz Páscoa
Romanian – Paşte Fericit
Russian – Schtsjastlivyje Paschi
Serbian – Hristos voskrese
Spanish – Felices Pascuas
Swedish – Glad Pask
Turkish – Mutlo (eller Hos) Paskalya

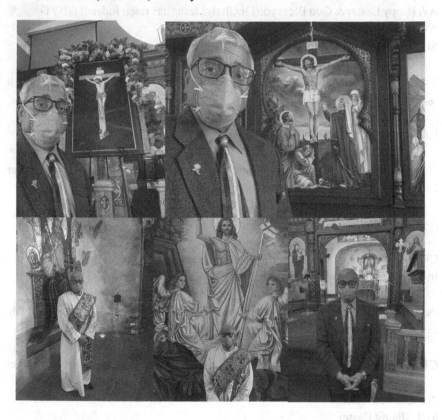

MA. Happy Easter God bless
NV. Happy Easter and God Bless you Doctor Ghaly 🙏
AB. Praise God! Wonderful words thank you sharing 🌷
DS. Happy Easter and May God Bless You and keep you safe 🙏❤️
JB. Have a blessed Easter Dr. G 🙏💝
SL. Happy Easter!!! May the Lord richly bless you today and always ❤️✝️
CG. Happy Easter and many blessings! ❤️🙏
VG. Srecan Uskrs i neka Vas Bog blagoslovi! 🙏❤️

SH. Happy Easter 🐣🙏

AP. Peace and reflection.

AG. Happy Easter

TG. Happy Easter God bless and many Blessings!!! 🙏

AP. Christ is Risen!

AP. Indeed He is Risen. Thank you father

JH. God's blessings to you always and strength for you to continue your kindness journey and soulful care

SS. Hristos Vaskrse, 🙏

AV. Happy Easter & God Bless you Dr.Ghaly! Jesus has risen indeed! GBYD 🐤🙏

AV. Beautiful photos! 🐤🙏

SP. Dr. Ramsis Ghaly

YOU WEREN›T TARTY YOU WERE ABSENT 😊 I›m glad you made it though 💜 Happy Easter ✝️

LA. John 3:16:

"For God so loved the world that He gave His only begotten Son, that whoever believes in Him should not perish but have everlasting life."

يوحنا ٣ : ١٦

١٦ لِأَنَّهُ هَكَذَا أَحَبَّ اللهُ الْعَالَمَ حَتَّى بَذَلَ ابْنَهُ الْوَحِيدَ لِكَيْ لَا يَهْلِكَ كُلُّ مَنْ يُؤْمِنُ بِهِ بَلْ تَكُونُ لَ الْحَيَاةُ الْأَبَدِيَّةُ.

Christ is risen from the dead; He who died trampled down death and upon those in the tombs bestowed eternal life.

Pekhrestos aftonf evol-khennee-ethmoot, fee-etaf-mo af-homy, ejen efmo owoh, nee etky khen-nee-emhaf, afer-ehmot no-oo empy-onkh en-eneh....

CR. Personal alone time with Jesus on Good Friday is a blessing of another kind ✝️

AS. Christ is risen!

MB. Happy Easter

DV. Vaistinu Vaskrese

My Orthodox Easter with COVID Patients!

Called to serve and honored to do so! And much blessing to be in this role as we pray for speed recovery to the victims of COVID-19!

I put on my PPE as we all by now have mastered the routine!

It is a virus ✹ from hell but soon be overpowered! The time must pass before it goes away! Be Ready for the Second waive and just know Lord our God is in Control!

No matter how virulent is the virus ✹, the virus ✹ remains a little tiny invisible virus ✹ and soon or later will fade away—-!

So regardless what might be, we are so ready for more knowing our will is strong and our faith is strong, soon in the Name of Jesus, our Risen God from death, we shall conquer COVID-19!!

"It is of the Lord's mercies that we are not consumed, because his compassions fail not. [23] They are new every morning: great is thy faithfulness. [24] The Lord is my portion, saith my soul; therefore will I hope in him. [25] The Lord is good unto them that wait for him, to the soul that seeketh him. [26] It is good that a man should both hope and quietly wait for the salvation of the Lord."

Lamentations 3:22-26 KJV

Ramsis Ghaly

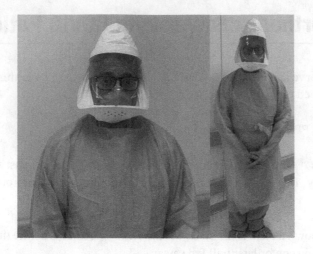

SS. Happy Easter Dr Ghaly

RH. Amen. Reading is a battle in itself. We are grateful for your love and protection. I Pray for our Sanity for all of us in our Activities!!!

AR. Amen and stay safe.

JB. I pray for you everyday.

TJ. DM. God bless and protect you always

SN. God Bless you Dr. Ghaly 🙏🙏🙏❤️

CG. You are always ready and willing to help when asked. Bless you! ❤️🙏

NA. The vaccine works.

Rz. Christ is Risen! Indeed He is Risen!

Easter 2021 with Victor and Gamal and Grandma 84 Years Old!

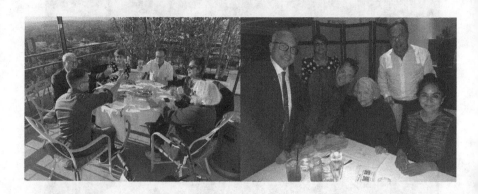

Happy Resurrection and happy Easter!

Happy Birthday Victor and congratulations

for all what you accomplished and just completed law school and the very best for more blessings.

Happy birthday 🎉🎂🎁 as well for your Grandma Ruth for 93 years old.

Thank you Gamal for your hospitality and great birthday party!

Ramsis Ghaly

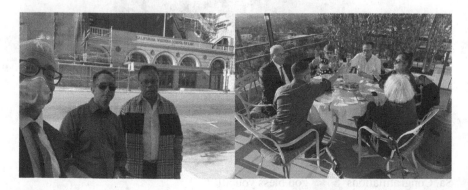

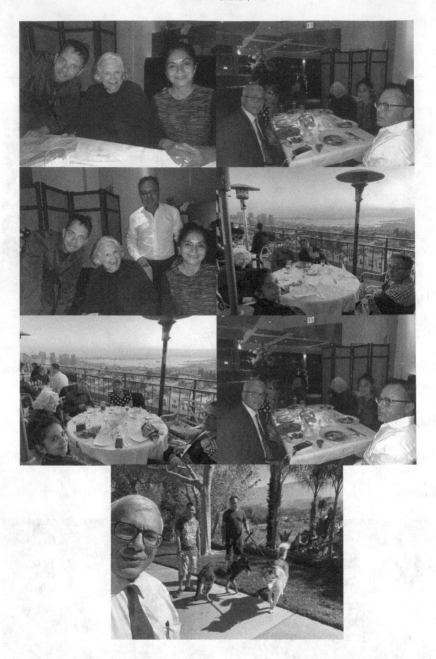

Ae. Happy Easter!
Sa. Congratulations 🌸🍀 god bless you all 🌸🌸
Av. That's awesome! Congratulations Happy Birthday 🎈🎉🎁
…

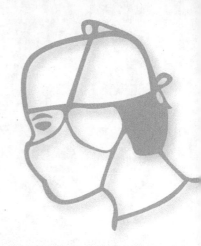

SECTION 9

To The Victims and Vulnerable of COVID 19

Through the Atrocities caused by COVID Surge and Political Unrest You are NOT Forgotten O Bravery Soldier of the Freedom!

A Poem in the Memory of All the Veterans In Veterans Day!
Written by Ramsis Ghaly

It was meant for me to sing with those who sacrificed their lives for us. As our Lord Jesus said there is no much love than someone put his life for another. He was our first Veteran that put His Life by his own will, for others in order for all of us to find life in Him. The same as all our veterans.

I meant to sing with them Happy Veteran's Day. I was joined by so many that wished to join. It is the love that deep rooted in each of them that made me do so.

It is the time for me and you to join them and do what they had done and carry on to the generations to come.

How much I wish this is not true! How much I wish that all things are fair!

When I looked at this photo and I read the caption my soul cried and I said: "it can't be and it must stop 🌑"!

I saw pictures of so many heroes we cherished with different colors, shapes and ethnicity under one roof America 🇺🇸 and one land called my sweet home my home United States 🇺🇸 of America 🇺🇸 under one flag of our home 🇺🇸!

As the Holy Trinity the Father, the Son and the Holy Spirit is One God so is the human race the spirit, soul and the flesh in one human being!

How much I wish this is not true!
How much I wish that all things are fair!
Wars see no color as death see no race
Crying is no difference between cultures as tears pour and heart aches when we loose a soul
To you up there, our love 💜 to you is the same!
To you up high our gratitude 🙏 to you is the same!

463

To you flying high, we salute 🏳️ you is the same to the last breathe!
How much I wish this is not true!
How much I wish that all things are fair!
One God One Spirit and one human race!
One country, One Nation and One flag 🏳️!
To you up there, our love 🖤 to you is the same!
To you up high our gratitude 🙏 to you is the same!
To you flying high, we salute 🏳️ you is the same to the last breathe!
How much I wish this is not true!
How much I wish that all things are fair!
Love 🖤 is One and God is the Love 🖤 but the haters of mankind are many demons Satan and satans!

MAY I SAY:
The tears 😭 are the same colorless and pure!
The bloodshed is the same red blood with agony from the heart!
The sorrows are the same of sadness of life being cut short!
The grieve is the same of heartbroken 😔 of human life no more!
The loss is the same of a human life forever is taken away from the loved ones and left behind in the world 🌐 we live in!
The spirit is the same; a breath from God the Lord!
The soul is the same; a life living within the flesh made from the ground dust.
The human heart 🖤 is the same; a life beating within the temple of the Lord!
The human brain 🧠 is the same; a glorious treasure within the bones!
The Love 🖤 is the same; a precious diamond within the soul!
The source of Love 🖤 is the same; a God gift to us all!
Jesus Christ is the same; The Savior of the World 📖, God in the flesh!
God the Creator is the same; The Most High of us all the Heavenly Father of all mankind!
The Cross ✝️ is the same; a sacrificed soul hanged in the flesh bleeding to death for others!
As the Very First Veteran of mankind that laid down His Life for the world, God in the flesh, the Redeemer of all people Jesus Christ Our Lord
Jesus; The Good Shephard said: "Greater love has no one than this, than to lay down one's life for his friends." (John 15:13)

I KNEW LONG AGO
We all are the same and equal, created by One God the Creator of all things and born of one father Adam and one mother Eve!
The male sperm has the same color among all nations as also the female ovum among the generations!

Moreover, the human compatibility for conception is the same among all cultures producing the same newborn baby breathing the air we share, the sun ☀ we enjoy, the moon 🌙 we look at as we all walk, run and race in one globe 🌍!

In all the colors, all have the same impact and the same effect: Battles devastate as fires 🔥 burns as bullets kill as explosives destroy any human flesh!

TODAY IS THE DAY

Today is the day to commemorate all the lives laid down for others!

Today is the day to pay respect for all those who sacrificed their gift of life for the freedom we all enjoy today and forever!

Today is the day to love one another for ever more as our veterans made the world better place for the generations to follow!

Let us remember the words of Love 💜 from Our Master and Savior said: "This is My commandment, that you love one another as I have loved you. 13 Greater love has no one than this, than to lay down one's life for his friends." (John 15:12-13)

So from now; Let us put our differences aside!

Let us cast out the divisions among us! And Let us love 💜 one another!

One God One Spirit and one human race!

One country, One Nation and One flag 🏴!

To you up there, our love 💜 to you is the same!

To you up high our gratitude 🙏 to you is the same!

To you flying high, we salute 🇺🇸 you is the same to the last breathe!

How much I wish this is not true!

How much I wish that all things are fair!

To you all: To each of You by name: To every soul sacrificed: Thank you and we all for ever grateful.

You all made for us the steps that we must follow and raised the bar we must reach higher and higher to be handed to our children and all the grandchildren to come!

May you all Rest In Peace in the hands of the Lord surrounded with the Divine Love and care until we see you again as we pray for you all today and tomorrow!!!!

Thank you all

CG. This is a beautiful tribute to all veterans living and deceased. Bless them all. 💜🙏

On 11/11/2020, we Remember President Trump: My poem to President Trump 2018 as he was Paying Respect visiting all alone Aisene Marne American Cemetery near Bellevue France 🇺🇸 at Veterans Day! Thank you Mr President!

On 11/11/2018 Poem:

A Poem Dedicated to the president Donald Trump and his visit to the
Aisne Marne American Cemetery near the Belleau France 💙🏴

Written by
Ramsis GHALY

I came across this photo of our president and it says it all!
I may be alone but I am with them 💙🏴!
I am all alone visiting the souls 💙🏴 I cherished most!
I may not be with you but I am with them 💙🏴!
I came thousands of miles away to pay tribute to them 💙🏴 and not for they!
I put the American flag over each bringing them love from my home and their
home America 💙🏴!
Friends, I made the journey for them 💙🏴 and not for they!
So, don't be judgmental because I am alone!
Thank you Mr. President Trump for visiting them the American Heroes at the
Marne American Cemetery, Belleau in France 💙🏴 and from home we salute
you and them sending our love and prayers 💙🏴 Amen!

++++

From the kings places, I excused myself to be with them 💙🏴; the American
heroes of World War I 💙🏴!
Thousands miles from home I flew in the freezing cold to visit the Aisne Marne
American Cemetery near the Belleau Wood battleground, in Belleau, France, 90
kilometers northeast of the capital 💙🏴!
It is the closest place to my heart where U.S. troops 💙🏴 had their breakthrough
battle by stopping a German push for Paris shortly after entering the war in 1917!

+++

In serenity, I took time to reflect!
In a solitude I walked the steps to visit the coffins one by one 💙🏴!
Barefooted, I kneeled to salute each and all the American veterans 💙🏴 with
sincere respect!
I put the American flag over each bringing them love from my home and their
home America 💙🏴!
Away from the world, I kneeled to the Lord of hosts praying for the comfort of
their souls 💙🏴!

+++

I may be alone but I am with them 🖤🇺🇸!

I may not be with you but I am with them 🖤🇺🇸!

I am all alone visiting the souls 🖤🇺🇸 I cherished most!

I came thousands of miles away to pay tribute to them 🖤🇺🇸 and not for they!

I put the American flag over each bringing them love from my home and their home America 🖤🇺🇸!

Friends, I made the journey for them 🖤🇺🇸 and not for they!

So, don't be judgmental because I am alone!

Thank you Mr. President Trump for visiting them the American Hero's in France 🖤🇺🇸 and from home we salute you and them sending our love and prayers 🖤 🇺🇸 Amen

Ramsis Ghaly

May I Enter unto thy Court O Lord my God!

To The Victims and Vulnerable of COVID-19

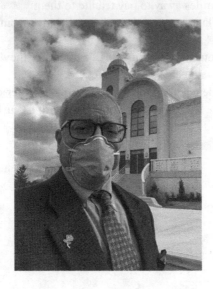

Ramsis GHALY
May I Enter unto thy Court O Lord my God!

Ramsis Ghaly

+ I am neither invited nor my name among the guest list; yet may I come to thy wedding!

+ I am not among thy faithful servant, may I come unto thy marriage!

+ I am not dressed with proper garment for thy wedding, may I come unto thy wedding!

+ I am neither articulate nor know how to talk, may I come unto thy marriage!

+ I am neither a royal nor a legend, may I come unto thy marriage! may I come unto thy wedding!

+ I am a lamp empty of oil, may I come unto thy wedding!

+ I am with no good deeds and didn't put my talents You have given me in the market, may I come unto thy wedding!

+ I have no coins and I earn no treasures, may I come unto thy wedding!

+ I am a homeless living by the crossroads and the freeways, my soul is among the bad and good and not one of thy guest, may I come unto thy marriage!

"Go ye therefore into the highways, and as many as ye shall find, bid to the marriage. [10] So those servants went out into the highways, and gathered together all as many as they found, both bad and good: and the wedding was furnished with guests." Matthew 22:9-10 KJV

+ I am not invited for thy Most Holy Wedding my King! I am not bidden to thy wedding, Behold, may I come unto thy marriage; thou prepared my dinner: my oxen and my fatlings are killed, and all things are ready: come unto the marriage.

"The kingdom of heaven is like unto a certain king, which made a marriage for his son, [3] And sent forth his servants to call them that were bidden to the wedding: and they would not come. [4] Again, he sent forth other servants, saying, Tell them which are bidden, Behold, I have prepared my dinner: my oxen and my fatlings are killed, and all things are ready: come unto the marriage. [5] But they made light of it, and went their ways, one to his farm, another to his merchandise:" Matthew 22:2-5 KJV

+ I am woman was a Greek, a Syrophenician by nation; I am lowly and eat of the crumbs which fall from their masters' table; May I come unto thy wedding!

"And, behold, a woman of Canaan came out of the same coasts, and cried unto him, saying, Have mercy on me, O Lord, thou Son of David; my daughter is grievously vexed with a devil. [23] But he answered her not a word. And his disciples came and besought him, saying, Send her away; for she crieth after us. [24] But he answered and said, I am not sent but unto the lost sheep of the house of Israel. [25] Then came she and worshipped him, saying, Lord, help me. [26] But he answered and said, It is not meet to take the children's bread, and to cast it to dogs. [27] And she said, Truth, Lord: yet the dogs eat of the crumbs which fall from their masters' table. [28] Then Jesus answered and said unto her, O woman, great is thy faith: be it unto thee even as thou wilt. And her daughter was made whole from that very hour." Matthew 15:22-28 KJV

+ Shew me thy ways, O Lord ; teach me thy paths. [7] Remember not the sins of my youth, nor my transgressions: according to thy mercy remember thou me for thy goodness' sake, O Lord. [11] For thy name's sake, O Lord, pardon mine iniquity; for it is great. [16] Turn thee unto me, and have mercy upon me; for I am desolate and afflicted. [20] O keep my soul, and deliver me: let me not be ashamed; for I put my trust in thee. Psalm 25:4,7,11,16,20 KJV

Psalm 25 "Unto thee, O Lord, do I lift up my soul. [2] O my God, I trust in thee: let me not be ashamed, let not mine enemies triumph over me. [3] Yea, let none that wait on thee be ashamed: let them be ashamed which transgress without cause. [4] Shew me thy ways, O Lord ; teach me thy paths. [5] Lead me in thy truth, and teach me: for thou art the God of my salvation; on thee do I wait all the day. [6] Remember, O Lord, thy tender mercies and thy lovingkindnesses; for they have been ever of old. [7] Remember not the sins of my youth, nor my transgressions: according to thy mercy remember thou me for thy goodness' sake, O Lord. [8] Good and upright is the Lord: therefore will he teach sinners in the way. [9] The meek will he guide in judgment: and the meek will he teach his way. [10] All the paths of the Lord are mercy and truth unto such as keep his covenant and his testimonies. [11] For thy name's sake, O Lord, pardon mine iniquity; for it is great. [12] What man is he that feareth the Lord ? him shall he teach in the way that he shall choose. [13] His soul shall dwell at ease; and his seed shall inherit the earth. [14] The secret of the Lord is with them that fear him; and he will shew them his covenant. [15] Mine eyes are ever toward the Lord ; for he shall pluck my feet out of the net. [16] Turn thee unto me, and have mercy upon me; for I am desolate and afflicted. [17] The troubles of my heart are enlarged: O bring thou me out of my distresses. [18] Look upon mine affliction and my pain; and forgive all my sins. [19] Consider mine enemies; for they are many; and they hate me with cruel hatred. [20] O keep my soul, and deliver me: let me not be ashamed; for I put my trust in thee. [21] Let integrity and uprightness preserve me; for I wait on thee. [22] Redeem Israel, O God, out of all his troubles."

+My name isn't written in thy Book of Life! I wasn't worthy and I didn't collect much of awards and. My soul deserves no reward! But I am Yours and You are mine my Beloved!!

+ There isn't life without You, please don't let me die the second death!! I beseech You let my soul in thy wedding O my Master!

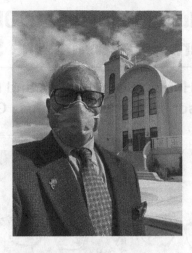

+ My life slept before my eyes! I didn't know You the way I should have! And now I come unto You empty hands but a heart full of love 🖤 to You O my Savior, may I come unto thy wedding!

+ I am neither invited nor my name among the guest list; yet may I come to thy wedding!

+ I am not among thy faithful servant, may I come unto thy marriage!

+ I am not dressed with proper garment for thy wedding, may I come unto thy wedding!

+ I am neither articulate nor know how to talk, may I come unto thy marriage!

+ I am neither a royal nor a legend, may I come unto thy marriage! may I come unto thy wedding!

+ I am a lamp empty of oil, may I come unto thy wedding!

+ I am with no good deeds and didn't put my talents You have given me in the market, may I come unto thy wedding!

KL. A wedding it will be when my Jesus I shall see! When I look upon his face, the one who saved me by his Grace!

MH. Love 🖤 this! I shall see him also with all the love 🖤 for him in my heart as well. He is always with me & answers my prayers as well.

JM. Beautiful

471

As a Human Flesh Gets Older It Withers Away While the Spirit

Within the Human Soul Bloweth and Blossoms!
Philosophy Written by Ramsis Ghaly

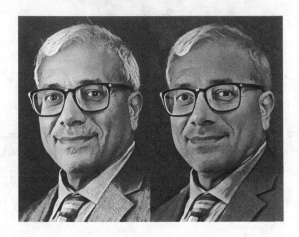

The nature is calling me "old", the people think I am "aged" and the government profiled me a a "senior citizen" and I have been pushed to the side and no longer of interest to the society that I was once living in and had been respected and ranked very high!!! None cared about my years of experiences, skills, knowledge and foresight! They are no longer important or even acknowledged or respected nowadays! As it is written: Titus 2:2 ESV Older men are to be sober-minded, dignified, self-controlled, sound in faith, in love, and in steadfastness.

But I am not old and I am Neither that person they drew nor the image they profiled me with! Let me explain:————-

As a Human Flesh Gets Older, It Withers Away, While the Spirit Within the Human Soul Bloweth and Blossoms! Indeed, as a human flesh gets older, the flesh withers away but the spirit revives more and more!

As a human flesh ages, it hits all of a sudden as other days slipped over night unnoticeable and the bodily aches are reminder of the age together with physical limitations climbing up one by one day by day!!

As a human flesh lives to the good old age, the soul is joyful with full of years gathered among own people!

As a Human Flesh Gets Older, the Earthly Senses Diminish While the Spiritual Senses Flourish!

As a human flesh gets older, the soul crowns as a queen full of glory, riches, honor, gratitude's and achievements of the years lived in faith, love sacrifice and service!

As a human flesh gets older, a man or a woman fills the earth with grace and increase the depth of humanity and establish the inheritance from generation to generation!

As a human flesh gets older, the love gets 🖤 deeper and real and the heartfelt emotions get plentiful!

As a human flesh gets older, life cherished more and more as everyday values tremendously!

As a human flesh gets older, the eyes become more tearful and the blessing are coming out abundantly!

As a human flesh gets older, being anxious 😟 is normal and worries about afterlife becomes genuine feeling close to the heart and the day of departure is no longer secret or unexpected!

As a human flesh get older, a man or a woman should be thankful that have lived a life that many didn't get chance to see!

Living one more day, it is another day to be saved indeed!

As a human flesh gets older, a man or a woman should be thankful that have lived a life that many didn't get chance to see!

As a human flesh gets older, a man or a woman actual get wiser but indeed gets closer to kiss goodbye!

As a human flesh gets older, a man or a woman loses the sensitivity of many human senses to the earthly matters to be able to sense the afterlife spirituality!

473

As a human flesh gets older, God opens the eyes to the heavenly and the unseen to prepare for what is beyond the world 🌑!

As a human flesh get older, it gets weaker, the desires subside and the passion to life goes down as the body gets more and more fragile!

As a human flesh gets older, the wishes for the seen, the hopes for the visible and the endeavors for material as they all be guided toward the life to come for the unseen!

As a human flesh gets older, the circle gets smaller and look closely many already had been gone and lost!

As a human flesh gets older, nonetheless, a man or a woman value life differently and has a different look at things around!

As you a human flesh gets older, the priorities absolutely get changed knowing the days ahead are counted!

As a human flesh gets older, there is no longer living the dream 🌝 but grasping the reality of life and the truth of the shadows of world!

As a human flesh gets older, a man or a woman lives more cautious not hastily and more thoughtful not to be heroic or patriotic but rather conservative!

As a human flesh gets older, a man or a Roman considers things haven't considered before, opens the eyes to things haven't acknowledge previously, opens the mind to things haven't accepted in the early days!

O friends, at the so called "old age", our father Abraham established our Lord covenant with humanity and give birth to the multitudes and innumerable future generations to fill the entire earth 🌍. And so many of the greatest fathers and mothers and various contributors did so one way or the other in history of mankind! In fact our Lord used the extreme age to establish His blessing and grace as with the newborn Samson and Samuel to the young boy David to the elder Moses and Abraham! Deuteronomy 34:7-8 KJV And Moses was an hundred and twenty years old when he died: his eye was not dim, nor his natural force abated. [8] And the children of Israel wept for Moses in the plains of Moab thirty days: so the days of weeping and mourning for Moses were ended.

God elected the weak and those rejected by man to show His grace and fill the earth with their hands-on experiences, touching hearts, kindness, mentorship, blessing, knowledge and wisdom in those believe in Him! As it is written: "That is why, for Christ's sake, I delight in weaknesses, in insults, in hardships, in persecutions, in difficulties. For when I am weak, then I am strong. "2 Corinthians 12:10 "My flesh and my heart may fail, but God is the strength of my heart and my portion forever." Psalm 73:26 "But he said to me, "My grace is sufficient for you, for my power is made perfect in weakness." Therefore I will boast all the more gladly about my weaknesses, so that Christ's power may rest on me." 2 Corinthians 12:9 "He gives strength to the weary and increases the power of the weak." Isaiah 40:29. "Come to me, all you who are weary and burdened, and I will give you rest." Matthew 11:28 "Cast all your anxiety on him because he cares for you." 1 Peter 5:7 "In the same way, the Spirit helps us in our weakness. We do not know what we ought to pray for, but the Spirit himself intercedes for us through wordless groans. Romans 8:26 "I can do all this through him who gives me strength. Philippians 4:13 "For the Spirit God gave us does not make us timid, but gives us power, love and self-discipline." 2 Timothy 1:71 "Watch and pray so that you will not fall into temptation. The spirit is willing, but the flesh is weak." Matthew 26:41 "A cheerful heart is good medicine, but a crushed spirit dries up the bones. Proverbs 17:22 "Speak up for those who cannot speak for themselves, for the rights of all who are destitute." Proverbs 31:8 "For we do not have a high priest who is unable to empathize with our weaknesses, but we have one who has been tempted in every way, just as we are—yet he did not sin." Hebrews 4:15 "Defend the weak and the fatherless; uphold the cause of the poor and the oppressed." Psalm 82:3

As a human flesh gets older, life gets different to be renewed to return to its origin not to its form!

Therefore, As a human flesh gets older, the flesh withers away but the spirit blossoms more and more! It is written: "But they that wait upon the Lord shall renew their strength; they shall mount up with wings as eagles; they shall run, and not be weary; and they shall walk, and not faint."

Isaiah 40:31 KJV
As a human flesh gets older, the flesh withers away but the spirit blossoms more and more! "The grass withereth, the flower fadeth: because the spirit of the Lord bloweth upon it: surely the people is grass. [8] The grass withereth, the flower fadeth: but the word of our God shall stand for ever." Isaiah 40:7-8 KJV And: "For to be carnally minded is death; but to be spiritually minded is life and peace. [9] But ye are not in the flesh, but in the Spirit, if so be that the Spirit of God dwell in you. Now if any man have not the Spirit of Christ, he is none of his. [10] And if Christ be in you, the body is dead because of sin; but the Spirit is life because of

righteousness. [13] For if ye live after the flesh, ye shall die: but if ye through the Spirit do mortify the deeds of the body, ye shall live." Romans 8:6,9-10,13 KJV And: John 3:6 "That which is born of the flesh is flesh, and that which is born of the Spirit is spirit." John 6:63 "It is the Spirit who gives life; the flesh profits nothing. The words that I speak to you are spirit, and they are life." And: "Watch and pray, that ye enter not into temptation: the spirit indeed is willing, but the flesh is weak." Matthew 26:41, KJV Watch ye and pray, lest ye enter into temptation. The spirit truly is ready, but the flesh is weak." Mark 14:38, KJV "That which is born of the flesh is flesh; and that which is born of the Spirit is spirit." John 3:6, KJV "It is the spirit that quickeneth; the flesh profiteth nothing: the words that I speak unto you, they are spirit, and they are life." John 6:63, KJV "For I know that in me (that is, in my flesh,) dwelleth no good thing: for to will is present with me; but how to perform that which is good I find not. For the good that I would I do not: but the evil which I would not, that I do." Romans 7:18-19, KJV "There is therefore now no condemnation to them which are in Christ Jesus, who walk not after the flesh, but after the Spirit . . . That the righteousness of the law might be fulfilled in us, who walk not after the flesh, but after the Spirit. For they that are after the flesh do mind the things of the flesh; but they that are after the Spirit the things of the Spirit. For to be carnally minded is death; but to be spiritually minded is life and peace . . . But ye are not in the flesh, but in the Spirit, if so be that the Spirit of God dwell in you. Now if any man have not the Spirit of Christ, he is none of his . . . For if ye live after the flesh, ye shall die: but if ye through the Spirit do mortify the deeds of the body, ye shall live." Romans 8:1, 4-6, 9, 13, KJV "Are ye so foolish? having begun in the Spirit, are ye now made perfect by the flesh?" Galatians 3:3, KJV "This I say then, Walk in the Spirit, and ye shall not fulfil the lust of the flesh. For the flesh lusteth against the Spirit, and the Spirit against the flesh: and these are contrary the one to the other: so that ye cannot do the things that ye would." Galatians 5:16-17, KJV "For he that soweth to his flesh shall of the flesh reap corruption; but he that soweth to the Spirit shall of the Spirit reap life everlasting." Galatians 6:8, KJV

As a Human Flesh Gets Older, It Withers Away, While the Spirit Within the Human Soul Bloweth and Blossoms! Indeed, as a human flesh gets older, the flesh withers away but the spirit revives more and more!

BIBLICAL VERSES OF ADVANCED AGE

Proverbs 16:31 ESV Gray hair is a crown of glory; it is gained in a righteous life.

Isaiah 46:4 ESV Even to your old age I am he, and to gray hairs I will carry you. I have made, and I will bear; I will carry and will save.

Job 12:12 ESV Wisdom is with the aged, and understanding in length of days.

Psalm 92:14 ESV They still bear fruit in old age; they are ever full of sap and green,

Psalm 71:18 ESV So even to old age and gray hairs, O God, do not forsake me, until I proclaim your might to another generation, your power to all those to come.

Psalm 71:9 ESV Do not cast me off in the time of old age; forsake me not when my strength is spent.

Leviticus 19:32 ESV "You shall stand up before the gray head and honor the face of an old man, and you shall fear your God: I am the Lord.

Proverbs 20:29 ESV The glory of young men is their strength, but the splendor of old men is their gray hair.

2 Corinthians 4:16 ESV So we do not lose heart. Though our outer self is wasting away, our inner self is being renewed day by day.

Proverbs 17:6 ESV Grandchildren are the crown of the aged, and the glory of children is their fathers.

Isaiah 40:31 ESV But they who wait for the Lord shall renew their strength; they shall mount up with wings like eagles; they shall run and not be weary; they shall walk and not faint.

Psalm 90:10 ESV The years of our life are seventy, or even by reason of strength eighty; yet their span is but toil and trouble; they are soon gone, and we fly away.

Psalm 37:25 ESV I have been young, and now am old, yet I have not seen the righteous forsaken or his children begging for bread.

Titus 2:2 ESV Older men are to be sober-minded, dignified, self-controlled, sound in faith, in love, and in steadfastness.

Job 5:26 ESV You shall come to your grave in ripe old age, like a sheaf gathered up in its season.

Job 32:7 ESV I said, 'Let days speak, and many years teach wisdom.'

Titus 2:3 ESV Older women likewise are to be reverent in behavior, not slanderers or slaves to much wine. They are to teach what is good,

Genesis 6:3 ESV Then the Lord said, "My Spirit shall not abide in man forever, for he is flesh: his days shall be 120 years."

Proverbs 23:22 ESV Listen to your father who gave you life, and do not despise your mother when she is old.

Deuteronomy 34:7 ESV Moses was 120 years old when he died. His eye was undimmed, and his vigor unabated.

Genesis 15:15 ESV As for yourself, you shall go to your fathers in peace; you shall be buried in a good old age.

Psalm 91:16 ESV With long life I will satisfy him and show him my salvation."

Job 11:17 ESV And your life will be brighter than the noonday; its darkness will be like the morning.

Philemon 1:9 ESV Yet for love's sake I prefer to appeal to you—I, Paul, an old man and now a prisoner also for Christ Jesus—

Isaiah 40:29 ESV He gives power to the faint, and to him who has no might he increases strength.

Ruth 4:15 ESV He shall be to you a restorer of life and a nourisher of your old age, for your daughter-in-law who loves you, who is more to you than seven sons, has given birth to him."

Psalm 71:17-18 ESV O God, from my youth you have taught me, and I still proclaim your wondrous deeds. So even to old age and gray hairs, O God, do not forsake me, until I proclaim your might to another generation, your power to all those to come.

Ecclesiastes 12:1-7 Remember also your Creator in the days of your youth, before the evil days come and the years draw near of which you will say, "I have no pleasure in them"; before the sun and the light and the moon and the stars are darkened and the clouds return after the rain, in the day when the keepers of the house tremble, and the strong men are bent, and the grinders cease because they are few, and those who look through the windows are dimmed, and the doors on the street are shut—when the sound of the grinding is low, and one rises up at the sound of a bird, and all the daughters of song are brought low— they are afraid also of what is high, and terrors are in the way; the almond tree blossoms, the grasshopper drags itself along, and desire fails, because man is going to his eternal home, and the mourners go about the streets— ...

1 Chronicles 29:28 ESV Then he died at a good age, full of days, riches, and honor. And Solomon his son reigned in his place.

Joel 2:28 ESV "And it shall come to pass afterward, that I will pour out my Spirit on all flesh; your sons and your daughters shall prophesy, your old men shall dream dreams, and your young men shall see visions.

Psalm 92:12-14 ESV The righteous flourish like the palm tree and grow like a cedar in Lebanon. They are planted in the house of the Lord; they flourish in the courts of our God. They still bear fruit in old age; they are ever full of sap and green,

Ecclesiastes 7:10 ESV Say not, "Why were the former days better than these?" For it is not from wisdom that you ask this.

Genesis 25:8 ESV Abraham breathed his last and died in a good old age, an old man and full of years, and was gathered to his people.

Luke 2:37 ESV And then as a widow until she was eighty-four. She did not depart from the temple, worshiping with fasting and prayer night and day.

Luke 2:36-38 ESV And there was a prophetess, Anna, the daughter of Phanuel, of the tribe of Asher. She was advanced in years, having lived with her husband seven years from when she was a virgin, and then as a widow until she was eighty-four. She did not depart from the temple, worshiping with fasting and prayer night and day. And coming up at that very hour she began to give thanks to God and to speak of him to all who were waiting for the redemption of Jerusalem.

Psalm 90:12 ESV So teach us to number our days that we may get a heart of wisdom.

Luke 1:36 ESV And behold, your relative Elizabeth in her old age has also conceived a son, and this is the sixth month with her who was called barren.

Deuteronomy 32:7 ESV Remember the days of old; consider the years of many generations; ask your father, and he will show you, your elders, and they will tell you.

1 Timothy 5:1-2 ESV Do not rebuke an older man but encourage him as you would a father, younger men as brothers, older women as mothers, younger women as sisters, in all purity.

Titus 2:2-3 ESV Older men are to be sober-minded, dignified, self-controlled, sound in faith, in love, and in steadfastness. Older women likewise are to be reverent in behavior, not slanderers or slaves to much wine. They are to teach what is good,

Job 12:20 ESV He deprives of speech those who are trusted and takes away the discernment of the elders.

Psalm 143:5 ESV I remember the days of old; I meditate on all that you have done; I ponder the work of your hands.

Job 42:17 ESV And Job died, an old man, and full of days.

1 Kings 12:6 ESV Then King Rehoboam took counsel with the old men, who had stood before Solomon his father while he was yet alive, saying, "How do you advise me to answer this people?"

Exodus 20:12 ESV Honor your father and your mother, that your days may be long in the land that the Lord your God is giving you.

Psalm 71:18-19 ESV So even to old age and gray hairs, O God, do not forsake me, until I proclaim your might to another generation, your power to all those to come. Your righteousness, O God, reaches the high heavens. You who have done great things, O God, who is like you?

Genesis 24:1 ESV Now Abraham was old, well advanced in years. And the Lord had blessed Abraham in all things.

Philippians 1:6 ESV And I am sure of this, that he who began a good work in you will bring it to completion at the day of Jesus Christ.

1 Kings 12:8 ESV But he abandoned the counsel that the old men gave him and took counsel with the young men who had grown up with him and stood before him.

Job 32:9 ESV It is not the old who are wise, nor the aged who understand what is right.

Genesis 47:9 ESV And Jacob said to Pharaoh, "The days of the years of my sojourning are 130 years. Few and evil have been the days of the years of my life, and they have not attained to the days of the years of the life of my fathers in the days of their sojourning."

Job 32:4 ESV Now Elihu had waited to speak to Job because they were older than he.

Deuteronomy 33:25 ESV Your bars shall be iron and bronze, and as your days, so shall your strength be.

Ephesians 6:1-3 ESV Children, obey your parents in the Lord, for this is right. "Honor your father and mother" (this is the first commandment with a promise), "that it may go well with you and that you may live long in the land."

James 4:14 ESV Yet you do not know what tomorrow will bring. What is your life? For you are a mist that appears for a little time and then vanishes.

1 Kings 3:14 ESV And if you will walk in my ways, keeping my statutes and my commandments, as your father David walked, then I will lengthen your days."

Exodus 7:7 ESV Now Moses was eighty years old, and Aaron eighty-three years old, when they spoke to Pharaoh.

1 Peter 1:24 ESV For "All flesh is like grass and all its glory like the flower of grass. The grass withers, and the flower falls,

Psalm 39:5 ESV Behold, you have made my days a few handbreadths, and my lifetime is as nothing before you. Surely all mankind stands as a mere breath! Selah

Isaiah 38:12 ESV My dwelling is plucked up and removed from me like a shepherd's tent; like a weaver I have rolled up my life; he cuts me off from the loom; from day to night you bring me to an end;

Psalm 23:1-6 ESV A Psalm of David. The Lord is my shepherd; I shall not want. He makes me lie down in green pastures. He leads me beside still waters. He restores my soul. He leads me in paths of righteousness for his name's sake. Even though I walk through the valley of the shadow of death, I will fear no evil, for you are with me; your rod and your staff, they comfort me. You prepare a table before me in the presence of my enemies; you anoint my head with oil; my cup overflows. ...

Genesis 37:3 ESV Now Israel loved Joseph more than any other of his sons, because he was the son of his old age. And he made him a robe of many colors.

Joshua 14:10 ESV And now, behold, the Lord has kept me alive, just as he said, these forty-five years since the time that the Lord spoke this word to Moses, while Israel walked in the wilderness. And now, behold, I am this day eighty-five years old.

Ecclesiastes 12:1-14 ESV Remember also your Creator in the days of your youth, before the evil days come and the years draw near of which you will say, "I have no pleasure in them"; before the sun and the light and the moon and the stars are darkened and the clouds return after the rain, in the day when the keepers of the house tremble, and the strong men are bent, and the grinders cease because they are few, and those who look through the windows are dimmed, and the doors on the street are shut—when the sound of the grinding is low, and one rises up at the sound of a bird, and all the daughters of song are brought low— they are afraid also of what is high, and terrors are in the way; the almond tree blossoms, the grasshopper drags itself along, and desire fails, because man is going to his eternal home, and the mourners go about the streets— ...

Ecclesiastes 12:1-3 ESV Remember also your Creator in the days of your youth, before the evil days come and the years draw near of which you will say, "I have no pleasure in them"; before the sun and the light and the moon and the stars are darkened and the clouds return after the rain, in the day when the keepers of the house tremble, and the strong men are bent, and the grinders cease because they are few, and those who look through the windows are dimmed,

Psalm 119:100 ESV I understand more than the aged, for I keep your precepts.

Ecclesiastes 9:10 ESV Whatever your hand finds to do, do it with your might, for there is no work or thought or knowledge or wisdom in Sheol, to which you are going.

Proverbs 10:27 ESV The fear of the Lord prolongs life, but the years of the wicked will be short.

1 Timothy 5:1 ESV Do not rebuke an older man but encourage him as you would a father, younger men as brothers,

Isaiah 47:6 ESV I was angry with my people; I profaned my heritage; I gave them into your hand; you showed them no mercy; on the aged you made your yoke exceedingly heavy.

Isaiah 46:3-4 ESV "Listen to me, O house of Jacob, all the remnant of the house of Israel, who have been borne by me from before your birth, carried from the womb; even to your old age I am he, and to gray hairs I will carry you. I have made, and I will bear; I will carry and will save.

Psalm 71:17 ESV O God, from my youth you have taught me, and I still proclaim your wondrous deeds.

Genesis 25:7-8 ESV These are the days of the years of Abraham's life, 175 years. Abraham breathed his last and died in a good old age, an old man and full of years, and was gathered to his people.

Proverbs 3:13 ESV Blessed is the one who finds wisdom, and the one who gets understanding,

Genesis 5:1-32 ESV This is the book of the generations of Adam. When God created man, he made him in the likeness of God. Male and female he created them, and he blessed them and named them Man when they were created. When Adam had lived 130 years, he fathered a son in his own likeness, after his image, and named him Seth. The days of Adam after he fathered Seth were 800 years; and he had other sons and daughters. Thus all the days that Adam lived were 930 years, and he died. ...

1 Timothy 5:17 ESV Let the elders who rule well be considered worthy of double honor, especially those who labor in preaching and teaching.

Lamentations 5:12 ESV Princes are hung up by their hands; no respect is shown to the elders.

Jeremiah 29:11 ESV For I know the plans I have for you, declares the Lord, plans for welfare and not for evil, to give you a future and a hope.

Psalm 103:5 ESV Who satisfies you with good so that your youth is renewed like the eagle's.

Deuteronomy 5:33 ESV You shall walk in all the way that the Lord your God has commanded you, that you may live, and that it may go well with you, and that you may live long in the land that you shall possess.

John 3:16-17 ESV "For God so loved the world, that he gave his only Son, that whoever believes in him should not perish but have eternal life. For God did not send his Son into the world to condemn the world, but in order that the world might be saved through him.

Deuteronomy 5:16 ESV "'Honor your father and your mother, as the Lord your God commanded you, that your days may be long, and that it may go well with you in the land that the Lord your God is giving you.

Revelation 1:1-20 ESV The revelation of Jesus Christ, which God gave him to show to his servants the things that must soon take place. He made it known by sending his angel to his servant John, who bore witness to the word of God and to the testimony of Jesus Christ, even to all that he saw. Blessed is the one who reads aloud the words of this prophecy, and blessed are those who hear, and who keep what is written in it, for the time is near. John to the seven churches that are in Asia: Grace to you and peace from him who is and who was and who is to come, and from the seven spirits who are before his throne, and from Jesus Christ the faithful witness, the firstborn of the dead, and the ruler of kings on earth. To him who loves us and has freed us from our sins by his blood ...

Isaiah 65:20 ESV No more shall there be in it an infant who lives but a few days, or an old man who does not fill out his days, for the young man shall die a hundred years old, and the sinner a hundred years old shall be accursed.

Psalm 148:12 ESV Young men and maidens together, old men and children!

Psalm 48:14 ESV That this is God, our God forever and ever. He will guide us forever.

Psalm 90:5 ESV You sweep them away as with a flood; they are like a dream, like grass that is renewed in the morning:

Job 15:10 ESV Both the gray-haired and the aged are among us, older than your father.

Numbers 8:25 ESV And from the age of fifty years they shall withdraw from the duty of the service and serve no more.

Zechariah 8:4 ESV Thus says the Lord of hosts: Old men and old women shall again sit in the streets of Jerusalem, each with staff in hand because of great age.

Psalm 92:12-15 ESV The righteous flourish like the palm tree and grow like a cedar in Lebanon. They are planted in the house of the Lord; they flourish in the courts of our God. They still bear fruit in old age; they are ever full of sap and green, to declare that the Lord is upright; he is my rock, and there is no unrighteousness in him.

James 4:4 ESV You adulterous people! Do you not know that friendship with the world is enmity with God? Therefore whoever wishes to be a friend of the world makes himself an enemy of God.

Psalm 71:9-10 ESV Do not cast me off in the time of old age; forsake me not when my strength is spent. For my enemies speak concerning me; those who watch for my life consult together

Psalm 71:1-24 ESV In you, O Lord, do I take refuge; let me never be put to shame! In your righteousness deliver me and rescue me; incline your ear to me, and save me! Be to me a rock of refuge, to which I may continually come; you have given the command to save me, for you are my rock and my fortress. Rescue me, O my God, from the hand of the wicked, from the grasp of the unjust and cruel man. For you, O Lord, are my hope, my trust, O Lord, from my youth. ...

Leviticus 19:1-37 ESV And the Lord spoke to Moses, saying, "Speak to all the congregation of the people of Israel and say to them, You shall be holy, for I the Lord your God am holy. Every one of you shall revere his mother and his father, and you shall keep my Sabbaths: I am the Lord your God. Do not turn to idols or make for yourselves any gods of cast metal: I am the Lord your God. "When you offer a sacrifice of peace offerings to the Lord, you shall offer it so that you may be accepted. ...

Proverbs 19:20 ESV Listen to advice and accept instruction, that you may gain wisdom in the future.

Psalm 139:1-24 ESV To the choirmaster. A Psalm of David. O Lord, you have searched me and known me! You know when I sit down and when I rise up; you discern my thoughts from afar. You search out my path and my lying down and are acquainted with all my ways. Even before a word is on my tongue, behold, O Lord, you know it altogether. You hem me in, behind and before, and lay your hand upon me. ...

Ecclesiastes 6:3 ESV If a man fathers a hundred children and lives many years, so that the days of his years are many, but his soul is not satisfied with life's good things, and he also has no burial, I say that a stillborn child is better off than he.

Joshua 14:10-11 ESV And now, behold, the Lord has kept me alive, just as he said, these forty-five years since the time that the Lord spoke this word to Moses, while Israel walked in the wilderness. And now, behold, I am this day eighty-five years old. I am still as strong today as I was in the day that Moses sent me; my strength now is as my strength was then, for war and for going and coming.

1 Peter 1:13 ESV Therefore, preparing your minds for action, and being sober-minded, set your hope fully on the grace that will be brought to you at the revelation of Jesus Christ.

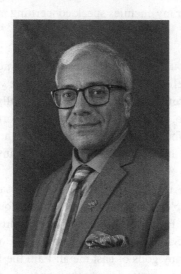

JM. Wonderful Writing 💕 Dr Ghaly 💕
KG. Very much needed words to see today! Thank you!

As we age, Society changes and those younger ones believe they KNOW it all and WE, with the foresight, knowledge and experience become labelled and pushed to the side. Yet, these younger ones born in the 80s haven't much needed life skills and once they marry only then seem to run back home to their parents for assistance. I've seen it so many times in the last 30 years. The world has lost respect for its gifted talented and most intelligent ones with experience. I predict it to become a huge life lesson when these know it all learn the hardest lesson and God Forbid lose someone they love close to them while they are off knowing it all.

Thank you so much for your wise words that bring great comfort in troubled times and daily life. Please stay safe, well and God Bless you Always for all you do! Xoxo

LR. Thank you for all these words of wisdom spoken and written down, from these reliable sources. Not only do I notice these words to be true, as I age, but have also noticed the loss of respect given to the AGED. I'm not sure why or where this comes from. Some are taken advantage of because of their age. Where did this begin? How did it get its start? Not everyone attempts this behavior, but it is very apparent that some DO. An AGING person needs more help, and may not ask. Shame on those who take advantage of anyone else, but especially the AGED. Wisdom is worth it's weight in gold from an aging person. No amount of money can buy it!

Thank you for these words that you spent so much time writing down for us. I will save and reread them as I age. They ARE a true 🎁 gift of wisdom from those that walked this world before us.

RH. A young girl. Just cause I have to pluck a few hairs on my chin once in a while
CG. Your words are right on point. I can't believe that older people are treated with disrespect. I haven't noticed this with younger people I have known, but I guess it can happen. You look very dapper in your photo.
SK. May God continue to bestow Blessings upon you!
MH. Well said & oh so true. Be safe out there. Time to relax & enjoy, travel & see your friends 😊 you look good.

487

It Is Not Death But It is New Beginning!

To The Victims and Vulnerable of COVID-19

Don't Cry 🙈 "the damsel is not dead, but sleepeth" "sorrow not, even as others which have no hope" "Be not afraid, only believe!! "To die is a gain—-to be with Christ which is far better"

Written by
Ramsis Ghaly

It isn't death 💀 but it is life!
It isn't death 💀 but it is a New Beginning with no end!
It isn't death 💀 but it is Grace to those honored to be the children of God in the Book of Life!
It isn't death 💀 but it is that time to be received to Jesus Christ!
It isn't death 💀 but meeting face-to-face with the Holy Lamb, the Savior of the world the Son of God!
It isn't death 💀 but it is union of the son and the daughter to the True Heavenly Father!
It isn't death 💀 but it is comfort to His own!
It isn't death, 💀 but the end of a test and beginning of the unimaginable awards!
It isn't death 💀 but it is step I to the step II results!
It isn't death 💀 but it is that step taken alone of no return!
It isn't death 💀 but entrance of saved souls to the Heavenly Castle 🏰!
It isn't death 💀 but it is a gain!
It isn't death 💀 but it is to be Christ which is far better!
It isn't death 💀 but it is the Heavenly Father call 📞 to come home!
It isn't death 💀 but it is invite of the Savior to His faithful servants!
It isn't death 💀 but it is departure!
It isn't death 💀 but it is sleepeth!
It isn't death 💀 but it is immediate transition from the seen to the unseen!
It isn't death 💀 but it is end of suffering and beginning of everlasting joy of the sheep!
It isn't death 💀 but it is the key to true freedom!
It isn't death 💀 but t is the final visit to the sacred secret closet taking off the old garment and dress with the most precious wedding holy garment!
It isn't death 💀 but it is final longtime waiting for goodbye 👋 to the world 🌍 tribulations!

488

It isn't death 💀 but it is removing the mortal flesh and liberating the immortal spirit!

It isn't death 💀 but it is a gate to eternity!

It isn't death 💀 but a flight ✈ lift over the clouds ☁ to dream life to come!

"Let not your heart be troubled: ye believe in God, believe also in me. [2] In my Father's house are many mansions: if it were not so, I would have told you. I go to prepare a place for you. [3] And if I go and prepare a place for you, I will come again, and receive you unto myself; that where I am, there ye may be also. [4] And whither I go ye know, and the way ye know. [6] Jesus saith unto him, I am the way, the truth, and the life: no man cometh unto the Father, but by me." John 14:1-4,6 KJV

Sadness and sorrows be transformed to joy and celebration!

Tears 😩 and cries 😩 be transformed to praises and exaltation!

Therefore, O weeping 😩 souls: Don't Cry 😩 the damsel is not dead, but sleepeth! Why make ye this ado, and weep???? So Do not laugh to scorn!!!

"And when he was come in, he saith unto them, Why make ye this ado, and weep? the damsel is not dead, but sleepeth. And they laughed him to scorn. But when he had put them all out, he taketh the father and the mother of the damsel, and them that were with him, and entereth in where the damsel was lying." Mark 5: 39-40 KJV

"As soon as Jesus heard the word that was spoken, he saith unto the ruler of the synagogue, Be not afraid, only believe." Mark 5:36 KJV

"And he took the damsel by the hand, and said unto her, Talitha cumi; which is, being interpreted, Damsel, I say unto thee, arise. [42] And straightway the damsel arose, and walked; for she was of the age of twelve years. And they were astonished with a great astonishment." Mark 5:41-42 KJV

Wherefore comfort one another with these words.

"But I would not have you to be ignorant, brethren, concerning them which are asleep, that ye sorrow not, even as others which have no hope. [14] For if we believe that Jesus died and rose again, even so them also which sleep in Jesus will God bring with him. [15] For this we say unto you by the word of the Lord, that we which are alive and remain unto the coming of the Lord shall not prevent them which are asleep. [16] For the Lord himself shall descend from heaven with a shout, with the voice of the archangel, and with the trump of God: and the dead in Christ shall rise first: [17] Then we which are alive and remain shall be caught up together with them in the clouds, to meet the Lord in the air: and so shall we ever be with the Lord. [18] Wherefore comfort one another with these words." 1 Thessalonians 4:13-18 KJV

It is a gain!
"For to me to live is Christ, and to die is gain. [22] But if I live in the flesh, this is the fruit of my labour: yet what I shall choose I wot not. [23] For I am in a strait betwixt two, having a desire to depart, and to be with Christ; which is far better:" Philippians 1:21-23 KJV

Don't Cry 😭 "the damsel is not dead, but sleepeth" "sorrow not, even as others which have no hope" "Be not afraid, only believe!! "To die is a gain—-to be with Christ which is far better"

"Now may the Lord of peace Himself continually grant you peace in every circumstance." 2 Thessalonians 3:16

Cg. Beautifully written representation of death to eternal life. 🖤🙏

America Acknowledged the Aremenian Christian Genocide 1915-1918

The Christians Armenian genocide 1915-1919 by the Islamic sword of Turks acknowledged and recognized formally 100 years later by America, President Biden. Despite the century of denial to the evilness of Ottoman Empire — so many years the Armenians are seeking justices and have never ever received justice. Congratulations to our Armenian American Christian community thank you for your perseverance and hardworking though decades!! Your ancestors together with all of us so proud of you!!

https://fb.watch/54icUh2ZC5/
https://fb.watch/54ihfesQFQ/

Thank you 🙏
APRIL 25, 2021

Let us remember the millions at least 34 million of Russian Mass Causalities in the turn of 20 century between world war II and the Dictator Joseph Stalin!!

Ramsis Ghaly

Estimates of the number of deaths attributable to the Soviet dictator Joseph Stalin vary widely. Some scholars assert that record-keeping of the executions of political prisoners and ethnic minorities are neither reliable nor complete[1] while others contend that archival materials declassified in 1991 contain irrefutable data far superior to sources used prior to 1991 such as statements from emigres and other informants.[2][3]

Exhumed mass grave of the Vinnytsia massacre

Prior to the dissolution of the Soviet Union and the archival revelations, some historians estimated that the numbers killed by Stalin's regime were 20 million or higher.[4][5][6] After the Soviet Union dissolved, evidence from the Soviet archives was declassified and researchers were allowed to study it. This contained official records of 799,455 executions (1921–1953),[7] around 1.7 million deaths in the Gulag,[8][9] some 390,000[10] deaths during the dekulakization forced resettlement and up to 400,000 deaths of persons deported during the 1940s,[11] with a total of about 3.3 million officially recorded victims in these categories. [12] The deaths of at least 5.5 to 6.5 million[13] persons in the Soviet famine of 1932–1933 are sometimes, but not always, included with the victims of the Stalin era.[2][14]

https://en.m.wikipedia.org/.../Excess_mortality_in_the...

Never forget the bravery of the 27 million Russians died in World War II

Let us remember the 27 million Brave men and women of Soviet Union Russia died during World War II against the Nazi Germany . The Soviet Union Russia paid the harshest price:

492

Hitler wanted not only to eradicate the Jews; he wanted also to destroy Poland and the Soviet Union as states, exterminate their ruling classes, and kill tens of millions of Slavs—

The Red Army was "the main engine of Nazism's destruction," writes British historian and journalist Max Hastings in "Inferno: The World at War, 1939-1945." The Soviet Union paid the harshest price: though the numbers are not exact, an estimated 26 million Soviet citizens died during World War II, including as many as

https://www.washingtonpost.com/.../dont-forget-how.../...
https://en.m.wikipedia.org/.../World_War_II_casualties_of...

EN.M.WIKIPEDIA.ORG
Excess mortality in the Soviet Union under Joseph Stalin - Wikipedia
Estimates of the number of deaths attributable to the Soviet dictator Joseph Stalin vary widely. Some scholars assert that record-keeping of the executions of political prisoners and ethnic minorities are neither reliable nor complete[1] while others contend that archival materials declassified in 1...

CG. ery sad time for both countries. When we visited these countries the people would tell how awful it was to be frighted of the Nazi's. They would show us bullet holes on the outside of the building where non believers were shot. I know it was like that in both countries. How very sad. 😥

Dedicated to My Patient Carmel Perino

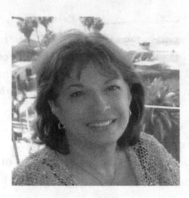

What a loss! My patient I have known for almost three decades just passed away!! We are crying heavily with running tears! You were just an eagle 🦅 flying full of love 🖤 always be in our hearts and homes! Rest in peace

Carmel Perino! This year need to end soon enough O lord we pray!!

Carmel Perino was the best in every aspect. She was our angel on earth and now she is joining the eternal paradise in Jesus hand in His bosom and St Mary.

Carmel served well her entire life and brought up gorgeous kids, and her children and grand children were all her life and love. They are grown and she always proud of them as we all are,

Onnie Richter, Angi and Louis. Her grand children are her testimony with her children, friends and all whoever met her.

I did Carmel surgery years ago and became so close to them all and became part of their family. In Christmas, in thanksgiving and many times, visits and phones. Her children are part of Me. I saw her two month ago and she was doing well.

Back then, many told her she won't recover from brain surgery and couldn't talk. Her two beautiful daughters Onni and Angi listen to no one and their love and Italian determination, Carmel lived two decades after surgery doing fantastic and got to see her grandchildren. Her own children continued to train her daily for two straight years when hospital and therapists said no hope until she regained her speech and ability to talk and converse! Never once her two daughters Angi and Onni left her sight. She loved them so much. What a strong woman was full of love. She did all by her own hands and her will took her thousands of Miles and her love 💜 filled the earth! I can't speak enough about you Carmel! You conquered the impossible during your earthly journey and now you are triumphant up high in heaven!

The death is all of a sudden, she was taken to Rush St Luke hospital and no much of information because of COVID mess! Michael was of great support to Carmel. So sorry Michael and all her friends and family members about your all loss!

Carmel your soul is in joy, you have done well and fought the good fight. We loved you so much and we will miss you much.

Onni, Angi and Louis no words that I could express our loss and deep sorrows and sadness. She was always proud of each of you and so we all are. She is in good comfort praying for us and holding our hearts always. Repose in peace Carmel with joy with the angels of our Lord Jesus, Amen we all pray

"I have fought a good fight, I have finished my course, I have kept the faith:8 Henceforth there is laid up for me a crown of righteousness, which the Lord, the righteous judge, shall give me at that day: and not to me only, but unto all them also that love his appearing."2 Timothy 4:7-8

Ramsis Ghaly

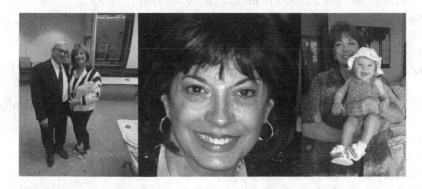

AK. So sorry for your loss, Doctor. 💜🙏
VA. Sorry
DM. So sorry for your loss
NP. So sorry for your loss 🙏 My deepest condolences for you and her family 🙏
JB. So very sorry for your loss! May she rest in the loving arms of her heavenly
   Father and may God grant comfort and peace to her family and friends.

LC. SO SORRY TO HEAR THIS She is flying with the Angels now R,I,P,AND GOD BLESS

CD. Lovely lady. I met her here at Silver Cross. RIP.

ml. Such a loss. I pray for her family during this time of grief. May her spirit live on in the hearts of her family. 🙏

Rp. My deepest condolences 🙏 such a beautiful woman.

Rf. I am so sorry. We know God has her now and is waiting for all of us to join her in Eternal Life.

Sr. She was such a beautiful lady!!

Kg. I am so very sorry for the loss of your patient and friend 😢

Db. Prayers for her family 🙏🙏

LB. Prayers for her family 🙏🙏

JJ, So sorry for your loss, prayers are sent for you, Carmel's whole family. Rip!

BB. So sorry

CN. So sorry to hear this. I got to know her through your foundation. She was a sweetheart.

LL. A dear friend gone too soon! Susie's bff and travel friend! Many hearty laughs with Carmie over the years. Oz and Michael and Chris often played together. Beautiful memories of the best of times. May you Rest In Peace Carmie! Our heartfelt sympathy to your family!

DL. Sincere condolences to all those who knew her and especially her family.

DE, So sorry for your loss 🙏

SK. May she Rest In Peace. I'm so grateful for our friendship, and will miss her dearly. She was a beautiful person inside and out! 🙏❤️😢

CG. My deepest condolences for you and her family. May she rest in peace. 🙏

KO. Prayers for her family 🙏🙏

KC. So sorry, Dr. Ghaly

MZ. I'm sorry for your loos my deepest condolences to you doctor God rest her soul in peace

AP. Memory Eternal to our sister in Faith - Carmel. Comfort and peace to family and friends. ✝️💐

NE. So sorry for your loss Dr. Ghaly! May her soul Rest In Peace!

TJ. I'm so sorry, Dr. Ghaly. Rest in Heaven, beautiful lady!

RN. Sorry for your loss Dr.Ghaly 🙏🙏

LM. So sorry for the loss of your friend sending condolences and prayers 🙏🙏🙏

BR. So sorry for your loss. May she rest in peace..

KW. Sorry for your loss. 🙏❤️

AV. Sorry to hear this! Praying for the family! 😢🙏

BC. May She Rest in Peace, Amen

RH. Sorry for your loss

RM. May you Rest in Peace God bless you and yours 😢🙏

BK. So sorry to hear this news Dr Ghaly. So very sad. Prayers for you and the family. 🙏🙏🙏

BD. So sorry for the loss of one you so blessed and cared for, sending prayers to you and the family. 🙏🙏🙏

AP. My sincerest and deepest condolences for your loss. May she R.I.P. 🙏😔🌷

BS. I am so sorry for your loss, Dr. Ghali

SM. Sorry for your loss Dr. Ghaly!

JM. A Beautiful Girl 🖤 Prayers For The Family 🖤

SS. I'm so sorry for your loss! All of you are in my prayers.

NL. So sorry for your loss. May the Lord comfort you and her family as you all grieve.

JM. So sorry 😢 our Deepest Condolences and prayers

MH. LM. My condolences to you and her family 🙏

RN. My condolences to you and to her family 🕯️✝️🙏😔

FL. Sorry it's never easy to loose friends

LP. So sad. I remember her when we were CINN

PH. I am so sorry. God has plans, but we never understand, do we.

MS. May she Rest In Peace 🕊️🙏

LH. So sorry for your loss 😞

PH. For you and her family 🙏❤️🙏❤️🙏❤️

MV. So sad! Prayers for all who loved her! 🙏🙏

JH. Sorry for your loss, Dr.Ghaly.

TC. ~ My condolences . . . 🖤

CS. So deeply sorry for your loss! May she RIP.

JD. So sorry, blessings to her family.

AA. Si sorry for your loss. Such a beautiful lady. May God guide her steps to Him.

SF. I'm so very sorry for the loss of your friend and patient. 🙏

TW. I'm so very sorry to hear of your dear friend/patient's passing. I know how much you care for your patient's.... you're such a loving, sweet and devoted Dr. I'm sending prayers up to our Heavenly Father to lift everyone up who loved your friend. Think…

JS. I'm so sorry for your loss Doc... 🙏🙏

KG. So sorry for your loss. Prayers to her family and friends

DU. Noooo, this is very sad news. What a beautiful person! 😔

AM. Oh Dr Ghaly, I am so very sorry. Praying for comfort for the family.

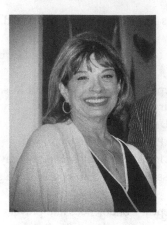

My mom

Carmel Perino

had complications early this morning and passed away at 5:53am. Thank you all so much for your kind words and prayers. She was such a strong, passionate, driven women that never stopped... NEVER STOPPED until God called her home. She will be missed dearly.

My brother

Louis Yangas

, sister (Ange), and I are navigating through this process and will keep you posted on the memorial service.

John 16:22

"You too have grief now; but I will see you again, and your heart will rejoice, and no one will take your joy away from you."

NS. I am 😢🙏 so sorry to read this. Your mom was a wonderful, kind person. You are all in my thoughts and 🖤🖤🖤 prayers DB. Onnie, sending you love & hugs! I am so sorry! She was a gem! I remember her well!

BE. Onnie, I am so sorry to hear this news and for the loss of your mother and your children's grandmother. Your family will continue to be in my prayers!

CB. I'm so sorry. I've known her since I was just in high school. She was always so energetic and outspoken. I never liked doing yard work or helping people move, but she was so fun to be around that I never minded doing it for her.

SC. So very loss, Onnie. Your Mom was simply amazing, a beautiful kind heart and a blessing to so many. My heart aches. God bless you all and may our beautiful Carmie rest in eternal peace.

FO, Dear Onnie, I am so very, very sorry about your mom. Carmie and I have been friends for a long time and I'm sorry I didn't meet you as an adult. I see she had complications, though I don't know what was wrong. My condolences to your entire family. Pl…

AM. I'm so sorry, Onnie. Nothing ever prepares you for the loss of your mom. Erik and I wish you peace as you navigate through this difficult time.

ST. Dearest Onnie, Louie, and Ange; I don't know how the world can possibly go on without your Mom's bubbly personality, friendly demeanor, kind heart, and dearest of all friends. I am beyond sorry for the entire family, and will miss my close friend until…

I'm so so sorry. She was the sweetest lady ever. She was a bright light and will never be forgotten. Condolences to your family. 🖤

JM. So very sorry for your loss 🐱 I will always remember your Mom 🖤 with beautiful memories 🐱 Keeping your entire family in my sincerest thoughts & prayers at this most sad time 🐱🙏🙏🖤

LM. I am very sorry to hear abt your Mom. She was a fantastic woman and a beautiful lady. My heart goes out to you, Angie and your brother. No words can take away your pain but please know we are all Sending prayers to you during this very difficult time…

DM, My heart breaks for you, Ange and Lou. May you all find peace during this difficult time. Many prayers sent across the pond from our family to yours

NM. I'm so sorry for your loss.

I went to grade school and high school with Carmel Ann and she was a special friend and a wonderful person.

My heart break for her family.

SC. I'm so sorry for your loss Onnie. I loved her so much she was the best women I have ever known I will miss you dearly..

JN. Lou Im so sorry for you loss and your entire family. Your mom was one of the most sweetest woman I have ever met. She was so kind and giving. She had a BIG heart. She will be missed by many. She always looked after my best friend Cheryl and I think…

DL. OMG - Just seeing this - please message me when you can with details for her so I can let this side of the Yangas clan know. I adored your Mom. Anything I can do please let me know

MN. Dear Onnie, Carm was one of our 'Soul Sisters' from her retreat group. We all became acquainted in 2014. Carm brought joy and laughter to us. We lover her dearly and share in your sorrow. Please know that she talked about you all the time and was …

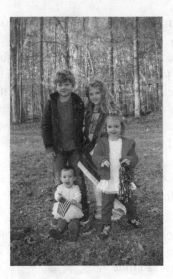

JW. Oh my God! I just talked to her when she got home from vacation. I'm so sorry 😭 My prayers are with you 🙏 and family.

BU. I am so so sorry for your loss Onnie! This is so sad news.

Love you dearly. I pray that the Lord will cover you with peace and comfort only He can give. 💙💙💙🙏🙏🙏 I'm so sorry to hear about loss: lots of prayers for your family. She will always be remembered as a great woman who raised wonderful children 💙🙏💙

AN. Onnie, Louis, Ange, I am so sorry to hear this news. She was always Aunt Carm to me and my biggest regret is not finding the time to get together with her to meet my children. We always tried to get together and it just never happened. Life is clearly …

JS. I am so sorry to hear this news Onnie. I have fond memories of your Mom in twin lakes when we were kids. She was always so kind to me. I wish your family peace in this time. Much love to you and yours. 💜

KB. I'm so sorry, Onnie. It just doesn't seem real. Some of my favorite earliest childhood memories were with you and your family. Your Mom was a bright light in a room, a friend when you needed one and always cared deeply about those around her. She will …

JW. I'm so sorry to hear this!!! Such a crazy difficult time already and now this huge loss. You are all in my prayers. I'm so sorry for this great loss. Thinking of you all. Sending our love.

SL. Onnie, so sorry to hear this. Your Mom was a special woman always full of energy, love, and life. I can't imagine what you and your family are going through. My deepest condolences. Stay strong, love you honey 💜

They Took Away my Son, my Man and my Only Brother!!!

Our Hearts are Mourning! My Soul in Mourns!
Written by Ramsis Ghaly

There is nothing worse than a mother burry her own baby, a father burry his own child, a newly wed burry her own husband, a younger sibling burry his own older only sibling, a friend burry his own friend and a country burry her own hero!!! Our deep condolences!!!

They didn't save my son, I am the mother dying with broken heart drowning in my tears!

They took my husband away, I am the wife just lost my life partner for ever debilitated, screaming in pains and grieving, my loss is severe!

Why you all didn't save my son, I am the father that just lost my flesh and heart, I am with deep sorrows and sadness, I can't believe I just lost him!

They didn't rescue my brother, I am the only brother to my brother and he was everything for me, I can't live without him, my heart is torn apart!

Why you let our American hero depart from us, we all his buddies; servicemen and women, five years with us and he was nominated the hero of the year!

Indeed much blessing to those unselfish healthcare workers whom care from hearts, dedicated sincerely to save lives, sincerely committed fully to rescue the sick, sacrificing to the last breath and consider their jobs sacred and holy and never ever business! Those faithful shall ripe grace and blessing from the Most High and miracles shall be performed through their hands saving lives and curing illnesses and nothing shall be impossible for them in Jesus Name, Amen 🙏!

O our Lord, we wish You take us all with him, the world is no longer livable without him!! Six weeks we didn't leave his sight and by hospital bed day and night! He was the healthiest one among us, never once complained, he was always smiling and joking bringing tenderness and love to our hearts! It all started by belly pain went to hospital and since then it was the beginning of the end! The first night was the last time we ever heard from him!

What we all didn't know that he always wish to go home with his Creator! In the midst of the night I heard his whispering words saying: "I will extol thee, O Lord ; for thou hast lifted me up, and hast not made my foes to rejoice over me. O Lord my God, I cried unto thee, and thou hast healed me"

I said Amen 🙏 our hero much love ❤️ and blessing to thy soul, we all praying day and night for our Almighty to heal soon!

He lifted his heart and opened his eyes looking up to heaven whispering with his lips as he was with fragile dying flesh: "O Lord, thou hast brought up my soul from the grave: thou hast kept me alive, that I should not go down to the pit"

Day by day his organs shut down one by one and his state deepened as his condition was in the red with multi organ failure! But every time I have looked at him, he was smiling with shining face never once cried! His soul was closer and closer to his Heavenly Father singing: "Sing unto the Lord, O ye saints of his, and give thanks at the remembrance of his holiness. For his anger endureth but a moment; in his favour is life:"

Overnight in the last night on earth he was weeping but in faith uttering the words of David: "weeping may endure for a night, but joy cometh in the morning. And in my prosperity I said, I shall never be moved. Lord, by thy favour thou hast made my mountain to stand strong: thou didst hide thy face, and I was troubled."

Yes indeed by the dawn early morning, his soul was lifted up from his feed and sick flesh saying: "I cried to thee, O Lord ; and unto the Lord I made supplication. What profit is there in my blood, when I go down to the pit? Shall the dust praise thee? shall it declare thy truth? Hear, O Lord, and have mercy upon me: Lord, be thou my helper"

As our hero was taking the last breath and his heart the last beating, his shinning faith looked brighter and his overnight agony vanished away! His words were: "Thou hast turned for me my mourning into dancing: thou hast put off my sackcloth, and girded me with gladness; To the end that my glory may sing praise to thee, and not be silent. O Lord my God, I will give thanks unto thee for ever."

I must say at that night, my eyes were drifted to Psalm30 and read it! To my ignorance, I though he is indeed will wake up that morning! But I didn't know that it was his time to come home to Jesus that morning! But who am I but a lost prodigal son!! Soon I saw a door was open and a spirit of comfort, glorious and bright! I starred but I couldn't see my Savior face! I knew He was there! The more I starred the more I saw the world that I couldn't take my eyes away! It was phenomenal, soft breeze, free of pains and constraints, atmosphere full of soothing quiescence! I kept reading in the psalm 30 all night and I text the mother and the wife. I said Psalm 30 is our beloved psalm!! I though he is indeed will wake up that morning! But I didn't know that it was his time to come home up high to Jesus that morning!

Amen 🙏 repose our hero, husband, son, brother, friend and everything in peace! My deep sympathy and condolences! Bless thy soul and my our Lord Jesus the Heavenly Father and the Holy Spirit comfort you all. Amen 🙏

"I will extol thee, O Lord ; for thou hast lifted me up, and hast not made my foes to rejoice over me. [2] O Lord my God, I cried unto thee, and thou hast healed me. [3] O Lord, thou hast brought up my soul from the grave: thou hast kept me alive, that I should not go down to the pit. [4] Sing unto the Lord, O ye saints of his, and give thanks at the remembrance of his holiness. [5] For his anger endureth but a moment; in his favour is life: weeping may endure for a night, but joy cometh in the morning. [6] And in my prosperity I said, I shall never be moved. [7] Lord, by thy favour thou hast made my mountain to stand strong: thou didst hide thy face, and I was troubled. [8] I cried to thee, O Lord ; and unto the Lord I made supplication. [9] What profit is there in my blood, when I go down to the pit? Shall the dust praise thee? shall it declare thy truth? [10] Hear, O Lord, and have mercy upon me: Lord, be thou my helper. [11] Thou hast turned for me my mourning into dancing: thou hast put off my sackcloth, and girded me with gladness; [12] To the end that my glory may sing praise to thee, and not be silent. O Lord my God, I will give thanks unto thee for ever." Psalm 30

Indeed much blessing to those unselfish healthcare workers whom care from hearts, dedicated sincerely to save lives, sincerely committed fully to rescue the sick, sacrificing to the last breath and consider their jobs sacred and holy and never ever business! Those faithful workers shall ripe grace and blessing from the Most High and miracles shall be performed through their hands saving lives and curing illnesses and nothing shall be impossible for them in Jesus Name, Amen 🙏!

Our Savior Promise to those workers: "And he said unto them, Go ye into all the world, and preach the gospel to every creature. [16] He that believeth and is baptized shall be saved; but he that believeth not shall be damned. [17] And these signs shall follow them that believe; In my name shall they cast out devils; they shall speak with new tongues; [18] They shall take up serpents; and if they drink any deadly thing, it shall not hurt them; they shall lay hands on the sick, and they shall recover." Mark 16:15-18 KJV

Amen 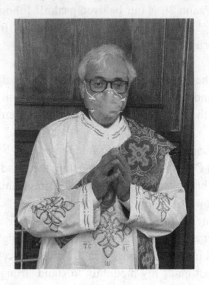 repose our hero, husband, son, brother, friend and everything in peace! My deep sympathy and condolences! Bless thy soul and my our Lord Jesus the Heavenly Father and the Holy Spirit comfort you all. Amen

AS. Amen

AB. Amen praise God Amen.

JB. Prayers.

CG. Bless all the front liners and those suffering from covid.

He Looked Up To Heaven Crying In Tears And Said: "O God Please Help Me And Look After My Dying Soul! Have mercy on me!!" Then, in the darkness of the night, he spend the entire night praying in tears while no one was seeing him!!

Written by Ramsis Ghaly

I was asked to write this living story close to your home worldwide:

An unknown man, walked all the way to find a sip of water to drink and little bite to eat and he didn't find! He Looked Up To Heaven Crying In Tears And Said: "O God Please Help Me And Look After My Dying Soul! Have mercy on me!!" Then, in the darkness of the night, he spend the entire night praying in tears while no one was seeing him!!

He searched all day long and I came back empty hand! He Looked Up To Heaven Crying In Tears And Said: "O God Please Help Me And Look After My Dying Soul! Have mercy on me!!" Then, in the darkness of the night, he spend the entire night, in the freezing cold, praying in tears while no one was seeing him!!

He wasn't clean and have no place to take a shower and my cloth is dirty and smelly! He was so poor waiting for someone with good heart 🖤! The Red Cross and Salvation Army haven't reached out to me and I have no to contact them! My look scared everyone come close to me and from my smell they run away from me! The police would like to have nothing with me. The churches and worshipping place resent me and they send me away at the doors! In fact, there are numerous court orders against him to come close to any of these places including malls, grocery stores, restaurants, shops, houses and many more! He Looked Up To Heaven Crying In Tears And Said: "O God Please Help Me And Look After My Dying Soul" Have mercy on me!!" Then, in the darkness of the night, in the freezing cold, he spend the entire night praying in tears while no one was seeing him!!

He went daily to the garage places search entire day for any food to eat, water to drink, canes to sell, or cloth to cover his nakedness or anything of value to earn a penny and buy a little bite to eat! Everyone around is sick of him and nothing left other than go to the cemetery and bury my flesh alive! He was neglected by many, bruised, despised and afflicted in all his days! He Looked Up To Heaven Crying In Tears And Said: "O God Please Help Me And Look After My Dying Soul! Have mercy on me!!" Then, in the darkness of the night, he spend the entire night, in the freezing cold praying in tears while no one was seeing him!!

He had no penny and no saving! My family and friends abandoned my many years ago! He was illiterate and his family had no money to support me. He was thrown out of school and his house and neighbors. He was raised among the gangs and the thieves in the streets! But he repented and followed Jesus in secret keeping the bible teaching in his heart all the time! His reputation never changed and he wasn't accepted by the people, the locals and the society! He Looked Up To Heaven Crying In Tears And Said: "O God Please Help Me And Look After My Dying Soul!" He Looked Up To Heaven Crying In Tears And Said: "O God Please Help Me And Look After My Dying Soul! Have mercy on me!" Then, in the darkness of the night, in the freezing cold, he spend the entire night praying in tears while no one was seeing him!!

He used to live in what his God send in my way and what the earth brings from fruits and vegetables and ever that became nil and rare nowadays! He Looked Up To Heaven Crying In Tears And Said: "O God Please Help Me And Look After My Dying Soul! Have mercy on me!" Then, in the darkness of the night, in the freezing cold, he spend the entire night praying in tears while no one was seeing him!!

Some of the Good Samaritans nearby used to bring him some food and drinks but they all moved away since the area has been hit lately with tornados and burglaries with high crimes! He Looked Up To Heaven Crying In Tears And Said: "O God Please Help Me And Look After My Dying Soul! Have mercy on me!!" Then, in the darkness of the night in the freezing cold, he spend the entire night praying in tears while no one was seeing him!!

In fact he got smacked, punched and attacked repeatedly because people thought he was one of thieves and criminals! He Looked Up To Heaven Crying In Tears And Said: "O God Please Help Me And Look After My Dying Soul! Have mercy on me!!" Then, in the darkness of the night in the freezing cold, he spend the entire night praying in tears while no one was seeing him!!

Many days; he keeps getting lost in the way back and he couldn't find his mobile home, he end by spending the nights by the nearby cemetery in a place no one knew but him! He Looked Up To Heaven Crying In Tears And Said: "O God Please Help Me And Look After My Dying Soul! Have mercy on me!!" Then, in the darkness of the night, he spend the entire night praying in tears while no one was seeing him!!

One day he arrived back to his mobile home, a heavy tornado took it with it! Since then, he was homeless wandering in remote areas! He Looked Up To Heaven Crying In Tears And Said: "O God Please Help Me And Look After My Dying Soul! Have mercy on me!!" Then, in the darkness of the night, he spend the entire night praying in tears while no one was seeing him!!

He filed for assistance, meal tickets, loans and stimulus checks —- He was still waiting! He knew no one to complete the paper work, or complete the computer forms! He had no address and his identity wasn't known! So if someone try to help, he would give up immediately! He was profiled as a running away criminal and sometimes as undocumented illegal thieve!!! He Looked Up To Heaven Crying In Tears And Said: "O God Please Help Me And Look After My Dying Soul! Have mercy on me!" Then, in the darkness of the night, he spend the entire night praying in tears while no one was seeing him!!

And when someone asked him: Why aren't getting help??" The first response he wasn't eligible and waiting for his turn! He Looked Up To Heaven Crying In Tears And Said: "O God Please Help Me And Look After My Dying Soul! Have mercy on me!!" Then, in the darkness of the night, he spend the entire night praying in tears while no one was seeing him!!

He was dying of poverty and no one is reaching out to his dying flesh! He Looked Up To Heaven Crying In Tears And Said: "O God Please Help Me And Look After My Dying Soul! Have mercy on me!!" Then, in the darkness of the night, he spend the entire night praying in tears while no one was seeing him!!

He was barefooted and maggots were eating his flesh and stuck all over his body! They were visible from fare! His texture was rough and his face full of wrinkles! He was skin over bones to the degree that his bones were eroding to the harsh dirty skin! His words were always full of blessing, harmless, thankful, content and obedient! He Looked Up To Heaven Crying In Tears And Said: "O God Please Help Me And Look After My Dying Soul! Have mercy on me!" Then, in the darkness of the night, he spend the entire night praying in tears while no one was seeing him!!

He went to the churches and he contacted charity organizations and all he received empty words and promise of prayers! He Looked Up To Heaven Crying In Tears And Said: "O God Please Help Me And Look After My Dying Soul! Have mercy on me!" Then, in the darkness of the night, he spend the entire night praying in tears while no one was seeing him!!

After giving up from finding a bite to eat or water to drink, he knocked the door of the first house he saw begging for a bite to eat or water to drink and he will leave. He would ask to leave something outside the door! But in humiliation they spit at his face and immediately the household called the police! He was arrested repeatedly and jailed overnight with felony charges in my file! In fact, he didn't have to knock the door for the neighbors to call the police! They all hated him and decided he didn't belong to this neighborhood. The court asked for someone to bailout from jail sentence but he had no one to come and help! So he stayed in jailed and he looked up to heaven and said: "O God please help me and look after my dying soul! Have mercy on me!!" Then, in the darkness of the night, he spend the entire night praying in tears while no one was seeing him!!

Nonetheless, toward later days of his life, he was spotted by a man with long beard dressed in white robe. No one knew this man or where he came from. Both will kneel for each other as if they knew each other for well. The man with white robe disappeared and he will continue this sojourn journey!

He got so sick in jail with high fever, the security guards thought he was making it up until his heart stopped beating and fainted over the cement! He lost my conscious and he was bleeding from his head profusely! 911 was called, CPR started and he began to catch his breath! He was taken to the closest hospital names St Mary and St Joseph! They diagnosed hi with brain hemorrhage and rushed him to surgery! But before the surgery, the nurses cleaned up from all the maggots that were eating my flesh! He Looked Up To Heaven Crying In Tears And Said: "O God Please Help Me And Look After My Dying Soul! Have mercy on me!" Then, in the darkness of the night, he spend the entire night praying in tears while no one was seeing him!!

He was in and out come in the first day after surgery! He saw the hospital chaplain standing before him! The chaplain introduced himself to him and said: "I am here per your call request" He hadn't call him at all but he was so happy to see him and he received a communion! Immediately, the chaplain started to tremble and star at him: O Lord Jesus O Lord Jesus O Lord Jesus forgive me! I didn't realize that this man is actually You! A voice came to the chaplain: "Go, be quiet, this is My son" I didn't know what has been transpired! I drifted back to coma!

As he recovered in his critical care unit, He Looked Up To Heaven Crying In Tears And Said: "O God Please Help Me And Look After My Dying Soul!" He raised his tremulous weak hands and for the first time he screamed and cries and whatever left of waters in his flesh ran out of his eyes! The walls of the rooms were shaking while he was praying: O my Lord and Savior who reached out to the poor Lazarus that was eating the remnants from the table of his master, send my father Abraham and take my soul: in thy hands I rest my soul!"

Indeed Jesus Himself descended down, reached out with His arms, wiped his tears and lift him up as he was taking his last breath! Immediately, the ICU staff saw lightening and smell of incense filling the man!

As they searched his body, they found a little tattoo cross and Our Heavenly prayers: "Our Father which art in heaven, Hallowed be thy name. [10] Thy kingdom come. Thy will be done in earth, as it is in heaven. [11] Give us this day our daily bread. [12] And forgive us our debts, as we forgive our debtors. [13] And lead us not into temptation, but deliver us from evil: For thine is the kingdom, and the power, and the glory, for ever. Amen. [14] For if ye forgive men their trespasses, your heavenly Father will also forgive you:" Matthew 6:9-14 KJV

A voce came from heaven: "This is my beloved son, he lived among you all and look how you all have treated him"

The news spread in the community and to all those that denied him: from the priests, pastors, ministers, charities, officials, shops, groceries, Neighbors, friends and they all cried in tears asking for forgiveness from the Lord of hosts. Yet the wrath of God swallowed the community with all its inhabitants!

I cried in humility and kneeled to my God and Savior: "O my Lord Jesus how many of those unknown saints around? We aren't worthy to their footsteps! We are so sorry and we have no excuse of our wickedness and inequities. Forgive our trespasses and my the unknown saint prayers and many of them be with us interceding before Your thrown, Amen 🙏"

"Then shall he say also unto them on the left hand, Depart from me, ye cursed, into everlasting fire, prepared for the devil and his angels: [42] For I was an hungred, and ye gave me no meat: I was thirsty, and ye gave me no drink: [43] I was a stranger, and ye took me not in: naked, and ye clothed me not: sick, and in prison, and ye visited me not. [44] Then shall they also answer him, saying, Lord, when saw we thee an hungred, or athirst, or a stranger, or naked, or sick, or in prison, and did not minister unto thee? [45] Then shall he answer them, saying,

Verily I say unto you, Inasmuch as ye did it not to one of the least of these, ye did it not to me. [46] And these shall go away into everlasting punishment: but the righteous into life eternal." Matthew 25:41-46 KJV

He Looked Up To Heaven Crying In Tears And Said: "O God Please Help Me And Look After My Dying Soul! Have mercy on me!!" Then, in the darkness of the night, he spend the entire night praying in tears while no one was seeing him!!

St Paul described them: "And others had trial of cruel mockings and scourgings, yea, moreover of bonds and imprisonment: [37] They were stoned, they were sawn asunder, were tempted, were slain with the sword: they wandered about in sheepskins and goatskins; being destitute, afflicted, tormented; [38] (Of whom the world was not worthy:) they wandered in deserts, and in mountains, and in dens and caves of the earth." Hebrews 11:36-38 KJV

Ramsis Ghaly

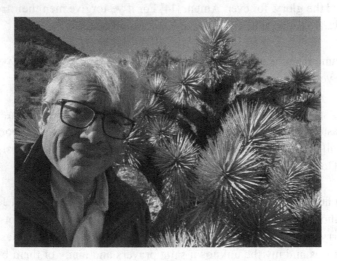

CG. Geat story that shows us to help all those who are in need, without having prejudice for anyone due to perceived differences. ♥🙏

PH. A true story of how people treat others unlike themselves, when they should be helping those in need. No matter the circumstances...as I always was taught and taught my kids and grandkids... because, you never know when it could be you or one of yours... ♥🙏

In the Memory of Isabella!

Poem dedicated to the heavenly soul of Isabella
Written by Ramsis Ghaly

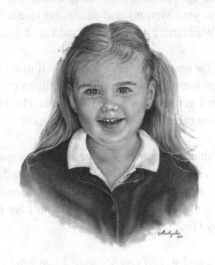

Mom I am a living angel among a crowd of angels dressed in pure white! Dad I am so busy getting know many of new friends! They are all angels like me!

Our Lord never left my sight! Jesus my God was with me all along my tumor journey! It was hard for me to describe Him back then but now I am with Him all the time!

Mom, Lord Jesus is so Awesome and kind! Remember that bed �, at that night He came and took me! First I heard a beautiful voice calling my name "Isabelle Isabelle Isabelle" three times!

Mom you know I was so tired 😴 and sick that night and I couldn't open my eyes! But at His voice, I woke up and I looked and here He is! I saw so many little angels coming with Him calling my name!

Dad, I just jumped full of joy regained all my health and more, from bed so happy and I realized I could fly! I am no longer sick or in pains but an angel wholly free in heaven!

511

My Lord Jesus stretched His arms and carried me to His chest and all of us flew so high! O mom it is so huge where I am, I can't described! It is so gorgeous! All are angels around! Do not be worried about me, my Heavenly Father is taking good care of me and no one can bother me at all. They are all holy angels!

O mom and dad, I love 🖤 you so much! I keep asking my Lord Jesus to keep you safe and watch over you! Mommy and daddy, my love to you I share up high above the clouds ☁️! Wait until I see you both and I shall tell you all about it!

I will never go far but for now I must introduce myself to all my new friends the little angels! I wish you are with me but it isn't the time yet! But my Lord Jesus promised me that after I get to know my new friends, He will let me help Him prepare a beautiful place for all of us together once more!

What can I say other than that tumor was the reason for me to be here by my Lord among the multitudes of heavenly hosts! We sing, we dance and learn new musicals! I now speak new language and wear a new dress 👗 and play new instruments! Mommy and day I miss you so much but I am not far! I love 🖤 it here the paradise of my God!

I didn't did! I am alive and well! I can see you! I can hear you! I love mommy and daddy!!

Rest with angels Isabella!!!

LA. I proudly post another beautiful portrait gifted by my Son, Vic - - - A gift from the heart . . 🖤

From Vic's Instagram account - - - Isabelle 🖤

On April 13th Michal and Jackie Borkowski received the unfortunate news. Their 3.5 year old daughter Isabelle was diagnosed with Diffuse intrinsic pontine glioma (DIPG). Diffuse intrinsic pontine glioma (DIPG) is a type of brain tumor found in the pons, which is part of the brainstem. DIPG primarily affects children, with most diagnoses occurring between 5 and 7 years of age. DIPG makes up 10-15% of all brain tumors in children, with about 100-300 new diagnoses per year in the United States and a similar number in Europe. Unlike many other pediatric cancers, there has been little progress in improving treatments and cure rates for DIPG over the last few decades. Unfortunately, fewer than 10% of children with DIPG survive two years from diagnosis. On Wednesday December 16th, at 10:50am Isabelle peacefully passed away. She fought so fiercely in her 8 month battle with DIPG that she didn't understand, while believing until the end that the doctors were going to fix her and make her feel better. It's absolutely heartbreaking. Even though we knew this was coming for 8 months now, it was impossible to prepare ourselves for the grief and emotions. Her smile, kindness toward others and mischievous personality will be with us for ever. She is terribly missed by her Mama, Dad, big brother and sister. It was my honor to draw her portrait for the family.

https://www.instagram.com/p/CKz34T9HXK2/
~~~~~~~~~~~~~~~~~~~~~~~~~

KS Beautiful child. Prayers for the family.

LA. Oh, Dr. Ramsis Ghaly, your poem is so very beautiful - a message directly from Heaven! I will make sure that Isabelle's Dad and Mom receive it. Thank you!! 💙 Many blessings to you as you continue to care for those in need. Your bright light so beautifully reflects the light of our Savior's love. 🖤

KG. Beautiful 🖤 child RIP Isabelle 🙏

IM. My deepest condolences and sympathy to her family She is now in peace Amen

CG. What a beautiful tribute to a beautiful child. Prayers for her family and may their pain ease with beautiful memories of their child. 🖤🙏

A Chicagoan's Mother from a Latino Descend!

Dedicated to her soul and all those fell victims to violence and by
their love donated their organs to give life to the sufferers!!

Written by Ramsis Ghaly

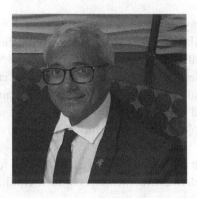

Long ago, I was on call in a level I Trauma hospital downtown Chicago where I
was asked to provide care to a "Gift of Hope" case for organ harvesting! I was so
traumatized going through it that it never left my mind! The story teared my heart
apart! At that time, the process was called: "Organ Harvesting" and the agency
was named the same "Organ Harvest" and the employed staff were considered
the "harvesters". Nowadays, the name changed to more appealing title: "Gift of
Hope".

The operating room was ready to go and so the nursing staff for the Gift of
Hope. I was amazed in minutes many surgeons and nursing staff showed up
from different medical centers at different universities from various States and
carrying their own favored surgical instruments and other boxes to carry the
organs in icy containers back to their facilities where the recipient patients are
ready in the operating room to receive the vital organs they have been waiting
for. One patient was in dire need of a heart, another of a kidney, a third of the
other kidney, a fourth of the lungs, a fifth of the liver, a sixth of the pancreas and
seventh of the intestines.

Two days ago, the patient was declared "Brain Dead". She died from her injury as the brain ⬤ hemorrhaged and swollen so severe within the skull to the degree that no longer blood, oxygen and nutrients made their way to the brain and hence strangulated and got killed! The patient actually never woke up since she got shot and all measures failed to regain her conscious back. Despite the tireless work in the critical care unit team to lower the pressure inside the skull, all were in vain and her brain proceeded to die but not all her other vital organs including the heart, the lungs, the liver, the kidneys, the intestines and the pancreas.

In almost thirty minutes in astonishing efficiency and in exact order, the surgery was about start as the patient moved to the operating room table in a huge operating theatre. I looked around, the patient was already prepped, draped and ready to go. I was stunned when I saw how in thirty minutes, the quiet operating room transformed unto a busy fast-speed factory opening up the patient and getting all the organs, soaking them with ice while freeing each organs from the body keeping the blood vessels intact and maintaining the integrity as much as possible. Then gently, the organs are handed over sterile to be placed securely in iced containers in freezing temperature. The ancillary staff were working non stop in their computers and phones, arranging for the immediate transportations of each organ accompanied by the surgeons and staff to arrive in time to their destiny while the recipient patient was already anesthetized in another state waiting to implant the donor organ. The data bank of the waiting recipient patients are in the thousands and must be screened in compatibility of the organs according to their priority list. The process is confidential, highly accurate and there is no room for mistakes as you can imagine! The fortunate ones are those receiving the compatible organs before they pass away while waiting for life saving organ! Indeed many of these recipients die while waiting!

Before the surgery began, complete silence in the room as "Time Out" is called and each introduce themselves, by name and who they were—. Then a senior staff from the "Gift of Hope" introduced the patient and what to remember about the patient. Then it was followed by a moment of silence in her memory and appreciation to donate the organs and where they were going and how many their lives would be saved!

However, not only no one knew the patient but also there was nothing mentioned about the patient in her memory. The patient never wrote a special note to be read and her children were so young to speak. There were no families around and only few things we were allowed to know from the police 🛡 investigating the murder. And those were: "A Chicagoan woman, a mother of five children from Latino descend"

I heard those words and I looked around in a freezing operating room as every person was concentrating to perform the duties and get the organs as fast, I cried in my heart and said: "Who will ever take the life of a mother of five children and shot her to death brutally and unconsciously?" I prayed and looked up to heaven while taking various organs from this great human being that not only she gave her life for her five children while living but her organs for the Seven very sick patients dying from their failed organs waiting for the life saving organ to flew out of state and bring life back to their souls and their families! I prayed and prayed from my broken heart and teared eyes: "O Lord can You please tell her how much she is loved, admired and in the behalf of humanity we all are in sorrows and sadness!!" At that time, how much I desired to reach out to her and her children and tell them all: "How special she was and how much her children will be cared for in her absence!!"

Our Savior Jesus described the True Love and no great Love than this to lay down thyself for others: "This is my commandment, That ye love one another, as I have loved you. [13] Greater love hath no man than this, that a man lay down his life for his friends." John 15:12-13 KJV. Jesus said: "I am the good shepherd, and know my sheep, and am known of mine. [15] As the Father knoweth me, even so know I the Father: and I lay down my life for the sheep. [16] And other sheep I have, which are not of this fold: them also I must bring, and they shall hear my voice; and there shall be one fold, and one shepherd. [17] Therefore doth my Father love me, because I lay down my life, that I might take it again. [18] No man taketh it from me, but I lay it down of myself. I have power to lay it down, and I have power to take it again. This commandment have I received of my Father." John 10:14-18 KJV

Why this magnificent patient be like all those of "Unknowns" with no voice or advocate?? I felt so bad and my soul became restless! I wasn't sure, if I was the only one emotionally very upset, saddened and in tears for her and her children. I tried to start a conversation of any of the staff around, but no one had interest since the goal was to take the organs and save the lives of those waiting for the organs. I proceeded to fall in depression and gloominess as I reached out to heaven writing her words as she wanted to be remembered. Suddenly, I felt obligated to speak in the patient behalf and acknowledge her soul and her selfless giving.! I shouted and said to all the staff saying: "As you all taking the organs of this lovely woman named "A Chicagoan mother of five children from the Latino descend" all listen as I will speak in her behalf reflecting in her journey and saying her words of how she would like to be remembered!!

A silence filled the operating room theatre and I started to utter her spoken words as follows: My soul said "yes" to harvest my organs to heal a dozen of the sick living! My spirit is so exalted to see those patients receiving my organs regaining their health and life back home to their families in joy!

I am a kind tender woman and a mother full of love 🖤! I am proudly a mother of five beautiful little children God Almighty has blessed me with!

If you wish to know my story!! I was raised in Chicago and always I wanted to be a good mom. I am from a Latino descend and raised in poverty!

I was struggled growing up! My childhood cut short and at some points of my life I questioned my life and living!

Finally I found a good man and father and I had five children! I gave all what I had to my children and I deprived them nothing! I made sure, their childhood won't be like mine!! I did all I can to protect them from the evil ones!

My neighborhoods weren't the best! I couldn't afford housing costs in other areas! We hear shots all the time and my children get shaken! I usually hugged them and took their minds away by letting them play with our lovely cat 🐈 and dog 🐕 ! I made wrong decisions in my life and no matter what I had done to reconcile things, I couldn't escape from the sequelae!

In a day of joy I was taking my children to buy some groceries, I heard gun shots around me all of the sudden! I reached out to my children to protect them taking them to my bosom! I was gunned down and they shot me dead 💀 🩸 🩸 🩸 !

They killed me 🩸 🩸 🩸 and I bled 🩸 🩸 🩸 to death! They took my life away leaving my children to be orphans! they cut my life short!

My beloved city Chicago is terrorized by the criminals and gangs! The innocents bystanders are always at risk! O men of the darkness why did you all gunned me down and shot me to death! I meant no harm and I cared much for my own children my flesh and blood! I heard screams from those men: "O woman you are in the wrong place at the wrong time! You aren't target! What made you come to this area at this time! We didn't mean to harm you! You are an innocent bystander! Our sorrows but we must run to escape for our lives while you are taking the last breath soaked in your own blood 🩸 🩸 🩸 !

https://en.m.wikipedia.org/wiki/Crime_in_Chicago
https://graphics.suntimes.com/homicides/

I had no family but my children and left no living will or living trust! I wasn't ready to go! I had nothing but my children! My children were everything for me and we lived from a meal tickets and those donors lovers of our Savior Jesus Christ!

My soul is shaking concerning about my children! Please take good care of them! They are my life and soul! Before my Lord Jesus, I kneel and cry asking for His forgiveness and extend His hand of mercy to the world of violence and darkness!

O my Lord Jesus God of earth and heaven overshadow my motherless kids! O mother of God surround my children with your motherhood love ♥! My love will never fail! May my Lord Jesus forgive you all!

Her words continued and filled the operating room theatre. Unbelievable scene, the organs were wrapped in boxes and taken away. The staff were gone with the organs and flew back to their destiny. The "Chicagoan woman a mother of five children from the Latino Descend" was left alone, her body was empty from the organs and the remains were the head and the skeleton. I was told to leave and no need for me anymore as the last person was sawing her skin before her body be delivered to the morgue. I was waived goodbye but for my soul it was never goodbye. I remained stunned and every time I remember the Chicagoan woman a mother of five children from the Latino descend, I cry and I kneel in tears with full respect and love praying to my and her Savior Jesus Christ to repose her soul and be with her children until the day He take my soul to meet her honorable soul face-to-face!

Let us pray for her soul and many like hers! The soul of the Chicagoan woman the mother of five children from the Latino descend uttering the words of Psalm 6: "O Lord, rebuke me not in thine anger, neither chasten me in thy hot displeasure. [2] Have mercy upon me, O Lord ; for I am weak: O Lord, heal me; for my bones are vexed. [3] My soul is also sore vexed: but thou, O Lord, how long? [4] Return, O Lord, deliver my soul: oh save me for thy mercies' sake. [5] For in death there is no remembrance of thee: in the grave who shall give thee thanks? [6] I am weary with my groaning; all the night make I my bed to swim; I water my couch with my tears. [7] Mine eye is consumed because of grief; it waxeth old because of all mine enemies. [8] Depart from me, all ye workers of iniquity; for the Lord hath heard the voice of my weeping. [9] The Lord hath heard my supplication; the Lord will receive my prayer. [10] Let all mine enemies be ashamed and sore vexed: let them return and be ashamed suddenly."

Psalm 116; "I love the Lord, because he hath heard my voice and my supplications. [2] Because he hath inclined his ear unto me, therefore will I call upon him as long as I live. [3] The sorrows of death compassed me, and the pains of hell gat hold upon me: I found trouble and sorrow. [4] Then called I upon the name of the Lord ; O Lord, I beseech thee, deliver my soul. [5] Gracious is the Lord, and righteous; yea, our God is merciful. [6] The Lord preserveth the simple: I was brought low, and he helped me. [7] Return unto thy rest, O my soul; for the Lord hath dealt bountifully with thee. [8] For thou hast delivered my soul from death, mine eyes from tears, and my feet from falling. [9] I will walk before the Lord in the land of the living. [10] I believed, therefore have I spoken: I was greatly afflicted: [11] I said in my haste, All men are liars. [12] What shall I render unto the Lord for all his benefits toward me? [13] I will take the cup of salvation, and call upon the name of the Lord. [14] I will pay my vows unto the Lord now in the presence of all his people. [15] Precious in the sight of the Lord is the death of his saints. [16] O Lord, truly I am thy servant; I am thy servant, and the son of thine handmaid: thou hast loosed my bonds. [17] I will offer to thee the sacrifice of thanksgiving, and will call upon the name of the Lord. [18] I will pay my vows unto the Lord now in the presence of all his people, [19] In the courts of the Lord's house, in the midst of thee, O Jerusalem. Praise ye the Lord."

Psalm 31: "In thee, O LORD, do I a put my trust; let me never be ashamed: deliver me in thy righteousness. [2] Bow down thine ear to me; deliver me speedily: be thou my strong rock, for an house of defence to save me. [3] For thou art my rock and my fortress; therefore for thy name's sake lead me, and guide me. [4] Pull me out of the net that they have laid privily for me: for thou art my strength. [5] Into thine hand I commit my spirit: thou hast redeemed me, O Lord God of truth. [6] I have hated them that regard lying vanities: but I trust in the Lord. [7] I will be glad and rejoice in thy mercy: for thou hast considered my trouble; thou hast known my soul in adversities; [8] And hast not shut me up into the hand of the enemy: thou hast set my feet in a large room. [9] Have mercy upon me, O Lord, for I am in trouble: mine eye is consumed with grief, yea, my soul and my belly. [10] For my life is spent with grief, and my years with sighing: my strength faileth because of mine iniquity, and my bones are consumed. [11] I was a reproach among all mine enemies, but especially among my neighbours, and a fear to mine acquaintance: they that did see me without fled from me. [12] I am forgotten as a dead man out of mind: I am like a broken vessel. [13] For I have heard the slander of many: fear was on every side: while they took counsel together against me, they devised to take away my life. [14] But I trusted in thee, O Lord: I said, Thou art my God. [15] My times are in thy hand: deliver me from the hand of mine enemies, and from them that persecute me. [16] Make thy face to shine upon thy servant: save me for thy mercies' sake. [17] Let me not be ashamed, O Lord ; for I have called upon thee: let the wicked be ashamed, and let them be silent in the grave. [18] Let the lying lips be put to silence; which speak grievous things proudly and contemptuously against the righteous. [19] Oh how great is thy goodness, which thou hast laid up for them that fear thee; which thou hast wrought for them that trust in thee before the sons of men! [20] Thou shalt hide them in the secret of thy presence from the pride of man: thou shalt keep them secretly in a pavilion from the strife of tongues. [21] Blessed be the Lord: for he hath shewed me his marvellous kindness in a strong city. [22] For I said in my haste, I am cut off from before thine eyes: nevertheless thou heardest the voice of my supplications when I cried unto thee. [23] O love the Lord, all ye his saints: for the Lord preserveth the faithful, and plentifully rewardeth the proud doer. [24] Be of good courage, and he shall strengthen your heart, all ye that hope in the LORD. ..."

"Return unto thy rest, O my soul; for the Lord hath dealt bountifully with thee. For thou hast delivered my soul from death, mine eyes from tears, and my feet from falling. I will walk before the Lord in the land of the living. I believed, therefore have I spoken: I was greatly afflicted:"

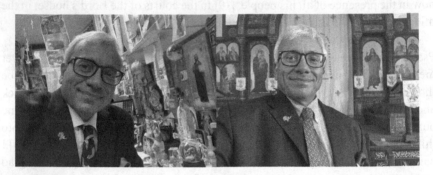

KG. God Bless you!!!

LW. Thank you for honoring this woman and praying for the children she leaves behind. As a parent of a Gift of Hope donor, I am comforted in reading your tribute. 💕

BH. What a beautiful memory honoring this mother. This was an amazing tribute to a victim of an awful tragedy. Bless you Dr. Ghaly for all you so selflessly do. Bless you for this wonderful testimony to a lost life and all the lost lives from unnecessary violence that then get forgotten with no regard to their outcome. Its a tragedy. Bless you for acknowledging this.

It hurts my heart letting it all sink in. I am crying and praying for her soul, your sweet soul and all the souls having to rely on the death of another so they may live.

You are an incredibly devoted, humble, loving and brilliant man. Thank you!

HE. Dr Ghaly do you ever rest?

CG. This is heartbreaking and yet so wonderful that she makes it possible for people waiting for lifesaving organs to have a second chance at life. Bless you for caring enough to share her story 🖤

AS. Amen

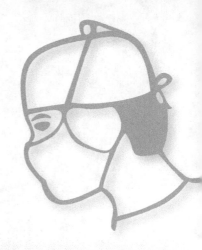

SECTION 10

Time To Live Outdoors and Run to the Mountains!

A Spiritual life by the Desert Surpass a Physical Life in Babylon by the Zion

In the midst of COVID, my soul said to me: A Spiritual life by the desert 🌵 surpass a physical life in Babylon by the Zion! Living in the Camp of David by the desert of Sinai excel living by the high Rise luxurious home by the city! Hear O my soul!

Written by Ramsis Ghaly

Living by Camp of David in the City of God and never again living by the great city of Babylon flooded with sins full of COVID-19!

O God, I had enough of COVID-19, please take my soul to thy wilderness by the desert of Sinai, let me live by the Camp ⛺ with children of Israel! Life with my Lord Jesus in the wilderness is a life in the heavenly kingdom by the Camp ⛺ of my father's Moses and David!

O Lord of Israel! Let me go and let me fly away from the world of sin full of COVID-19! No more masks or gowns or curfew or restrictions Thou shall liberate my soul free in the thy desert of Sinai by Camp David!

There, by mount Sinai, my soul is comforted knowing thou there and so are Your children! Let me go to the house of the Lord, Jerusalem on earth, the Camp ⛺ of David and attend to His Tabernacle: "I was glad when they said unto me, Let us go into the house of the Lord. [2] Our feet shall stand within thy gates, O Jerusalem. [3] Jerusalem is builded as a city that is compact together: [4] Whither the tribes go up, the tribes of the Lord, unto the testimony of Israel, to give thanks unto the name of the Lord. [5] For there are set thrones of judgment, the thrones of the house of David. [6] Pray for the peace of Jerusalem: they shall prosper that love thee. [7] Peace be within thy walls, and prosperity within thy palaces. [8] For my brethren and companions' sakes, I will now say, Peace be within thee. [9] Because of the house of the Lord our God I will seek thy good." Psalm 122

After what I went through with COVID-19, a living under a tent ⛺ with the Lord triumph a living in the high rise by the major US cities!

Look at the world now! First COVID wave is already followed by a second COVID wave full force dying in thousands with many new variants are coming in the way! It is all lockdown! Lock in lock out indoor house arrest hard to breath with face covers! All the worshipping places and the churches are closed! The shops and gathering no more! The law of the land enforced cover up and stand away and be alone by the walls! The pandemic is going through the entire world's population with no mercy! No more graves or burial places! Their bodies are stored by the freezing trucks! This is the world that one more a world of glory!!

I learned through my Journey of COVID-19, I No longer wish to live in the most civilized world but I'd rather be with my Lord at mount Sinai!

Living in the world by the Spirit according to the Grace of God and the laws of His land is the way to excel! The world is indeed "Vanity of vanities, saith the Preacher, vanity of vanities; all is vanity." Ecclesiastes 1:2 KJV

I wish the old days come back and please take away the modem days! Living in civilized world took away the originality and purity of our souls! My soul said to me: "My Partner, So much loss with technology but so much gain with nature!"

It came the time to experience the beauty of the desert primitive culture and send me away from the man-made architecture 2020!

I'd rather be in the desert 🏜️🌵🐪 with my Lord and Not to be in the king's houses 🏚️ !! I will get know more and more my Savior! My eyes will begin to see what I couldn't see and to hear what I couldn't hear when I was in the world!

With the Lord nothing else matters, none of the politics, rankings, social accomplishments, figures and images!

At mount Sinai, under the tent 🎪 of Israel neither the freezing nights nor the heat of the sun ☀️ matters!

Under the tent 🎪, I will rest in peace and deep in the desert I will obtain much blessings! The love and harmony by the deserts are further away from the hate and hostility in the world!

The glory of God and the richness by the mountains of the Lord fulfill the hearts and souls! My soul adores His presence at His mountains 🏔️!

My Savior is indeed much transparent by the desert as there is no more cloudiness of the world!

Under the tent by the holy mountain I heard the voice of my God for the first time saying: "Hear therefore, O Israel, and observe to do it ; that it may be well with thee, and that ye may increase mightily, as the Lord God of thy fathers hath promised thee, in the land that floweth with milk and honey. [4] Hear, O Israel: The Lord our God is one Lord: [5] And thou shalt love the Lord thy God with all thine heart, and with all thy soul, and with all thy might. [13] Thou shalt fear the Lord thy God, and serve him, and shalt swear by his name. [14] Ye shall not go after other gods, of the gods of the people which are round about you; [15] (For the Lord thy God is a jealous God among you) lest the anger of the Lord thy God be kindled against thee, and destroy thee from off the face of the earth. [16] Ye shall not tempt the Lord your God, as ye tempted him in Massah. [17] Ye shall diligently keep the commandments of the Lord your God, and his testimonies, and his statutes, which he hath commanded thee. [18] And thou shalt do that which is right and good in the sight of the Lord: that it may be well with thee, and that thou mayest go in and possess the good land which the Lord sware unto thy fathers," Deuteronomy 6:3-5,13-18 KJV

By mount Sinai, I received God's Ten Commandments directly from Him as by the holy mountain of Jerusalem my soul received the Aptitudes as it is written: Exodus 20:1-17 KJV [1] And God spake all these words, saying, [2] I am the Lord thy God, which have brought thee out of the land of Egypt, out of the house of bondage. [3] Thou shalt have no other gods before me. [4] Thou shalt not make unto thee any graven image, or any likeness of any thing that is in heaven above, or that is in the earth beneath, or that is in the water under the earth: [5] Thou shalt not bow down thyself to them, nor serve them: for I the Lord thy God am a jealous God, visiting the iniquity of the fathers upon the children unto the third and fourth generation of them that hate me; [6] And shewing mercy unto thousands of them that love me, and keep my commandments. [7] Thou shalt not take the name of the Lord thy God in vain; for the Lord will not hold him guiltless that taketh his name in vain. [8] Remember the sabbath day, to keep it holy. [9] Six days shalt thou labour, and do all thy work: [10] But the seventh day is the sabbath of the Lord thy God: in it thou shalt not do any work, thou, nor thy son, nor thy daughter, thy manservant, nor thy maidservant, nor thy cattle, nor thy stranger that is within thy gates: [11] For in six days the Lord made heaven and earth, the sea, and all that in them is, and rested the seventh day: wherefore the Lord blessed the sabbath day, and hallowed it. [12] Honour thy father and thy mother: that thy days may be long upon the land which the Lord thy God giveth thee. [13] Thou shalt not kill. [14] Thou shalt not commit adultery. [15] Thou shalt not steal. [16] Thou shalt not bear false witness against thy neighbour. [17] Thou shalt not covet thy neighbour's house, thou shalt not covet thy neighbour's wife, nor his manservant, nor his maidservant, nor his ox, nor his ass, nor any thing that is thy neighbour's.

Quiescence replaces the noisy cities, horns, peeps and the psalms instead of loud songs!

I prefer to eat from the manna bread 🥖 from heaven than from the most Delicious meal 🍽 made by the best chef cook!

By the desert 🌵 of the Lord God send me quails to cover the camp and in the morning the dew round about! The wilderness with the Lord is a heavenly kingdom by the Camp! "And it came to pass, that at even the quails came up, and covered the camp: and in the morning the dew lay round about the host. [14] And when the dew that lay was gone up, behold, upon the face of the wilderness there lay a small round thing, as small as the hoar frost on the ground. [15] And when the children of Israel saw it, they said one to another, It is manna: for they wist not what it was. And Moses said unto them, This is the bread which the Lord hath given you to eat." Exodus 16:13-15 KJV

The True light of God of Israel is much much more luminous than the artificial light 💡 of this world 🌐!

By the desert 🐐, My Lord was so kind to my soul! He put before me by day in a pillar of a cloud, to lead me the way; and by night in a pillar of fire, to give give light; to go by day and night: He took not away the pillar of the cloud by day, nor the pillar of fire by night, from before my soul! Exodus 13:21-22 KJV

I love to be by the mountains 🏔 of God mount Sinai and not by the Babylon tower of Zion!

At night I count the stars 🌠🌠🌠 and praise the Lord of hosts! At the early dawn, I pray at the tabernacle of the Lord and provide my offering! During the day I labor in the court of my God!

By the Sinai mount, my Heavenly Father gives me Peace in my soul, the breeze of fresh air, the divine nurtures to my bones and beating heart 💜 of an eagle 🦅!

No more shall my soul get mislead by the fake world and it's glamorous look! I'd rather live all my life close to nature of God creation as it was created thousands of years ago!

Barefooted simple life content in my ways and no more hectic life racing my finance and increase my saving competing in material wealth!

By the desert 🌵 I followed my father Moses with the children of Israel and I stood from far off! It was so magnificent, I couldn't come close from its glory!! I saw God presence by His mountain the thundering, the smoke, noise of trumpet as it is written: "And all the people saw the thunderings, and the lightnings, and the noise of the trumpet, and the mountain smoking: and when the people saw it, they removed, and stood afar off. [19] And they said unto Moses, Speak thou with us, and we will hear: but let not God speak with us, lest we die. [20] And Moses said unto the people, Fear not: for God is come to prove you, and that his fear may be before your faces, that ye sin not. [21] And the people stood afar off, and Moses drew near unto the thick darkness where God was. [22] And the Lord said unto Moses, Thus thou shalt say unto the children of Israel, Ye have seen that I have talked with you from heaven." Exodus 20:18-22 KJV And: "And seeing the multitudes, he went up into a mountain: and when he was set, his disciples came unto him: [2] And he opened his mouth, and taught them, saying, [3] Blessed are the poor in spirit: for theirs is the kingdom of heaven. [4] Blessed are they that mourn: for they shall be comforted. [5] Blessed are the meek: for they shall inherit the earth. [6] Blessed are they which do hunger and thirst after righteousness: for they shall be filled. [7] Blessed are the merciful: for they shall obtain mercy. [8] Blessed are the pure in heart: for they shall see God. [9] Blessed are the peacemakers: for they shall be called the children of God. [10] Blessed are they which are persecuted for righteousness' sake: for theirs is the kingdom of heaven." Matthew 5:1-10 KJV What did I gain when I ran away from my home by mount Sinai and the holy desert 🌵 of the Lord and moved to the big city 🏙️ working day and night through computers and machines and spoke through smart phones and I attending virtual meeting through zoom in and out technology??

By the wilderness with the Lord, I found His church! I immediately kneeled to the ground and worshiped my Lord! I looked around the desert of Sinai and up the mountain ⛰️ of the Lord and from far I saw Camp David! I screamed in exaltation as I ran in joy to enter my Lord Tabernacle! I sang with David saying: "How amiable are thy tabernacles, O Lord of hosts! [2] My soul longeth, yea, even fainteth for the courts of the Lord: my heart and my flesh crieth out for the living God. [3] Yea, the sparrow hath found an house, and the swallow a nest for herself, where she may lay her young, even thine altars, O Lord of hosts, my King, and my God. [4] Blessed are they that dwell in thy house: they will be still praising thee. Selah. [5] Blessed is the man whose strength is in thee; in whose heart are the ways of them. [6] Who passing through the valley of Baca make it a well; the rain also filleth the pools. [7] They go from strength to strength, every one of them in Zion appeareth before God. [8] O Lord God of hosts, hear my prayer: give ear, O God of Jacob. Selah. [9] Behold, O God our shield, and look upon the face of thine anointed. [10] For a day in thy courts is better than a thousand. I had rather be a doorkeeper in the house of my God, than to dwell in the tents of wickedness. [11] For the Lord God is a sun and shield: the Lord will give grace and glory: no good thing will he withhold from them that walk uprightly. [12] O Lord of hosts, blessed is the man that trusteth in thee." Psalm 84

I replied to my soul yes indeed!!! In the midst of COVID, my soul said to me: A Spiritual life by the desert 🌵 super pass a physical life in Babylon by the Zion! Living in the Camp of David by the desert of Sinai excel living by the high Rise luxurious home by the city! Hear O my soul!

Image taken from Ghislaine Labre. Thank you

PP. Happy New Year Dr. Ramsis Ghaly
FA, I agree Dr Ghaly
GL. Oh! Je suis très touchée et émue par vos mots inspirés de ma photo 🙏🙏 🙏 Je vous dis un infini MERCI, pour tant d'Amour et de Conscience, pour tant d'inspiration et de Justesse! Bénédictions Cher Ramsis 🙏🙏🙏🌿✨ 🌺🌊🌊🌊
CG. Well written with much thought and love of our Lord. Bless you. ❤️🙏
JM. "Beautiful Text" Magnificent Visual 💕

Author
Ghislaine Labre

Oh, oh! Oh! I am very touched and moved by your words inspired by my photo I say an infinite THANK YOU, for so much Love and Consciousness, for so much inspiration and Justness! Blessings Dear Ramsis 🙏🙏🙏🌿✨🌺🌊🌊🌊

As There is No Coronavirus in the Mountains, There isn't also in the freezing crispy snow mountains!!

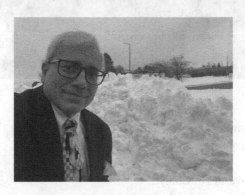

If COVID pandemic taught us a lesson, it is to go away to the remote places and not just to enjoy but to actually live by the nature to get to know Him away from the noisy distracted world 🌐 condensed population compacted with man-made technology!!

Run away with thy life and breath fresh air not polluted with viruses and harmful particles of the world!

Chicagoan's Fresh crispy cold air taking an early break from face mask after a heavy hospital on call caring for both COVID and non COVID patients Giving thanksgiving to the Lord and praying 🙏 for His mercy!

Instead of a beautiful sunny mountains 🏔, stormy 🌥 snow mountains and freezing crispy cold 🥶 and more new news in few hours of brittle icy 🥶 cold and roads!

Despite all of these crispy news, we look to the warmth and love 💜 and life eternity the unseen and invisible! In fact my Savior offered me a peaceful office full of blessing and a practice full of His grace for my soul!

You all stay warm, safe and be at peace, our Savior is our God and Heavenly Father for ever and ever Amen 🙏

Ramsis Ghaly
Www.ghalyneurosurgeon.com

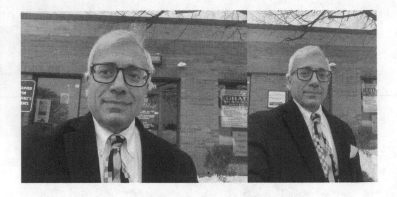

GV. Brrr! It looks cold! Awesome tie, by the way!

CP. Very nice pictures. ☺

RC. Continue to stay safe.

AL. Amén

JD. Stay safe and warm Dr. Ghaly !!

CR. Thanks Dr Ghaly, you brighten my day.

SB. Thank you Dr. Ghaly for all you do!
I will be making an appointment with you soon!
I pray you know about Chiari Malformation

KG. Its healing and refreshing to see that smiling face. God Bless.

CG. Be careful driving later and be safe. Love the pictures and especially your colorful tie and pocket square.

KO. Enjoy the fresh air Dr Ghaly, being out there for a break, even for 15 min, does a world of good, be safe in yours travels, Lord bless you

AV. Stay warm & safe!! 😊🐾🙏

JM. I love your words

SJ. "Run away with thy life and breath fresh air..." - I love those words. They are both poetic and necessary 🖤

BCD. I agree,. I was born at home in my mother's four poster bed. We had cows, pigs, chickens, sunshine and fresh air.

But I prefer to Stay That Way!

Ramsis Ghaly

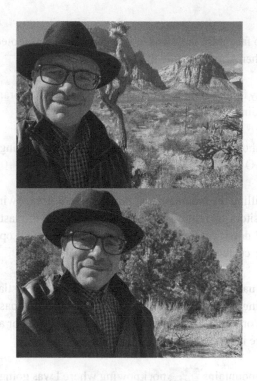

I want once to feel natural and walk causal with no tracking or mocking letting myself go! O lord leave me here with the unknowns!

I asked myself what industry had brought us other than pollution and what science had done to mankind other than loss of simplicity and what civilization had brought the world 🌐 other than corruption!

A voice came to me out of dungeon pit; "Escape for thy soul!" I rose up and locked my door 🚪 behind!

I prayed to my Lord: "Take wherever You wish lead my way and hold my hand bring me to You"

I don't know 🧎 where I am? But I do prefer to stay that way!

I let my soul go up the trail while my form went down to the Canyon! I am lost in the Forest!

I thought for today I just disappear to a desert 🌵 place with no signal or in-line connection!

For once, I put no facemask or gowns or gloves walked barefooted holding a cane as during my father Abraham time thousands of years ago!

There are so many innocent trees with pale leaves and broken branches but at least with trunks standing straight!

I walked among those trees 🌳 🌲 not knowing where I was going! But I preferred to stay that way! O lord leave me here with the unknowns!

The fresh air is filling the mountains 🏔 and the winds are blowing left and right! There are no visitors or requests and as the churches, monasteries and many places are closed down yet the deserts and mountains are all open 24/7 with no set regulations or curfews!

I have no map or navigation system! There are no stars of celestial body to follow but sun ☀ shining all over the mountains! There is no compass and I couldn't follow the winds or birds! I realized there are no street signs or any directions of some sort as there is no sextant or chronometer!

I climbed up the mountains 🏔🏔 not knowing where I was going! But I preferred to stay that way! O lord leave me here with the unknowns!

I needed to run away! It was so much going on in the nation! I could only pray since I had no voice or fame!

It is the time to remove the cables and wires around me and let no phone ring or alarm scream at me! I took off all the wireless signals out of my way!

Let me go back to the nature not knowing where I am going and what I am doing!

I want once to feel natural and walk causal with no tracking or mocking letting myself go! O lord leave me here with the unknowns!

I feel much valuable where I am since I am the only one around here! The birds 🐦 are looking at me amazed and so are the trees 🌲!

Other than to be in the watch for the hidden snakes and scorpions and the crazy hunters, I feel safe! I don't know anybody here since neither google map nor MapQuest made it here yet!

No layers or complexity and no competition or arguments! Everything here is simple and free! We all treated the same as the Holy Spirit all over the canyon!

There were no news or dues and neither scales or measures! The land had no end and I didn't know when to stop ● or take a rest!

It started by exploration and fears as I am all alone but with my Savior! It ended to be a life to live with my soulmate my Beloved!

I went up to hills and down to the valleys, it was so quiet and peaceful! The sky has no limit and the mountains had no boundaries! I flew like a bird and rejuvenated line an eagle!

I started to make a tent for myself as the night is approaching! I collected some wood sticks and took a little nap z^z! There was no way for me to slaughter an animal to eat or pick up a fruit out of a tree 🌲! I looked around for waters! I wished to find a well!

However there was some fires 🔥 and signs of living human being! I can only guess there is a military Base further away! I found some solars spread away!

I finally found my soul and surfaced my identity! It was one of my best journey to come close to my Master! My soul get to open to my Heavenly Father as He came close to me! Before I reached up to Him He reached out to me and just before I said Abba He called me "My son"

O my gosh, I screamed! My soul touched the Spirit! Instantly I found myself in a Canyon with no base and a Forest with no end and a mountain with no top! I kneeled down to my Lord and said hallelujah hallelujah hallelujah to my Savior and my Master!

I sang to the Lord psalms 98-100:

Psalm 98
[1] O sing unto the Lord a new song; for he hath done marvellous things: his right hand, and his holy arm, hath gotten him the victory. [2] The Lord hath made known his salvation: his righteousness hath he openly shewed in the sight of the

heathen. [3] He hath remembered his mercy and his truth toward the house of Israel: all the ends of the earth have seen the salvation of our God. [4] Make a joyful noise unto the Lord, all the earth: make a loud noise, and rejoice, and sing praise. [5] Sing unto the Lord with the harp; with the harp, and the voice of a psalm. [6] With trumpets and sound of cornet make a joyful noise before the Lord, the King. [7] Let the sea roar, and the fulness thereof; the world, and they that dwell therein. [8] Let the floods clap their hands: let the hills be joyful together [9] Before the Lord ; for he cometh to judge the earth: with righteousness shall he judge the world, and the people with equity.

Psalm 99

[1] The Lord reigneth; let the people tremble: he sitteth between the cherubims; let the earth be moved. [2] The Lord is great in Zion; and he is high above all the people. [3] Let them praise thy great and terrible name; for it is holy. [4] The king's strength also loveth judgment; thou dost establish equity, thou executest judgment and righteousness in Jacob. [5] Exalt ye the Lord our God, and worship at his footstool; for he is holy. [6] Moses and Aaron among his priests, and Samuel among them that call upon his name; they called upon the Lord, and he answered them. [7] He spake unto them in the cloudy pillar: they kept his testimonies, and the ordinance that he gave them. [8] Thou answeredst them, O Lord our God: thou wast a God that forgavest them, though thou tookest vengeance of their inventions. [9] Exalt the Lord our God, and worship at his holy hill; for the Lord our God is holy.

Psalm 100

[1] Make a joyful noise unto the Lord, all ye lands. [2] Serve the Lord with gladness: come before his presence with singing. [3] Know ye that the Lord he is God: it is he that hath made us, and not we ourselves; we are his people, and the sheep of his pasture. [4] Enter into his gates with thanksgiving, and into his courts with praise: be thankful unto him, and bless his name. [5] For the Lord is good; his mercy is everlasting; and his truth endureth to all generations.

I wish I had taken this journey long ago! But let me reach out to you and invite to leave the mud of the world and come here where you don't know where are you going! But let it be that way!

I want once to feel natural and walk causal with no tracking or mocking letting myself go! O lord leave me here with the unknowns!

Amen 🙏

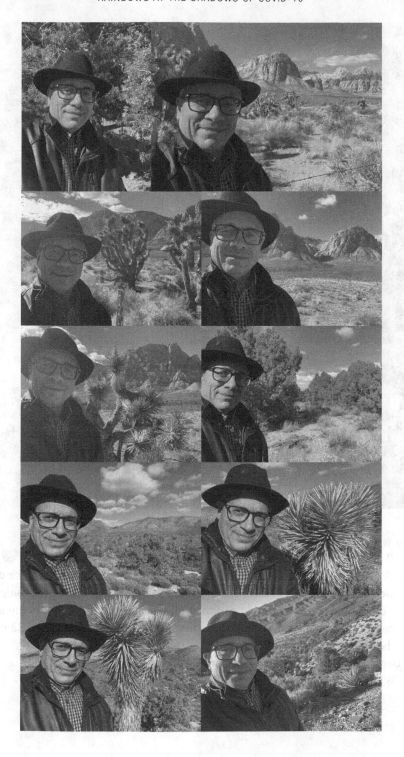

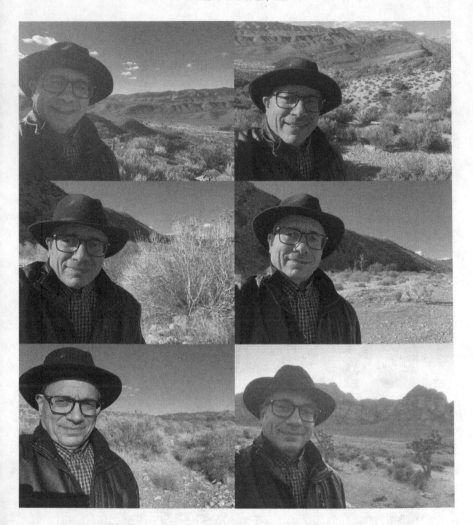

LKI wish I could be walking with you in nature. Thinking of you! 🖤
CG, Wouldn't it be wonderful if we could all take that journey. Great photos! 🖤🙏
TM. A beautiful poem, Ramsis, and I see Red Rock Canyon behind you. One day
   we will walk there together.......thank you, my friend, for calling me tonight.
   You did more for me in that call than all the other doctors here in months
   and I thank you from the bottom of my heart. God bless you, dear Ramsis
   the Great! 🖤
rc. Great photos, great nature, great journey, great all good man like you
Jm. What A Wonderful Feeling Dr. Ghaly 💕

Run Away for thy Life!
The Divine Calling Following COVID-19

Written by
<u>Ramsis Ghaly</u>

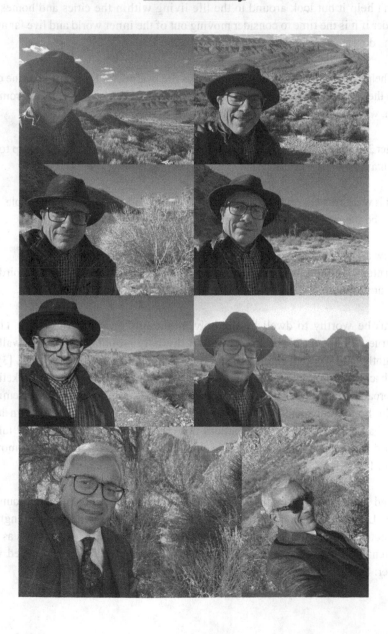

A Divine Calling: To the mountains 🏔️🏔️ I shall go to spend the 2020 Christmas! I got dressed with my best fashionable suit, luxurious Christmas tie and pocket square and cuff link dressy white shirt and classy black shoe to receive Baby Jesus at the manager by the holy mountain of the Lord in a remote desert place! It is that time!!

I can't help it but look around to the life living within the cities and homes but wonder if it is the time to consider moving out of the inner world and live far away by the desert 🏜️🐫🌵 and mountains 🏔️🏔️!

Our help is coming from the mountain says the psalmist; "I will lift up mine eyes unto the mountains, from whence cometh my help. [2] My help cometh from the Lord, which made heaven and earth." Psalm 121:1-2 KJV

In fact 2020 COVID-19 is a Renewal for God calling to His people: "go up to the mountains—"

As it is written: "Go up to the mountains, bring wood and rebuild the temple, that I may be pleased with it and be glorified," says the Lord." Haggai 1:8

Renew a Divine calling to human soul to flee as a bird to mountains 🏔️🏔️ as it is written: "In the Lord put I my trust: how say ye to my soul, Flee as a bird 🦅 to your mountain?" Psalm 11:1 KJV

Let us be worthy to dwell by the holy mountains 🏔️🏔️ of the Lord! Those the true worshipers of the Lord dwell in thy holy mountain 🏔️ Lord, walketh uprightly, and worketh righteousness, and speaketh the truth in his heart. [3] He that backbiteth not with his tongue, nor doeth evil to his neighbour, nor taketh up a reproach against his neighbour. [4] In whose eyes a vile person is contemned; but he honoureth them that fear the Lord. He that sweareth to his own hurt, and changeth not. [5] He that putteth not out his money to usury, nor taketh reward against the innocent. He that doeth these things shall never be moved. Psalm 15:1-5 KJV

Indeed listen to the psalmist: Psalm 24:3 Who may ascend into the mountain of the Lord? And who may stand in His holy place? God setteth His strength in the mountains and human souls rejoice by the pastures of tge wilderness as it is written: "Which by his strength setteth fast the mountains; being girded with power: Psalm 65

The righteousness is mighty by mountains 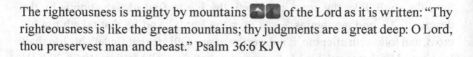 of the Lord as it is written: "Thy righteousness is like the great mountains; thy judgments are a great deep: O Lord, thou preservest man and beast." Psalm 36:6 KJV

The Almighty foundation is in the holy mountains 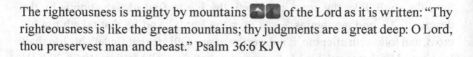 as it is written: "His foundation is in the holy mountains." Psalm 87:1 KJV

The Lord is our trust and the mountains 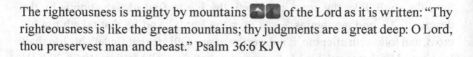 of our souls cannot be removed or shaken and for ever abode and all around us and within the souls as it is written: "They that trust in the Lord shall be as mount Zion, which cannot be removed, but abideth for ever. [2] As the mountains are round about Jerusalem, so the Lord is round about his people from henceforth even for ever." Psalm 125:1-2 KJV

Let us then flee to deserts 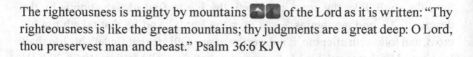 and mountains 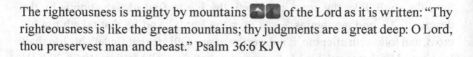 while they are around before the mountains 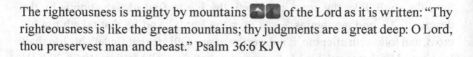 will be taken away in those days as it is written: "And every island fled away, and the mountains were not found." Revelation 16:20 KJV

Indeed, I heard a voice for thy people to begin moving out and rebuild churches for the Lord and Temples to serve His Name! Run away to find thy soul

The mountains 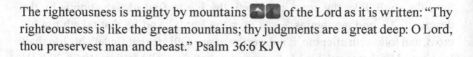 are rising as the cities are falling and the shut down of the inner world whereas the blooming of deserts and blossoming of the mountains 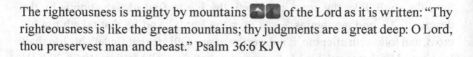 as it is written: Psalm 104:8 The mountains rose; the valleys sank down To the place which You established for them.

People are running away already to the parks, deserts 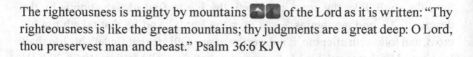 and mountains 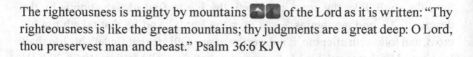 seeking freedom, fresh air and no restriction!

Have you ever stopped for a second and reflect in how people of the inner cities are living under?? They are in doors, in terrors and fears to go out or mix with others or live a life of freedom, restrained in house arrest and many didn't leave their homes for months, what kind of life is this?

In the meantime, those living sole out of the city by much acres of lands in a solitude are enjoying much freedom with least infection!

In fact, I hear many families are moving away and buying big home to live and work virtually!

I wonder if it is the time to Reform the way modern mankind is living and reconsider life away from the sin cities!

541

Save thy soul! Take thy cross and loseth thy life to find it! Salvation is by the deserts 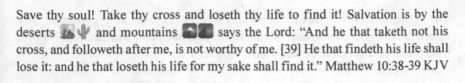 and mountains says the Lord: "And he that taketh not his cross, and followeth after me, is not worthy of me. [39] He that findeth his life shall lose it: and he that loseth his life for my sake shall find it." Matthew 10:38-39 KJV

The deserts and mountains are contagious for righteousness and good well among people!

The Holy Spirit is roving over the mighty deserts and the mountains of the Lord!

In the deserts and mountains where the soul is at serenity, the human brain at tranquility, the eyes sees and ears hear what is of the Lord as the world is casted out and not allowed to enter unto The deserts and mountains !

The mountains are known to be the seat of the Lord and they are the Lord's. Satan and corruption didn't invade the deserts and the mountains of the Lord! God said to Moses: Exodus 19:3 Moses went up to God, and the Lord called to him from the mountain, saying, "Thus you shall say to the house of Jacob and tell the sons of Israel:"

Furthermore, as man go out to the deserts and climb up to the mountains , God comes down to His mountains as it is written: Exodus 19:20 The Lord came down on Mount Sinai, to the top of the mountain; and the Lord called Moses to the top of the mountain, and Moses went up.

In the deserts and the mountains God will teach His ways and guide the people in His paths! Micah and Isiah predicted these days and said many nations will come and say, "Come and let us go up to the mountain of the Lord That He may teach us about His ways And that we may walk in His paths." Micah 4:2 Many nations will come and say, "Come and let us go up to the mountain of the Lord And to the house of the God of Jacob, That He may teach us about His ways And that we may walk in His paths." For from Zion will go forth the law, Even the word of the Lord from Jerusalem." And: Isaiah 2:3

In the mountains where God spoke to His children and handed Moses the very first Commandments written with fingers: Exodus 24:12 Now the Lord said to Moses, "Come up to Me on the mountain and remain there, and I will give you the stone tablets with the law and the commandment which I have written for their instruction."

542

In the deserts 🏜️🌵 and the mountains ⛰️🏔️, where the Good Shepherd find the astry souls to save: "How think ye? if a man have an hundred sheep, and one of them be gone astray, doth he not leave the ninety and nine, and goeth into the mountains, and seeketh that which is gone astray?" Mathew 18: 12

In the deserts 🏜️🌵 and the mountains ⛰️🏔️ live the consecrated human souls for Jesus dying from the world but living in the spirit living as angels on earth but in the flesh: They were stoned, they were sawn asunder, were tempted, were slain with the sword: they wandered about in sheepskins and goatskins; being destitute, afflicted, tormented; [38] (Of whom the world was not worthy:) they wandered in deserts, and in mountains, and in dens and caves of the earth. Hebrews 11:37-38 KJV

The mountains where at the end of days the mighty inhabitants of earth will run to and hide themselves in the dens and in the rocks of the mountains as it is written: "And the kings of the earth, and the great men, and the rich men, and the chief captains, and the mighty men, and every bondman, and every free man, hid themselves in the dens and in the rocks of the mountains;" Revelation 6:15 KJV

Lord says to the Modern man exposed to COVID-19 Pandemic go up to the mountains 🏔️⛰️

Exodus 34:2 So be ready by morning, and come up in the morning to Mount Sinai, and present yourself there to Me on the top of the mountain. Exodus 34:4 So he cut out two stone tablets like the former ones, and Moses rose up early in the morning and went up to Mount Sinai, as the Lord had commanded him, and he took two stone tablets in his hand. Exodus 24: 2 Then He said to Moses, "Come up to the Lord, you and Aaron, Nadab and Abihu and seventy of the elders of Israel, and you shall worship at a distance.

In fact, we thank our Lord because of the deserts 🌵🏜️ and mountains ⛰️🏔️ since at the end of days, the mountains won't be found as it is written: "And the great city was divided into three parts, and the cities of the nations fell: and great Babylon came in remembrance before God, to give unto her the cup of the wine of the fierceness of his wrath. [20] And every island fled away, and the mountains were not found. [21] And there fell upon men a great hail out of heaven, every stone about the weight of a talent: and men blasphemed God because of the plague of the hail; for the plague thereof was exceeding great." Revelation 16:19-21 KJV

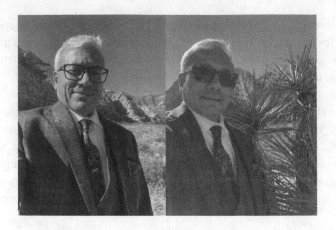

Run Away for thy Life!

The Divine Calling Behind COVID-19

I can't help it but look around to the life living within the cities and homes but wonder if it is the time to consider moving out of the inner world and live far away by the desert 🏚️ 🐪 🌵 and mountains ⛰️ ⛰️!

In fact 2020 COVID-19 is a Renewal for God calling to His people: "go up to the mountains—"

As it is written: "Go up to the mountains, bring wood and rebuild the temple, that I may be pleased with it and be glorified," says the Lord." Haggai 1:8

The Lord ask each human soul to flee as a bird 🐦 to mountains ⛰️ ⛰️ as it is written: "In the Lord put I my trust: how say ye to my soul, Flee as a bird to your mountain?" Psalm 11:1 KJV

Let us be worthy to dwell by the holy mountains ⛰️ ⛰️ of the Lord! Those the true worshipers of the Lord dwell in thy holy mountain ⛰️ Lord, walketh uprightly, and worketh righteousness, and speaketh the truth in his heart. [3] He that backbiteth not with his tongue, nor doeth evil to his neighbour, nor taketh up a reproach against his neighbour. [4] In whose eyes a vile person is contemned; but he honoureth them that fear the Lord. He that sweareth to his own hurt, and changeth not. [5] He that putteth not out his money to usury, nor taketh reward against the innocent. He that doeth these things shall never be moved. Psalm 15:1-5 KJV

Indeed listen to the psalmist: Psalm 24:3 Who may ascend into the mountain of the Lord? And who may stand in His holy place?

God setteth His strength in the mountains and human souls rejoice by the pastures of tge wilderness as it is written: "Which by his strength setteth fast the mountains; being girded with power: [7] Which stilleth the noise of the seas, the noise of their waves, and the tumult of the people. [12] They drop upon the pastures of the wilderness: and the little hills rejoice on every side. [13] The pastures are clothed with flocks; the valleys also are covered over with corn; they shout for joy, they also sing." Psalm 65:6-7,12-13 KJV

The righteousness is mighty by mountains 🔺 🔺 of the Lord as it is written: "Thy righteousness is like the great mountains; thy judgments are a great deep: O Lord, thou preservest man and beast." Psalm 36:6 KJV

The Almighty foundation is in the holy mountainsas 🔺 🔺 it is written: "His foundation is in the holy mountains." Psalm 87:1 KJV

The Lord is our trust and the mountains 🔺 🔺 of our souls cannot be removed or shaken and for ever abode and all around us and within the souls as it is written: "They that trust in the Lord shall be as mount Zion, which cannot be removed, but abideth for ever. [2] As the mountains are round about Jerusalem, so the Lord is round about his people from henceforth even for ever." Psalm 125:1-2 KJV

The lord laid the foundation of the earth and established the mountains 🔺, valleys and habitation for His people and treasures the waters, the springs, the valleys, greens and herbs, fowels, birds and nests, cattle and goats, lions, the trees and branches, fruits, and much more to praise the Lord as it is written: "Who laid the foundations of the earth, that it should not be removed for ever. [6] Thou coveredst it with the deep as with a garment: the waters stood above the mountains. [8] They go up by the mountains; they go down by the valleys unto the place which thou hast founded for them. [10] He sendeth the springs into the valleys, which run among the hills. [12] By them shall the fowls of the heaven have their habitation, which sing among the branches. [13] He watereth the hills from his chambers: the earth is satisfied with the fruit of thy works. [14] He causeth the grass to grow for the cattle, and herb for the service of man: that he may bring forth food out of the earth; [16] The trees of the Lord are full of sap ; the cedars of Lebanon, which he hath planted; [17] Where the birds make their nests: as for the stork, the fir trees are her house. [18] The high hills are a refuge for the wild goats; and the rocks for the conies. [21] The young lions roar after their prey, and seek their meat from God. [22] The sun ariseth, they gather themselves together, and lay them down in their dens. [24] O Lord, how manifold are thy works! in wisdom hast thou made them all: the earth is full of thy riches. [32] He looketh on the earth, and it trembleth: he toucheth the hills, and they smoke. [33] I will sing unto the Lord as long as I live: I will sing praise to my God while I have my being." Psalm 104:5-6,8,10,12-14,16-18,21-22,24,32-33 KJV

Let us flee to deserts 📖 🌱 and mountains ⛰ ⛰ while they are around before the mountains ⛰ ⛰ will be taken away in those days as it is written: "And every island fled away, and the mountains were not found." Revelation 16:20 KJV

Indeed, I heard a voice for thy people to begin moving out and rebuild churches 🏠 for the Lord and Temples to serve His Name! Run away to find thy soul

The mountains ⛰ ⛰ are rising as the cities are falling and the shut down of the inner world whereas the blooming of deserts and blossoming of the mountains ⛰ ⛰ as it is written: Psalm 104:8 The mountains rose; the valleys sank down To the place which You established for them.

People are running away already to the parks, deserts 🌱 📖 and mountains ⛰ ⛰ seeking freedom, fresh air and no restriction!

There is always fresh high flow of winds, air, sun and nature to cleanse the human body from bad viruses 🦠 🦠 and microbes!

Have you ever stopped for a second and reflect in how people of the inner cities are living under?? They are in doors, in terrors and fears to go out or mix with others or live a life of freedom, restrained in house arrest and many didn't leave their homes for months, what kind of life is this?

In the meantime, those living sole out of the city by much acres of lands in a solitude are enjoying much freedom with least infection!

In fact, I hear many families are moving away and buying big home to live and work virtually!

I wonder if it is the time to Reform the way modern mankind is living and reconsider life away from the sin cities!

God wants the human soul not preoccupied with the world but a tabernacle for the Holy Spirit! In the world the children of God shall leave their worries, bank accounts, properties, wealth and all materials and come with virgin empty heart starving for the Lord of Lords and Nis Salvations!

Save thy soul! Take thy cross and loseth thy life to find it! Salvation is by the deserts 📖 🕊 and mountains ⛰ ⛰ says the Lord: "And he that taketh not his cross, and followeth after me, is not worthy of me. [39] He that findeth his life shall lose it: and he that loseth his life for my sake shall find it." Matthew 10:38-39 KJV

Leave the world behind, take up his cross, and follow Jesus the Savior of the world, For what is a man profited, if he shall gain the whole world, and lose his own soul? or what shall a man give in exchange for his soul? Matthew 16:24-26 KJV [24] Then said Jesus unto his disciples, If any man will come after me, let him deny himself, and take up his cross, and follow me. [25] For whosoever will save his life shall lose it: and whosoever will lose his life for my sake shall find it. [26] For what is a man profited, if he shall gain the whole world, and lose his own soul? or what shall a man give in exchange for his soul?

It is customary when the anger of the Lord arise that reformation of man occurs and the only places to cleanse are those of purity by the desert 📖 🕊 🐪 and the mountains ⛰ ⛰!

The deserts 🕊 📖 and mountains ⛰ ⛰ are contagious for righteousness and good well among people!

The Holy Spirit is roving over the mighty deserts 📖 🕊 and the mountains ⛰ ⛰ of the Lord!

In the deserts 🕊 📖 and mountains ⛰ ⛰ where the soul is at serenity, the human brain at tranquility, the eyes sees and ears hear what is of the Lord as the world is casted out and not allowed to enter unto The deserts 🕊 📖 and mountain ⛰ ⛰!

The mountains are known to be the seat of the Lord and they are the Lord's. Satan and corruption didn't invade the deserts 🕊 📖 and the mountains ⛰ ⛰ of the Lord! God said to Moses: Exodus 19:3 Moses went up to God, and the Lord called to him from the mountain, saying, "Thus you shall say to the house of Jacob and tell the sons of Israel:"

Furthermore, as man go out to the deserts 🕊 📖 and climb up to the mountains ⛰ ⛰, God comes down to His mountains ⛰ ⛰ as it is written: Exodus 19:20

547

The Lord came down on Mount Sinai, to the top of the mountain; and the Lord called Moses to the top of the mountain, and Moses went up.

With the ongoing Pandemic, I wonder if It is a Divine Calling to follow Moses steps and run out of the Corrupted cities unto Mount Sinai!

There is a Recall for the people of Lord to leave the corruption and re-enter the uncontaminated deserts away from the infected world!

It perhaps that time where the city people move out to live by the deserts 🕌 🏕️!

Man had made sin cities and now is the time to cleanse by the purity of the mountains ⛰️ ⛰️!

It is the time to move the city to desert 🏕️ 🌵 🐪!

As God asked Moses to take His people out of the world to mount Sinai and lived for 40 years, so it is now!

Since COVID-19, there is a constant calling; run with thy life and stay away from gathering, closed spaces and stay by the open spaces with winds and fresh air circulating all the time!

I toured the deserts 🏕️ 🕌 and the mountains and find only few Temples for the Lord!

In the deserts and 🏕️ 🕌 the mountains ⛰️ ⛰️ God will teach His ways and guide the people in His paths! Micah and Isiah predicted these days and said many nations will come and say, "Come and let us go up to the mountain of the Lord That He may teach us about His ways And that we may walk in His paths." Micah 4:2 Many nations will come and say, "Come and let us go up to the mountain of the Lord And to the house of the God of Jacob, That He may teach us about His ways And that we may walk in His paths." For from Zion will go forth the law, Even the word of the Lord from Jerusalem." And: Isaiah 2:3 And many peoples will come and say, "Come, let us go up to the mountain of the Lord, To the house of the God of Jacob; That He may teach us concerning His ways And that we may walk in His paths." For the law will go forth from Zion And the word of the Lord from Jerusalem.

In the mountains ⛰️ ⛰️ where God spoke to His children and handed Moses the very first Commandments written with fingers: Exodus 24:12 Now the Lord said to Moses, "Come up to Me on the mountain and remain there, and I will give you the stone tablets with the law and the commandment which I have written for their instruction."

n the deserts 🏚 🌳 and the mountains ⛰ ⛰, where the Good Shepherd find the astray souls to save: "How think ye? if a man have an hundred sheep, and one of them be gone astray, doth he not leave the ninety and nine, and goeth into the **mountains**, and seeketh that which is gone astray?" Mathew 18: 12

In the deserts 🏚 🌳 and the mountains ⛰ ⛰ live the consecrated human souls for Jesus dying from the world but living in the spirit living as angels on earth but in the flesh: They were stoned, they were sawn asunder, were tempted, were slain with the sword: they wandered about in sheepskins and goatskins; being destitute, afflicted, tormented; [38] (Of whom the world was not worthy:) they wandered in deserts, and in mountains, and in dens and caves of the earth. Hebrews 11:37-38 KJV

In the deserts 🏚 🌳 and the mountains ⛰ ⛰, where the human souls shall run at the end of days from satan inhabitants of the inner world 🌑: Then let them which be in Judaea flee into the **mountains**: Mathew 24:16 and But when ye shall see the abomination of desolation, spoken of by Daniel the prophet, standing where it ought not, (let him that readeth understand,) then let them that be in Judaea flee to the **mountains**: Mark 13: 14 Then shall they begin to say to the **mountains**, Fall on us; and to the hills, Cover us. Luke 23:30

The mountains where at the end of days the mighty inhabitants of earth will run to and hide themselves in the dens and in the rocks of the mountains as it is written: "And the kings of the earth, and the great men, and the rich men, and the chief captains, and the mighty men, and every bondman, and every free man, hid themselves in the dens and in the rocks of the mountains;" Revelation 6:15 KJV

Lord says to the Modern man exposed to COVID-19 Pandemic

Haggai 1:8 Go up to the mountains, bring wood and rebuild the temple, that I may be pleased with it and be glorified," says the Lord.

Psalm 104:8 The mountains rose; the valleys sank down

To the place which You established for them.

Micah 4:2 Many nations will come and say, "Come and let us go up to the mountain of the Lord

And to the house of the God of Jacob, That He may teach us about His ways And that we may walk in His paths." For from Zion will go forth the law, Even the word of the Lord from Jerusalem.

Exodus 24:15 Then Moses went up to the mountain, and the cloud covered the mountain.

Isaiah 2:3 And many peoples will come and say, "Come, let us go up to the mountain of the Lord, To the house of the God of Jacob; That He may teach us concerning His ways And that we may walk in His paths." For the law will go forth from Zion And the word of the Lord from Jerusalem.

Exodus 19:20 The Lord came down on Mount Sinai, to the top of the mountain; and the Lord called Moses to the top of the mountain, and Moses went up.

Exodus 34:2 So be ready by morning, and come up in the morning to Mount Sinai, and present yourself there to Me on the top of the mountain.

Exodus 34:4 So he cut out two stone tablets like the former ones, and Moses rose up early in the morning and went up to Mount Sinai, as the Lord had commanded him, and he took two stone tablets in his hand.

Exodus 24: 2 Then He said to Moses, "Come up to the Lord, you and Aaron, Nadab and Abihu and seventy of the elders of Israel, and you shall worship at a distance.

Exodus 24:12 Now the Lord said to Moses, "Come up to Me on the mountain and remain there, and I will give you the stone tablets with the law and the commandment which I have written for their instruction."

Deuteronomy 10:1 "At that time the Lord said to me, 'Cut out for yourself two tablets of stone like the former ones, and come up to Me on the mountain, and make an ark of wood for yourself.

Exodus 24:18 Moses entered the midst of the cloud as he went up to the mountain; and Moses was on the mountain forty days and forty nights.

Exodus 19:3 Moses went up to God, and the Lord called to him from the mountain, saying, "Thus you shall say to the house of Jacob and tell the sons of Israel:

Exodus 24:13 So Moses arose with Joshua his servant, and Moses went up to the mountain of God.

Exodus 24:9 Then Moses went up with Aaron, Nadab and Abihu, and seventy of the elders of Israel,

Exodus 19:23 Moses said to the Lord, "The people cannot come up to Mount Sinai, for You warned us, saying, 'Set bounds about the mountain and consecrate it.'"

Exodus 19:24 Then the Lord said to him, "Go down and come up again, you and Aaron with you; but do not let the priests and the people break through to come up to the Lord, or He will break forth upon them."

Numbers 20:25 Take Aaron and his son Eleazar and bring them up to Mount Hor;

Numbers 20:27 So Moses did just as the Lord had commanded, and they went up to Mount Hor in the sight of all the congregation.

Deuteronomy 3:27 Go up to the top of Pisgah and lift up your eyes to the west and north and south and east, and see it with your eyes, for you shall not cross over this Jordan.

Deuteronomy 32:49 "Go up to this mountain of the Abarim, Mount Nebo, which is in the land of Moab opposite Jericho, and look at the land of Canaan, which I am giving to the sons of Israel for a possession.

1 Samuel 10:3 Then you will go on further from there, and you will come as far as the oak of Tabor, and there three men going up to God at Bethel will meet you, one carrying three young goats, another carrying three loaves of bread, and another carrying a jug of wine;

Psalm 24:3 Who may ascend into the hill of the Lord? And who may stand in His holy place?

Jeremiah 31:6 "For there will be a day when watchmen On the hills of Ephraim call out, 'Arise, and let us go up to Zion, To the Lord our God.'"

In fact, we thank our Lord because of the deserts 🏜️ 🏞️ and mountains ⛰️ 🏔️ since at the end of days, the mountains won't be found as it is written: "And the great city was divided into three parts, and the cities of the nations fell: and great Babylon came in remembrance before God, to give unto her the cup of the wine of the fierceness of his wrath. [20] And every island fled away, and the mountains were not found. [21] And there fell upon men a great hail out of heaven, every stone about the weight of a talent: and men blasphemed God because of the plague of the hail; for the plague thereof was exceeding great." Revelation 16:19-21 KJV And: "And the kings of the earth, and the great men, and the rich men, and the chief captains, and the mighty men, and every bondman, and every free man, hid themselves in the dens and in the rocks of the mountains; [16] And said to the mountains and rocks, Fall on us, and hide us from the face of him that sitteth on the throne, and from the wrath of the Lamb: [17] For the great day of his wrath is come; and who shall be able to stand?" Revelation 6:15-17 KJV

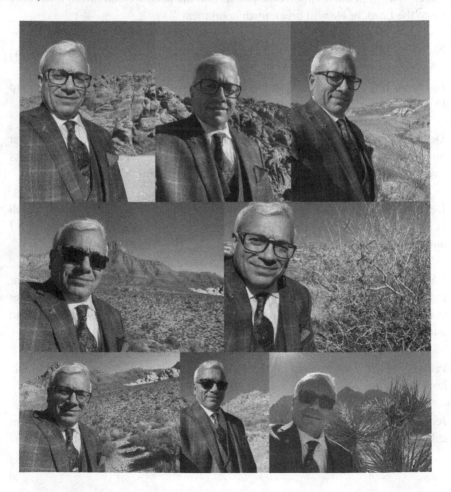

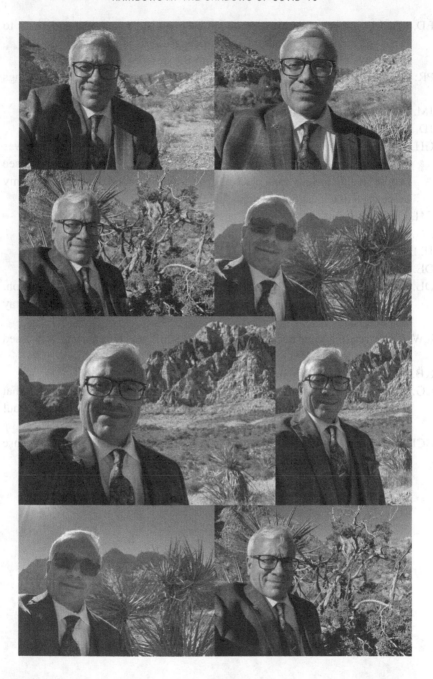

BK. The desert looks good on you Dr Ghaly.
MH. We have beautiful mountains here in Idaho.

ED. I find living in the desert surrounded by beautiful mountains and vistas to be so spiritual. The air, nature, quiet, peacefulness is all very liberating 🌲 I can drive two miles out of my city into the desert.

PR. Excellent my friend, may the day bring new wonderful light and the evenings be good upon you, may you always be safe.

JM. Blessings doctor you have great faith

JD. Merry Christmas Dr. Ghaly!

GH. Yes, my mother said before she died, you must get out of the cities. She was an evangelical Christian, very well read on politics and Christianity! I see people fleeing the city for a place to grow your own food. I love and miss my hometown of Chicago, but am not being led by God to return.

GH. I love your suit!

KG. Have a very Merry Christmas and a happy, healthy New Year, Dr. Ghaly 🎄

JJ. Enjoy your well deserved break.

DE. Merry Christmas 🌲🎄

DL. Merry Christmas Dr. Ramsis Ghaly. Enjoy your well deserved vacation. Enjoy all your photos and writings. May God continue to bless you. Stay safe and healthy.

KW. I love reading your beautiful writings. Thank you for sharing. A blessed Christmas to you, D

KB. Merry Christmas Dr. Ghaly.

CG. It would be wonderful to get away from the pandemic and everything that it brings but unfortunately we have to stay here and deal with it. Bless you! Great picture

BCD. Excellent. Get dressed in your finest garments and take some Frankense and Myrrh essential oils with you. Great ritual.

Even for Just Few! I Found Comfort Running Away to the Desert During Unfolding of COVID!

Written by Ramsis Ghaly

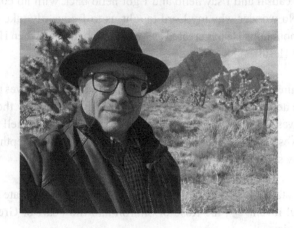

It is that time to run away for few hours of the day in a solitude with nature deep in the desert 🌵 by the mountain of my Lord Jesus!! Even if for just few!

If I just take of myself out of the world 🌐 even if for few, my soul might listen to the voice of my beloved and hear His voice!

Indeed, the mountains 🏔 and the surroundings all the time call His Name and worship His glory and therefore His presence always manifested by the Nature He has created! It is the time of my ailing soul to attend for prayers and vigil in the midst of His Divine Radiance!

My soul applauded the special tranquility and the sounds of the winds, the smell of fresh air and purity all around. Indeed there isn't any distractions or disputes but healing to the soul and praises to my Lord!

It didn't take much to leave my belongings, politics and worldly things behind, put the world behind and jump in the wagon to travel for few! The craziness of what is going on around in the world is becoming unbearable to my fragile form! So glad I took some time away at my special happy place, at the citadel of Joy! It is that time to recharge and rejuvenate in the beautiful desert!

I heard the Coronavirus says to me: "I am not coming" and I saw the viruses are running away at the highways! The mountains are too holy for them to come close and the deserts are too harsh for them to consider! So I took my facemask with me just in case and I put it on and off in the road! Don't be crazy my soul says and look forward to see the Lord" I replied Amen 🙏!

I took off my fake layers of the world, remove the shadows and be real and surface me! I became causal and I say hello and I got hello back with no cost or burden of thoughts! No wonder why my Lord taught us to frequently take a break and attend to the mountains He has created as My Savior had done when He was living with us by the flesh!

By the mountains 🏔 of the Lord, my soul regain strength and revives powers from above! By the deserts, my soul received peace and hope! And by the loneliness, my soul receives Love 🖤 from my Heavenly Father! By the smell of fresh air, my soul receives nourishment and hydration! The nature gives depth to my roots and faith to my soul!

I am all alone standing in a boundless arena, but with my Soulmate my Beloved whom my soul loveth 🖤, the Rose of Sharon and the Pearl of Great price the Only Silver Coin 🪙!

Here by the deserts 🌵 of my heavenly fathers, the light and the glory, the freedom and supreme majesty of holiness and divinity! The Spirit of the Lord is all around me is vibrant and full of fervent warmth and loyalty! The Lord is My pride and my greatness!

In my Lord land, I put my footlings as I feel the priceless harmony and robust energy! There is no moment of sadness or dwindling!

During the Transition of powers, the uprise snd unrest in our nation, I wish for you all to distance your souls away by the nature so you may find peace in His Name! Our Lord Jesus us indeed In Control! Amen 🙏

Psalm 86
"Bow down thine ear, O Lord, hear me: for I am poor and needy. [2] Preserve my soul; for I am holy: O thou my God, save thy servant that trusteth in thee. [3] Be merciful unto me, O Lord: for I cry unto thee daily. [4] Rejoice the soul of thy servant: for unto thee, O Lord, do I lift up my soul. [5] For thou, Lord, art good, and ready to forgive; and plenteous in mercy unto all them that call upon thee. [6] Give ear, O Lord, unto my prayer; and attend to the voice of my supplications.

[7] In the day of my trouble I will call upon thee: for thou wilt answer me. [8] Among the gods there is none like unto thee, O Lord; neither are there any works like unto thy works. [9] All nations whom thou hast made shall come and worship before thee, O Lord; and shall glorify thy name. [10] For thou art great, and doest wondrous things: thou art God alone. [11] Teach me thy way, O Lord ; I will walk in thy truth: unite my heart to fear thy name. [12] I will praise thee, O Lord my God, with all my heart: and I will glorify thy name for evermore. [13] For great is thy mercy toward me: and thou hast delivered my soul from the lowest hell."

Ramsis Ghaly

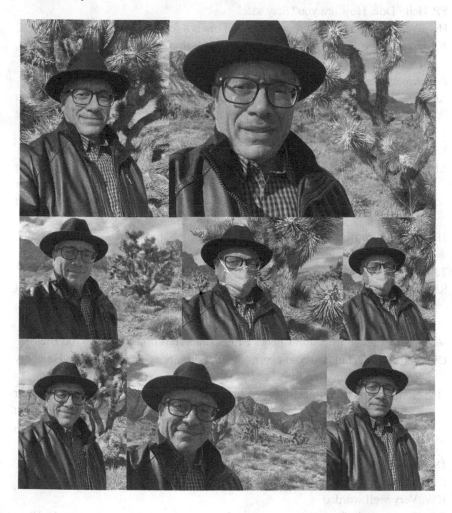

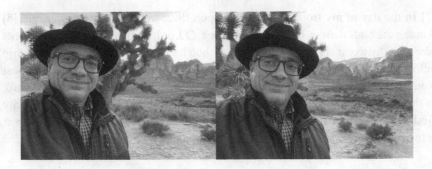

PP. Hello Doc. How are you? Stay safe!

HC. We all need a break now and again. This is a lot.

JC. I would take a break where you are in this! Is that the Joshaua tree behind you, I was there once! You look great 🙏🙏

AB. Amen praise God! Good words

AC. ... when I look at Your pictures and read Your words, I understand, that You are very sensitive Human and I understand that God inspires You to do great things ... 🎃🎃💜💜

KE. Handsome* Wish We didn't need the masks anymore May God Bless*

ED. Amen Doctor. Today we ventured out to the beautiful desert for a long peaceful walk. It does the soul good to be with our Savior and restoring our spirits. I saw a beautiful huge owl. For some reason that made me feel that the Lord is right here protecting us. God bless.

JB. So glad you have some time away at your happy place, at your citadel. Recharge and rejuvenate in the beautiful desert Dr. G.

TJ. Beautiful scenery - enjoy your peace! God bless you always.

SJ. Your written words took me out to the mountains and deserts, and there I experienced the quiet loneliness where my heart prayed - thank you for the momentary reprieve from this world.

VM. Enjoy the nature'$ atmosphere BFF. Looks so relaxing place. God Bless

CR. Your words and how you express your faith are so inspiring. Yes He is my Rose of Sharon.

DK. So glad you got a much needed break. Bask in the love and beauty of our Lord for as long as needed to recharge! You are a refreshing and bright light in such a dark and chaotic world 🌑 Thank you for sharing your gift from God with us!!

JM. Amen Dr. Ghaly 💕

CC. Amen 🙏

KW. Very well worded

CG. Great words from a great person. I enjoy your writings very much. Bless you! 💜🙏

I Found Comfort Running Away to the Desert During Unfolding of COVID

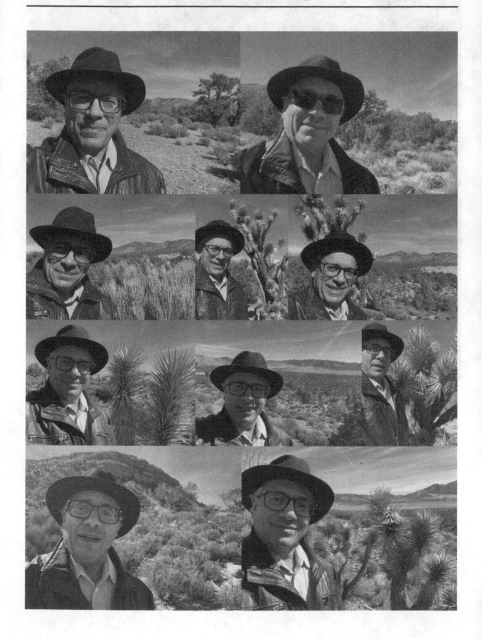

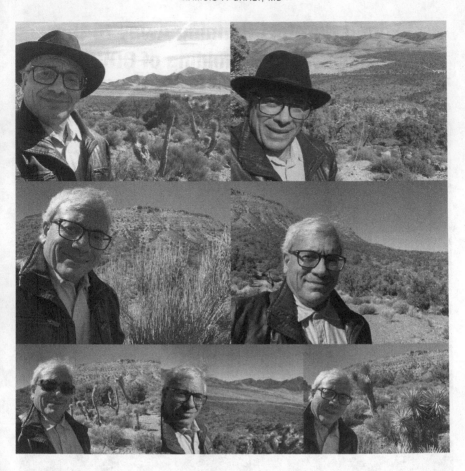

Sunday the Day of the Lord by the White Mountains!!

Written by Ramsis Ghaly

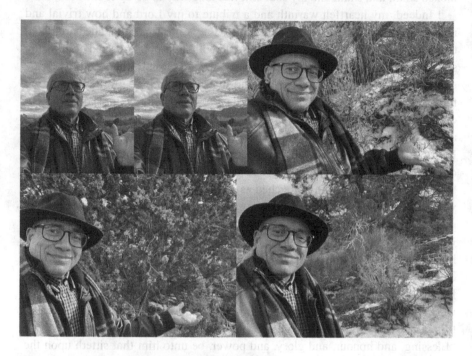

It was a regular Sunday Dawn and feeling down with COVID-19 lockdown and shutting the doors ▊ of the church of the Lord! I was aroused with a soft whisper voice! My soul said to my spirit: "let us be alone with our Creator and get away it is Sunday the Day of the Lord! I heard a voice: "Come and join me"! Let us climb 🌲 the mountains ⛰! Let me show the white snow in My Mountains and the ice covering the deserts! Look at what I found: the mountains ⛰⛰ tanned pure white like snow! Let us together hid by the white mountains ⛰! Let us sit by the ice! The pure white ICE 🧊 and snow covering the mountains ⛰⛰! The frozen waters 💧 all over in the remote God's creation! Some of trees 🌳🌲 are still green! The waters transformed to white rounded crystals all over the mountain ⛰ ! I was touched with aroma smell erupts from the icy land! As I kept climbing 🌲 , it appeared endless and I felt free walking 🚶 in a boundless land! There was no evidence of human hand ✋ or man feet 👣 made it thus far but me! There was no phone signal or electronic wiring but only the Holy Spirit descending from above! O my Lord I am unworthy of Your gratitude 🙏 to me and my soul is honored

561

and privileged to be here with You! The mountain 🔺 Pinacle was further away as the prayers and songs to the Lord pouring heavily! As I climbed Higher and higher, My soul and spirit got warmer and warmer with my Lord! The sun ☀ was shining in and out made the treat blessed and holy! My soul and spirit were humbled to look at the world from up high by the mountain 🔺 top! The world looked small and small and my soul still has long way to go up to the mountains 🔺! Indeed, my heartfelt warmth and a tribute to my Lord and how trivial and minute is the deceiving world! Thank You 🙏 my Lord finally I made barefooted to the peek! Now I sat on the top of the world with my Lord Jesus and nothing my soul in need of the world 🌑 of darkness! I was so close to the clouds ☁ wide open vision to the heaven incredible and marvelous to be with the Lord at the top of the mountain 🔺! I ran out of words and stood before Him speechless but only to find myself staring and up hauling! I had no fear and filled with courage and adventure as in the days of pilgrimage of my fathers Abraham and Elijah m! My Lord Jesus made my soul feel triumphing over the self and taste the victory over the world in His Name! Gorgeous and great to be with my Savior all alone by the white icy mountain untouched as He had formed for my soul millions of years ago before I was born! I raise my arms up to heaven from the top of the mountain 🔺 saying: "… Holy, holy, holy, Lord God Almighty, which was, and is, and is to come. And when those beasts give glory and honour and thanks to him that sat on the throne, who liveth for ever and ever, [10] The four and twenty elders fall down before him that sat on the throne, and worship him that liveth for ever and ever, and cast their crowns before the throne, saying, [11] Thou art worthy, O Lord, to receive glory and honour and power: for thou hast created all things, and for j thy pleasure they are and were created." Revelation 4:8-11 KJV "Blessing, and honour, and glory, and power, be unto him that sitteth upon the throne, and unto the Lamb for ever and ever." Revelations 5:13. And I concluded with Father's Prayer "—Our Father which art in heaven, Hallowed be thy name. [10] Thy kingdom come. Thy will be done in earth, as it is in heaven. [11] Give us this day our daily bread. [12] And forgive us our debts, as we forgive our debtors. [13] And lead us not into temptation, but deliver us from evil: For thine is the kingdom, and the power, and the glory, for ever. Fir thine the power the glory and kingdom fur ever and ever, Amen 🙏" Mathhews 6:9-13. Silence and tranquility! Peace and love 🖤! Truth and Spirit sprouting 🌱! Neither virus 🦠 nor science! Neither face-masking nor pollution! Neither distraction nor misleading! It is the time to pray and open my heart 🖤 to my Heavenly Father! Let us sing to the Lord new song 🎵 🎶 by the white mountains! Praise the Lord praise the Lord of hosts! Let us nourish the soul with the virgin land as it was created millions of years ago by the hand of Almighty! The sun ☀ Was going away as the clouds ☁ covered the sky! I saw a huge tree 🌳 on the top of the mountain 🔺 similar to the pictures of the tree of life! It was a divine calling to rest for a little while!

I sat by the tree 🌲 full of the mighty grace and grasping the fresh air before my feet take the steps back to the ground! I wasn't in need of any food or drinks, my soul was just thirst with my Lord and hungry for the Bread of Life! I didn't want to go down and return to where I came before! I prayed for God to let me stay with Him even for just an overnight stay! O the voice came out of the clouds ☁: "Go back son and tomorrow is at hand. Let the darkness come down as the daylight vanishes away from the mountain for the time being" it is indeed fearful to be present without the True Light of God as the entire white mountain was getting covered with dark clouds and face the darkness with blowing winds of the night all alone"! Goodbye 👋 goodbye 👋 goodbye 👋 to mountain 🏔 of the Lord and solitude with my Beloved and soulmate! From the bottom God took me with His hands up to the top! From down in the dungeon and pit, the Almighty lifted my soul up to the top of mountain 🏔 and sit with Him! A spiritual vision resembles a beautiful heavenly dream where the human soul visit with the Lord and liveth for little while in His Grace! Amen 🙏 my Lord Jesus the God above all gods!

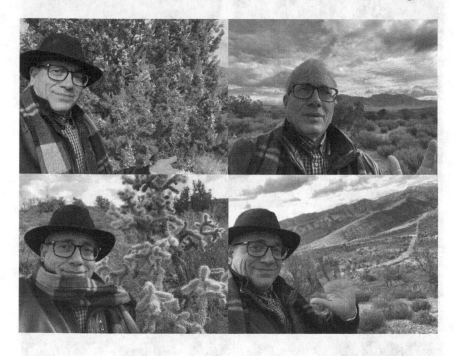

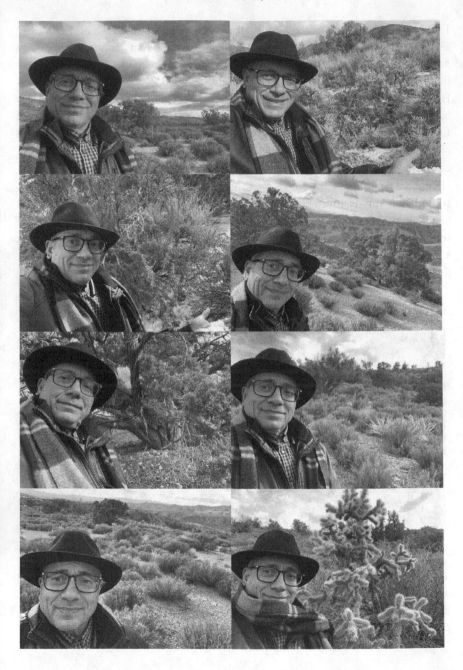

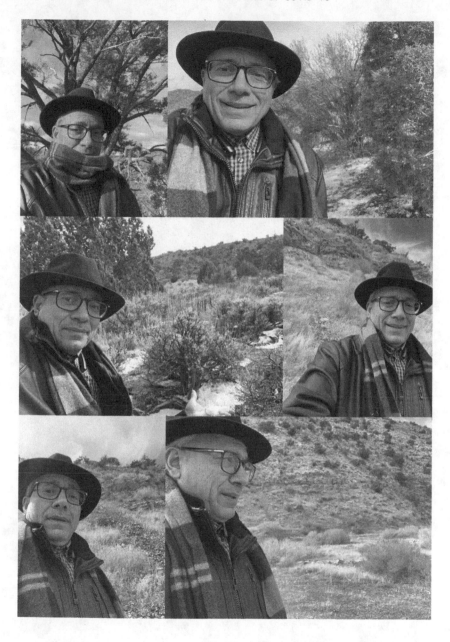

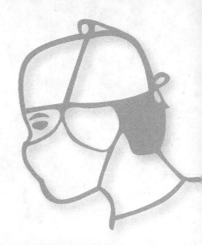

SECTION 11

Author and COVID-19

My God Brought me all the Way From Egypt 36 Years Ago to Care for COVID Victims!

My God brought me all the way from Egypt 36 years ago and has blessed me to be His servant for all these years at Cook County hospital Chicago, learning, saving lives and teaching generations and generations! And as much Left, I am proud to continue to serve as As a Neurosurgeon, as an anesthesiologist, as an Intensivist and as pain specialist.

And His mercy never ceased and now God has blessed me to see the day of our ancient hospital is being renovated and turning it's blue lights joining the entire nation and the world 🌐 to show gratitude to the healthcare workers and to the first responders!

I lived to care through the days of Chicago trauma victims of gangs, mobs, violence and all the waives of epidemics and endemic over the years and now I am living the days of COVID pandemic to care for our fellow men and women.

Not Not Not me but My Lord Jesus took me from my hands in 1980's when I was scared knowing that I will never make it for one more day to be a professor and teacher reaching the top that I have never dreamed of. And now I am an author of 17 books writing all of what My Lord Jesus has done for me and with me since I was conceived in my mom womb.

"I am crucified with Christ: nevertheless I live; yet not I, but Christ liveth in me: and the life which I now live in the flesh I live by the faith of the Son of God, who loved me, and gave himself for me." Galatians 2:20 KJV

May our Lord Jesus bless our Country America and bless the world and conquer COVID soon, Amen 🙏

Ramsis Ghaly

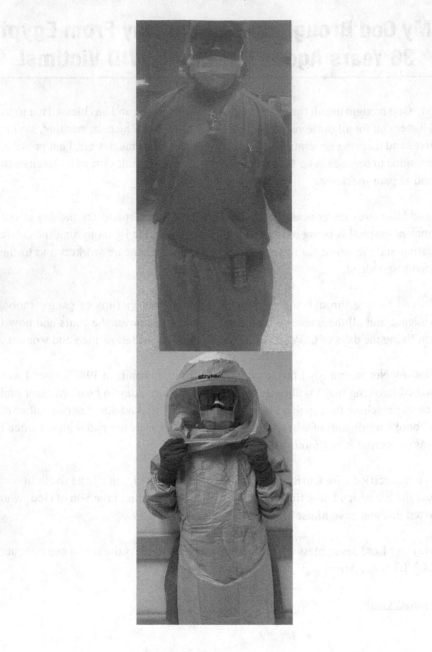

January 20, 2020 was My very first post to warm the world against the imminent COVID -19 pandemic and called upon worldwide chain of prayers —-

https://www.facebook.com/1150861349/posts/10221108146470558/?d=n

Let us call upon worldwide chain of prayers to Our Lord Jesus to put stop ⬤ the Coronavirus virus 🦠 outbreak pandemic. We pray for China 🏴 and our beloved Chinese people through this tough time

Ramsis Ghaly

We are behind our supplication to the Most High to have mercy upon His handmaid and come down and save His people from that Coronavirus virus 🦠 outbreak pandemic.

Coronavirus live updates: China says death toll hits 213, confirmed cases rise to 9,692

How vulnerable is man just overnight the virus Coronavirus spread across the continents and soon United Nations is calling it Emergency epidemic. And so we all should call upon emergency prayers to Lord our God Jesus.

With all the man grandiose and high level of healing, man and science cannot even stop a virus 🦠 only one type of virus 🦠. How nothing is man and could be destroyed in seconds!

My brethren let us all ask for a global prayer 🙏 to our Lord Jesus to stop ⬤ that virus outbreak and rescue His children in China and worldwide. How much my heart 💜 is aching, please Lord Jesus You are the Only One that can heal the sick, rescue thy people and put a stop ⬤ to the Coronavirus virus outbreak. In Jesus Name, Amen 🙏🙏🙏

No one, no medicine, no leadership, no earthly ⬤ treatment, no money, no science and no nothing exist to neither cure nor put a stop ⬤ to that virus 🦠 outbreak but the Lord of glory.

Let us all form chains of prayers pleading to our Lord Jesus. Let the church 🏛 doors be open and raise incense with unceasing prayers. Let us fast and bow down to our Lord Jesus to have mercy upon the world and conquer that Coronavirus virus ✹ outbreak pandemic.

Our Lord Jesus told us to ask Him and now we do O Lord Jesus: "23And in that day ye shall ask me nothing. Verily, verily, I say unto you, Whatsoever ye shall ask the Father in my name, he will give it you. 24Hitherto have ye asked nothing in my name: ask, and ye shall receive, that your joy may be full.25These things have I spoken unto you in proverbs: but the time cometh, when I shall no more speak unto you in proverbs, but I shall shew you plainly of the Father. 26At that day ye shall ask in my name: and I say not unto you, that I will pray the Father for you: 27For the Father himself loveth you, because ye have loved me, and have believed that I came out from God. 28I came forth from the Father, and am come into the world: again, I leave the world, and go to the Father." (John 16: 23-28)

Our Lord Jesus promise is: "19Again I say unto you, That if two of you shall agree on earth as touching any thing that they shall ask, it shall be done for them of my Father which is in heaven. 20For where two or three are gathered together in my name, there am I in the midst of them." (Matthew 18:19-20)

Jesus said: "13And whatsoever ye shall ask in my name, that will I do, that the Father may be glorified in the Son. 14If ye shall ask any thing in my name, I will do." John 14:13

So let us all O people get together and pray to our Lord: "7Ask, and it shall be given you; seek, and ye shall find; knock, and it shall be opened unto you: 8For every one that asketh receiveth; and he that seeketh findeth; and to him that knocketh it shall be opened. 9Or what man is there of you, whom if his son ask bread, will he give him a stone? 10Or if he ask a fish, will he give him a serpent? 11If ye then, being evil, know how to give good gifts unto your children, how much more shall your Father which is in heaven give good things to them that ask him?" Matthew 7:7-11

Our Lord Jesus said to His children: "They shall take up serpents; and if they drink any deadly thing, it shall not hurt them; they shall lay hands on the sick, and they shall recover." Mark 16:18

Jesus ask of us" "And as ye go, preach, saying, The kingdom of heaven is at hand.8 Heal the sick, cleanse the lepers, raise the dead, cast out devils: freely ye have received, freely give." Matthew 10:7-8

Our Lord is the True Bread of life from heaven if any man eat of this bread, he shall live for ever:

"Verily, verily, I say unto you, He that believeth on me hath everlasting life.48 I am that bread of life.49 Your fathers did eat manna in the wilderness, and are dead.50 This is the bread which cometh down from heaven, that a man may eat thereof, and not die.51 I am the living bread which came down from heaven: if any man eat of this bread, he shall live for ever: and the bread that I will give is my flesh, which I will give for the life of the world.52 The Jews therefore strove among themselves, saying, How can this man give us his flesh to eat?53 Then Jesus said unto them, Verily, verily, I say unto you, Except ye eat the flesh of the Son of man, and drink his blood, ye have no life in you.54 Whoso eateth my flesh, and drinketh my blood, hath eternal life; and I will raise him up at the last day.55 For my flesh is meat indeed, and my blood is drink indeed.56 He that eateth my flesh, and drinketh my blood, dwelleth in me, and I in him.57 As the living Father hath sent me, and I live by the Father: so he that eateth me, even he shall live by me.58 This is that bread which came down from heaven: not as your fathers did eat manna, and are dead: he that eateth of this bread shall live for ever." (John 6:48-58)

Let us call upon worldwide chain of prayers to Our Lord Jesus to put stop ⬤ the Coronavirus virus 🦠 outbreak pandemic.

We pray for China 🇨🇳 and our beloved Chinese people through this tough time

Amen Lord Jesus have mercy upon us and rescue thy people. You are the Only One we know and we don't known anyone else but You because You all our True Love 💚 and Savior. And through You we live, move and do. Our being is You and our life is You. Amen 🙏

RAMSIS GHALY FACEBOOK POST
MARCH 16, 2020
During COVID-19, I am Searching for Whom my soul loveth!
A Poem dedicated to the World During the Journey of COVID-19
Written by
Ramsis Ghaly

During COVID-19: O daughters of Jerusalem, if ye find my Beloved, tell Him, I am sick of love 💚!

The world 🌐 has COVID-19, but I have my Savior Jesus Christ in the Cross died for me and the salvation of the world 🌐 in the Name of the Father, the Son and the Holy Spirit One God Amen! 🙏

As COVID-19 keep spreading all over the world 🌐, the Love of the Father, Grace of the Son and the Communion of the Holy Spirit overshadow the inhabitants of Earth, His handmaid!

During COVID-19, my soul is on journey, O daughters of Jerusalem, if ye find my Beloved, tell Him, I am sick of love 💜! I need my Love during COVID-19 please find my Beloved: I charge you, O daughters of Jerusalem, if ye find my beloved, that ye tell him, that I am sick of love." (Song of Songs 5:8)

As COVID-19 keep spreading all over the world 🌐, the Love of the Father, Grace of the Son and the Communion of the Holy Spirit overshadow the inhabitants of Earth, His handmaid!

As COVID 19 is trying to divide us away and remove us from the house of the Lord, but our Lord Jesus strengthen us and prayed to His Father to save our souls at that day as He told Simon Peter: "31And the Lord said, Simon, Simon, behold, Satan hath desired to have you, that he may sift you as wheat: 32But I have prayed for thee, that thy faith fail not: and when thou art converted, strengthen thy brethren." (Luke 22:31-32)

While the world around me is COVID-19, hunkering down and imposing social curfew and extreme restrains, but my soul is free and is lifted up to heaven and my mouth is opened and singing to the Lord of Heaven and Earth!

While my people are distancing away from me, my Lord Jesus is coming closer and closer to my soul: let me kiss Him with kisses and Let him kiss me with the kisses of his mouth: for thy love is better than wine. Because of the savior of thy good ointments thy name is as ointment poured forth, therefore do the virgins love thee. Draw me, we will run after thee: the king hath brought me into his chambers: we will be glad and rejoice in thee, we will remember thy love more than wine: the upright love thee." (Song of Songs 1:2-4)

Although I am black with COVID-19, but I am comely and my soul is white like a snow in my Savior, the sun ☀ hath looked upon my me: I am black, but comely, O ye daughters of Jerusalem, as the tents of Kedar, as the curtains of Solomon.6 Look not upon me, because I am black, because the sun hath looked upon me: my mother's children were angry with me; they made me the keeper of the vineyards; but mine own vineyard have I not kept." (Song of Songs 1:5-6)

The world is busy with COVID-19, but My soul is busy to find Whom my soul loveth: so Tell me, O thou whom my soul loveth, where thou feedest, where thou makest thy flock to rest at noon: for why should I be as one that turneth aside by the flocks of thy companions?8 If thou know not, O thou fairest among women, go thy way forth by the footsteps of the flock, and feed thy kids beside the shepherds' tents." (Song of Songs 1:7-8)

You might be COVID-19 the pandemic of 2020 as I called you back on January 30, but my Lord of Hosts is the King of Glory until the End of ages and from ages unto ages!

https://www.facebook.com/1150861349/posts/10221108146470558/?d=n

You COVID-19 intent to do evil against the inhabitants of earth, but my Lord God MRA t it unto good to bring to pass, as it is this day, to save much people alive as my father Joseph once said: "But as for you, ye thought evil against me; but God meant it unto good, to bring to pass, as it is this day, to save much people alive." (Genesis 50:20)

You Intend to destroy my flesh with COVID-19, But my Lord intent to manifest Himself and be glorified through COVID-19 as long as it is day with our Heavenly Father as He told His disciples about the man born blind "Neither this man nor his parents sinned," said Jesus, "but this happened so that the works of God might be displayed in him. 4 As long as it is day, we must do the works of him who sent me. Night is coming, when no one can work. 5 While I am in the world, I am the light of the world." (John 9:3)

The world ⬤ has COVID-19, but I have my Savior Jesus Christ in the Cross died for me and the salvation of the world ⬤ in the Name of the Father, the Son and the Holy Spirit One God Amen 🙏!

While all things are in the hid and locked in, my soul is exalted with the Lord of hosts!

While the world around me is shutting down, my soul is opening up to my Beloved!

While the countries around me are locking down, my spirit is rising up to the heaven!

While the cities around me are closing their walls, my soul is flying high stretching its wings up to the heaven!

While the world activities are silenced, my tongue is singing to Lord new songs and melodies

While my enemy is ailing my flesh and taking my breath away, my Savior reviving my soul to fly as an Eagle 🦅 among His hosts!

While the darkness overwhelming the face of the earth, my Lord Jesus, in the fourth watch, is walking on the sea pulling me with His arms saying: "Be of good cheer; it is I; be not afraid." (Matthew 14:27)

While the sadness spreading the globe, my soul is joyful in the Lord God the Glory!

While the doubts and worries are abundant in these days, the faith and hope in my Savior is overshadowing my soul!

While the horrific news are bombarding all over, my elated mouth unceasing praising my Heavenly Father!

While I am with heavy laden and heavy burden, my soul is drawn to Beloved calling me: Come unto me, all ye that labour and are heavy laden, and I will give you rest.29 Take my yoke upon you, and learn of me; for I am meek and lowly in heart: and ye shall find rest unto your souls.30 For my yoke is easy, and my burden is light." (Matthew 11:28-30)

While the fears and terrors are everywhere, my spirit is at Peace in my Lord the King of Peace is widoeting in my ears saying: "Peace I leave with you, my peace I give unto you: not as the world giveth, give I unto you. Let not your heart be troubled, neither let it be afraid." (John 14:27)

While the earth is in suffering and in mourning, my spirit praising my Lord God with the sound of the trumpet: praise him with the psaltery and harp!

While the stores, offices, shops, and Resturants are closing down, the sanctuary of the Lord is open for me praising Him in the firmament of His power!

While the schools and working places are locked down, my heart ♥ is praising the Lord of Heaven and Earth with the timbrel and dance: praise him with stringed instruments and organs!

While I have no more visitors or friends around, my soul is complete in the Lord praising Him upon the loud cymbals: praise him upon the high sounding cymbals!

While everything around me gloomy and dreadful, everything within my soul that hath breath praise the LORD. Praise ye the LORD!

While the world is crying 😭 in tears in aches and pains, my soul is singing 🎤 with David the Psalmist: "Praise ye the LORD. Praise God in his sanctuary: praise him in the firmament of his power.2 Praise him for his mighty acts: praise him according to his excellent greatness.3 Praise him with the sound of the trumpet: praise him with the psaltery and harp.4 Praise him with the timbrel and dance: praise him with stringed instruments and organs.5 Praise him upon the loud cymbals: praise him upon the high sounding cymbals.6 Let every thing that hath breath praise the LORD. Praise ye the LORD." (Psalm 150)

While the outside is full of sadness and darkness, the inside my soul is full of Joy and light!

While the sickness is spreading fast, the grace of God is filling faster my heart ♥ healing my soul!

While the pandemic is moving in and its destruction is settling in for the days to come, the Holy Spirit is rejuvenating my soul in holiness!

While COVID-19 threatening my life, The LORD is my shepherd; I shall not want.2 He maketh me to lie down in green pastures: he leadeth me beside the still waters.3 He restoreth my soul: he leadeth me in the paths of righteousness for his name's sake.4 Yea, though I walk through the valley of the shadow of death, I will fear no evil: for thou art with me; thy rod and thy staff they comfort me.5 Thou preparest a table before me in the presence of mine enemies: thou anointest my head with oil; my cup runneth over.6 Surely goodness and mercy shall follow me all the days of my life: and I will dwell in the house of the LORD for ever." (Psalm 23)

+During COVID-19: O daughters of Jerusalem, if ye find my Beloved, tell Him, I am sick of love ♥!

"I charge you, O daughters of Jerusalem, if ye find my beloved, that ye tell him, that I am sick of love." (Song of Songs 5:8)

I hear my Beloved voice, my Lord: The voice of my beloved! behold, he cometh leaping upon the mountains, skipping upon the hills." (Song of Songs 2:8)

I drift to sleep but my heart waketh: it is the voice of my beloved that knocketh, saying, Open to me, my sister, my love, my dove, my undefiled: for my head is filled with dew, and my locks with the drops of the night." (Song of Songs 5:2)

My Lord is calling me, I must answer! My Beloved is stretching His arms toward me, I am eager to see Him! "My beloved is mine, and I am his: he feedeth among the lilies." (Song of Songs 2:16)

My Heavenly Father is coming to take me, I must be ready! 3 I am my beloved's, and my beloved is mine: he feedeth among the lilies." (Song of Songs 6:3)

"I am my beloved's, and his desire is toward me." (Song of Songs 7:10) Nothing shall quench my love to my Savior: Many waters cannot quench love, neither can the floods drown it: if a man would give all the substance of his house for love, it would utterly be contemned." (Song of Songs 8:7)

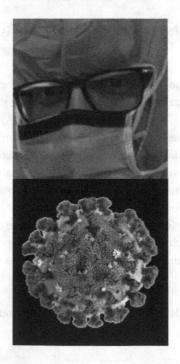

This Post of Mine about the Beginning of COVID in Chicago, is so Close to my Heart!

Ramsis Ghaly March 14, 2021

The true story behind this post that was shared 83 times and commented upon by 206 comments and interested so many people, yet I was harshly attacked by American corporates for saying the truth about COVID-19! It will be forever a memorable for my soul!

It was my very first eye opening to what COVID-19 would bring to mankind and to our nation while so many weren't aware! My Lord opened my eyes to foresee what our nation and the world about face!!!

This was my very first Post to warn alert Chicago and Chicagoans that Coronavirus is in our city! I was just intubated the very first patient and i could see the evil virus destroying the individual and no was any relationship of the flu virus. At that time, I felt obligated to put another post to warn Chicago and the nation and the world!

O my gosh, the post put me in serious troubles with hospitals and media at that time! I was accused by spreading rumors and sending false alarms to the people of Chicago and politicians and how can I dare write such a post!

I suffered so much because of this post no matter what I tried to say---! i was in a major and serious trouble! I cried and prayed to my Lord at that time. It did not take more than a week and it was reality all over the city of Chicago!

The same as my post in January 31, 2020, when I warned the world of the impending pandemic and many accused me for spreading false rumors and it was just a type of flue!!

Let us reflect at those moments and never be enslave to politicians or threatened by self-absorbed corporates!

But instead, Be yourself honest before God and the people. Be a listening vessel to the voice of God!

Thank you Lord Jesus for letting us reflect in Your repeated visitations!

Ramsis Ghaly
updated his status.
March 14, 2020 ·
Shared with Public

Ramsis Ghaly March 14, 2020

Chicago coronavirus in our town: let us pray for the sick and those in the front line
O my Lord Jesus for Your children we pray in Your Holy Name. Amen
Psalm 51

1   Have mercy upon me, O God, according to thy lovingkindness: according
    unto the multitude of thy tender mercies blot out my transgressions.
2   Wash me throughly from mine iniquity, and cleanse me from my sin.
3   For I acknowledge my transgressions: and my sin is ever before me.
4   Against thee, thee only, have I sinned, and done this evil in thy sight: that thou
    mightest be justified when thou speakest, and be clear when thou judgest.
5   Behold, I was shapen in iniquity; and in sin did my mother conceive me.
6   Behold, thou desirest truth in the inward parts: and in the hidden part thou
    shalt make me to know wisdom.
7   Purge me with hyssop, and I shall be clean: wash me, and I shall be whiter
    than snow.
8   Make me to hear joy and gladness; that the bones which thou hast broken
    may rejoice.
9   Hide thy face from my sins, and blot out all mine iniquities.
10 Create in me a clean heart, O God; and renew a right spirit within me.
11 Cast me not away from thy presence; and take not thy holy spirit from me.
12 Restore unto me the joy of thy salvation; and uphold me with thy free spirit.
13 Then will I teach transgressors thy ways; and sinners shall be converted
    unto thee.
14 Deliver me from bloodguiltiness, O God, thou God of my salvation: and my
    tongue shall sing aloud of thy righteousness.
15 O Lord, open thou my lips; and my mouth shall shew forth thy praise.
16 For thou desirest not sacrifice; else would I give it: thou delightest not in
    burnt offering.
17 The sacrifices of God are a broken spirit: a broken and a contrite heart, O
    God, thou wilt not despise.
18 Do good in thy good pleasure unto Zion: build thou the walls of Jerusalem.
19 Then shalt thou be pleased with the sacrifices of righteousness, with burnt
    offering and whole burnt offering: then shall they offer bullocks upon thine
    altar.

Charlene Mentzer Glowaty It's sad when you, an intelligent doctor, cannot share what you believe to be true and proven as true. Whatever happened to freedom of speech? 🖤🙏

LR. The truth will set you fre

KA. Wow

MP. May God be with us as he always is. Let us learn the lessons, and become a better world. Dear Lord, please protect the Good and innocent, and have mercy on the sinners, we all sin, some worse than others, no human is perfect Lord. Thank you for you sacrifice. Praying for you and patients

MA. Praying for you Dr. Ghaly and for God to guide your hands to help that patient and you and all those administering help to him or her And everybody else that needs it. 🙏🙏🙏🙏🙏 And May god keep you and all your staff safe as well as the patients, thank you for everything that you do.

JM. I'm praying for you. You were an answer to my prayer years ago when I was in severe pain. May the blood of Jesus cover and protect you and your co-workers.

DD. May God watch over all of the patients, family and selfless caregivers of all the future Covid 19 patients! God have mercy, in Jesus name!

CB. God bless you and all your residents and fellows. Are prayers with you all 🙏🙏🙏

KW. Your in my prayers-You are an inspiration and example for all of us in healthcare!

LG. Praying with you and for you. Please be safe.

TA. The Lord bless you and keep you safe.

CK. God bless you and your work, Dr. Ghaly. May the Lord keep you safe from this virus.

TR. You are such a special man!!

JA. God bless your good heart Dr. Ramsis Ghaly... May the Lord keep you safe always

ED. God Bless you Doctor. These patients are in the best care possible with you. 🙏

MA. Sending love and prayers 🖤🙏 Stay safe and well.

IS. We'll pray for you Dr. Ghaly 🙏🌷

MK. "He that dwelleth in the secret place of the most High shall abide under the shadow of the Almighty. I will say of the Lord, He is my refuge and my fortress: my God; in him will I trust. Surely he shall deliver thee from the snare of the fowler, and fr...

MP. Prayers for all our healthcare providers. Dear God bless and protect these brave people, keep them safe as they do your work. Amen. Psalm 91 for your protection Sir. Blessings. Have no fear.

RJ. A Blessing for Physicians May you always heal and be healed....

LS. God be with you

DM. Dr Ghaly, praying always that you and the rest of our medical personnel be safe

JC. Dr. Ghaly asking God for His help and miracle to continously guide and bless you and your team.

TR. Thank you so very much for your daily post. I truly hope that you know just how much they have help so many of us with intelligent medical 😊 information, sincere spiritual support. May the good Lord continue to bless you and assist you on this path he ...

AB. Amen

CA. God bless you and keep you well Dr.

TJ. AMEN!

SH. Amen/thanks/remaining in prayer. S.H. 🖤

DL. I believe that snow yesterday was God cleansing us

BM. Many 🙏🙏 for you Ramsis Ghaly and your staff. You›re such a blessing to many people!

CC. Amen. Thank you

CR. Amen

TL. Now you just need God to protect you from JB Pritzger.

MC. Amen. God bless us all.

SE, Amen

MA. Amen

RH. Grateful for your Grace. Amen

AV. Amen! 🐢🙏

COVID Mystery Revealed!

Lately, as thorough investigation on COVID-19 ongoing, COVID-19 Mystery revealing with it!! I am so thankful to my Lord and gift of intuition that whatever I wrote in my three books covering COVID-19 pandemic is turning to be very true!

It wasn't easy since unknowing what the future, a year later, will reveal. It wasn't easy to be against the media and come up with the uncommon!

The mainstream was exposed to listen to tremendous doubts and the uprise of false, misleading and conflicted information!

I was accused to be paranoia and spread rumors——It was many days and nights of more than a year of external hardships, threats and intimidation!

Thank you for reading my posts and books!

https://books.google.com/.../Coronavirus_the_Pandemic_of...
Ramsis Ghaly

BOOKS.GOOGLE.COM

Coronavirus the Pandemic of the Century and the Wrath of God

Towards the end of 2019, I started to feel that the Lord, our God, had had enough of the stubborn and stiff necked people as their wickedness, rebellion, and disobedience continued against him and his son. These actions were a resemblance of the days of Noah, Sodom, Gomorrah, and Nineveh. I felt tha...

Bg. Congratulations on your bold integrity in the midst of censorship and shaming. DM. I believe you always speak the truth

583

Nomination and Awarded Notable Healthcare Award hero In Crain's Chicago March 8, 2021 Thank you Chicago's Crain's March 2021

Ramsis Ghaly

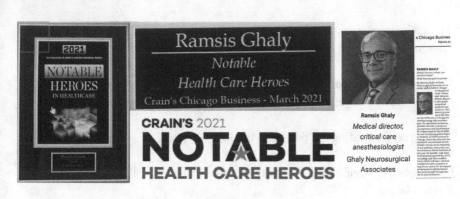

I went over my emails and I found this surprise email with nomination---Whoever nominated me, I am not worthy but the patients, nursing frontliners, students and residents --are! thank you, I just do my Job in my Savior Jesus Name, Thank you!!

Dear Ramsis,
We received a nomination on your behalf for Crain's upcoming Notable Healthcare Heroes list. We found your nomination very compelling ---

Thank you,

Notables Team
Crain's Chicago Business
www.ghalyneurosurgeon.com
GHALYNEUROSURGEON.COM
www.ghalyneurosurgeon.com

YR. Congratulations Ramsis Ghaly! Thank you for doing God's work. We are so blessed to have you in our lives!

ET. DM. You SOOOOOO.....deserve this. 💚 You are The Best of the Best with a Heart of Gold

MD. f course you deserve it 😊

LM. That's awesome!!

SA. Congratulations!

KO. Yes you deserve it, I'm not your patient, but from all I have heard and read what you say and all the love and care you give your pts and everyone, you are very deserving of this award. Congradulations kind and giving man

RP. DL. You are so humble Dr. Ramsis Ghaly. Awards for everyone. Congratulations.

MS. Good deal take it 😘👍

AL. Wow! That's awesome!

ZC. You are the man Dr.Ghally,

CR. You exceeds beyond expectation. Dr. Gahly you deserve the award.

MR, AV. Congratulations 💚💚💚 You are a blessing to so many! 🐾🙏

ME. Oooray! You deserved the Honor, My Dr Ghaly!

JB. ore than well deserved Dr. Ghaly!! This is wonderful!!

BP. You are worthy 🙏

RH. Making sure the Glory is JESUS. AmenGC. You're a hero for sure!

BH, Couldn't find a more worthy and deserving person, congratulations!!

KG. You ARE a healthcare hero, Dr. Ghaly!!!

SA. Congratulations Dr. Ghaly, you deserve it!

MW. Hooray!!!S 💚 M. Congratulations Dr Ghaly. You are amazing and do gods work. I am so happy for you.

CR. You deserve this on every level.

BM. Congratulations 🎊🥂

ID, Congratulations Ghaly! You are the most worthy surgeon I know! I have seen your amazing surgical work first hand. You change the lives of everyone that crosses your path. You have been given a gift from God. The talent is in your mind and in your hands...

SCG. Congratulations on your well-deserved nomination. You are a wonderful, caring doctor who is always comforting to your patients and a blessing. 💚🙏

SB. Congrats! 🎊🎊 Dr. Ghaly. You so deserve this honor.

LW. I cannot think of anyone who deserves it more than you....

PH. Outstanding!! Congratulations 👏

ML. You are my Saint!

JD. That's awesome! Congratulations!

DM. You deserve it!

CG. Congratulations! 🎉

LL. Congratulations!!!! You so deserve this, in Jesus name. 💚💚💚🙏🙏🙏

FA. YOU DESERVE IT DR GHALY.. THE SURGEON WITH A HEART OF GOLD 🤍

VW, Awesome...congratulations! You've earned it!

RC. Definetily you are worth an deserve all the good in the world!

VG. Congratulations!! You deserve the NAME of medicine, good doctor, good man, with a big heart. God bless you!!! 🙏🙏🙏🙏🙏

AS. Congratulations ‼️ That's awesome you Deserve it 👏🙏

SS. Congratulations on your nomination!!

MN. Congrats you are so worthy..

CP. Congrats Dr. Ghaly!!! 🌸🌸🌸

MP. You deserve it!

Sn. You certainly deserve it. 🖤

KM. Wonderful!

FA. YOU DESERVE IT DR GHALY.. THE SURGEON WITH A HEART OF GOLD

SC. you are so very worthy whomever did it knows all too well

BL. You are very worthy and loved for being the phenomenal person you are!

CH. You definitely deserve it!

JO. My neurosurgeon has been on the front lines of Covid in Chicago saving lives and innovating as he goes. Truly a man with God given talent, he's also extremely spiritual and prayerful in all of the work he performs. 💙💙💙

YC. Dr. Ghaly was part of our coffee club back in a Wheaton. He has served tirelessly during the COVID crisis and saved many lives. I'm so happy that he has received much-deserved recognition. I can't help but think of those medical professionals who don't get public praise. Last week, when we ran our Spartan race in Florida, I met a young RN from the Mayo Clinic. She's been in the profession for just two years. Nothing had prepared her for the reality of COVID. When I thanked her for her bravery and selflessness, she cried. This serves as a reminder to keep our first responders in our hearts and prayers. A simple word of thanks, a smile, or a meal go a long way to show that we care.

MD. Our wonderful friend and Neurosurgeon in Chicago who helped me to get the right diagnosis when I was in pain. There is nothing more important in life than good friends. Thank you Ramsis for all you do.

MN. To me you are the best you saved my live Dr.Ghaly and all Ways kept in touched to see how i was. Many other doctors you don't here from on less you call there office and all you talk to is the doctor incident. God Bless Dr.Ghaly

DL. This Dr. Is AMAZING!!! IF you know anyone that needs help with ANYTHING MEDICAL CALL DR. G. He is the BEST!! WE HAVE REFERRED HIM TO A LOT OF OUR FRIENDS!! WE GOT THE HELP AND ANSWERS WE NEEDED!!!!!

BJ. Congrats dr Ghaly this is beyond deserved and sooo much more! You have no ideal how many lives you have touched let alone saved! God bless you and all that you do!

DL. Simply the best. Better than all the rest. Please don't retire. I may need you.

HH. Congratulations my Best Doctor of the World. BRAVO my Friend Dr.Ramsis Ghaly. ! !

SC. you have earned this a million times over! good things come to all that wait and now you have gotten your moment job well done dr

AM. That is incredibly awesome my dear friend!! I am so very happy that they recognize and honor what we, who are blessed to be called "Ghaly Patients" already know of you. I thank God daily for bringing you into our lives. May God continue to bless you and continue working through you with each patient you touch. We LOVE you Dr Ghaly.

SS. Ah you see this does not surprise me. Because being one of your patience and having met so many of your other patience we know one thing. You are simply the best!!! But most of all for the reason of giving your true unconditional love to everyone. You say you are just a servant but anyone who you have helped would say different. Congratulations

SD. Thank you Doctor Ghaly for all that you do, saving so many lives with such precision and dedication. 🖤🖤🙏

YR. Congratulations Ramsis Ghaly! Thank you for doing God's work. We are so blessed to have you in our lives!

KM. You deserve this. Your belief that your skill was amplified with God's help & never take credit. You helped save my life. I'm so thankful we met & became friends. I respect you & care for you. I pray for you especially with Covid still digging in its nasty claws in people.

DH. Hero isn't even a good enough word...Congrats, Dr Ramsis Ghaly, you certainly deserve it!

KG/ Mabrouk and God Bless you from Egypt with love.

GS. You're an amazing physician and teacher!

TB. You are an awesome physician 🖤

NE. Congratulations and Alef Mabrouk!!

JC. Congratulations you are amazing 🌼

BH. An angel amongst us.

LR. Congratulations 🎉

KS. Congratulations, Dr. Ghaly!

BK. Huge recognition Dr Ghaly!! Congratulations!!!

RS. Well deserved! Congrats

GS. Congratulations

JB. Congratulations

ND. So awesome! Congratulations

CR. Congratulations!!! Well deserved. 👏

587

SM. Congrats

SS. Congrats Doc!!!

JW. Congratulations

BT. The Best Dr....... !!!!!!!

BV. Congratulations

SI. Very well deserved Dr. Ghaly

RP. Thank you for your service 🙏❤️🙏❤️🙏

CP. Very nice. 🙂

KE. You are an exceptional doctor! May God bless you!

YC. Congratulations, Dr. Ghaly! Thank you for your tireless efforts to serve your
   fellow man.

MG. Congratulations

BV. In His care in your care....Thankyou

CP. Congrats Dr. Ghaly!!! 🎉🎉🎉

PH. You definitely deserved that. You are the best.

LM. Congratulations

RM. Congrats Dr Ghaly

SH. Congratulations! You are amazing and such a blessing to so many!

NM. That's amazing, congratulations and well deserved! 🎉🎉🎉

Karen Bazzell McGinnis

You deserve this. Your belief that your skill was amplified with God's help &
never take credit. You helped save my life. I'm so thankful we met & became
friends. I respect you & care for you. I pray for you especially with Covid still
digging in its nasty claws in people.

DE. Congrats 👍

YY. Great 👍

PT. Wow Dr Ghaly. That is an awesome and well-deserved honor! Congrats

KC. Congratulations!! Well deserved!!

LV. Congratulations!

JU. Congratulations Dr Ghaly!

BB. Congrats Dr. Ghaly!

JC. Congratulations!

CB. Congratulations Dr. Ghaly! So proud of you. God bless.

SA. Thank you Dr Ghaly for your dedication, faith and the gift of healing. Well
   deserved! 🙏

PW. Outstanding !!

SS. Congratulations Dr. Ghaly. Well deserved.

RS. Congratulations

BP. Congrats dr Ghaly this is beyond deserved and sooo much more! You have no ideal how many lives you have touched let alone saved! God bless you and all that you do!

ME. Congratulations Dr Ghaly! Proud to work alongside you @Stroger.

ML. This is wonderful! So very proud of you! Thank you for saving so many lives. 😊

SC. Ah you see this does not surprise me. Because being one of your patience and having met so many of your other patience we know one thing. You are simply the best!!! But most of all for the reason of giving your true unconditional love to everyone. You say you are just a servant but anyone who you have helped would say different. Congratulations

VA. Congratulations

CM. Excellent!!! Congratulations 🔴

RH. Congratulations

RC. Thanks for all tour efforts!

DC. Congratulations, awesome to see!

BC. Congratulations!

DM. Congratulations

GV. Congratulations! No one deserves it more!

CA. Thank you Doctor Ghaly for all that you do, saving so many lives with such precision and dedication. 🖤🖤🙏

DL. Congratulations Dr!

LK. Great news, Dr. Ghaly!! Congratulations!!

JT. Congratulations! 🎉 Well deserved! It's been a long year for you. May God Bless you!

AP. Congratulations 🥂

ZC. Congratulations

Dr.Ghally. God blesses you so you can be a blessing to others.

DM. Congrats And God bless you more

IR. Congratulations Uncle! What a huge honor!

ZQ. Congratulations!

BM. Congratulations!!!!

RE. Congratulations

LH. Congratulations

ES. Congratulations Ramsis

HC. Congrats, well deserved

RD. Congratulations!!!!!

AG. Congratulation Dear Ramsis Ghaly 🌷

ER. Congratulations Dr. Ramsis !!!

NE. Congrats Dr. Ghaly, we are so proud of you!

GR. CONGRATULATIONS

RS. Congratulations! الف مبروك

589

DL. Simply the best. Better than all the rest. Please don't retire. I may need you.

AA. So very proud of you my Brother!

AM. Congratulations! A very well deserves recognitions!!

HH. Congratulations my Best Doctor of the World. BRAVO my Friend Dr.Ramsis Ghaly. ! !

SS. Congratulations, thank you for your care for patients. 💛

TM. Well deserved. Congratulations

GS. Congrats Dr! We miss you at Starbucks!

SC. proud of you dr 👍

SC, you have earned this a million times over! good things come to all that wait and now you have gotten your moment job well done dr

LT. U r the best!

VG. Čestitam

JR. Well done Dr Ramsis! Congratulations!!

DB. Congratulations and thank you for your devotion to your patients.

MW. Congratulations

CC. Congratulations Dr. Ghaly. Sooo well deserved

TC. Congrats &god bless always

NV. SC. Congratulations Dr. Ghaly!!! So proud of you and your accomplishments.

JW. congratulations

FA. Agree well deserved the Doctor with a heart of 🤍

SM. You are truly amazing Dr Ghaly.

JV. You are a incredible Doctor. And we thank you for that

RS. Congrats

TJ. Congratulations! Well deserved - God bless you.

GM. 🎉 congratulations. Well deserved

NP. Congratulations! Well deserved

BH. Congratulations, so well deserved you amazing man! 🖤

TS. Well deserved! Thank you for all of the great work Dr Ghaly!

LD. Congratulations Dr. Ghaly!! So much respect and love we have for u!! 🖤

AB. Excellent service to those in need! Congratulations!!! Dr Ghaly you are truly a wonderful person with tremendous talent and an ability to connect with your patients! You go above and beyond!!! Forever grateful!!! Aeschylus Bryant!!! 🙏

LW. You are The Best my friend!!

BM. Congratulations

TB. CONGRATULATIONS WELL DESERVED!!!

bl. Congratulations
🖤

Jb. Such well deserved recognition!!! Congratulations Dr.G.!!!

DS. Congrats

I went over my emails and I found this surprise email with nomination--- Whoever nominated me, I am not worthy but the patients, nursing frontliners, students and residents --are! thank you, I just do my Job in my my Savior Jesus Name, Thank you!!

2/2/2021

Dear Ramsis,

We received a nomination on your behalf for Crain's upcoming Notable Healthcare Heroes list. We found your nomination very compelling ---

Thank you,

Notables Team

Crain's Chicago Business

CR. www.ghalyneurosurgeon.com

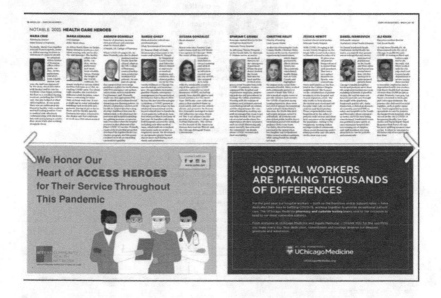

RAMSIS GHALY

Medical director, critical care
anesthesiologist
Ghaly Neurosurgical Associates

Dr. Ramsis Ghaly of Ghaly
Neurosurgical Associates is on
senior staff at John H. Stroger
Jr. Hospital of
Cook County
and Advocate
Illinois Mason-
ic and teach-
es medical
students and
residents. He's
clinical profes-
sor at the Uni-
versity of Illinois at Chicago for
anesthesiology and neurosurgery. He specializes in trauma,
gunshot wounds, emergency
management and resuscitation.
He believes that in March 2020
he was the first anesthesiologist
to intubate a COVID patient in
Chicago. Since the onset, he has
intubated, resuscitated and delivered critical care to hundreds
of sick patients, with peak numbers between March and June of
last year. He handles calls from
both hospitals around the clock,
including code blue notifica-
tions, which indicate a medical
emergency such as cardiac or
respiratory arrest. He developed
an inexpensive plastic barrier
that protects staff during anesthesia and intubation.

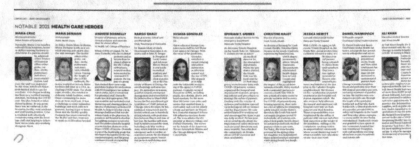

Another Day in the Paradise taking appropriate caution with PPE and multiple layers!!!

Ramsis Ghaly

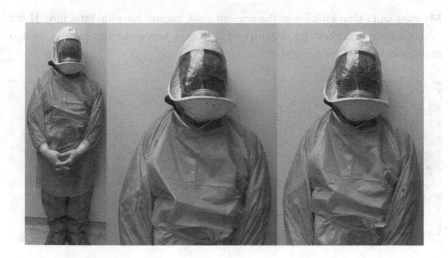

KG. Awesome 👊

CG. Be safe! 🖤🙏

TJ. Stay safe & God bless you for your service.

KE. Stay safe! May God Bless You

RC. Thank you for all your services! God bless you, bless all an be with you

LD. Praying for you and your patients! Stay safe!

JM. "Excellent"

AU. God bless you Dr G!

CT. God bless

Early Morning Leaving my Place of Service the Famous JSH of Cook County Hospital!

As I journey during the second wave surge of COVID-19, I remember the years of my service at Cook County Hospital since 1986.

My eyes can't stop looking at the ancient cook county hospital (and now Hyatt hotel) where I worked for 35 thirty five years servicing the great Chicago metropolitan and Chicagoans!

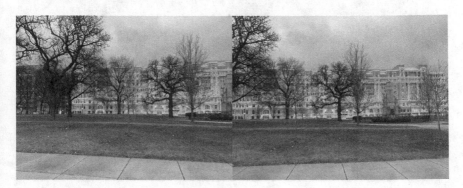

CG. Beautiful build

PP. Amazing!

JB. You made an incredible impact on so so many people there Dr. Ghaly. They were truly blessed to have you there.!

RH. Magnificent

JP. I took my pediatric affiliation there when I was in nurses training in the late 50s

MD. Is the cook Hospital is a hotel now?
How many rooms there, it looks beautiful 👍👍

JZ. Worked next door at rush. It was sad when it was vacant. Haven't seen the inside since the redo. Glad they didn't tear it down.

AL. You are a great doctor... God bless you more.

MB. That place is huge and beautiful, as so many other buildings in the windy city. ☺

DM. great memories

HH. Wonderful Pictures, Congratulations Dr. Ramsis Ghaly. ! !

RP. It looks absolutely beautiful! 😌

It is Not My Daily Adventure But Rather My Daily Joy!

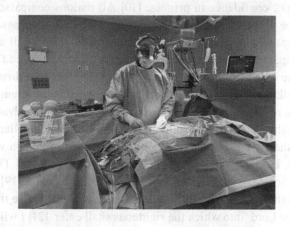

It isn't my daily Adventures, but rather my life journey and constant joy in my Lord Jesus serving His people yet performing my duties!!!

Between brain and spine surgeries, COVID intubation ventilator and anesthetic supports to teaching residents and dining with me!! And all these are done in joy and honor praising my Savior Lord Jesus Christ praising His Name above all names For thine the power, glory and kingdom forever and ever Amen!!

And I consider all these are nothing for the Love 🖤 of my Lord Jesus, Amen 🙏!

As it is written: "Who shall separate us from the love of Christ? shall tribulation, or distress, or persecution, or famine, or nakedness, or peril, or sword? [36] As it is written, For thy sake we are killed all the day long; we are accounted as sheep for the slaughter. [37] Nay, in all these things we are more than conquerors through him that loved us. [38] For I am persuaded, that neither death, nor life, nor angels, nor principalities, nor powers, nor things present, nor things to come, [39] Nor height, nor depth, nor any other creature, shall be able to separate us from the love of God, which is in Christ Jesus our Lord." Romans 8:35-39 KJV

Psalm 118
"O give thanks unto the Lord ; for he is good: because his mercy endureth for ever. [2] Let Israel now say, that his mercy endureth for ever. [3] Let the house of Aaron now say, that his mercy endureth for ever. [4] Let them now that fear the Lord say, that his mercy endureth for ever. [5] I called upon the Lord in distress:

the Lord answered me, and set me in a large place. [6] The Lord is on my side; I will not fear: what can man do unto me? [7] The Lord taketh my part with them that help me: therefore shall I see my desire upon them that hate me. [8] It is better to trust in the Lord than to put confidence in man. [9] It is better to trust in the Lord than to put confidence in princes. [10] All nations compassed me about: but in the name of the Lord will I destroy them. [11] They compassed me about; yea, they compassed me about: but in the name of the Lord I will destroy them. [12] They compassed me about like bees; they are quenched as the fire of thorns: for in the name of the Lord I will destroy them. [13] Thou hast thrust sore at me that I might fall: but the Lord helped me. [14] The Lord is my strength and song, and is become my salvation. [15] The voice of rejoicing and salvation is in the tabernacles of the righteous: the right hand of the Lord doeth valiantly. [16] The right hand of the Lord is exalted: the right hand of the Lord doeth valiantly. [17] I shall not die, but live, and declare the works of the Lord. [18] The Lord hath chastened me sore: but he hath not given me over unto death. [19] Open to me the gates of righteousness: I will go into them, and I will praise the Lord: [20] This gate of the Lord, into which the righteous shall enter. [21] I will praise thee: for thou hast heard me, and art become my salvation. [22] The stone which the builders refused is become the head stone of the corner. [23] This is the Lord's doing; it is marvellous in our eyes. [24] This is the day which the Lord hath made; we will rejoice and be glad in it. [25] Save now, I beseech thee, O Lord: O Lord, I beseech thee, send now prosperity. [26] Blessed be he that cometh in the name of the Lord: we have blessed you out of the house of the Lord. [27] God is the Lord, which hath shewed us light: bind the sacrifice with cords, even unto the horns of the altar. [28] Thou art my God, and I will praise thee: thou art my God, I will exalt thee. [29] O give thanks unto the Lord ; for he is good: for his mercy endureth for ever."

Ramsis Ghaly
www.ghalyneurosurgeon.com

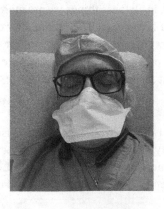

BRAIN SURGERIES

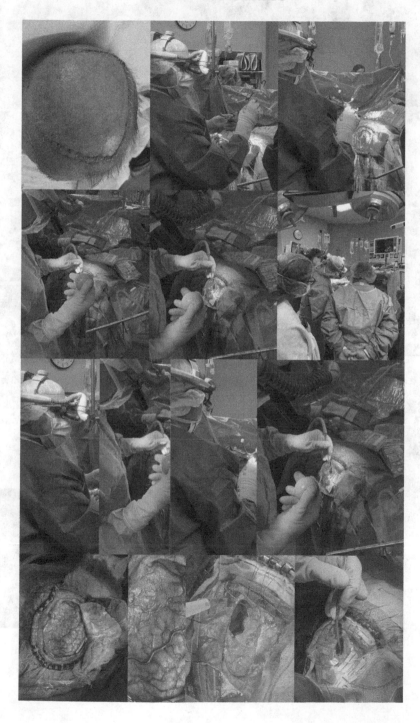

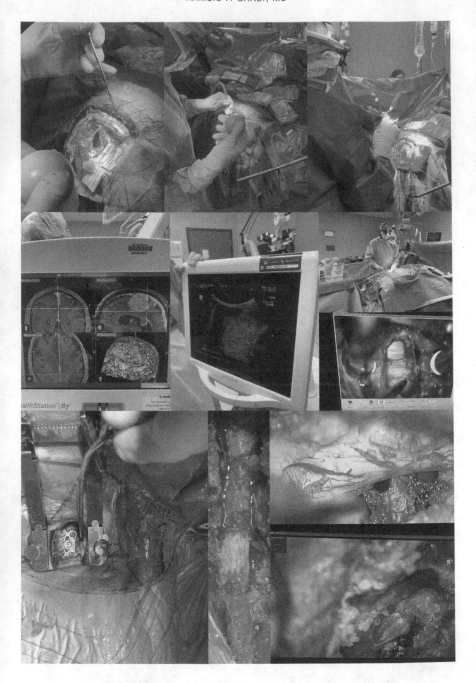

SPINAL SURGERIES

INTUBATE COVID PATIENTS AND PROVIDE ANESTHESIA AND VENTILATORY CARE

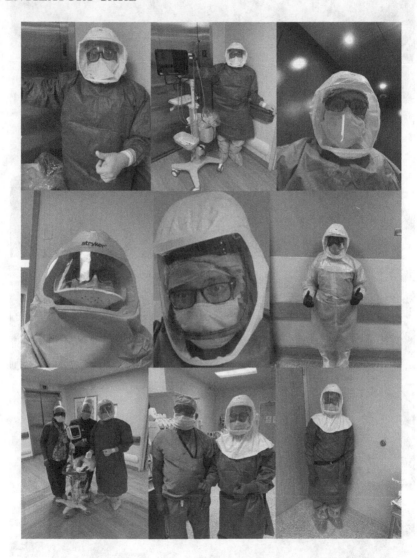

DINNING WITH MY RESIDENTS

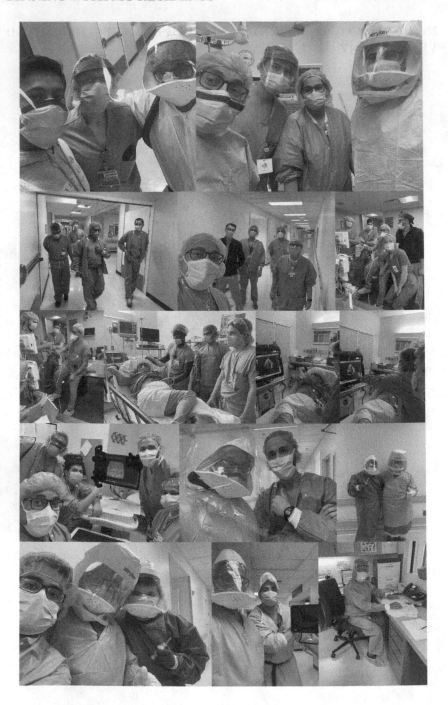

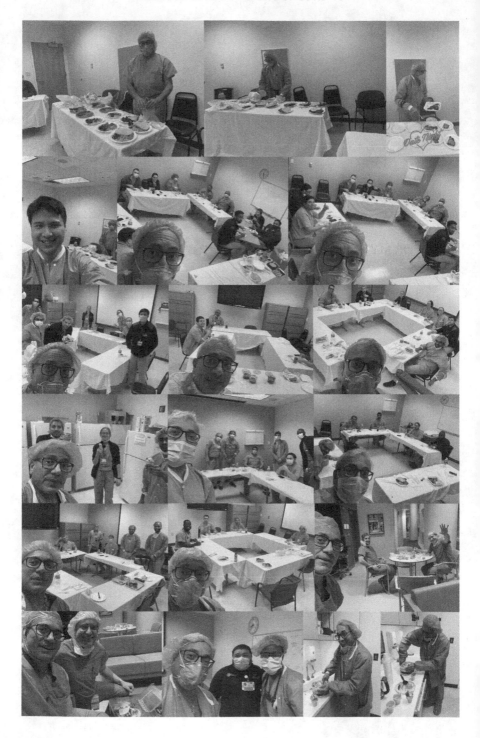

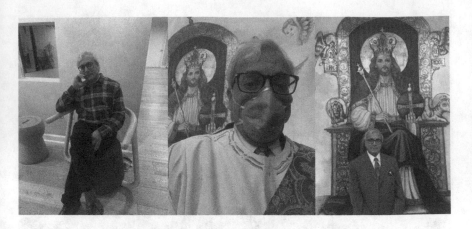

PRAY FOR MY PATIENTS AND RESIDENTS

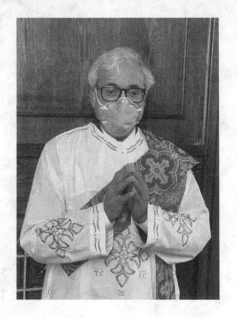

JOY AND LOVE OF WHAT GOD HAVE GIVEN ME TO DO!!

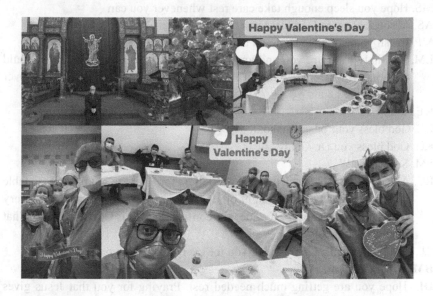

EP. You are such a blessing as you allow The Lord to guide your heart and hands.

DC. Thank you for all you do. We were all blessed when God gave you to us.

LG. Amen.

MO. Not sure if you saw but you were identified as a Crane's top provider Dr. Ghaly. Thank you for being a pillar of the medical community https://www.chicagobusiness.com/.../crains-2021-notable...

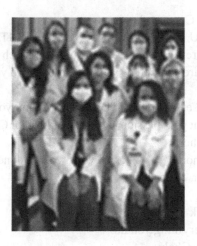

CHICAGOBUSINESS.COM
Crain's 2021 Notable Health Care Heroes
Crain's 2021 Notable Health Care Heroes

MB. God protect you Doctor

MS. Hope you sleep enough take care rest whenever you can 🌷😴💜

AS. Absolutely agree God bless you.

MP. I wish you would come down to St Louis sometime!

LM. Dr.Ghaly I admire you and any person in the health care position I could never have the strength that you have may god bless you always and look over your healing hands ✝️💜

KE. Amen

CL. God bless your beautiful soul. 🙏🙏🙏

KG. God bless you Dr. Ghaly 🙏

SM. Superhero!!!!

RC. Amen to that! He is worthy! All our labors for Him are but our "reasonable service" (Romans 12:1) in light of all He's done for us. And one day every knee will bow and every tongue will confess that Jesus Christ is Lord. What a day that will be!

SJ.. God bless you Dr.Ghaly thank you for everything that you do 🙏🙏🙏

BM. Amen and Amen!

DL. Hope you are getting much needed rest. Praying for you that Jesus gives strength and good health. Stay safe. Thank you for all you do. You are so appreciated.

JV. To God be the glory! Amen, Dr Ghaly 🕊️🙏

SD. I am so blessed by the way you give God all the glory! You are amazing doctor! God bless you!

LB. I really like all the different pictures of you in different scenarios! Very interesting!

JH. I am proud of you Congratulations

FA. GOD BLESS YOU DR GHALY THE DOCTOR WITH A HEART OF 💜

CG. You are such a great.caring doctor. You do so much here on earth to help others that I am sure you will be well rewarded when you see our Lord. Bless you! 💜🙏

SJ. You are a beloved servant of God, Dr. Ghaly. Thank you for being you 💜

LS. I love reading about your passion and sold out love for Christ plus your tireless efforts to serve others.

MH. You are to be honored 🙏💜 for all your work is done for the communities. You are a great Dr. & Teacher as well.

ML.. My hero!

RC. Proud of tour work

AP. Thank you for everything you do.

JJ. God Bless You! Dr. Ghaly

Every Day Serving with Many Front liners Looking Forward for Better Days Ahead!

More and more COVID Victims in dire need to ventilators and intubations!

Unrelenting but never give up, in distress but always joyful servant to our Lord and in deep sorrows and sadness but never despair!

Soon help in the way in Faith and Hope for Our Lord Jesus our Savior to intervene appealing to His mercy and love 🖤!

It shall take it course and one day it shall all go away!

At that time, it will open up 🆙 and we will be no longer in fear racing in the open and not concern to be close to each other again! Laughing 😄 and talking loud showing our true smiley 😊 face with our lips 👄 and celebrating each other in hugs and kisses!!

It is my toast cheers when I threw these PPE, PARR, masks, gowns, gloves faraway!

I can't wait 😄 for that day when we all praise our Lord Jesus and fulfill our vows! Thanksgiving to you all!

"In my distress I cried unto the Lord, and he heard me. [2] Deliver my soul, O Lord, from lying lips, and from a deceitful tongue. [3] What shall be given unto thee? or what shall be done unto thee, thou false tongue? [4] Sharp arrows of the mighty, with coals of juniper. [5] Woe is me, that I sojourn in Mesech, that I dwell in the tents of Kedar! [6] My soul hath long dwelt with him that hateth peace. [7] I am for peace: but when I speak, they are for war." Psalm 120:1-7 KJV "I will lift up mine eyes unto the hills, from whence cometh my help. [2] My help cometh from the Lord, which made heaven and earth. [3] He will not suffer thy foot to be moved: he that keepeth thee will not slumber. [4] Behold, he that keepeth Israel shall neither slumber nor sleep. [5] The Lord is thy keeper: the Lord is thy shade upon thy right hand. [6] The sun shall not smite thee by day, nor the moon by night. [7] The Lord shall preserve thee from all evil: he shall preserve thy soul. [8] The Lord shall preserve thy going out and thy coming in from this time forth, and even for evermore." Psalm 121:1-8 KJV

Ramsis Ghaly
Www.ghalyneurosurgeon.com

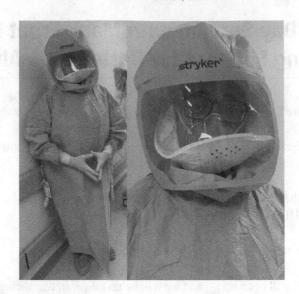

KN. Happy Thanksgiving Dr. Ghaly

KG. Love and prayers 🙏

CJ. God bless you

RC. Love and prayers gol all, including you

JB. Prayers Dr. G. 💜

CG. I can imagine you and all the front liners are looking forward to when this pandemic is over for good. Bless you all for being our heroes. I look forward to the day when the whole world opens up again. When we can go to church and sing to our hearts content. When we can go out to eat or fly wherever we want. I look forward to the day I can come to your office without a mask and give you a hug and say thank you for being the best. 💜🙏

KB. Happy Thanksgiving Dr. Ghaly.

JT. Happy Thanksgiving Dr. Ghaly.

VG. Srecan dan zahvalnosti dr.Gali 🙏🙏

VV. May Our God always protect and guide you dr. <u>Ramsis Ghaly</u>

AS YOu continue to serve the severely ill and desperate patients

ND. Thank you for your hard work and dedication!!!! We appreciate you!

AS. Be safe

My Medical Mission

Once I was asked What is the medical profession??

I replied: It is an oath, it is a commitment, it is a responsibility, it is a life in trust but most of all it is MY LOVE

Ramsis Ghaly
www.ghalyneurosurgeon.com

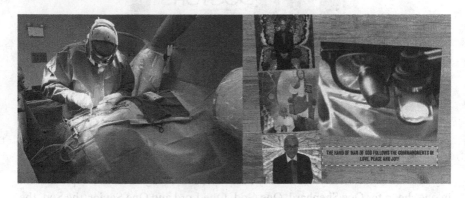

Cg. It is an oath you uphold with much love. 🖤🙏
SJ. The above describes you to a T 🖤🖤🖤
RC. Blessings for you
AM. Perfectly said!

America's Most Honored Doctors award 2021

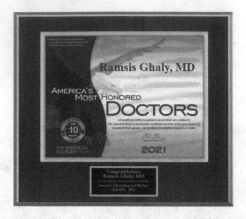

All thanks go to my Savior and Lord Jesus and to you America and my patients! My parents are joyful!!

My success is you all success and my accomplishment is you all accomplishment, in one sheep for One Shephard, One God, One Lord and One Savior, the Son, the Father and Holy Spirit, Amen 🙏

Indeed, Nothing impossible with my Savior and Love Jesus!

From a busboy working in a restaurant in 1984 and 1985 to America's Most Honored Doctors!

From a rejected medical graduate 🧑🏻‍🎓 because of my intimate and vocal Egyptian Coptic orthodox Christian faith to free and accepted America's Most Honored Doctors!

From being thrown unto one of the very poorest remote villages in Egypt 🇪🇬 because of being Christian, poor and have no connection to one of the America's Most Honored Doctors!

From lowly and poverty all my early years of life until adulthood to abundance and flourishing by Jesus my Lord and America!

Biblical verses:

1.) But Jesus looked at them and said, "With man this is impossible, but with God all things are possible." ~ Matthew 19:26 ESV

2.) For nothing will be impossible with God. ~ Luke 1:37

3.) I can do all things through him who strengthens me. ~ Philippians 4:13

4.) Jesus looked at them and said, "With man it is impossible, but not with God. For all things are possible with God." ~ Mark 10:27 ESV

5.) He said to them, "Because of your little faith. For truly, I say to you, if you have faith like a grain of mustard seed, you will say to this mountain, move from here to there, and it will move and nothing will be impossible for you." ~ Matthew 17:20 ESV

6.) And the LORD said, Behold, the people [is] one, and they have all one language; and this they begin to do: and now nothing will be restrained from them, which they have imagined to do. ~ Genesis 11:6 KJV

7.) I know that thou canst do every [thing], and [that] no thought can be withholden from thee. ~ Job 42:2 KJV

8.) For God so loved the world, that he gave his only begotten Son, that whosoever believeth in him should not perish, but have everlasting life. ~ John 3:16 KJV

9.) Therefore I say unto you, What things soever ye desire, when ye pray, believe that ye receive [them], and ye shall have [them]. ~ Mark 11:24 KJV

10.) Fear thou not; for I [am] with thee: be not dismayed; for I [am] thy God: I will strengthen thee; yea, I will help thee; yea, I will uphold thee with the right hand of my righteousness. ~ Isaiah 41:10 KJV

11.) Ah Lord GOD! behold, thou hast made the heaven and the earth by thy great power and stretched out arm, [and] there is nothing too hard for thee: ~ Jeremiah 32:17 KJV

12.) What then shall we say to these things? If God is for us, who can be against us? ~ Romans 8:31 ESV

13.) In all your ways acknowledge him, and he will make straight your paths. ~ Proverbs 3:6

14.) No temptation has overtaken you that is not comman to man. God is faithful, and he will not let you be tempted beyond your ability, but with the temptation he will also provide a way of escape, that you may be able to endure it. ~ 1 Corinthians 10:13 ESV

15.) Behold, I am the Lord, the God of all flesh. Is there anything too hard for me? ~ Jeremiah 32:27 ESV

All thanks go to my Savior and Lord Jesus and to you America and my patients! My parents are joyful!!
Ramsis Ghaly
Www.ghalyneurosurgeon.com

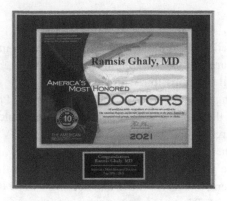

CW. I wouldn't be alive today if it wasn't for Dr Ramsis Ghaly!
❤️❤️❤️❤️❤️❤️❤️❤️❤️❤️❤️❤️❤️❤️❤️❤️

KD. Congratulations
Dr Gahly! Yes you are America's most honored doctors, but most importantly, our families' most honored doctor!

Aunt of CW! Bless you, and THANK YOU! Congratulations Dr Gahly!! We honor you also! Aunt of your patient Chrissy!

BV. Feel the mutual respect and love....
TV. You will get through this once again Chrissy. Prayers will never stop. Hug Eric so hard. Squeeze the construction out of him. Only for the love. 😂❤️🙏
AC. Congratulations our most Beloved Dr Ghaly
SS. Congratulations Doc!
MW. ❤️❤️❤️ Awesome News!!! ❤️❤️❤️
DC. Congratulations
VV. Congratulations 🎊 God bless
SP. Congratulations
🎉🎊👏
AN. Congratulations
ML. Congratulations
Dr. Ghaly!
LS. That's awesome! Congratulations!
DE. Congratulations! ❤️
NV. Congratulations and God Bless Doctor Ghaly, you are the best 🙏
NV. Well deserved! Congratulations
DYT. Congrats 🎊🎉👏 Doc!!
BC. Congratulations!!!!
FC. Congratulations
BG. That's awesome!!!

610

JH. Awesome! Congratulations!

HR. Congratulations

LM. That's awesome! Congratulations and MUCH DESERVED!!! 🖤

AG. Awesome. Congratulations

LL. Congratulations

CC. Well deserved

RC. Congratulations!

MR. That's awesome! Congrats!

HK. That's awesome! Congratulations!

SJ. Congratulations, Dr. Ghaly 🖤🖤🖤

NC. Congratulations

CG. Congratulations! You more than deserve this. Blessings! 🖤🙏

CS. Congratulations 👏

OS. Congratulation!

BM. That's awesome! Congrats

JC. Congratulations you have earned it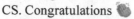

CP. Congratulations

DC. Congratulations 🖤 Well deserved! God Bless you Doctor Ghaly 🙏🖤
    Awesome! Congratulations

GR. CONGRATULATIONS !!!

PF. Outstanding!! Congrats! Well deserved. 🖤🎉🍾🎁

CB. So happy and proud of you Dr. Gahly. Congratulations! You deserve it. God
    bless.

DD. Congrats! Very Blessed...

LR. Highly honored

VW. Congratulations 🖤

AB. Congratulations!

MM. Congratulations!!! 🎉

OC. Congratulations

MD. Congratulations!!

ET. Congratulations 🖤🖤

AS. Congratulations 🍾🎉

SC. Outstanding!!! not surprised proud of you my friend never cease to amaze
    me but well deserved!

SA Outstanding!!! congratulations

MY. Congratulations

LW. justly deserved! such a kind heart! congratulations

ID. Well deserved!!

SC. Congratulations !!!!

SC. That's awesome! Congrats!

JM. Congratulations Doctor Ghaly.

AC. Wooow, Congratulations 😊, I am so so happy for You Dear Dr. Ramsis Ghaly ❤️

RH. Congratulations

DM. Outstanding You Certainly Deserve this. 👏👏👏

KN. 💕⭐✨👍🍾💃🎉🍻💐🌷🍻🥂🎀🎁 Wishing YOU the VERY BEST AND...

KW. Congratulations!

LE. Thrilled for you...it is well deserved. May God bless and keep you.

RM. Congratulations 🎊🎉 Dr Ghaly There is no doubt about it, the world would be a better place if there were more men like you in it 🙏🙏🙏 VS. Congratulations Dr Ghaly

NS. Congratulations!

FA. Well deserved congratulations Dr Ghaly

AB. وانا شاهد علي تاريخ الكفاح

KS. Congratulations

MO. Congratulationsto you on a well deserved honor!! 🙏🙏🙏❤️❤️❤️

CR. OMG!!! I felt like crying!!!! You do deserve it!!!!! How nice must be to stay in the hearts of all your grateful patients and students!!Thanks forever my dear Doctor.

LW. Wish more doctors could be like you Dr Ghaly!

BCD. Awesome, yes you are

ZC. Congratulations! That's awesome! Your kindness Dr.Ghally makes you the most beautiful person in the world.

MS. Congratulations

AG. Congratulations

KS. Congratulations!

WP. Congratulations!!

HM. Congratulations Dr. Ghaly! Well deserved!

SG. Congratulations!!!

CG. Congratulations Dr Ghaly!

RS. Congratulations dear friend! الف مبروك

SN. You are blessed and you bless many. thanks be to our Lord for you. You deserve this honor 🙏🙏🙏❤️

EP. Congratulations!

PH. Congratulations

LS. Congratulations - you deserve it!!

AK. Excellent, congratulations

WP. Bravo Doc!!

AL. You're the BEST 🙏

VG. Congratulations Dr Ghaly!!!

JD. Congratulations

LK. So proud of you Dr Ramsis Ghaly. Well deserved indeed.

JM. Congratulations Dr. Ghaly!

CH. Congratulations Dr. Ghaly!

TS. Congratulations

NE. Congrats Sir!

VS. Congratulations Dr.Ghaly!

EH. Congratulations to a superb human being!!!!

EM. Congratulations Dr Ramsis Ghaly God bless

DL. Congratulations

KE. Very deserving! Congratulations!!!

MD. Congratulation to our wonderful friend and Neuro Surgeon Ramsis Ghaly
in Chicago. His quotations of the Bible are great and make understand who
was on his side. You can read about his fascinating life in his first book. "A
Christian from Egypt". Yes he had a very tough start and never gave up.

KE. Very deserving! Congratulations!!!

YF. Congratulations that is awesome huge accomplishment !!! God is good !!!!!

ED. Congratulations Dr.Ghaly! Well done sir.

CY. Keep it up..God bless u doctor 🙏🖤

JM. Congratulations Dr.Ghaly!

AS. Congratulations!!!Very well deserved! 👏👏👏

LM. And Most Honored People!

JH. Congratulations

BS. Congratulations

ND. You are one of a kind, Dr. Ramsis Ghaly! Congratulations.

SG. Congratulations

CR. You certainly are well deserving of this award. And we all know that you
give all the glory to God!

CR. Well deserving! Congratulations

NW, Congratulations!!

TR. I couldn't agree more!!! 🖤🖤

JC. You definitely deserve it'

OT. If you offer yourself to the Great Lord and His sick children... this is His
reward to u, Doc...

MN. Amazing! Thank you for sharing your journey! May God continue to
bless you!

SP. Well deserved 👏

EB. Congratulations in order y'a Dr

JZ. Congrats!

LA. Congratulations, Dr. Ghaly, on your well-deserved award!!The fruit of your
labor is sweet, and sweeter still to those who have been blessed by it....

LH. Congratulations

SK. Congratulations!

DM. Thank you Dr. Ramsis Ghaly !!! May or Lord and Savior continue to bless those hands of yours!

AF. الف مليون مبروك د. رمسيس .تستاهل كل خير .

SN. Congratulations Dr. Ghaly 🎉!!

DD. Congrats, so we'll deserved.

LM. Congratulations

BK. Congratulations! You deserve this! Praise God for all you do, Dr Ghaly. 🖤

MN. Congratulations

MG. Congratulations! I am sure deserved!!!

LL. Congratulations Dr Ghaly!

EH. God guided you along the way, to bless the world with your gift of healing. Well done Dr. Ghaly! Congrats!!!

MG. SHINE! Congratulations 🎊🎉🥂🍾

BL. Congratulations Dr Ghaly!

RS. Well deserved, congratulations

JB. You certainly deserve this honor, Dr. Ghaly 🎈

MK. Congratulations

HS. Congratulations!!!

RN. Congratulations

GS. Congratulations

DM. Congratulations Dr. Ghaly, Well deserved!

SJ. Congratulations

RS. Very well deserved, congratulations

JE. Congratulations! God be with you brother!

TJ. DR Ghaly, you are so deserving of this honor. God bless you on your journey.

KG. Congratulations 🎊🍾🎉

VG. Congratulations!!!

AB. Dr Ghaly!!! You're the best!!!

LA. Congrats! You deserve it!

GR. Amen!

JL. Congratulations DOC

JW. Keep up the amazing work Doc! Thank you for all you do!

SA. Congratulations!!! Thank you for the wonderful care of all my patients over past 20 years!!! Well deserved! 🖤

NM. You ROCK

KP. Big congrats you are so deserving 🖤

LV. Congratulations Dr.Ghaly. 👏👏 you're the BEST 🏆

JC. Congratulations 🌷🌷🌷

DS. So well deserved!! Congrats Dr. Ramsis Ghaly!!

DH. Congrats Dr Gahly!

MW. Congratulations

Five Stars!!

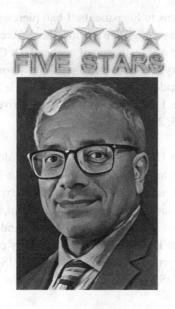

Dr. Ramsis Ghaly, MD
Neurosurgery
Healthgrades
Dr. Ghaly's Reviews 2020
4.8 out of 5

Thank you so much to my patients for taking the time and write comprehensive reviews in my behalf and giving me the Five Star Award 4.8 in healthgrades. Thank you

Dr. Ghaly is an exceptional doctor! For several years, I have suffered from lower back pain that was getting progressively worse. My niece had corrective back surgery and highly recommended that I meet with her doctor, Dr. Ghaly. This was the best advice! After a couple of visits, he scheduled surgery to correct the damage to my spine that was caused by arthritis. During each visit, he explained the procedure to me and to my family in terms that were easy to understand. His level of care and patience increased my comfort level with having the optional surgery. He was very thorough, kind, and ready to answer all of my questions. Having him perform the surgery was one of the best decisions that I have ever made. I am so glad to have received the recommendation from my niece! Currently, I am in my second week of recovery from the surgery and I feel great! I just cannot say enough good things about Dr. Ghaly; he is an outstanding professional. Juana P – Jul 19, 2020

This is a doctor that listens to his patients. I had piercing pain on the top of my head. I was told that is was a migraine. I know the difference between a migraine and the stabbing pain that was on the top of my head. Dr Ghaly was very thorough in asking about my history and listening to my description of my pain. I had some tests done and it was decided that I needed surgery. He removed the tumor that put pressure on my nerve. I am now pain-free and can live a "normal" life. Mercy in Saint Charles – Feb 05, 2019

I am so impressed with Dr.Ghaly, I have seen any doctors in my life and I have never felt that a doctor really cares about me but Dr.Ghaly. He makes me feel special and not just another one patient. He is extremely smart, talented, professional, gifted, extraordinarily competent, skillful, makes you feel like you are in the best hands, but also he is sweet, loving and COMPASSIONATE. I wish this world had more Dr.Ghalys! He was the only one Dr. who gave me an accurate diagnosis. I am proud of him! n MIRIAM CRISTINA RUTKOWSKI in BRACEVILLE, ILLINOIS – May 11, 2018

Dr Ghaly did what no one else could he is guided by our lord Jesus Christ He took my pain away he is the most caring human being as a person and dr Thank you Jesus for guiding me to him Praise to you Jesus and to Dr Ghaly! Robert Coyne in Bourbonnais illinois – Aug 05, 2017

Dr. Ghaly is an Awesome surgeon he is patience and kind loving he has wonderful bedside manors. Its hard to find doctors like this in this day and age. Please do not change. Kenyata Jackson – Oct 02, 2020

FA. You deserve 5 ⭐ 5 💎
AB. Praise God
LM. Much deserved 💗
VW. Awesome! Congratulations
TS. congratulations
CB. You are an instrument of God with a heart full of love and compassion. Congratulations and God bless.
SM. 5 stars is not enough!!!!! The best!!!!
EB. Well done, you make us all proud.
RM. Congratulations You deserve it and more 🎁
AL. 10 out of 5

RH. Very handsome paining. Congratulations Dr. the world is a better place with you in it. God's blessings to you and everyone that you take care of. Amen

JM. "Excellent" Dr. Ghaly 💕 Thank You For All You Do For Mankind 💕 Amen

LA. x10!!!

CG. You certainly deserve those 5 stars and more. You are a healer through Gods' guidance and are such a caring doctor. 🖤🙏

SC. yes you are but in my book you are 1000000 stars not surprised

AK. Dr Ghaly, I was so happy to meet you. You are an amazing man. God bless you

KO. Of course... you are the best!

MS. Congratulations Dr.G

DM. You deserve all the stars in heaven

CS. U r a Godsend!

DM. You deserve all the stars in heaven

BM. You are a Servant of God!

MH. You deserve it! Your one of the Best! DRS. Ever! Great teacher! You have a great gift in healing people. Thanks to you always praising the Lord & giving him the thanks for working threw you to heal his people. You are definitely someone to look up too.

CCC. Well deserved.

Jd. Simply the best. He is in the business of helping people. That's it.

JC. The best!

TM. Amen. Ramsis Ghaly, M.D., has hands guided by our Lord, and also a heart filled with the love of our Lord. Congratulations, dearest Ramsis. You deserve this and so much more. Your grateful friend, Terry 🖤

GR. !!! My dear friend !!! You are an Angel in human body ... God chose you from among the Egyptian Copts and He did it on purpose, because the mainstream of Jesus' true teachings is cultivated by the Copts. Your abilities, intellect, faith, noble heart allow you to save human life...I am very proud of you and I congratulate you !!! Jesus is very close to you ...

Allie Larson
Ramsis Ghaly
March 30 at 4:44 PM ·

Happy doctor's day, Dr. Ghaly. Thank you for your hard work and dedication to your patients. You make a difference in each person's life that you touch.

JC. Happy Doctors Day Dr. Ghaly! Thank you for all that you do!! 🙏🧸🤍
   Ramsis Ghaly
FA. Happy Dr's Day Dr Ghaly

NE. Happy Dr. day! Dr. Ramsis Ghaly

Cristina Rojas-Rutkowski

March 30 at 3:16 PM ·

When there are tears you are a shoulder; when there is pain you are a medicine; when there is a tragedy, you are hope...

You are more than just a doctor, you are a friend, guide and example of love.

Thank you so much Dr.
Ramsis Ghaly

HAPPY NATIONAL DOCTOR'S DAY!!!!

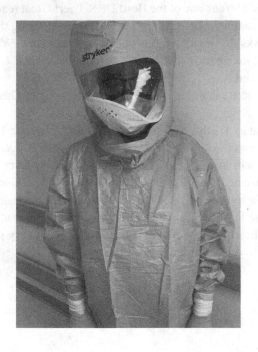

The "Journey of no Return" from Egypt to America at the hope of "Journey of Return": A story from the heart must tell to the second generation and future generations

Written from my heart by Ramsis Ghaly

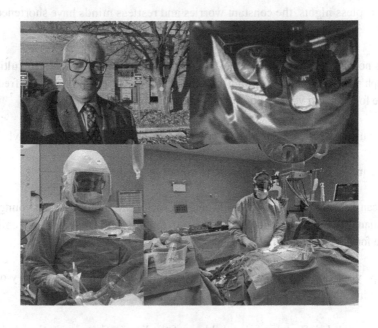

As my sincere colleagues are resting in heaven currently after a long journey from Egypt to America, I felt obligated to tell briefly our story of journey of no return.

O our children it is so painful to talk about our experiences throughout our journey!

It is indeed bring tears to my eyes and heartfelt emotions mixed between sadness and pride!

O our children, if you just now what your dads and moms had went through! It shall make you cry and lose your sleep!

The story must be told as God made sure His people the Israelites remember with Mighty hand He rescued them from the slavery in Egypt and the brutal hand of Ramsis the Pharaoh. So you all the children of and the descendant of the first generation must know your dads and moms "Journey of no Return"

Your dads and moms were subjected through so much, yet they pursued the dreams and made home for you all in a great country USA!

God the Almighty, Jesus the Lord overshadowed their journey despite in many times, it appeared He was far!

The sleepless nights, the constant worries and restless minds have shortened our lives!

It was not joyful to go through horrific and repeated struggles, but the ultimate triumph was God in heaven and you the children on earth, America free and secure for you and your children and grandchildren!

The "Journey of no return" has never left my mind, as if it was yesterday!

I wrote many books and many more to come!

How can I forget the tortuous roads and the rocky mountains we the youngsters Christians of Egypt climbed to pursue our dreams and to secure our children future for decades to come!

Perhaps your dad didn't have a chance to tell the children the true story of our sojourning journey to America!

Let me speak briefly to you the children of the heroic first generation dads and moms:

A group of us, first generation, flew thousands of miles away from home to come to America knowing it is a journey of no return. The doors were shut before us in our homeland Egypt. Discrimination against Christians, the Coptic natives orthodoxy was unreal and continued to be regardless of the news in the media. Nonetheless, at that time, the Islamic gulf countries were pouring money in Egypt targeting the youth and college students early on. Egypt at that time like now, a group is so wealthy and everybody else was poor.

The money from the Islamic gulf countries were in dire need. The Muslim brotherhood was born and allocated themselves in silence in each university including my medical school, Ain Shams university, El Abbasia Square Cairo. The Muslims were helping each other extremely well. The teachers and professors of the colleges and universities were all indirectly part of the Muslim organization supporting them blindly for simple reason, they were also Muslim brotherhood. There was no one Christian teacher or professor except one and he was rich and belong to a very wealthy family. Christians were not allowed in many sites and even examining Muslim women or be ranked academically tenure rank. They distributed their own books, examinations, conducted in private their own meeting and planning raids and rages against Christians in the schools. Despite, the news media, the Muslim brotherhood movements were integral part since they invaded our beloved Coptic country Egypt in the fifth century. But by 1970's and 1980's, the political move was to sell Egypt and its historic pyramids to the richness of the Islamic gulf countries especially Saudi Arabia.

We the Coptic Christians of Egypt, the native of the land and the descendant of the pharaohs were helpless and exposed to much mocking and humiliation. The Muslims, our highly educated college friends called us blasphemers, defilers and adulterous because we claim our God has a mother and son and father. Therefore, we the Christians deserve death and inferior treatment. As a matter of survival, the Christians formed their own group tutoring each other and sympathizing with each other. For instance, I used my gift to teach myself and be able to teach others. Some of our Christian friends had relatives in Immigrant countries America, Australia and England and started to distribute the medical books, assays and examination courses in preparation to leave abroad.

We, the Coptic Christians of Egypt, had no representation in the government and Coptic Head quarter had no authority or power to assist us except through their prayers. The administration of Christians Coptic of Egypt has never been of strong voice or politically strong. I remember the best we the Coptic Christians could do, is to plea to the Vatican Pope in Italy or president of America to help. But all our cries went in vain. At that time, as now, the Vatican was busy for the Vatican and the West. The political machine in the Middle east at that time, was all centered about Israel and Arabs. We all were raised, Israel must go and the Arabs must fight Israel. Therefore the Christian discrimination and the ongoing atrocities against the Christians by the Muslims buried under the carpet stepping their shoes to buried even more and more and deny that ever existed.

As we the Christians became senior in our school, the struggle got worse and worse to the degree that soon we all realized, we had no future to pursue our academic career. The best specialties were taken by the Muslims, the best admirable places across Egypt were also taken by them. Many of us were thrown into villages and working in chemical planets. We, the Christian students were humiliated, received demotions in our scores and ended unto justification for the medical school dean office to hand us poor graduation ranks. I was told that I was so stupid and do not deserve to be a doctor. Every night, I went home crying. My parents were poor, I had no place to study. The food was rare in these days. There was no money to take private tutoring or bribe someone since the entire culture were established in bribery. Who you know was very important and many of us didn't know many influential politicians or connecting to so called "movers and shakers" under the table. In fact, it wasn't uncommon to falsify papers, passports and credentials to leave the country. My dad was rightly so very restricted in doing the right thing and never take the short cut or depend on man but only God. My dad never believed in giving exchanging favor for favor and certainly our poor family weren't connected at all. We have lived in a poor community far away from Cairo and my grand dad was the first native of the community. In fact, a street was name after him.

Among many of my Christian colleagues, I was forced to work unto a remote village with no water or electricity of hospital set up for a year and afterward, I was ordered to work in a military chemical planet. I was as many of us felt angered, suffocated and reached dead ends. Some of the Christians were lucky had some relatives abroad and got help and left in journey of no return and many like myself had no money and had no much of help. The miracle of its time occurred and president Sadat made the peace deal with Israel and Europe and America opened the doors to the youth of Egypt in 1981. It was our heavenly wagon. With no hesitation, we the Coptic Christians joined the thousands of lines to get Visas and begin our "journey of no return". O my God, it was a true miracle, came from nowhere. The economy was so poor in Egypt. The poverty got worse and worse. We borrowed money from each other. We spend sleepless nights find ways to leave and airplanes to go. It was unreal. I could not imagine that my turn would be coming. Many of us had never ride a car, only public transportation buses and trains waiting in lines for hours to go from point A to point B.

Nonetheless, None of us have ever left Egypt or any member of our families. We always lived like close to Nile river and all our relatives lives close to each other and shared the heritage from on generation to another. Therefore, travelling abroad was so revolutionary and scary in our times and never before over 5000 years. Every house, one of our colleagues travelled abroad and took "journey of no return" left a crying parents in exceedingly sorrows and sadness. The parents and families were heartbroken. Many lived by the house door waiting for the mail man to come and knock the door for a letter from their sons and daughters. Many others went to their neighbor phones waiting for a long distance call. The fortunate ones were able to bring their loved ones to America and many others like myself could not and lost my parents departed to heaven without being there for them. It almost like a dream journey deep in our heart it was a "Journey of No Return" yet it was our hope to be a "Journey of Return"

What was strange, that one day we were together, next day, we hear one of our friends already left the country abroad and took the "journey of no Return". I certainly did not know to where and how. The competition was high and the secrets were kept in the hearts so that nothing would go wrong. This was the common esteem at that time. I lost my Christian colleagues one by one including my brothers left one by one. Many unlucky ones like myself, we could not find loop holes or external assistance like the smart ones of us. We waited in lines and never gave up. Many flew to other countries using them as transition to enter America and others stayed kept sending letters to hospitals in America. The letter weren't cheap, they were very expensive knowing my dad salary was 50 pounds a month and each envelope close one pound and average number of letters were minimum of 800 letters. My day and family used to say I am crazy waiting for the impossible. My close friend was the post mail man every day, I was looking for him. The American center of the Middle east was my aspiration and the staff were so kind but their hands were tight--

Early Days in America

O our children, early days in America, weren't easy our children. We had to proof ourselves. We had established no credit yet. We didn't know the system. There was no social media or cell phones or computers. Everything cost money and long distance. Many trips we took in Grey Hound bus and barefooted. We had work any job to make living and support our families. We worked in jobs available to make living, clean the floors, washed dishes, worked in gas stations, boss boys, chiefs in restaurants and many others. Our daily schedule was 24/7 with no minute for luxury. Working these jobs, while studying for medical American examinations and sending letters pleading for hospital job interviews. The church was a place to share. But also a place to connect and try to get married to someone to help you and family to support. But the church was also a place to belittle many new comers and laugh at their struggles. If you did not have a relative or marry one of their daughters, you had received no help but your story of struggle was an entertainment in their dining table. Many Egyptians were well established in America and rich. After showing off their richness, the maximum you get out of them was a brief letter of reference that worth nothing. Otherwise, we have received many open messages to leave and go back to Egypt, why we were here, no spots available, we committed the biggest mistake to come to America. The other conversations were derogatory and belittling. Many early on got the message and started to mix up with outside people and ask for help from other cultures and ethnicities. Some fought the way to deny the truth and got burned out with reality that many established families would also jok about the new comers and offer no help but rather obstacles. However, the fortunate ones found medical residency in a public hospital usually. It became a start to help each other's. We used to sneak in and share the beds, bathrooms and many of us slept in the floors. We sneaked into the cafeteria with fake ID to eat for free, or through the elevators to hid in a place to rest for a little. We shared books and entry to libraries. At that time, there was no ID required or rigid security in hospitals.

We had to multitask and make many compromises especially in the medical and surgical specialties we chose. Surgery general and subspecialties, Ophthalmology, dermatology, and major prestige American hospitals and universities were no way a choice for us the foreigners. There was a common saying among us, the established doctors and congregation in the church mostly were of no help in our career as if "America was only open for them and closed afterward" The maximum help you get is a free meal and prayers, unless you were part of the family. In those tough days, we began to open to the non-Egyptians and melt well with what America and Americans and immigrants could offer. In my story, the non-Egyptians had helped me most. This is America, a land of the free and brave, the land of opportunity and dreams. America was worth fight for and everyone of us established his or her career. It was a wake call and essential lesson to all of us; Egypt wasn't the only country on earth and the Christians of Egypt weren't the only good Christians of the world. We came out of the closets, counting our gains and loses became Americans in every meaning of it respect and share with all, open and never be prejudice or discriminate or be opinionated. And many moved on raising family and had the heritage children raised in freedom and awards for our labors in an established home and luxury that we were deprived back in our homeland Egypt.

Marriages weren't easy at that time. The new comers believed that Egyptian Christians born and raised from the Egypt were the way to go and others felt Egyptian Coptic Christians raised in America were the way to go and few believed Americans and other nationalities were the way to go. The results were painful as so many fell apart and domestic disputes became unreal. There was no good guide or marital council or expectation set to know the pros and cons. The real solid Egyptian Christians demanded the wife or the husband must be from Egypt unaltered by the West culture. The flexible ones said they all the daughters and sons of Adam and Eve and Christ is One all over the world. At the end of the day, only few had successful marriages for life and many were broken apart.

Sometimes I wish my early days of struggle were shortened or better guided by heartfelt people. Instead, some of us had some sort of help in early days but many of us were taking advantage by the established the traffickers and opportunistic. There are so many stories to tell many unpleasant but the most important story to tell our children of the new comers, we did it and with the grace of God, we were very successful and raised you all out of nothing.

Psalm 121

1 I will lift up mine eyes unto the hills, from whence cometh my help.2 My help cometh from the LORD, which made heaven and earth.3 He will not suffer thy foot to be moved: he that keepeth thee will not slumber.4 Behold, he that keepeth Israel shall neither slumber nor sleep.5 The LORD is thy keeper: the LORD is thy shade upon thy right hand.6 The sun shall not smite thee by day, nor the moon by night.7 The LORD shall preserve thee from all evil: he shall preserve thy soul.8 The LORD shall preserve thy going out and thy coming in from this time forth, and even for evermore.

The End

Now after I told briefing about the real story of the "Journey of no return" that your dads and moms carried through, be proud of them, rank them always highly in your heart, keep the memory from generation to generation.

They were so special people, suffered much, struggled tremendously, deprived from so many things to save the penny for you for tomorrow They weren't complainers. They kept in their hearts. They never told you how much dreadful roads they took to raise you. The Nobel reason is not to let you worry or take the smile away.

O children, your dads and mom were true heroes, kept the Coptic Christian faith strong in their hearts, handed you the ancient Coptic Christian faith unaltered to you and your children. O children of your dads and moms of first immigrants, remember them kindly, pray for them and visit their graves. The roses you buy mixed with incense and prayers. Keep their comfort by knowing you are successful and following their steps in faith. Instead of crying, please go do something noble for another person in need. There are so many like us new comers were crying for help and waiting for you. Celebrate your dad and moms by being successful, raise your kids in the Christian faith and carry on the mission. You help your dads and moms by helping strangers and new comers regardless.

And now, after they fought the good fight, they are resting in comfort with Lord Jesus joining their families singing the praises of triumph with the heavenly hosts. And most importantly, praying for you all and wish for you all to know, you have saints representing you all before the Holy Lamb of God. Amen

As it is written: (2 Timothy 4:7-8) "7 I have fought the good fight, I have finished the race, I have kept the faith. 8 Now there is in store for me the crown of righteousness, which the Lord, the righteous Judge, will award to me on that day—and not only to me, but also to all who have longed for his appearing."

Let us utter the words with King David to our dearest friend the Soul of my colleague as it ascends up to its comfort:

"5Gracious is the Lord, and righteous; Yes, our God is merciful.6The Lord preserves the simple; I was brought low, and He saved me.7Return to your rest, O my soul, For the Lord has dealt bountifully with you.8For You have delivered my soul from death, My eyes from tears, And my feet from falling.9I will walk before the LordIn the land of the living.10I believed, therefore I spoke,'" (Psalm 116)

Amen 🙏
Ramsis Ghaly www.ghalyneurosurgeon.com

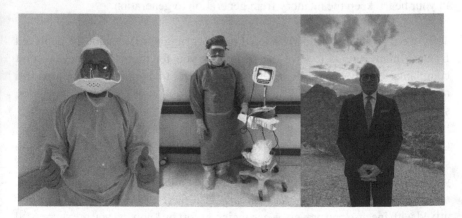

Medical profession to me?
written by
Ramsis Ghaly

Once I was asked What is the medical profession??
I replied: It is an oath, it is a commitment, it is a responsibility, it is a life in trust but most of all it is MY LOVE,
I am one of you and I will do it again and again,
My years are between the hospitals and the clinics,
Racing between emergencies and surgeries,
From patient to another and from a hospital room to the next,
So many times I wish I could fly to come faster to you my patients,
You are my priority, you are my first and nothing will stand the way,

++++

My life is yours and your comfort is my dream,
Allow me to care for your wounds, let me help you to ease your suffering,
I have the science together with the hand of the Almighty,
My Lord is Jesus and He is the God that can do the Impossible,
(Matthew 19:26) "But Jesus beheld them, and said unto them, With men this is impossible; but with God all things are possible."
I strive to cure since the hope is endless here and life eternal is to come,
Together let us pray and ask the Most High to heal as He said:
(Luke 11:5-13)
(Matthew 7:6-8) "7Ask, and it shall be given you; seek, and ye shall find; knock, and it shall be opened unto you: 8For every one that asketh receiveth; and he that seeketh findeth; and to him that knocketh it shall be opened."

++++++

I can not take off my mind from my patients and the loved ones,
I keep thinking and thinking and ask myself what else I can and should do,
As I listen to my patient, I wander what it can be the challenge,
As I examine the patient, I pray to the Most High to point for me the area of trouble,
As I summarize the condition and come up with the diagnosis and next steps,
I stop for a second and I take the blessing from Him my Savior,
As I perform the surgery, I realize I am working in the temple of my Lord in His patient,
With respect and sincere humility, I handle the human tissue as I extract the illness,

I know it is the hand of God, the body is anesthetized but the spirit is awaken and roaming around me,
As I look at the human anatomy, I see the hand of God and His treasure,
Jesus Hand is guiding, the two angels of my patient are all around,
My patient, the temple of God is sleeping but the heavenly hosts together praising with me,
The operating room I find the Glory of my God, by the examining bed is His presence and His hand is extended to heal,
My ultimate joy when the disease is conquered and my patient is recovered,
Until then I can not recover and my concerns keep building up,
So many times, I wish I could do more and more for you all,
I pray more and more and ask the Lord of Grace to guide me and do what is right for His children,

+++++

My friend, If you do not find me in the hospital, I am in the clinics,
When I have a time off you will find me at the Medical library,
The patients are the gifts, they are my life treasure,
My day is night and my night is day,
My clock is reversed as my day and night is mixed up,
I drive in the dark and back in the dark,
I miss the sun all the time to see my patients,
I count the stars as I drive back and as soon as I get in, I am again back in the road,
Nothing else I see myself do except caring for my patients,

++++++++

It was at night back in 1979, when I saw a vision and my Lord Jesus opened the door for me,
I answered the call from heaven as I was in the high school,
Since then my eyes are steadfast in the medical field I am,
I am eager to serve as I look forward to healing,
The day I was born to the day I go, my life is for you all,
It is an honor and a sincere treasure to be chosen to do what my Lord Jesus asks of me,
He is the Healer, I am the maid and you all are His chosen children,
My patients are blessing and my Lord love them,
My Lord allows the sickness for them to be His sons and daughters,
As my patients go through the illness together I suffer with them,
My pains are their pains and I can hardly lay in my bed resting my head over my billow,
Many times, I wish it was me so I can see the smile on them once more,

I learn so much from you as I see my Lord Jesus through you all,
I pray for you all as you pray for me too,

++++

Blessing to you all the doctors of the universe,
My Lord Jesus love you so much, you sacrifice your soul to the fellow men and women,
There is no price to pay you back except to say thank you: may our Lord Jesus reward you much in His Kingdom,
As He healed the sick, He ask you to do the same,
My Lord Jesus bless the doctors: the physicans and surgeons everywhere,
Keep your sacred mission up high and our Lord Jesus is writing your names in His Book of Life

+++

Once I was asked What is the medical profession??
I replied: It is an oath, it is a commitment, it is a responsibility, it is a life in trust but most of all it is MY LOVE,
Lord Jesus you said: "Heal the sick, cleanse the lepers, raise the dead, cast out devils: freely ye have received, freely give." (Matthew 10:8)
Lord Jesus as you healed all sickness please use me and my colleagues to heal whoever thou send in our way----Thank you Lord. Amen
Respectfully
Ramsis Ghaly, www.ghalyneurosurgeon.com

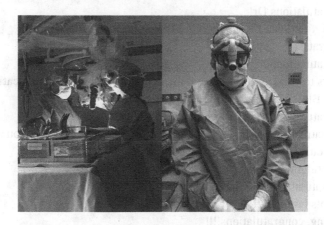

Cg. You are not only a doctor who heals those who are suffering but you also heal your patients spiritually through your writings.. 🖤🙏
Ko. So true with every word, Char

Cr. Wish there were more doctors like you 😊 God has given you the best of gifts and yet you depend totally and completely on Him for all that you do.
As. You are a wonderful Dr for all that you

My Four Board Certifications Renewed in Four Different Disciplines
Neurosurgery since 1998
Anesthesiology since 1993
Neurocritical Care since 2008
Pain Management since 1997

I would like you all to know that I just passed my recertification in Neurocritical Care. I have been preparing for sometime and I just received the news that I obtained 96%. Neurocritical care completes my Neurosurgery and Anesthesia/ Neuro and Pain Managment board certifications extremely well.

Praise our Lord Jesus

DE. Congrats 🙏
ML. Congratulations Dr Ramsis Ghaly! You truly are, Heaven sent. Much love and gratitude for all that you do for the ill.
KC. Congratulations, Dr. Ghaly!!
RVV. Amen 🙏✝️🙏😊 Congratulations 🙏🙏🙏✝️🙏🙏🙏❤️❤️❤️
AV. Congratulations! 💖🙏
EB. Congratulations
DS. Congratulations Dr!
AG. Congratulations, Dr. Ghaly! God Bless you always and forever 🙏❤️
MR. Congrats!
GS. Congratulations
GC. Cheers to you Dr. Ghaly! Amazing accomplishments and dedication.
CD. God's Blessings to a truly special Doctor
JW. Congratulations! You are a very talented physician.
CG. Congratulations! Dr Ghaly May our Lord continue to Bless you and watch over you. ❤️🙏
JS. Congratulations !!!
CG. Congratulations Dr Ghaly!!
BJ. Congrats brainiac!!!! Very impressive
SF. Amazing, congratulations!!!!
JH. Congratulations Doc!!!!
CS. Wonderful! Congratulations & thank you for your dedication.
AN. Congrats
AE. Congratulations! Great job!!!

JM. Congratulations

NL. Congratulations!

ZC. Congrarulations Dr.Ghaly, you are one of a kind doctors. 👍

MD. Ramsis 🙏🙏

JB. Congratulations Dr. Ghaly!! Many physicians narrow their scope of practice in different specialties but don't take the extra training and then testing for board certification. Your board certifications in four specialties is amazing. This is more of what makes you the incredible physician you are!!

EA. Definitely could have used you but hopefully I am in good hands now

EA. Yay Congrats Dr!!

VG. Čestitam dr.Ghalu!! Vi ste ime medicine. Bog vas blagoslovio!! 🙏🙏❤️ 🖤 Doctor Ghaly je jedan od najboljih doctora što se jako brine za njegove pciente. On je operisao i brinio za moju mamu Zoru kad je imala stroke in 2004. Neznam da još ima takvih doctora na svetu kao je Doctor Ghaly!

VG. Gospođo Nado, dr.Ghalu samo divne reči, o njemu može da se govori.Veliki doktor, veliki čovek, velikog srca, posvecen pacijentima.Vašoj mami Zori želim dobro zdravlje, srecu i dug život.Pozdrav, vama i vašoj porodici, Sa velikim poštovanjem! 🖤🖤🖤 Congratulations!!!

CB. Congratulations Dr. Gahly! You are so blessed because you have a big heart. So proud of you. May the Lord continue to give you good health, happiness and more blessings. God bless you.

AC. Congratulation on the continuing medical gift you are to so many! 🖤🎉🌷

MA. Congratulations Dr Ramsis Ghaly God bless

CE. Congratulations Dr Ghaly. I wouldn't expect anything less. May God continue to bless u. 🖤

DK. Congratulations Dr. 🎊

CG. Congratulations; you are a brilliant person! Great job!

NV. Congratulations 🎊🖤 Doctor Ghaly you are the best! God Bless you 🙏

BD. You are an inspiration to us all, thank you for being you, and if you didn't know is a gift to all.

TEW. You are a wise, talented, hard-working, intelligent and caring child of God and you are a gift to us all! Thank you for helping me and so many others! Love, hugs and prayers sent your way!

MY. الرب يحفظك ويحميك وشكرا لرب المجد يسوع المسيح ابن الله اللحى آمين الذى يقود موكب نصرتك اٍد البروفسير رمسيس

LS. Congratulations. You are truely a blessing to all.

JS. Congratulations 🎊🖤🎉

DC. Your the best

CT. You are a rare individual, you are brilliantly blessed, I'm so very proud of you, kudos my Friend ✨👊✨

LL. LR. A jack of all trades!

AS. Congratulations!

EH. Congratulations 👏

DL. Congratulations Doc

AF. Congratulations

PH. Congratulations!! That's fantastic 👍😄

CP. Congratulations Dr. G. ‼️ We're very proud of you. 😊💕

KG. DB. Way to go!!!!

JJ. Awesome way to use the gifts God has blessed you with!! Thank you.

DM. Jack of all traits ..faithful servant of Jesus with a big heart for humanity

KC. Congrats Dr. Ghaly!!!! This is amazing!

MH. Wow! Very impressive so very proud of you.

HC. Praise the Lord!!

SN. JZ. Congrats!

BD. Very impressive

MO. Congratulations! We are so blessed and proud to know you! God's Blessing pour onto you.

AS. Congratulations

KE. Awesome

BD. Congratulations!! You deserve it!!

KH. Congratulations!

SM. Some people!! 😂😂😂😂 Just in case you felt that your 1 residency was an accomplishment, 💩💩💩💩. Haha! Super duper proud of you, Dr. Ramsis Ghaly! He's the only one out there like this....And a spine surgeon. I'll never forget how you answered me when I asked you, "How did you do all that?" You're so humble....saying it's easier than remaining chaste (virgin)! You made me feel super special!!! I value all your insight and wisdom. You're one of a kind and God truly works in you! Thank you for always being there for me, whenever I needed a true friend! You're super motivational and amazing!!!! Congrats! God bless you always! 🎉

SJ. Praise our Lord Jesus 💜 A well deserved recognition to our one and only Dr. Ghaly, our Earth angel who is our Gift from God. Congratulations 🎉 and Thank YOU 🙏💜

CB. "Ramsis, you are an amazing and gifted surgeon and a person everyone should know. God bless you 🙏"

rb. Congratulations!

Cr. CONGRATULATIONS!!!!!

Ab. You're Awesome Dr.Ghaly!!

Kc. Big congrats 💜

The sacred place that means much to many!

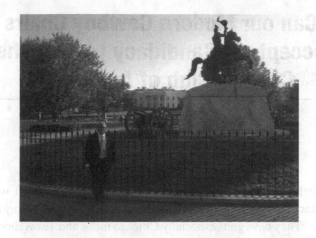

While I was walking Lonely in the desert, I found the Mother of my Lord the Theotokos St Mary. I called upon her name and I didn't hesitate to ask if I can take a selfi together with the mother of Jesus. She smiled at me as I came closer and I took several. I kept them in my heart as She intercede for all of us continuously before Her Son Lord Jesus. She blessed my soul. Amen

Ramsis Ghaly

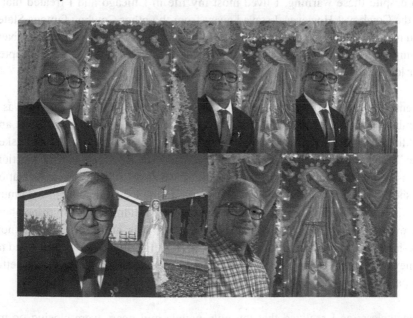

Can our Modern Cowboy Chairs accept my Candidacy to Join The Cowboy Club of America??

Written by
Ramsis Ghaly

I never thought one day, I will write a post about this!! In fact I was warned repeatedly back in Egypt and through many of my early years to stay away from the Cowboys! They have guns especially Chicago mobs and Texas shooters! They are Red Necks and they do not accept any foreigners or strangers! Stay away they will kill you, reject you and discriminate big time against you! They aren't warm people like Middle Eastern but rather cold and care much about their own and the mighty dollar!!! I was always reminded with horrific movies of gun shotting of the Wild West and whenever I watched those films, I went to bed dreaming about the killing but admired by the strength and legacy of those cowboys!

So despite these warning, I lived most my life in Chicago and I treated many of the Cowboys! However, I stayed away from the other Cowboy famous States and regions such as Texas, Carolinas, Oklahoma, Dakotas, Idaho Montana, New Hampshire— But I still reached a stage back then that I will never be accepted nor looked up upon by a cowboy or cowgirl!!!

I remember 10 years ago I attended a rodeo and convinced myself as I was a hombre. But a Cowboy and his girl and friends looked at me with surprise and holding the tip of his cowboy hat 🤠 down covering almost his eyes and asked me: " What are you doing here?? I trembled and I wasn't expecting the question. I was sitting next to him in the same row and we never started any conversation or show interest. So I said: "My travel agent told me I should go it is fun" i must admit I was with my norm custom tie and suit and I didn't know anything about the event or wear jeans 👖 with Polo tie and denim shirt and boots. I didn't know yee-haw yeeeee haw partener or gitty up or HOWDY PODNER either. I had no boney or Partner 🐎. Perhaps I should have learned before I attended to be better prepared!! I was the only one and I didn't belong so I left!

Nonetheless, as I realized that my own people and peers were closing on me and weren't of much help and many mocked me and took advantage of me and made fool out of nativity, I started to reach out and open up to others and look at all people regardless to what I was told about other cultures and ethnicity. The way we were raised was in a closed society reading only Egyptian newspapers, watching only Egyptian national news and learning in public school what the government wanted us to know. It was to the degree that I am still suffering in trying to believe that the world wasn't only Egypt and Jesus the God wasn't only for the Middle East!

My mom was my inspiration to the West. She loved the West and America. I know she is happy to read this post in heaven giving her the tribute she never heard before but it ran in my blood since I was her child in her bosom. I knew one thing loud and clear my mom loved the Wild West and the Cowboys especially John Wayne and Marline Monroe. I also knew from St Paul, if I want to live in America, I should live as an American and not as an Egyptian. If I want to be a doctor, I must learn from Americans and treat them all equally. As Egypt persecuted me for my Christian faith all my life with no dignity or respect and cut all opportunities because of my faith in Jesus, America became my new immigrant home forever. I never believed in living in America and call it home but keep my heart in Egypt. I took all what I have from heart, mind and soul to my new home America sweet home!

It wasn't easy especially after decades and centuries of living only in Egypt and see the world and God as Egypt only! It took time for me to see the world as one, the people as one and Jesus the Lord wasn't only for Egypt 🇪🇬!

But as I came across many of them and I treated some, I fell in love with them! They are honest and no nonsense. I realized in short time they are the back bone of America and Christianity!

I immediately saw on the Cowboy and cowgirl of America 🇺🇸, the pure faith in the land! The real and originals!!

****

Friends;
Cowboys and Cowgirls will never betray Jesus for another God!
Cowboys and girls will never betray the Gospel for another book or doctrine!
Cowboys and Cowgirls will never betray America for another country!
Cowboys and Cowgirls will never betray their families and inheritance for bureaucracy!
Cowboys and Cowgirls will never betray hardworking for laziness and short cuts!
Amen to American 🇺🇸 Cowboys/ Cowgirls and the Cowboys and Cowgirls of America!

*****

But I never saw the Cowboy part of my Egyptian king Ramsis III Version!!

I wonder if the Modern Cowboy 🤠 chairs will accept me since I have little to offer of my English slang! I have no ranch or cow! In fact I do not know how to ride a horse 🐎 or drink beer or wear jeans 👖 and I will never claim that I am as a strong as they are!

But I share much of their values—- Let us examine those—
But I am a public Servant love 💜 very much my Savior Jesus and my new home country USA!

I believe in the Holy Trinity the Heavenly Father, the Son and the Holy Spirit One God, Amen. I believe in the Holy Bible and strive to do good! I do not depend in government to support me but rather I sweat 💧 😅 day and night to help many according to my calling from my Heavenly Father!

I believe in the Truth, Morals and hardworking! I love America and the well-being of USA! I believe I must work hard for every penny and earn my degrees! I do not once believe in living by someone else including my parents or loved ones or even the government wealth but my own through the works of my own hands given to me by God the Almighty!

I believe mankind established as one human race created from God and our parent Adam and Eve the children of the Most High!

I believe in Jesus the Lord in the flesh incarnated and became man and give Himself in the cross to die for us all people and save us from death to once again earn to be His own children and life Eternity with Him! Jesus our Redeemer who died for us and through His salvation, He opened the gate for the faithful believers to enter from the valley of death to the green pasture with Him!

I am a doer and not a politician! I depend on my Lord Jesus and the gifts that He has entrusted my soul with Abd Bever ever in lip service or cheap talks!

I believe that my life in earth is a journey that determine my eternal destiny! I never once thought that the world is my destiny or my goal after death as my ancestors the pharaohs believed!

I believe in serving and not to be servant as my Master taught me! I believe in the Aptitudes and the Creed and My Lord Jesus until the last breath!

636

I believe in Jesus Christ second coming and the Judgment day at which every soul shall give account in his and her deeds! Those who had done good and believe in Him the Son of God and Savior be with Him in His Kingdom forever and ever more!

I was born in Cairo from an ancient family with 7000 years pharaoh inheritance! None of my blooded family ever left the Nile River region and I am together with my brothers are the first ever!

I am one of the Ancient Christian of Africa named Coptic Orthodox Church ⛪ established in the very first church of Christ before any of the Christian division by St Mark the apostle and Evangelist disciple of our Savior first hand!

"For though I be free from all men, yet have I made myself servant unto all, that I might gain the more. [20] And unto the Jews I became as a Jew, that I might gain the Jews; to them that are under the law, as under the law, that I might gain them that are under the law; [21] To them that are without law, as without law, (being not without law to God, but under the law to Christ,) that I might gain them that are without law. [22] To the weak became I as weak, that I might gain the weak: I am made all things to all men, that I might by all means save some. [23] And this I do for the gospel's sake, that I might be partaker thereof with you. [24] Know ye not that they which run in a race run all, but one receiveth the prize? So run, that ye may obtain. [25] And every man that striveth for the mastery is temperate in all things. Now they do it to obtain a corruptible crown; but we an incorruptible. [26] I therefore so run, not as uncertainly; so fight I, not as one that beateth the air: [27] But I keep under my body, and bring it into subjection: lest that by any means, when I have preached to others, I myself should be a castaway." 1 Corinthians 9:19-27 KJV

Perhaps we can meet half way, I will wear a Cowboy hat 🤠🎩 and instead of wearing Jeans 👖 I wear a fashionable suit with luxurious tie and pocket and pocket square with nice whit shirt and cufflinks!! In addition, I will definitely wear both hats boldly and proudly and joining my cowboy and girls club in my charisma loon good!!

So 36 years later living in America as I take off my hat and extend my hands asking: Can our Modern Cowboy Chairs accept my Candidacy to Join The Cowboy Club of America??

Respectfully
Ramsis Ghaly

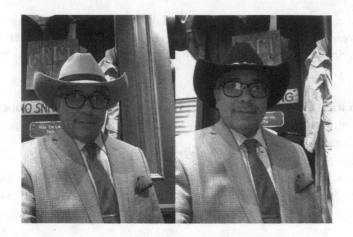

PP. Absolutely yes! Love the cowboy hats
KG. Love these. So true and you are a true cowboy. Black hat!
AR. Love it, love the cowboy hat. Love the ancestry you shared.
JC. How handsome you are in that black 🤠 hat 🙏🙏
CC. Yee Hah!
DR. Looking good!
VG. Looking good!!
DC. Looking good hombre.
RC. Wonderful! You look great wearing both cowboy hats!
BJ. Hey there cowboy
KG. You look mighty fine in that cowboy hat!!!
ML. Look at you wearing that Cowboy hat. You resemble JR Ewing.
TC. You look great Dr. Ghaly!
TH. That is an awesome look for you Dr.!!!
KJ. .... Dr. needs to get on a horse! this could be arranged! I am well assured a
    mutual friend of mine and the Dr's would smile down from the heavens.
MP. You just need a bolo tie and a denim shirt, Pardner
KW. I grew up with Roy Rodgers and Dale Evans and Gene Autry. Living in the
    Midwest state of Illinois, that's who I thought were real cowboys. Growing
    up in a family of six kids, we never traveled, let alone went on vacations.

Then once married the love of my life and had two children of our own, we would
travel all over North America, and saw the Wild West, camped the Big Horn
National Forest and saw the real Cowboys and the REAL ORIGINAL Americans,
the brave Indian Tribes.

I LOVE AMERICA.

SA. You should come visit Texas. It's like no other place in the US.

TB. Love That Look On U

RH. That's one fine hat you have on doctor. Did you go with the white one or the black one.?

CR. Yee haw!!

CR. Never seen an egiptian cowboy but you look so so good!! Stay safe.

CB. You look great Dr. Gahly.

VM. You look great my friend.

JD. YeeHaw there cowboy. Gitty up and get to Texas. They say everything is bigger in Texas. I have 3 brothers, nieces and nephews that live there. But be careful because in Texas they are ALL packing. (Guns). You will fit right in with your cowboy hat 🤠 indeed we are !!!! 👍😊

JP. I thoroughly enjoyed your post today. We are all on the road to our heavenly, eternal home. God doesn't care about our outer appearance, only our heart appearance. You have a beautiful heart and I am blessed to call you my Facebook friend. God bless you on your journey back to Him.

FA, Love it Dr

CE. You look good in that hat. All you need now is a horse!

AS. I like the black hat best

NS. HOWDY PODNER.

GP. Dr **Ramsis Ghaly** you look so cute 🖤🖤

MR. You're definitely a white hat kind of guy!

BCD. Black hat. Pardner

RB. You should definitely be writing and publishing books, for all to enjoy the fascinating readings! Your true faith and love for God is what carries you through each day. And with such charisma, I might add!!! You are absolutely a beautiful soul. Trust me, I know them when I meet or come across them! You will most certainly hear from our Heavenly Father, "Well done, my good and faithful servant!"

Both hats loon great! Wear them boldly and proudly!! 👍 Shout out from this Cowgirl in Houston, Texas!

RM. Looking good Partner

DM. looks good on you

JM. "Awesome"

LM. Where your pony

MA. Very handsome Dr God bless

SC. yeeeee haw partener

SC. hopefully you have some cowboy boots

SB. The tan hat looks the best and I agree with

SC. - you need boots to go with the hat! 😋

KS. If you ever want to learn to ride a horse, let me know. ☺

KM. Great look! I can't imagine anyone that is around you not accepting you! You're amazing! God has definitely blessed you 🙏🙏

DK. Beautiful. You are such an inspiration and have a gift for healing from God and a great heart!! Gods continued blessings over your life 🙏💜

CT. The look fits you Doc 🤠

KC. You look great, Dr. Ghaly!

MS. I like the beige hat on you better 😊

NA. Go cowboy! Go cowboy!

Ma. I love it! Join the cowboy club! 😈 kv.

Kv. Awesome Ramsis :)

Cs. Wonderful.

Ms. Very handsome dude 🌷😊

Tg. First time i see you dressed cowboy, you look great, I love it !!

Cg. I like the black hat. You are a cowboy in your own way. Instead of taking care of cattle, you take care of patients. Cowboys often perform a multitude of other ranch-related tasks, similar to you and your multitasking. You meet the qualifications for a cowboy. 🖤

Ap. The look is good on you hope you have boots too

Writing While Walking and Looking Around

Real Story

I was told if I walk alone and keep writing in my iPod while walking is sending a suspicious and criminal body language signal!

I was in the middle of finalizing my Post focusing and ignoring the surrounding as always, and out of no where three policemen and a policewoman stopped me, surrounded me and question me and checked my ID, interrogating me as they didn't believe me——! She grasped my ID, she took with her hand and moved her hand behind her to give it to next police officer. I was Trapped as they were talking among themselves. I felt really bad because I made them feel uncomfortable and suspicious of me. I tried to help and said; "whatever you need of me!! Then they ask me how to pronounce your name. Then, Are you from Egypt? What are you doing here???——-Your behavior are very suspicious??? I said I have my facemask on obeys all the rules!! I spelled my name —I told my address—I googled myself —I told them I a physician!! The more I talked the more they become more suspicious and they didn't want to leave me! People coming and going and they are starring as if they caught a great fish!

Then a policewomen 👮 👮 👮 after checking me, they told me "they are doing their job" Then, while the policemen investigating my ID and making their phone calls, the policewoman 👮 said "Sometimes weird people as Artists and writers could be confused with criminals. You were looking around and writing. Your behavior and body signals are very suspicion" I said: "No problem this who I am and these are my writings. I want you all to feel comfortable and do their job." They continued to make phone calls and kept checking while their numbers increased ——but then they let me go!!

I was proud of myself, I didn't lose it but I wanted really to tell them about what I write, perhaps I can recruit them to my page! But they had no interest! They really didn't believe me as they were busy investigating!!

Then she said, perhaps you need to stop writing while walking alone and looking around? I said: "This what I had done all my life. I study while walking and I keep walking and writing since I was a child. Back in Egypt I had no desk or chair. I always carried my books and notes while I was walking, or working or in bus or train and I did all my studying and writing! When I came to US, I continued to

641

do the same! Never a minute passes by without learning! This what I promised myself since childhood!

Guess what I continued to write and I didn't let them threaten of intimidate me! And they continued to watch me while I was walking so slow since I must write before what I want to write goes away!!! Now I am walking writing a post about the incident!!

O my gosh our ancient ways are being dinosaurs 🦕🦖🦕 and being profiled suspicious nowadays.

Ramsis Ghaly

DC. You handled it very well.

DBH. Good job doc. America the free is fading away 😦

DE. I'm so sorry that happened to you 😿🙏

CJ. Wow. If that's the case everyone would be suspicious. Everyone does it

KG. I'm so sorry that happened to you there! Great job you handled it so well. Please take care and yes, the system now seems all are suspicious and profiled if not a certain ethnicity, sad to say. God Bless you and stay safe and well!

KW. Good point! I wish they could have read your important writings! Chicago needs enlightening right now! So, be safe, be happy & keep living your good life, Ramsis!

GH. They owe you an apology! So sorry you experienced that! God Bless You! I was interrogated in Naples, Italy by a policewoman I couldn't understand a thing she said in Italian. She still kept talking. Something about me buying a counterfeit designer bag?

GV. I'm so sorry you had to endure that!

VA. Ignorance is horrible waste of a brain

KG. Good for you, Dr. Ghaly!!!

BT. That's an odd way to be profiled. I'm sorry you had to go through such an event.

JD. So sorry that happened to you !!! If they only knew who you are and the lives you have saved !!!

CG. Oh my!! Being the gentleman you are, you handled that situation very well. Sorry it happened at all. 🖤🙏

MA. So angry that that happened to you Dr.. When was this? Where was this? Shame on them, but proud of you for keeping your cool. 😡❤️🙏🙏

AP. I'm sorry. What can we do to support you. So sad this happened.

AR. I'm sorry this happened to you. How horrible! Keep your head high and do what you do best.

GS. I can certainly understand them harassing you for looking suspicious! Your intelligent, educated, professional doctor & renowned surgeon! And your not dressed up as ANTIFA or BLM! VERY SUSPICIOUS INDEED! Ps, your such a kind & loving human being, I'm truly sorry for the CHICAGO POLICE BEHAVIOR!

RN. I'm so sorry you had to experience 😖 that but I believe everything is for a reason, you might not have had the opportunity to talk to them about your writings at that moment, but I'm sure they won't forget you 😊 God was just giving them an introduction to Dr. Ramsis Ghaly - they probably went back to the squad car to look you up 😉 you never know 🙇

GS. Dear Doctor, you need to learn to blend in when your out in public, never wear a suit & tie, it alarms people you may be some type of weirdo! Get some dirty jeans & get a coat from salvation army. Then get a big belligerent looking nose pierce, put some holes in your ears, surgecically split your tongue, & a few facial tattoos, shows your really radical. Next work on your street creds by participating in a "mostly peaceful" protest,,, aka riot! Get in with a group of arsonist burning looters, & snag your self a tv set, & a pair of gym shoes. Then for some real street creds, tear down a statue & urinate on it while being video to proudly show your children one day!

SS. Your comment is just as racist as what was done to him. Just because we look different doesn't give us the right to judge someone else. Some of the nicest people have tattoos. You can't judge a book by it's cover. Not every protester of color does the awful things you just said. Some white people do the same things. You can't judge a whole race on other People's actions.

LW. Unbelievable but still interesting.......Ignorance at its best.

SS. I'm so sorry that happened to you. I look around me all the time. It's called looking to know what is going on around me and being aware of what is going on around me so I don't get robbed in Chicago. Where were you at Chicago or Aurora. I'm going to complain. If it was my white self it would not have happened. Them asking if you were Eyption is down right racial and they won't stop the behavior if they never get in trouble. I have been racial when I dated someone who had black foster children. A woman in a grocery store who happened to be black stopped me and the children to say your not their mother they're are either your boyfriends children or foster children. The boyfriend wasn't there or she would have seen he was white too. It didn't matter to me what color the children were. I wouldn't have been upset with her if the oldest child hadn't heard her talk like that and asked me what did she say again. He was upset by it. He loved me as much as I loved him. The second time I experienced racism was when I was told they would like to hire me but could not because I was the wrong color. Racism in any form is wrong.

rp. Dr. Ghaly you handled it well! They have no idea what you do every day by giving people back their quality of life pain free- and throw COVID-19 in and the care you provide! Thank you for all you do you are a fine Physician and god works through you to heal your patients! 🙏💙😌

Ju, I'm sorry that you hat to go through. Exactly same 💩 we experienced on daily basis by communist back than.

Ap. This is wrong -

Jb. Oh Dr. G!!!! We are so sorry to hear this. You are relaxing and writing in the place that gives you the most peace, and now this. You handled it so well, but this would be very unnerving for anyone. We all understand your walking and writing, but please always be aware of your surroundings, we don't want you to get hurt either. May the rest of your time there give you peace and contentment!!! 💬💬💟💟🙏🙏

JU, Everyone should read this how far everything is going.

CR. Stupid people. They let the real criminals go lose. This is supposed to be "the land of the free".

JM. That's Creepy, Be Careful Dr. Ghaly!!!

CL. This is wildly inappropriate!! Keep writing and keep walking!! Continue to be safe!! We love you and your work!! Where did this happen?

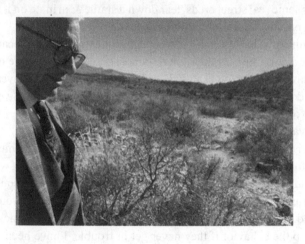

What I Do at the End of My Clinic?

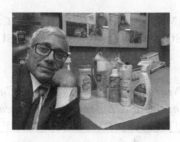

I make sure all messages and all patients are well taking care off leaving nothing behind!

Seal the charts and computers while keep thinking about my patients well being!!

While the air purifier with ultraviolet rays blowing fresh and clean air, I spray the entire office, the tables, desks, chairs, exam tables, medical exam tools, carpets with all kind of antibacterial and viral sprays!

I water the plants while thanking my Lord for healing my patients and praising His Name for a day full of gifts, blessing and grace!

Ramsis Ghaly

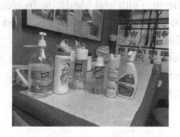

ML. You are so very special Dr. **Ramsis Ghaly!** 🤎🤎🖤

RA. Dr. Clean

CG, That is what makes you such a caring doctor. Making sure your patients have a clean and sanitized office to wait in. 🖤🤎

MH. Your an "Awesome Dr!"

RP. God Bless you 🙏

LA, You're a great dr!

AC. God Bless You Dear **Ramsis**

645

BOOK AUTHORED BY DR RAMSIS F. GHALY

RAMSIS F. GHALY, M.D., F.A.C.S.
PROFESSOR OF NEUROLOGICAL SURGERY
AND ANESTHESIOLOGY

*Board Certified in Neurosurgery, NeuroCritical Care, Anesthesiology
& Pain Management & Independent Medical Examiner*
BOOK AUTHORED BY DR RAMSIS F. GHALY
www.ghalyneurosurgeon.com

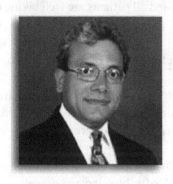

Books Authored by Dr. Ramsis F. Ghaly:

1-Christianity and The Brain: Faith and Medicine in Neuroscience
 Christianity and the Brain: Volume I: Faith and Medicine in
 Neuroscience Care
 ISBNs: Softcover: **9780595424931**
  Hardcover: **9780595884940**
  E-Book: **9780595868278**
Iuniverse
1663 Liberty Drive
Bloomington, IN 47403
P: 800.288.4677
customer.service@iuniverse.com

2- Christianity and The Brain: The Human Brain and Illness Journey Between
Earth and Heaven
 Christianity and the Brain Volume II: The Christian Brain and
 the Journey between Earth and Heaven
 ISBNs: Softcover: **9780595424955**

Hardcover **9780595884957**

E-Book: **9780595868292**

Iuniverse

1663 Liberty Drive

Bloomington, IN 47403

P: 800.288.4677

customer.service@iuniverse.com

3- Christianity and The Brain: Last Hour Journey

Christianity and the Brain: Volume III

ISBNs: Softcover: **9780595424962**

Hardcover **9780595884964**

E-Book: **9780595868308**

Iuniverse

1663 Liberty Drive

Bloomington, IN 47403

P: 800.288.4677

customer.service@iuniverse.com

4- Christianity and The Brain: Stories of 100 Patients1. CHRISTIANITY AND THE BRAIN: PATIENTS STORIES: Subtitle: 100 STORIES OF HOPE, FAITH AND COURAGE

ISBNs: Softcover: **9781450240437**

Hardcover **9781450240420**

E-Book: **9781450240444**

Iuniverse

1663 Liberty Drive

Bloomington, IN 47403

P: 800.288.4677

customer.service@iuniverse.com

5- A Christian from Egypt, a Life Story of a Neurosurgeon Pursuing The Dreams For Quintuple Board Certifications: Volume I of III My Journey in Egypt

Ebook: 9781499080520, Softcover: 9781499080537, Hardcover: 9781499080544 PID 537164

XLIBRIS

1663 Liberty Drive

Bloomington, IN 47403

P: 888.795.4274

F: 610.915.0294 / 812.355.4079

www.Xlibris.com

6- A Christian from Egypt, a Life Story of a Neurosurgeon Pursuing The Dreams For Quintuple Board Certifications: Volume II of III My American Journey

Ebook: 9781503534551,
   Softcover: 9781503534568,
   Hardcover: 9781503538092 PID 704437
XLIBRIS
1663 Liberty Drive
Bloomington, IN 47403
P: 888.795.4274
F: 610.915.0294 / 812.355.4079
www.Xlibris.com

7- A Christian from Egypt, a Life Story of a Neurosurgeon Pursuing The Dreams For Quintuple Board Certifications: Healthcare Experiences, Views and Patients Testimonials
   Ebook: 9781503521438,
      Softcover: 9781503521452,
      Hardcover: 9781503521445 PID 634031
XLIBRIS
1663 Liberty Drive
Bloomington, IN 47403
P: 888.795.4274
F: 610.915.0294 / 812.355.4079
www.Xlibris.com

8- The Persecuted Human Brains in the Way to The Cross
   Ebook: 9781524543112,
      Softcover: 9781524543129,
      Hardcover: 9781524543136 PID749887
XLIBRIS
1663 Liberty Drive
Bloomington, IN 47403
P: 888.795.4274
F: 610.915.0294 / 812.355.4079
www.Xlibris.com

9- The Spirit of Christ in the Human Brain and Neurosurgery: Personal Views
   Ebook: 9781543449099,
      Softcover: 9781543449105,
      Hardcover: 9781543449112 PID 766755
XLIBRIS
1663 Liberty Drive
Bloomington, IN 47403
P: 888.795.4274
F: 610.915.0294 / 812.355.4079
www.Xlibris.com

10- Divinity and Satanism in the Human Brain: A Reflection of a Coptic Christian Brain Surgeon
      Ebook: 9781543449075,
          Softcover: 9781543449075,
          Hardcover: 9781543449082 PID 766757
XLIBRIS
1663 Liberty Drive
Bloomington, IN 47403
P: 888.795.4274
F: 610.915.0294 / 812.355.4079
www.Xlibris.com

11- The Spiritual Journey of a Coptic Christian Brain Surgeon: View and Reflections
      ISBN: 1532059647, 9781532059643
2018
Iuniverse
1663 Liberty Drive
Bloomington, IN 47403
P: 800.288.4677
customer.service@iuniverse.com

12- Touching Stories of My Life in Journey to Christian Holiness and Hands on Patients Care in a Weeping Healthcare: Volume 1 (2019) Touching stories of my Life in Journey to Christian Holiness and Hands- on Patient Care in a Weeping Healthcare: The Brain of Man of God and the Hand of Man of God Reflection of a Coptic Christian Neurosurgeon (Volume I)
      Ebook: 9781796035087,
          Softcover: 9781796035094,
          Hardcover: 9781796035100 PID 795541
XLIBRIS
1663 Liberty Drive
Bloomington, IN 47403
P: 888.795.4274
F: 610.915.0294 / 812.355.4079
www.Xlibris.com

13- Touching Stories of My Life in Journey to Christian Holiness and Hands on Patients Care in a Weeping Healthcare: Volume 2 (2019)
Touching stories of my Life in Journey to Christian Holiness and Hands- on Patient Care in a Weeping Healthcare: The Brain of Man of God and the Hand of Man of God Reflection of a Coptic Christian Neurosurgeon (Volume II)
      Ebook: 9781796038903,
          Softcover: 9781796038910,
          Hardcover: 9781796038927 PID 795542

XLIBRIS
1663 Liberty Drive
Bloomington, IN 47403
P: 888.795.4274
F: 610.915.0294 / 812.355.4079
www.Xlibris.com

14- My Journey Volume I (2020)
XLIBRIS
1663 Liberty Drive
Bloomington, IN 47403
P: 888.795.4274
F: 610.915.0294 / 812.355.4079
www.Xlibris.com

15- **My Journey Volume II xlibrius (2020)**
Ebook: 9781796081824,
Softcover: 9781796081831,
Hardcover: 9781796081848 PID 803494
XLIBRIS
1663 Liberty Drive
Bloomington, IN 47403
P: 877.775.7551 ext: 7117
F: 812.355.4079
tami.seno@authorsolutions.com
XLIBRIS
1663 Liberty Drive
Bloomington, IN 47403
P: 888.795.4274
F: 610.915.0294 / 812.355.4079
www.Xlibris.com

16- **Coronavirus the Pandemic of the Century and the wrath of God**
xlibris 2020) 978-1-9845-8166-2
1663 Liberty Drive
Bloomington, IN 47403
P: 888.795.4274
F: 610.915.0294 / 812.355.4079
www.Xlibris.com

To order:
https://www.amazon.com/s?k=books+by+ramsis+ghaly&dc&qid=1567370930&ref=aw_s_fkmr0

Publishers:

www.amazon.com
www.xlibris.com +1 (888) 795-4274
www.iuniverse.com +1 (800) 288-4677

17- **The Roses of Love Bloom in my Christianity and Neurosurgery Patients**
xlibris 2021)
1663 Liberty Drive
Bloomington, IN 47403
P: 888.795.4274
F: 610.915.0294 / 812.355.4079
www.Xlibris.com

To order:
https://www.amazon.com/s?k=books+by+ramsis+ghaly&dc&qid=1567370930&ref=aw_s_fkmr0

Publishers:
www.amazon.com
www.xlibris.com +1 (888) 795-4274
www.iuniverse.com +1 (800) 288-4677

18- Unfolding COVID-19: Thoughts, Memories and Patients' Stories
xlibris (2021)
1663 Liberty Drive
Bloomington, IN 47403
P: 888.795.4274
F: 610.915.0294 / 812.355.4079
www.Xlibris.com

To order:
https://www.amazon.com/s?k=books+by+ramsis+ghaly&dc&qid=1567370930&ref=aw_s_fkmr0

Publishers:
www.amazon.com
www.xlibris.com +1 (888) 795-4274
www.iuniverse.com +1 (800) 288-4677

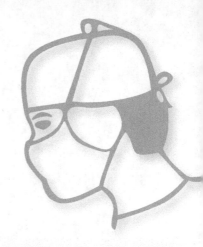

SECTION 12

PERSONAL VIEWS ON COVID-19

A Nation Shall Mourn!

1/5/2021
A Post written by Ramsis Ghaly October 9, 2020

From COVID-19 to Politics-20, no one could escape the deleterious impact in our Nation! A Nation Shall Mourn!

From California COVID-19 surge is getting out of control to Washington Capitol demonstrations is getting out of control! No one could escape the deleterious impact in our Nation! A Nation Shall Mourn!

From South to North, the uprising is getting out of control and from East to West the unrest is getting out of control! No one could escape the deleterious impact in our Nation! A Nation Shall Mourn!

The gap between the people and the leaders is getting out of control and the mistrust between the American people and the politicians is getting out of control! No one could escape the deleterious impact in our Nation! A Nation Shall Mourn!

The imposed restrictions upon the public is getting out of control and the auscultating politics are getting out of control! No one could escape the deleterious impact in our Nation! A Nation Shall Mourn!

The lost jobs are getting out of control and the crashing economy is getting out of control! No one could escape the deleterious impact in our Nation! A Nation Shall Mourn!

Ramsis Ghaly
October 9, 2020 ·
Shared with Public
Nation shall Mourn!!

Rams is Ghaly
Isaiah 24:4 "The earth mourns and withers, the world fades and withers, the exalted of the people of the earth fade away."
Isaiah 33:9 "The land mourns and pines away,
Lebanon is shamed and withers;
Sharon is like a desert plain,

655

And Bashan and Carmel lose their foliage."

Jeremiah 4:28 "For this the earth shall mourn
And the heavens above be dark,
Because I have spoken, I have purposed,
And I will not change My mind, nor will I turn from it."

Lamentations 1:4 "The roads of Zion are in mourning
Because no one comes to the appointed feasts.
All her gates are desolate;
Her priests are groaning,
Her virgins are afflicted,
And she herself is bitter."

Isaiah 3:26 "And her gates will lament and mourn,
And deserted she will sit on the ground."

Lamentations 2:8 "The Lord determined to destroy
The wall of the daughter of Zion.
He has stretched out a line,
He has not restrained His hand from destroying,
And He has caused rampart and wall to lament;
They have languished together."

Joel 1:10 "The field is ruined,
The land mourns;
For the grain is ruined,
The new wine dries up,
Fresh oil fails."

Amos 1:2 "He said,
"The Lord roars from Zion
And from Jerusalem He utters His voice;
And the shepherds' pasture grounds mourn,
And the summit of Carmel dries up."

Isaiah 24:7 "The new wine mourns,
The vine decays,
All the merry-hearted sigh."

Isaiah 29:2 "I will bring distress to Ariel,
And she will be a city of lamenting and mourning;
And she will be like an Ariel to me."
Ezekiel 32:16 "This is a lamentation and they shall chant it. The daughters of the nations shall chant it. Over Egypt and over all her hordes they shall chant it," declares the Lord God."

Zechariah 12:11 "In that day there will be great mourning in Jerusalem, like the mourning of Hadadrimmon in the plain of Megiddo."

Matthew 13:42
Verse Concepts
and will throw them into the furnace of fire; in that place there will be weeping and gnashing of teeth.

Revelation 18:8 "For this reason in one day her plagues will come, pestilence and mourning and famine, and she will be burned up with fire; for the Lord God who judges her is strong."

Amos 8:10 "Then I will turn your festivals into mourning
And all your songs into lamentation;
And I will bring sackcloth on everyone's loins
And baldness on every head.
And I will make it like a time of mourning for an only son,
And the end of it will be like a bitter day."

Amos 5:16-17 "Therefore thus says the Lord God of hosts, the Lord,
"There is wailing in all the plazas,
And in all the streets they say, 'Alas! Alas!'
They also call the farmer to mourning
And professional mourners to lamentation.
"And in all the vineyards there is wailing,
Because I will pass through the midst of you," says the Lord."

Joel 1:8-13 "Wail like a virgin girded with sackcloth
For the bridegroom of her youth.
The grain offering and the drink offering are cut off
From the house of the Lord.
The priests mourn,
The ministers of the Lord.
The field is ruined,

The land mourns;
For the grain is ruined,
The new wine dries up,
Fresh oil fails.
read more."

Amos 5:17 "And in all the vineyards there is wailing,
Because I will pass through the midst of you," says the Lord."
"Therefore humble yourselves under the mighty hand of God, that He may exalt you at the proper time, casting all your anxiety on Him, because He cares for you." 1 Peter 5:6-7

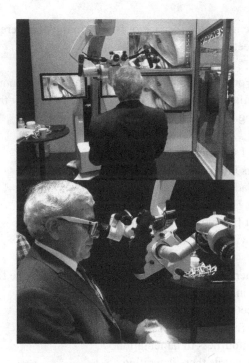

JM. Yes doctor a nation shall mourn.
AV. Praying for our country!! 💔🙏
CG. So very heartbreaking is all I can say. 😢
AV/. Amen! 💔🙏🇺🇸🧑
ED. Amen. 🙏 Praying for our nation, our world.
SC. We have to humble ourselves as a nation. Hearts are turning to stone. We have broken the laws of our God.

The Second Wave of COVID

**COVID is back in Chicago with vengeance like early
days. Intensive Care units are getting busier and busier
and my calls intubating the COVID VICTIMS!!**

O my God, here again we start to don and doff flashing back to the tough early days of COVID servicing the public and saving lives.

I am the crying soul! I am the voice of reality! Please put an end to COVID the pandemic and heal the people! Please O World 🌍 please O leaders put differences to the side and run the race to find the cure and rescue thy people! I beg you all crying 😰 in tears for the sake of our race and our children do so now!!

The numbers are up but we the Frontliners are really down and fatigued working in a system without awarding or Fair recognition. We are getting the blame but yet we aren't the cause!

The cause is that there is neither vaccine nor treatment and the year is almost over ten months later since the COVID Pandemic has started!

The people are starving while millions of jobs are lost and the lockdown is all over for so long with no stimulus money and thus far no hope other than empty words!

I turn on the TV, I listen to the radio and I read the newspaper and there is absolutely nothing about hope but much of politics, disputes, talks, outing, and riots!!!!!

I am the crying soul! I am the voice of reality! Please put an end to COVID the pandemic and heal the people! Please O World 🌍 please O leaders put differences to the side and run the race to find the cure and rescue thy people! I beg you all crying 😰 in tears for the sake of our race and our children do so now!!

"O Lord my God, in thee do I put my trust: save me from all them that persecute me, and deliver me: [2] Lest he tear my soul like a lion, rending it in pieces, while there is none to deliver. [3] O Lord my God, if I have done this; if there be iniquity in my hands; [4] If I have rewarded evil unto him that was at peace with me; (yea, I have delivered him that without cause is mine enemy:) [5] Let the enemy persecute my soul, and take it ; yea, let him tread down my life upon the earth, and lay mine honour in the dust. Selah. [6] Arise, O Lord, in thine anger, lift up

thyself because of the rage of mine enemies: and awake for me to the judgment that thou hast commanded. [7] So shall the congregation of the people compass thee about: for their sakes therefore return thou on high. [8] The Lord shall judge the people: judge me, O Lord, according to my righteousness, and according to mine integrity that is in me. [9] Oh let the wickedness of the wicked come to an end; but establish the just: for the righteous God trieth the hearts and reins. [10] My defence is of God, which saveth the upright in heart. [11] God judgeth the righteous, and God is angry with the wicked every day. [12] If he turn not, he will whet his sword; he hath bent his bow, and made it ready. [13] He hath also prepared for him the instruments of death; he ordaineth his arrows against the persecutors. [14] Behold, he travaileth with iniquity, and hath conceived mischief, and brought forth falsehood. [15] He made a pit, and digged it, and is fallen into the ditch which he made. [16] His mischief shall return upon his own head, and his violent dealing shall come down upon his own pate. [17] I will praise the Lord according to his righteousness: and will sing praise to the name of the Lord most high." Psalm 7:1-17 KJV

Please you all be safe in Jesus our Healer Name, Amen 🙏!

Ramsis Ghaly

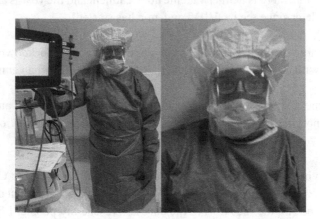

JD. Stay safe!
KK. Amen! 🙏
MS. Stay safe please 🌹😷
RN. Take care Dr.Ghaly, you are always in my prayers 🖤🖤🙏🙏
DE. Please stay safe with all that you do for so many people 🙏
JC. Take care of yourself also, a lot of people count on you 🙏🙏🙏
TA. Take care and stay safe 🙏🙏🙏

MO. Stay safe! We have had a big increase in numbers too. We are tired but we know more now than we did back in March. We will get through this! Thank you for your dedication during this difficult time

DS. Be safe Dr. Ghaly..God Bless you 🙏❤️

PA. Please stay safe...the world needs you very much

KL. Jesus is out only hope!

TW. Be safe Dr. Ghaly! God Bless You 🙏❤️🙏

CS. Please stay safe! May God continue use you for healing 🙏

KB. Amen

RB. Be safe! God bless you!

KM. Take care, and be safe!

ML. Love you Dr. Ghaly! You are heaven sent. I want to thank you for all that you do. Please stay safe!

CR. Stay safe Doctor Ghaly, we need you ❤️❤️❤️❤️

CR. May the Lord continue to protect you in all that you do and give you his continued grace, wisdom and strength.

CD. Be safe. 🙏🙏🙏

CG. Amen! Praying that the Heavenly Father place his arms of protection around you and all of the front line workers! Hear our cry Lord! In Jesus name we pray!

CG. Bless you and all the front line workers. May our Lord continue to protect you all. 🙏❤️

CE. Stay safe Dr Ghaly. May god rest his hands on u and continue to bless u and heal everyone u encounter. Prayers with u always!

MR. Be safe 🙏🙏🙏

DM. My prayers that you and the rest of chicagoans be covered wiith the blood of Jesus

LM. Oh my gosh Dr. Ghaly numbers are so HIGH worse than spring just awful pray, pray, praying for this all to go away my heart goes out to the sick and the ones tending to the sick. God Bless 🙏🙏🙏🙏🙏🙏

TM. Thank you

MY. خلى بالك من نفسك ربنا يرحم برحمته الواسعة حبيبي الغالي

JB. O Lord please please I pray so so hard to stop the plaque.

JJ. May Jesus be with you and fill you with his peace.

MN. Amen

JM. AMEN

UNFOLDING COVID

Gratitude to all the Essentials: Thank You!

Through this political heat and disputes, we must recognize in action and appreciate the continuing hardworking frontlines since February 2020 and ongoing tremendous sacrifice to do their work in person exposing themselves in the harms way.

Instead, many of the essentials received demotion, cut benefits and salaries and none was awarded or got raises despite repeated promises!

We can't thank you enough all essentials including but not limited to healthcare as nurses, paramedics, physicians and hospitals, teachers and schools and colleges and universities, law enforcement, military troops, navy, homeland, FBI, CIA, Cyber Security and all other security agents, food and grocery, farmers, Restaurants, construction workers, plumbing and repairs, manufacturers, businesses, IT informatics,——-and many others! Thank you 🙏 thank you 🙏 thank you 🙏 from our hearts and souls !!

Ramsis ghaly
Www.ghalyneurosurgeon.com

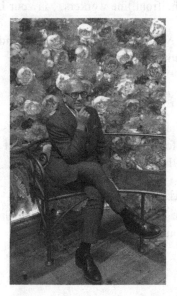

CT. Well put my Friend, and Awesome picture, so distinguished ✨👍✨
AR. Thank you
RA. Great photo and a loving doctor.

Don't Be Fearful But Joyful! The Second
Wave Isn't As Bad As The First Wave!

Dear Brethren: St Paul is sending you all the following message: "Be anxious for nothing, but in everything by prayer and supplication with thanksgiving let your requests be made known to God." Philippians 4:6

Looking back as a since the very beginning until the end as a Very First Frontliner caring for Chicagoans and Illinoisans COVID victims back on March, April and May 2020, there is no comparison and not even close!

Yes there is increase in the positivity rates and many of us are getting infected with COVID but to-date, yet to hear among my circle that a single person got so sick and needed an ICU bed or getting intubated!

Don't Be Fearful But Joyful! Let us Help Each Other in This Tough Time and Support One Another!

The Second Wave Isn't As Bad As The First Wave!

Brethren, Stay Strong Against the Second Wave and Arm Yourself with Faith and Mask to Defeat it as You Defeated the First Wave!

The Second Wave Isn't As Bad As The First Wave! Praise Lord Jesus but praise neither man made vaccine nor treatment nor Medicine nor Science nor intellectual intelligence nor Modern Frontiers nor vaccine research Lab nor WHO nor NIH nor CDC nor Google nor Microsoft nor Facebook nor Twitter nor Linkin nor so called "Experts"! But Who to praise is Lord Jesus and his creation to human Natural Immunity that stood thousands of years against all kind of human enemies!

Therefore, Be Vigilant and Put your Mask and Keep Going:
1) *Don't surrender!*
2) *Don't lose hope!*
3) *Don't hid in the dark!*
4) *Don't be gloomy!*
5) *Don't isolate yourself!*
6) *Don't burden yourself!*
7) *Don't overwhelm yourself!*
8) *on't tangle yourself in the mud—-!*
9) *Don't stop ● living!*
10) *Don't let it intimidate you!*

11) *Don't trust everything you hear!*
12) *Don't be pessimistic and look at half full!*
13) *Don't lose faith in God the Lord of earth and heaven!*
14) *Don't lose focus!*
15) *Don't be down in ourselves!*
16) *Don't overcome by evil!*
17) *Don't cry 😭 or she'd any tears!*
18) *Don't Be Fearful but Joyful!*

The Second Wave Isn't As Bad As The First Wave!

Brethren, Stay Strong Against the Second Wave and Arm Yourself with Faith and Mask to Defeat it as You Defeated the First Wave!

The Almighty provided His children with Natural Vaccine called "Autoimmunity" within our flesh and blood to combat viruses, weaken them and ultimately kill them!

God knows our weak nature and the grandiose fake minds of our scientists and the powerless so called "Modern Medicine", and the clueless of so called "Artificial Intelligence" and stupidity of so called "Digital Informatics"

In fact God laughs at them saying; "He that sitteth in the heavens shall laugh: the Lord shall have them in derision. Then shall he speak unto them in his wrath, and vex them in his sore displeasure. Yet have I set my king upon my holy hill of Zion. I will declare the decree: the Lord hath said unto me, Thou art my Son; this day have I begotten thee. Ask of me, and I shall give thee the heathen for thine inheritance, and the uttermost parts of the earth for thy possession. Thou shalt break them with a rod of iron; thou shalt dash them in pieces like a potter's vessel. Be wise now therefore, O ye kings: be instructed, ye judges of the earth. Serve the Lord with fear, and rejoice with trembling-"

As it is written: *"Why do the heathen rage, and the people imagine a vain thing? [2] The kings of the earth set themselves, and the rulers take counsel together, against the Lord, and against his anointed, saying, [3] Let us break their bands asunder, and cast away their cords from us. [4] He that sitteth in the heavens shall laugh: the Lord shall have them in derision. [5] Then shall he speak unto them in his wrath, and vex them in his sore displeasure. [6] Yet have I set my king upon my holy hill of Zion. [7] I will declare the decree: the Lord hath said unto me, Thou art my Son; this day have I begotten thee. [8] Ask of me, and I shall give thee the heathen for thine inheritance, and the uttermost parts of the earth for thy possession. [9] Thou shalt break them with a rod of iron; thou shalt dash them in pieces like a potter's vessel. [10] Be wise now therefore, O ye kings: be instructed, ye judges of the earth. [11] Serve the Lord with fear, and rejoice with trembling. [12] Kiss the Son, lest he be angry, and ye perish from the way, when his wrath is kindled but a little. Blessed are all they that put their trust in him."*

Psalm 2:1-12 KJV
Therefore, Don't Be Fearful but Joyful! The Second Wave Isn't As Bad As The First Wave! Stay Strong Against the Second Wave and Arm with Faith and Mask to Defeat it as the First Wave was Conquered!

Now let us all praise our Lord Jesus the Conquer of all our enemies and the True Healer against all pandemics singing increase the praises to Christ with our tongues, lift up Jesus with our hearts and sing to our savior with our tunes saying with those Middle East Arabic Christians:

https://www.facebook.com/WheyJeremiah/videos/629162931062183/?vh=e&d=n

Our Savior has triumphed over the darkness and it's authority and lit up our days and give them joyful colors and the light of day is increasing:

https://www.facebook.com/WheyJeremiah/videos/629162931062183/?vh=e&d=n

Psalm 147
Praise ye the Lord: for it is good to sing praises unto our God; for it is pleasant; and praise is comely. The Lord doth build up Jerusalem: he gathereth together the outcasts of Israel. He healeth the broken in heart, and bindeth up their wounds. He telleth the number of the stars; he calleth them all by their names. Great is our Lord, and of great power: his understanding is infinite. The Lord lifteth up the meek: he casteth the wicked down to the ground. Sing unto the Lord with thanksgiving; sing praise upon the harp unto our God: Who covereth the heaven with clouds, who prepareth rain for the earth, who maketh grass to grow upon the mountains. He giveth to the beast his food, and to the young ravens which cry. [10] He delighteth not in the strength of the horse: he taketh not pleasure in the legs of a man. The Lord taketh pleasure in them that fear him, in those that hope in his mercy. Praise the Lord, O Jerusalem; praise thy God, O Zion. For he hath strengthened the bars of thy gates; he hath blessed thy children within thee. He maketh peace in thy borders, and filleth thee with the finest of the wheat. He sendeth forth his commandment upon earth: his word runneth very swiftly. He giveth snow like wool: he scattereth the hoarfrost like ashes. He casteth forth his ice like morsels: who can stand before his cold? He sendeth out his word, and melteth them: he causeth his wind to blow, and the waters flow. He sheweth his

word unto Jacob, his statutes and his judgments unto Israel. He hath not dealt so with any nation: and as for his judgments, they have not known them. Praise ye the Lord.

Psalm 148

Praise ye the Lord. Praise ye the Lord from the heavens: praise him in the heights. Praise ye him, all his angels: praise ye him, all his hosts. Praise ye him, sun and moon: praise him, all ye stars of light. Praise him, ye heavens of heavens, and ye waters that be above the heavens. Let them praise the name of the Lord: for he commanded, and they were created. He hath also stablished them for ever and ever: he hath made a decree which shall not pass. Praise the Lord from the earth, ye dragons, and all deeps: Fire, and hail; snow, and vapour; stormy wind fulfilling his word: Mountains, and all hills; fruitful trees, and all cedars: Beasts, and all cattle; creeping things, and flying fowl: Kings of the earth, and all people; princes, and all judges of the earth: Both young men, and maidens; old men, and children: Let them praise the name of the Lord: for his name alone is excellent; his glory is above the earth and heaven. He also exalteth the horn of his people, the praise of all his saints; even of the children of Israel, a people near unto him. Praise ye the Lord.

We must move forward as a nation to learn from the fatal mistakes and shortcoming in order to recruit the true Doers and scientists to combat Bioweapons and Bioterrorism using such viruses and other danger species to humanity. The failure is huge to prevent early on and to find prompt treatment in the beginning of pandemic before the spread of COVID!

Amen

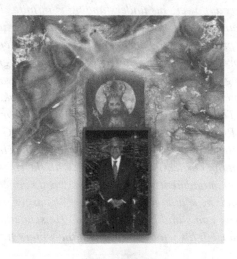

JM. Thank you

SA. ربنا يفرحك د. رمسيس ويبارك حياتك 🤲🤲

CG. You always offer positive words and thoughts in a troubled world. Thank you! Bless you always! 🖤🙏

SC. Thank you, Dr. Ghaly.

America 🇺🇸 Resume Your Life Back! Let us walk in the Vine! Let Us Rise Up and Smell the Roses 🌹🥀 Once More!

Written by Ramsis Ghaly

America 🇺🇸 2020 was a nightmare dream and envy of satanism! Come out of your homes and hidden places America 🇺🇸! Start to walk in the light 💡 in daytime before the darkness takes away and swallow you alive!

Our Lord Jesus words you you America 🇺🇸 and the World 🌏 today: "Are there not twelve hours in the day? If any man walk in the day, he stumbleth not, because he seeth the light of this world. [10] But if a man walk in the night, he stumbleth, because there is no light in him." John 11:9-10 KJV

The Coronavirus is not as strong and the caysakitues aren't as bad!

America 🇺🇸 take hold of yourself and stand up and begin to run the global race as you used to be leading the world in success!

The COVID numbers are up but the critical Intensive Care Unit is not as used to be!

The COVID is much weaker and the symptomatic patients aren't as sick!

America 🇺🇸 start to normalize your life cautiously and enough surrender your precious life!

It will take much for you America 🇺🇸 to recondition yourself!

It won't easy because leaving your homes, your nest and your remote hid out aren't that simple!

To return back and expose yourself to the outside world and start to interact with people in person isn't that trivial!

To resume Ore-COVID era, it will need years!

Furthermore wireless jobs and technologies may not be of help in the transition or supporting change!

In fact, the existing state of affairs and status quo is very attractive to continue since there is no much of hardworking, sweeting, accountability and much of exposure with no more excuses of cover up!!!

America 🇺🇸 Take your first step, wash 🧼 out the past and cheer, fear not be of good courage!

Matthew 14:27 But straightway Jesus spake unto them, saying, Be of good cheer; it is I; be not afraid.

Psalm 31:24 ESV Be strong, and let your heart take courage, all you who wait for the Lord!

Psalm 27:14 ESV Wait for the Lord; be strong, and let your heart take courage; wait for the Lord!

Joshua 1:9 ESV Have I not commanded you? Be strong and courageous. Do not be frightened, and do not be dismayed, for the Lord your God is with you wherever you go."

Acts 23:11 ESV The following night the Lord stood by him and said, "Take courage, for as you have testified to the facts about me in Jerusalem, so you must testify also in Rome."

Isaiah 40:31 ESV But they who wait for the Lord shall renew their strength; they shall mount up with wings like eagles; they shall run and not be weary; they shall walk and not faint.

America 🇺🇸 Resume Your Life Back! Let us walk in the Vine! Let Us Rise Up and Smell the Roses 🌹🎵 Once More!

Psalm 68:1-35
Let God arise, let his enemies be scattered: let them also that hate him flee before him. [2] As smoke is driven away, so drive them away: as wax melteth before the fire, so let the wicked perish at the presence of God. [3] But let the righteous be glad; let them rejoice before God: yea, let them exceedingly rejoice. [4] Sing

unto God, sing praises to his name: extol him that rideth upon the heavens by his name Jah, and rejoice before him. [5] A father of the fatherless, and a judge of the widows, is God in his holy habitation. [6] God setteth the solitary in families: he bringeth out those which are bound with chains: but the rebellious dwell in a dry land. [7] O God, when thou wentest forth before thy people, when thou didst march through the wilderness; Selah: [8] The earth shook, the heavens also dropped at the presence of God: even Sinai itself was moved at the presence of God, the God of Israel. [9] Thou, O God, didst send a plentiful rain, whereby thou didst confirm thine inheritance, when it was weary. [10] Thy congregation hath dwelt therein: thou, O God, hast prepared of thy goodness for the poor. [11] The Lord gave the word: great was the company of those that published it. [12] Kings of armies did flee apace: and she that tarried at home divided the spoil. [13] Though ye have lien among the pots, yet shall ye be as the wings of a dove covered with silver, and her feathers with yellow gold. [14] When the Almighty scattered kings in it, it was white as snow in Salmon. [15] The hill of God is as the hill of Bashan; an high hill as the hill of Bashan. [16] Why leap ye, ye high hills? this is the hill which God desireth to dwell in; yea, the Lord will dwell in it for ever. [17] The chariots of God are twenty thousand, even thousands of angels: the Lord is among them, as in Sinai, in the holy place. [18] Thou hast ascended on high, thou hast led captivity captive: thou hast received gifts for men; yea, for the rebellious also, that the Lord God might dwell among them. [19] Blessed be the Lord, who daily loadeth us with benefits, even the God of our salvation. Selah. [20] He that is our God is the God of salvation; and unto God the Lord belong the issues from death. [21] But God shall wound the head of his enemies, and the hairy scalp of such an one as goeth on still in his trespasses. [22] The Lord said, I will bring again from Bashan, I will bring my people again from the depths of the sea: [23] That thy foot may be dipped in the blood of thine enemies, and the tongue of thy dogs in the same. [24] They have seen thy goings, O God; even the goings of my God, my King, in the sanctuary. [25] The singers went before, the players on instruments followed after; among them were the damsels playing with timbrels. [26] Bless ye God in the congregations, even the Lord, from the fountain of Israel. [27] There is little Benjamin with their ruler, the princes of Judah and their council, the princes of Zebulun, and the princes of Naphtali. [28] Thy God hath commanded thy strength: strengthen, O God, that which thou hast wrought for us. [29] Because of thy temple at Jerusalem shall kings bring presents unto thee. [30] Rebuke the company of spearmen, the multitude of the bulls, with the calves of the people, till every one submit himself with pieces of silver: scatter thou the people that delight in war. [31] Princes shall come out of Egypt; Ethiopia shall soon stretch out her hands unto God. [32] Sing unto God, ye kingdoms of the earth; O sing praises unto the Lord; Selah: [33] To him that rideth upon the heavens of heavens, which were of old; lo, he doth send out his voice, and that a mighty voice. [34] Ascribe ye strength unto God: his excellency is over Israel, and his strength is in the clouds. [35] O God, thou art terrible out of thy holy places: the God of Israel is he that giveth strength and power unto his people. Blessed be God.

America 🇺🇸 Resume Your Life Back! Let us walk in the Vine! Let Us Rise Up and Smell the Roses 🌹🌷 Once More!

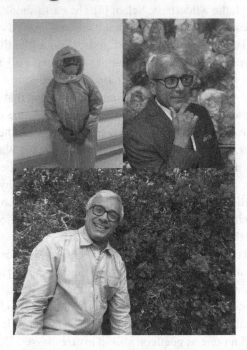

AV. Thank u so much Dr Ghaly for these wonderful verses of truth & encouragement! SC. You prayers fill me with hope and tears of joy!
SC. You prayers fill me with hope and tears of joy!

Morning 11/12/2020 to you all and to our Lord Jesus and the earth and heaven above and to all our God creation though the darkness of political wars and gloominess of COVID Surge!

Thank you 🙏 Lord and our Savior Jesus for the gift of today's early morning sun rise!

Daniel said, "Let the name of God be blessed forever and ever, for wisdom and power belong to Him." Daniel 2:20

You all have blessed day and go looking up to our Lord in heaven and be safe to be His will and not our will in earth as in heaven Amen 🙏

"After this manner therefore pray ye: Our Father which art in heaven, Hallowed be thy name. [10] Thy kingdom come. Thy will be done in earth, as it is in heaven. [11] Give us this day our daily bread. [12] And forgive us our debts, as we forgive our debtors. [13] And lead us not into temptation, but deliver us from evil: For thine is the kingdom, and the power, and the glory, for ever. Amen. [14] For if ye forgive men their trespasses, your heavenly Father will also forgive you:" Mathew 6:9-14 KJV

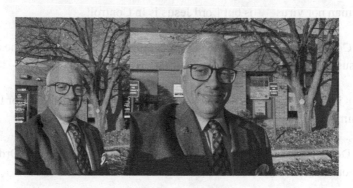

LS. Amen 🙏

AV. Good Morning Dr Ghaly! Thank you for precious words of truth! GBYD 🐾🙏

TN. Looking great Dr. Ghaly! Have a wonderful day 🤍

KM. Be safe Dr CG. Amen! Stay safe!

MB. Nice morning Dr.Ghaly. 🖤🙏

AC. And Blessings on YOUR day Dr. 🖤🌻🌷

TH. Your posts always start my day with a positive attitude!!

BC. The start of a good day! See you soon.

VD. Stay safe Dr. AS. God bless you have a wonderful day

DL. Amen 🙏

CG. Good morning and what a beautiful morning it is. Hope you have a wonderful day. Bless you! 🖤🙏🇺🇸

RW. Good morning Dr. Ghaly, have a great day

JC. You always have that wonderful smile, Good morning Dr. 🙏

RM. Good Morning and God bless you 🙏🙏 Be safe 🐚

KE. Praying

MN. Amen

KZ. Someone got a haircut!

MR. Looking great doctor God bless you 😍😍

RS. God Bless You Dr. Ghaly! Stay safe! 🖤

God Almighty Our Lord Jesus is in Control!

Written by Ramsis Ghaly

In the midst of the widespread tribulation and fears, let us remember that God Almighty Our Lord Jesus is in Control!

Neither man nor virus 🦠 is but Lord Jesus is In Control!

Neither Coronavirus nor Pandemic nor epidemic nor illnesses nor sickness is but Lord Jesus is In Control!

Neither Kings nor Queens, Presidents nor Prime Minister nor Rulers, nor Leaders nor Commanders nor Giants are but Lord Jesus is In Control!

Neither Doctrine nor Supreme Court nor Court nor Law nor worldly Orders nor Regulations are but Lord Jesus is In Control!

Neither political party nor COVID virus 🦠 is but Lord Jesus is In Control!

Neither Chinese High Tech Virology Lab nor the scientists are but Lord Jesus is In Control!

Neither the wise of this world nor the rich but Lord Jesus is In Control!

Neither the haters of mankind nor the haters of good are but Lord Jesus is In Control!

Neither the opportunistic nor the wicked is but Lord Jesus is In Control!

Neither the anti-godly nor the ungodly is but Lord Jesus is In Control!

Neither Facebook nor Twitter nor Google nor Linkin nor Wikipedia or any social media is but Lord Jesus is In Control!

Neither CNN nor FOX nor MSNBC nor CNBC nor Bloomberg nor Headline nor ABC nor BBC nor any News is but Lord Jesus is In Control!

Neither Washington Post nor Wall Street nor New York Times, USA Today nor Herald nor Tribune nor any Newspapers are but Lord Jesus is In Control!

Neither the millionaires nor the Billionaires nor the most affluent but Lord Jesus is In Control!

Neither satan nor darkness is but Lord Jesus is In Control!

Neither wars nor earthquakes or hurricanes are but Lord Jesus is In Control!

Neither global warming nor flooding are but Lord Jesus is In Control!

Neither bioweapons nor terrors nor army nor machine guns nor sonic bombs nor explosives nor any weapon of evils are but Lord Jesus is In Control!

Biblical Verses
Isaiah 35:4 say to those with fearful hearts, "Be strong, do not fear; your God will come, he will come with vengeance; with divine retribution he will come to save you."

Isaiah 43:1 But now, this is what the LORD says— he who created you, Jacob, he who formed you, Israel: "Do not fear, for I have redeemed you; I have summoned you by name; you are mine.

Joshua 1:9 Have I not commanded you? Be strong and courageous. Do not be afraid; do not be discouraged, for the LORD your God will be with you wherever you go."

Matthew 6:34 Therefore do not worry about tomorrow, for tomorrow will worry about itself. Each day has enough trouble of its own.

John 14:27 Peace I leave with you; my peace I give you. I do not give to you as the world gives. Do not let your hearts be troubled and do not be afraid.

Psalm 23:4 Even though I walk through the darkest valley, I will fear no evil, for you are with me; your rod and your staff, they comfort me.

Psalm 34:4 I sought the LORD, and he answered me; he delivered me from all my fears.

Psalm 94:19 When anxiety was great within me, your consolation brought me joy.

Romans 8:38-39 For I am convinced that neither death nor life, neither angels nor demons, neither the present nor the future, nor any powers, neither height nor

673

depth, nor anything else in all creation, will be able to separate us from the love of God that is in Christ Jesus our Lord.

Psalm 27:1 The LORD is my light and my salvation— whom shall I fear? The LORD is the stronghold of my life— of whom shall I be afraid?

1 Peter 5:6-7 Humble yourselves, therefore, under God's mighty hand, that he may lift you up in due time. Cast all your anxiety on him because he cares for you.

Psalm 118:6 The LORD is with me; I will not be afraid. What can mere mortals do to me?

Psalm 115:11 You who fear him, trust in the LORD— he is their help and shield.

Romans 8:28 ESV
And we know that for those who love God all things work together for good, for those who are called according to his purpose.

Isaiah 41:10 ESV
Fear not, for I am with you; be not dismayed, for I am your God; I will strengthen you, I will help you, I will uphold you with my righteous right hand.

Proverbs 19:21 ESV
Many are the plans in the mind of a man, but it is the purpose of the Lord that will stand.

Proverbs 16:9 ESV
The heart of man plans his way, but the Lord establishes his steps.

1 Corinthians 10:13 ESV
No temptation has overtaken you that is not common to man. God is faithful, and he will not let you be tempted beyond your ability, but with the temptation he will also provide the way of escape, that you may be able to endure it.

Joshua 1:9 ESV
Have I not commanded you? Be strong and courageous. Do not be frightened, and do not be dismayed, for the Lord your God is with you wherever you go."

Matthew 6:34 ESV
"Therefore do not be anxious about tomorrow, for tomorrow will be anxious for itself. Sufficient for the day is its own trouble.

Jeremiah 29:11 ESV

For I know the plans I have for you, declares the Lord, plans for welfare and not for evil, to give you a future and a hope.

Ephesians 1:11 ESV

In him we have obtained an inheritance, having been predestined according to the purpose of him who works all things according to the counsel of his will,

Psalm 27:1 ESV

Of David. The Lord is my light and my salvation; whom shall I fear? The Lord is the stronghold of my life; of whom shall I be afraid?

Psalm 115:3 ESV

Our God is in the heavens; he does all that he pleases.

Matthew 19:26 ESV

But Jesus looked at them and said, "With man this is impossible, but with God all things are possible."

2 Timothy 1:7 ESV

For God gave us a spirit not of fear but of power and love and self-control.

Isaiah 45:6-7 ESV

That people may know, from the rising of the sun and from the west, that there is none besides me; I am the Lord, and there is no other. I form light and create darkness, I make well-being and create calamity, I am the Lord, who does all these things.

Isaiah 45:7 ESV

I form light and create darkness, I make well-being and create calamity, I am the Lord, who does all these things.

Isaiah 14:24 ESV

The Lord of hosts has sworn: "As I have planned, so shall it be, and as I have purposed, so shall it stand,

Proverbs 21:1 ESV

The king's heart is a stream of water in the hand of the Lord; he turns it wherever he will.

Psalm 94:19 ESV
When the cares of my heart are many, your consolations cheer my soul.

Psalm 46:1 ESV
To the choirmaster. Of the Sons of Korah. According to Alamoth. A Song. God is our refuge and strength, a very present help in trouble.

John 14:27 ESV
Peace I leave with you; my peace I give to you. Not as the world gives do I give to you. Let not your hearts be troubled, neither let them be afraid.

Philippians 4:6-7 ESV
Do not be anxious about anything, but in everything by prayer and supplication with thanksgiving let your requests be made known to God. And the peace of God, which surpasses all understanding, will guard your hearts and your minds in Christ Jesus.

Psalm 22:28 ESV
For kingship belongs to the Lord, and he rules over the nations.

Proverbs 16:4 ESV
The Lord has made everything for its purpose, even the wicked for the day of trouble.

Luke 12:22-26 ESV
And he said to his disciples, "Therefore I tell you, do not be anxious about your life, what you will eat, nor about your body, what you will put on. For life is more than food, and the body more than clothing. Consider the ravens: they neither sow nor reap, they have neither storehouse nor barn, and yet God feeds them. Of how much more value are you than the birds! And which of you by being anxious can add a single hour to his span of life? If then you are not able to do as small a thing as that, why are you anxious about the rest?

Isaiah 55:8-11 ESV
For my thoughts are not your thoughts, neither are your ways my ways, declares the Lord. For as the heavens are higher than the earth, so are my ways higher than your ways and my thoughts than your thoughts. "For as the rain and the snow come down from heaven and do not return there but water the earth, making it bring forth and sprout, giving seed to the sower and bread to the eater, so shall my word be that goes out from my mouth; it shall not return to me empty, but it shall accomplish that which I purpose, and shall succeed in the thing for which I sent it.

Job 12:10 ESV
In his hand is the life of every living thing and the breath of all mankind.

1 Peter 5:6-7 ESV
Humble yourselves, therefore, under the mighty hand of God so that at the proper time he may exalt you, casting all your anxieties on him, because he cares for you.

1 John 4:18 ESV
There is no fear in love, but perfect love casts out fear. For fear has to do with punishment, and whoever fears has not been perfected in love.

1 Chronicles 29:11-12 ESV
Yours, O Lord, is the greatness and the power and the glory and the victory and the majesty, for all that is in the heavens and in the earth is yours. Yours is the kingdom, O Lord, and you are exalted as head above all. Both riches and honor come from you, and you rule over all. In your hand are power and might, and in your hand it is to make great and to give strength to all.

Psalm 118:6-7 ESV
The Lord is on my side; I will not fear. What can man do to me? The Lord is on my side as my helper; I shall look in triumph on those who hate me.

Revelation 1:17 ESV
When I saw him, I fell at his feet as though dead. But he laid his right hand on me, saying, "Fear not, I am the first and the last,

Psalm 23:4 ESV
Even though I walk through the valley of the shadow of death, I will fear no evil, for you are with me; your rod and your staff, they comfort me.

Psalm 56:3 ESV
When I am afraid, I put my trust in you.

Psalm 23:1-6 ESV
A Psalm of David. The Lord is my shepherd; I shall not want. He makes me lie down in green pastures. He leads me beside still waters. He restores my soul. He leads me in paths of righteousness for his name's sake. Even though I walk through the valley of the shadow of death, I will fear no evil, for you are with me; your rod and your staff, they comfort me. You prepare a table before me in the presence of my enemies; you anoint my head with oil; my cup overflows. ...

Psalm 103:19 ESV
The Lord has established his throne in the heavens, and his kingdom rules over all.

1 Timothy 6:15 ESV
Which he will display at the proper time—he who is the blessed and only Sovereign, the King of kings and Lord of lords,

Jeremiah 32:27 ESV
"Behold, I am the Lord, the God of all flesh. Is anything too hard for me?

Hebrews 1:3 ESV
He is the radiance of the glory of God and the exact imprint of his nature, and he upholds the universe by the word of his power. After making purification for sins, he sat down at the right hand of the Majesty on high,

Genesis 50:20 ESV
As for you, you meant evil against me, but God meant it for good, to bring it about that many people should be kept alive, as they are today.

Psalm 55:22 ESV
Cast your burden on the Lord, and he will sustain you; he will never permit the righteous to be moved.

Philippians 4:13 ESV
I can do all things through him who strengthens me.

Daniel 4:35 ESV
All the inhabitants of the earth are accounted as nothing, and he does according to his will among the host of heaven and among the inhabitants of the earth; and none can stay his hand or say to him, "What have you done?"

2 Chronicles 20:6 ESV
And said, "O Lord, God of our fathers, are you not God in heaven? You rule over all the kingdoms of the nations. In your hand are power and might, so that none is able to withstand you.

Job 42:2 ESV
"I know that you can do all things, and that no purpose of yours can be thwarted.

Lamentations 3:37 ESV
Who has spoken and it came to pass, unless the Lord has commanded it?

1 Peter 5:7 ESV
Casting all your anxieties on him, because he cares for you.

Psalm 135:6 ESV
Whatever the Lord pleases, he does, in heaven and on earth, in the seas and all deeps.

Matthew 10:29 ESV
Are not two sparrows sold for a penny? And not one of them will fall to the ground apart from your Father.

John 16:33 ESV
I have said these things to you, that in me you may have peace. In the world you will have tribulation. But take heart; I have overcome the world."

Isaiah 14:27 ESV
For the Lord of hosts has purposed, and who will annul it? His hand is stretched out, and who will turn it back?

Psalm 34:7 ESV
The angel of the Lord encamps around those who fear him, and delivers them.

Psalm 46:10 ESV
"Be still, and know that I am God. I will be exalted among the nations, I will be exalted in the earth!"

Mark 6:50 ESV
For they all saw him and were terrified. But immediately he spoke to them and said, "Take heart; it is I. Do not be afraid."

Revelation 1:1-20 ESV
The revelation of Jesus Christ, which God gave him to show to his servants the things that must soon take place. He made it known by sending his angel to his servant John, who bore witness to the word of God and to the testimony of Jesus Christ, even to all that he saw. Blessed is the one who reads aloud the words of this prophecy, and blessed are those who hear, and who keep what is written in it, for the time is near. John to the seven churches that are in Asia: Grace to you and peace from him who is and who was and who is to come, and from the seven spirits who are before his throne, and from Jesus Christ the faithful witness, the firstborn of the dead, and the ruler of kings on earth. To him who loves us and has freed us from our sins by his blood ...

Isaiah 43:1 ESV
But now thus says the Lord, he who created you, O Jacob, he who formed you, O Israel: "Fear not, for I have redeemed you; I have called you by name, you are mine.

Zephaniah 3:17 ESV
The Lord your God is in your midst, a mighty one who will save; he will rejoice over you with gladness; he will quiet you by his love; he will exult over you with loud singing.

Amos 3:6 ESV
Is a trumpet blown in a city, and the people are not afraid? Does disaster come to a city, unless the Lord has done it?

Mark 5:36 ESV
But overhearing what they said, Jesus said to the ruler of the synagogue, "Do not fear, only believe."

Genesis 1:1 ESV
In the beginning, God created the heavens and the earth.

Psalm 34:4 ESV
I sought the Lord, and he answered me and delivered me from all my fears.

Romans 8:38-39 ESV
For I am sure that neither death nor life, nor angels nor rulers, nor things present nor things to come, nor powers, nor height nor depth, nor anything else in all creation, will be able to separate us from the love of God in Christ Jesus our Lord.

Daniel 2:21 ESV
He changes times and seasons; he removes kings and sets up kings; he gives wisdom to the wise and knowledge to those who have understanding;

1 Peter 3:14 ESV
But even if you should suffer for righteousness' sake, you will be blessed. Have no fear of them, nor be troubled,

Proverbs 16:33 ESV
The lot is cast into the lap, but its every decision is from the Lord.

Isaiah 41:2 ESV

Who stirred up one from the east whom victory meets at every step? He gives up nations before him, so that he tramples kings underfoot; he makes them like dust with his sword, like driven stubble with his bow.

Isaiah 43:9 ESV

All the nations gather together, and the peoples assemble. Who among them can declare this, and show us the former things? Let them bring their witnesses to prove them right, and let them hear and say, It is true.

Psalm 24:1 ESV

A Psalm of David. The earth is the Lord's and the fullness thereof, the world and those who dwell therein,

2 Timothy 1:6 ESV

For this reason I remind you to fan into flame the gift of God, which is in you through the laying on of my hands,

Isaiah 35:4 ESV

Say to those who have an anxious heart, "Be strong; fear not! Behold, your God will come with vengeance, with the recompense of God. He will come and save you."

John 14:5 ESV

Thomas said to him, "Lord, we do not know where you are going. How can we know the way?"

Psalm 91:4 ESV

He will cover you with his pinions, and under his wings you will find refuge; his faithfulness is a shield and buckler.

Deuteronomy 31:6 ESV

Be strong and courageous. Do not fear or be in dread of them, for it is the Lord your God who goes with you. He will not leave you or forsake you."

1 Chronicles 29:11 ESV

Yours, O Lord, is the greatness and the power and the glory and the victory and the majesty, for all that is in the heavens and in the earth is yours. Yours is the kingdom, O Lord, and you are exalted as head above all.

Psalm 66:7 ESV
Who rules by his might forever, whose eyes keep watch on the nations— let not the rebellious exalt themselves. Selah

Ephesians 1:11-12 ESV
In him we have obtained an inheritance, having been predestined according to the purpose of him who works all things according to the counsel of his will, so that we who were the first to hope in Christ might be to the praise of his glory.

Romans 13:1 ESV
Let every person be subject to the governing authorities. For there is no authority except from God, and those that exist have been instituted by God.

Matthew 6:12 ESV
And forgive us our debts, as we also have forgiven our debtors.

Ephesians 1:4 ESV
Even as he chose us in him before the foundation of the world, that we should be holy and blameless before him. In love

Zechariah 4:6 ESV
Then he said to me, "This is the word of the Lord to Zerubbabel: Not by might, nor by power, but by my Spirit, says the Lord of hosts.

Revelation 1:8 ESV
"I am the Alpha and the Omega," says the Lord God, "who is and who was and who is to come, the Almighty."

1 Corinthians 13:12 ESV
For now we see in a mirror dimly, but then face to face. Now I know in part; then I shall know fully, even as I have been fully known.

John 6:37 ESV
All that the Father gives me will come to me, and whoever comes to me I will never cast out.

Psalm 27:14 ESV
Wait for the Lord; be strong, and let your heart take courage; wait for the Lord!

John 13:7 ESV
Jesus answered him, "What I am doing you do not understand now, but afterward you will understand."

Romans 3:23 ESV
For all have sinned and fall short of the glory of God,

Hebrews 11:1-40 ESV
Now faith is the assurance of things hoped for, the conviction of things not seen. For by it the people of old received their commendation. By faith we understand that the universe was created by the word of God, so that what is seen was not made out of things that are visible. By faith Abel offered to God a more acceptable sacrifice than Cain, through which he was commended as righteous, God commending him by accepting his gifts. And through his faith, though he died, he still speaks. By faith Enoch was taken up so that he should not see death, and he was not found, because God had taken him. Now before he was taken he was commended as having pleased God. ...

Philippians 4:19 ESV
And my God will supply every need of yours according to his riches in glory in Christ Jesus.

Psalm 91:1-16 ESV
He who dwells in the shelter of the Most High will abide in the shadow of the Almighty. I will say to the Lord, "My refuge and my fortress, my God, in whom I trust." For he will deliver you from the snare of the fowler and from the deadly pestilence. He will cover you with his pinions, and under his wings you will find refuge; his faithfulness is a shield and buckler. You will not fear the terror of the night, nor the arrow that flies by day, ...

Revelation 1:1 ESV
The revelation of Jesus Christ, which God gave him to show to his servants the things that must soon take place. He made it known by sending his angel to his servant John,

Romans 9:21 ESV
Has the potter no right over the clay, to make out of the same lump one vessel for honorable use and another for dishonorable use?

Isaiah 8:1-22 ESV
Then the Lord said to me, "Take a large tablet and write on it in common characters, 'Belonging to Maher-shalal-hash-baz.' And I will get reliable witnesses, Uriah the priest and Zechariah the son of Jeberechiah, to attest for me." And I went to the prophetess, and she conceived and bore a son. Then the Lord said to me, "Call his name Maher-shalal-hash-baz; for before the boy knows how to cry 'My father' or 'My mother,' the wealth of Damascus and the spoil of Samaria will be carried away before the king of Assyria." The Lord spoke to me again: ...

John 3:16-17 ESV
"For God so loved the world, that he gave his only Son, that whoever believes in him should not perish but have eternal life. For God did not send his Son into the world to condemn the world, but in order that the world might be saved through him.

Hebrews 11:3 ESV
By faith we understand that the universe was created by the word of God, so that what is seen was not made out of things that are visible.

John 19:11 ESV
Jesus answered him, "You would have no authority over me at all unless it had been given you from above. Therefore he who delivered me over to you has the greater sin."

Acts 17:10-11 ESV
The brothers immediately sent Paul and Silas away by night to Berea, and when they arrived they went into the Jewish synagogue. Now these Jews were more noble than those in Thessalonica; they received the word with all eagerness, examining the Scriptures daily to see if these things were so.

Genesis 8:22 ESV
While the earth remains, seedtime and harvest, cold and heat, summer and winter, day and night, shall not cease."

Jonah 1:4 ESV
But the Lord hurled a great wind upon the sea, and there was a mighty tempest on the sea, so that the ship threatened to break up.

James 1:13 ESV
Let no one say when he is tempted, "I am being tempted by God," for God cannot be tempted with evil, and he himself tempts no one.

Romans 8:29-30 ESV

For those whom he foreknew he also predestined to be conformed to the image of his Son, in order that he might be the firstborn among many brothers. And those whom he predestined he also called, and those whom he called he also justified, and those whom he justified he also glorified.

Psalm 9:10 ESV

And those who know your name put their trust in you, for you, O Lord, have not forsaken those who seek you.

VW. Amen!

VG. Amin!

MY. God bless you Dr Ramses Amen

Through the Atrocities caused by COVID Surge and Political Unrest, You aren't Forgotten O Bravery Soldier of the Freedom!

A Poem in the Memory of All the Veterans In Veterans Day!
Written by Ramsis Ghaly

It was meant for me to sing with those who sacrificed their lives for us. As our Lord Jesus said there is no much love than someone put his life for another. He was our first Veteran that put His Life by his own will, for others in order for all of us to find life in Him. The same as all our veterans.

I meant to sing with them Happy Veteran's Day. I was joined by so many that wished to join. It is the love that deep rooted in each of them that made me do so.

It is the time for me and you to join them and do what they had done and carry on to the generations to come.

How much I wish this is not true! How much I wish that all things are fair!

When I looked at this photo and I read the caption my soul cried and I said: "it can't be and it must stop ⬤"!

I saw pictures of so many heroes we cherished with different colors, shapes and ethnicity under one roof America 🏴 and one land called my sweet home my home United States 🏴 of America 🏴 under one flag of our home 🏴!

As the Holy Trinity the Father, the Son and the Holy Spirit is One God so is the human race the spirit, soul and the flesh in one human being!

How much I wish this is not true!
How much I wish that all things are fair!
Wars see no color as death see no race
Crying is no difference between cultures as tears pour and heart aches when we loose a soul
To you up there, our love 💜 to you is the same!
To you up high our gratitude 🙏 to you is the same!
To you flying high, we salute 🇺🇸 you is the same to the last breathe!
How much I wish this is not true!
How much I wish that all things are fair!
One God One Spirit and one human race!
One country, One Nation and One flag 🇺🇸!
To you up there, our love 💜 to you is the same!
To you up high our gratitude 🙏 to you is the same!
To you flying high, we salute 🇺🇸 you is the same to the last breathe!
How much I wish this is not true!
How much I wish that all things are fair!
Love 💜 is One and God is the Love 💜 but the haters of mankind are many demons Satan and satans!
MAY I SAY:
The tears 😢 are the same colorless and pure!
The bloodshed is the same red blood with agony from the heart!
The sorrows are the same of sadness of life being cut short!
The grieve is the same of heartbroken 😔 of human life no more!
The loss is the same of a human life forever is taken away from the loved ones and left behind in the world 🌍 we live in!
The spirit is the same; a breath from God the Lord!
The soul is the same; a life living within the flesh made from the ground dust.
The human heart 💜 is the same; a life beating within the temple of the Lord!
The human brain 🧠 is the same; a glorious treasure within the bones!

The Love 💜 is the same; a precious diamond within the soul!
The source of Love 💜 is the same; a God gift to us all!
Jesus Christ is the same; The Savior of the World 📖, God in the flesh!

God the Creator is the same; The Most High of us all the Heavenly Father of all mankind!

The Cross ✝ is the same; a sacrificed soul hanged in the flesh bleeding to death for others!

As the Very First Veteran of mankind that laid down His Life for the world, God in the flesh, the Redeemer of all people Jesus Christ Our Lord

Jesus; The Good Shephard said: "Greater love has no one than this, than to lay down one's life for his friends." (John 15:13)

I KNEW LONG AGO

We all are the same and equal, created by One God the Creator of all things and born of one father Adam and one mother Eve!

The male sperm has the same color among all nations as also the female ovum among the generations!

Moreover, the human compatibility for conception is the same among all cultures producing the same newborn baby breathing the air we share, the sun ☀ we enjoy, the moon 🌙 we look at as we all walk, run and race in one globe 🌐!

In all the colors, all have the same impact and the same effect: Battles devastate as fires 🔥 burns as bullets kill as explosives destroy any human flesh!

TODAY IS THE DAY

Today is the day to commemorate all the lives laid down for others!
Today is the day to pay respect for all those who sacrificed their gift of life f
or the freedom we all enjoy today and forever!
Today is the day to love one another for ever more as our veterans made the world better place for the generations to follow!
Let us remember the words of Love 💜 from Our Master and Savior said: "This is My commandment, that you love one another as I have loved you. 13 Greater love has no one than this, than to lay down one's life for his friends." (John 15:12-13)
So from now; Let us put our differences aside!
Let us cast out the divisions among us! And Let us love 💜 one another!
One God One Spirit and one human race!
One country, One Nation and One flag 🏳!
To you up there, our love 💜 to you is the same!
To you up high our gratitude 🙏 to you is the same!
To you flying high, we salute 🏳 you is the same to the last breathe!

How much I wish this is not true!
How much I wish that all things are fair!
To you all: To each of You by name: To every soul sacrificed: Thank you and we all for ever grateful.
You all made for us the steps that we must follow and raised the bar we must reach higher and higher to be handed to our children and all the grandchildren to come!
May you all Rest In Peace in the hands of the Lord surrounded with the Divine Love and care until we see you again as we pray for you all today and tomorrow!!!!

Thank you all

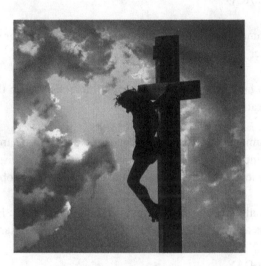

CG. This is a beautiful tribute to all veterans living and deceased. Bless them all. 🖤🙏

On 11/11/2020, we Remember President Trump: My poem to President Trump 2018 as he was Paying Respect visiting all alone Aisene Marne American Cemetery near Bellevue France 🎌 at Veterans Day! Thank you Mr President!

On 11/11/2018 Poem:

A Poem Dedicated to the president Donald Trump and his visit to the
Aisne Marne American Cemetery near the Belleau France 🖤🇺🇸
Written by
Ramsis Ghaly

I came across this photo of our president and it says it all!
I may be alone but I am with them 🖤🇺🇸!

I am all alone visiting the souls 💜🇺🇸 I cherished most!
I may not be with you but I am with them 💜🇺🇸!
I came thousands of miles away to pay tribute to them 💜🇺🇸 and not for they!
I put the American flag over each bringing them love from my home and their home America 💜🇺🇸!
Friends, I made the journey for them 💜🇺🇸 and not for they!
So, don't be judgmental because I am alone!
Thank you Mr President Trump for visiting them the American Heroes at the Marne American Cemetery, Belleau in France 💜🇺🇸 and from home we salute you and them sending our love and prayers 💜🇺🇸 Amen!

++++

From the kings places, I excused myself to be with them 💜🇺🇸; the American heroes of World War I 💜🇺🇸!
Thousands miles from home I flew in the freezing cold to visit the Aisne Marne American Cemetery near the Belleau Wood battleground, in Belleau, France, 90 kilometers northeast of the capital 💜🇺🇸!
It is the closest place to my heart where U.S. troops 💜🇺🇸 had their breakthrough battle by stopping a German push for Paris shortly after entering the war in 1917!

+++

In serenity, I took time to reflect!
In a solitude I walked the steps to visit the coffins one by one 💜🇺🇸!
Barefooted, I kneeled to salute each and all the American veterans 💜🇺🇸 with sincere respect!
I put the American flag over each bringing them love from my home and their home America 💜🇺🇸!
Away from the world, I kneeled to the Lord of hosts praying for the comfort of their souls 💜🇺🇸!

+++

I may be alone but I am with them 💜🇺🇸!
I may not be with you but I am with them 💜🇺🇸!
I am all alone visiting the souls 💜🇺🇸 I cherished most 💜🇺🇸!
I came thousands of miles away to pay tribute to them and not for they!
I put the American flag over each bringing them love from my home and their home America 💜🇺🇸!
Friends, I made the journey for them 💜🇺🇸 and not for they!
So, don't be judgmental because I am alone!

Thank you Mr President Trump for visiting them the American Hero's in France 💚🇺🇸 and from home we salute you and them sending our love and prayers 💚🇺🇸 Amen

Ramsis Ghaly

In So Many Ways---

Written By Ramsis Ghaly

In so many ways, we share what we go through in our journeys.

Let us live together the life worthy in love and service one to another----

The good that we do, the bad that we do not mean to do and the ups and downs that we always face in our days.

Our minds wonders of when we began, where are we going and why should it be this way???

Friends, what matters are what we do for others and the fruits we leave behind.

In the meanwhile, we continue living, learning from the past and stronger we get and wiser we become.

In the morning, we renew our vows to the God of goodness and looking up to heavens for a better day ahead.

So my friends, today is coming to an end, yesterday is behind and tomorrow is at hand together we shall share.

Let us live together the life worthy in love and service one to another----

Respectfully
Ramsis Ghaly www.ghalyneurosurgeon.com

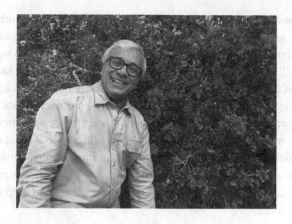

AK. Beautiful 😊💜

JC. You look very happy there, nice smile 🙏

KM. Keep smiling & shinning 💜🙏

MR. Great picture Dr. Ghaly! It shows your inner light!

LB. Looking very dapper!!!

RC. This is wonderful. Can I share it? Love your smile!

MS. Beautiful flowers behind you.

KC. Great picture!

CG. Such beautiful thoughts! Bless you! Nice picture. Miss that smile!

AB. Amen praise God

MN. Dr Ghaly your write as aways you have a great day and stay safe.

SW. Beautiful heart, Beautiful smile. 😃

SC. Yes!

RN. Beautiful 💜💜

KO. Amen, what we do for others, without asking for anything in return, is what really counts in life.

My Previous Write up about Ebola Pandemic 2014!

Ramsis Ghaly
October 15, 2014 ·
Shared with Public

EBOLA

I am do sorrowful and upset about the nursing staff got no sufficient protection and attention needed from the Dallas hospital officials. I have said it for years, it should no longer be surprise. The "cook Book" is run by no cooks or customers and forced to follow on the people that matters most. We, all healthcare providers,

691

must protect ourselves and voice our concerns. We are not just numbers to follow protocols. We are the providers. I am so proud of the nursing union voicing the concerns and frightening for the nurses even the non Dallas union staff. Good job nursing union!!!!. No one interviewed the nurses or the providers. I am sadden for the sickness of the staff. EBOLA continue grow, it is fatal and the way patients die is unimaginable, bleeding and blood running from each office. We isolated the virus 30 years ago but we did not develop vaccine or treatment for it. The reason "it was not cost effective" based on the business model that does not care about individual life lost and companies that not interested if financial profit is marginal from such a project. Life us priceless and I ask for return of the good medicine for each and for all. May God heal the victims and help us to provide cure to His children

Ramsis Ghaly
October 16, 2014 ·

EBOLA: the need of designated hospital in Each state
We going more in wrong direction. Hospitals cannot and will not be able to perfect a highly contagious and fatal disease. Please, designate one hospital in each State and put all the resources, isolation, treatment and research. Please do not subject the public and staff to more---.

October 16, 2014
Ramsis Ghaly

EBOLA
In my "last hour journey "book of Christianity and the brain back in 2010. I reflected from the Revelation that at the end of days, the wrath will come in a different non conventional forms such as viruses and mutated strains. But also in biologic and at the cell levels rather than the known old fashion. Man went beyond to areas should not go. It is the sane when man from the right and wrong tree. It is the same as man did in the time of Babylon. The revelation said to go back and stand from where man fallen. Be humble and pray in faith doing the utmost what is right.

HD. Words that become more clear as time passes. 𝗝𝗝𝗝
CG. This can certainly apply to the current pandemic.
CG. I totally agree!!!

The Year of 2021 Shall Be All About COVID 2021!!

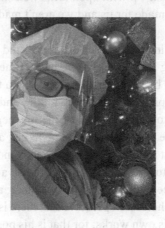

Be ready and be patient! Don't listen to false promises! The 2021 undoubtedly will be all about COVID 2021 and Politics!

As the man chases the Virus 🦠! So the virus 🦠 chases the man! So the opportunistic and the corruption chase the man! And much more surprises waiting at the door! Don't wait for either stimulus check or COVID relief! There were so much drama and confusion in 2020! let it not be that way in 2021!

It is the time for more storms and struggles! Tribulations are meant to be! Therefore, take one day at a time, cherich each minute and value the time putting things in a new prospective! Life is a gift!

The time of relief isn't yet close but you all can do it! Vaccine or no vaccine but put your hope in God and not in princes!! "Put not your trust in princes, nor in the son of man, in whom there is no help. [4] His breath goeth forth, he returneth to his earth; in that very day his thoughts perish. [5] Happy is he that hath the God of Jacob for his help, whose hope is in the Lord his God: [6] Which made heaven, and earth, the sea, and all that therein is: which keepeth truth for ever:" Psalm 146:3-6 KJV

Be in good courage and not in fear! The Lord of Lords is In Control! COVID never changed God's love to mankind or Lord's Promises to His inheritance! Thank God Up high in His kingdom no COVID and no sickness but wholeness and holiness and nothing can overcome the Spirit!

693

Our Journey on earth 🌑 is going according what is written for each of the living soul!

So let us stand up and Mask Up with open arms welcome 🔺 2021! The coming year 2021 is made for us and we aren't made for 2021!

To everything under the sin there is a season and an end so is for COVID says the preacher: "To every thing there is a season, and a time to every purpose under the heaven: [2] A time to be born, and a time to die; a time to plant, and a time to pluck up that which is planted; [3] A time to kill, and a time to heal; a time to break down, and a time to build up; [4] A time to weep, and a time to laugh; a time to mourn, and a time to dance; [6] A time to get, and a time to lose; a time to keep, and a time to cast away; [7] A time to rend, and a time to sew; a time to keep silence, and a time to speak; [8] A time to love, and a time to hate; a time of war, and a time of peace. [20] All go unto one place; all are of the dust, and all turn to dust again. [22] Wherefore I perceive that there is nothing better, than that a man should rejoice in his own works; for that is his portion: for who shall bring him to see what shall be after him?" Ecclesiastes 3:1-4,6-8,20,22 KJV

O inhabitants of earth 🌑!! So what COVID 2021, we are so ready to face reality and face the Truth! Our ancestors went though much more and so we have done so and much more for years and years!

Let us face it! We are already getting used to the change in our lives to be virtual as the technology is picking up in the digital science!

Smile and take selfi! Say hello from a distance while texting! Tun in for more zooms and drive through while the on-line will be the main stream!

The human brain 🧠 has so much potentials to carry you up through the hills! Adapt and be innovative and line-up the ideas for success!

O brethren, guess what, this Christmas 🌲 many of us including myself got virtual cakes, virtual cloth, virtual cards and virtual greetings. All of these are stored wireless in virtual hard drive despite the fact that our hands and homes are empty and never actual received any of those virtual Christmas 🌲 gifts 🎁 and greetings!

So start to adjust your daily living to COVID 2021 and be virtual and thank our Lord Jesus for 2021 in everything of everything and for everything!

Indeed, it could have been worse and many of us could have not made it thus far!

Fear Not! Let us not be troubled but ready for the Second or the Third Watch when the Master comes: "Fear not, little flock; for it is your Father's good pleasure to give you the kingdom. [33] Sell that ye have, and give alms; provide yourselves bags which wax not old, a treasure in the heavens that faileth not, where no thief approacheth, neither moth corrupteth. [34] For where your treasure is, there will your heart be also. [35] Let your loins be girded about, and your lights burning; [36] And ye yourselves like unto men that wait for their lord, when he will return from the wedding; that when he cometh and knocketh, they may open unto him immediately. [37] Blessed are those servants, whom the lord when he cometh shall find watching: verily I say unto you, that he shall gird himself, and make them to sit down to meat, and will come forth and serve them. [38] And if he shall come in the second watch, or come in the third watch, and find them so, blessed are those servants. [39] And this know, that if the goodman of the house had known what hour the thief would come, he would have watched, and not have suffered his house to be broken through. [40] Be ye therefore ready also: for the Son of man cometh at an hour when ye think not." Luke 12:32-40 KJV

Listen to our Father Daniels the thousand three hundred and five and thirty days!! Blessed is he that waiteth, and cometh to the thousand three hundred and five and thirty days: "Blessed is he that waiteth, and cometh to the thousand three hundred and five and thirty days. [13] But go thou thy way till the end be: for thou shalt rest, and stand in thy lot at the end of the days." Daniel 12:12-13 KJV

Listen to revealed Words! Bless those waithth for the Day of God: "When the Lamb broke the fifth seal, I saw underneath the altar the souls of those who had been slain because of the word of God, and because of the testimony which they had maintained; and they cried out with a loud voice, saying, "How long, O Lord, holy and true, will You refrain from judging and avenging our blood on those who dwell on the earth?" And there was given to each of them a white robe; and they were told that they should rest for a little while longer, until the number of their fellow servants and their brethren who were to be killed even as they had been, would be completed also." Revelation 6:9-11

+Biblical Verses of Waiting for the Lord;

Hosea 12:6 "Therefore, return to your God, Observe kindness and justice, And wait for your God continually." Isaiah 51:5 "My righteousness is near, My salvation has gone forth, And My arms will judge the peoples; The coastlands will wait for

Me, And for My arm they will wait expectantly." Micah 7:7 "But as for me, I will watch expectantly for the Lord; I will wait for the God of my salvation. My God will hear me." Isaiah 8:17 "And I will wait for the Lord who is hiding His face from the house of Jacob; I will even look eagerly for Him." Lamentations 3:24-26 "The Lord is my portion," says my soul, Therefore I have hope in Him." The Lord is good to those who wait for Him, To the person who seeks Him. It is good that he waits silentlyFor the salvation of the Lord."

Psalm 5:3 "In the morning, O Lord, You will hear my voice; In the morning I will order my prayer to You and eagerly watch." Psalm 27:14 "Wait for the Lord; Be strong and let your heart take courage; Yes, wait for the Lord." Psalm 33:20 "Our soul waits for the Lord; He is our help and our shield. Psalm 130:5 I wait for the Lord, my soul does wait, And in His word do I hope." Psalm 37:7 "Rest in the Lord and wait patiently for Him; Do not fret because of him who prospers in his way, Because of the man who carries out wicked schemes." Psalm 39:7 "And now, Lord, for what do I wait? My hope is in You." Psalm 123:2 "Behold, as the eyes of servants look to the hand of their master, As the eyes of a maid to the hand of her mistress, So our eyes look to the Lord our God, Until He is gracious to us." Psalm 25:5 "Lead me in Your truth and teach me, For You are the God of my salvation; For You I wait all the day. Psalm 145:15-16The eyes of all look to You, And You give them their food in due time. You open Your handAnd satisfy the desire of every living thing."

James 5:7-8 "Therefore be patient, brethren, until the coming of the Lord. The farmer waits for the precious produce of the soil, being patient about it, until it gets the early and late rains. You too be patient; strengthen your hearts, for the coming of the Lord is near."

1 Corinthians 4:5 "Therefore do not go on passing judgment before the time, but wait until the Lord comes who will both bring to light the things hidden in the darkness and disclose the motives of men's hearts; and then each man's praise will come to him from God." Titus 2:13 "looking for the blessed hope and the appearing of the glory of our great God and Savior, Christ Jesus," Hebrews 9:28 "so Christ also, having been offered once to bear the sins of many, will appear a second time for salvation without reference to sin, to those who eagerly await Him." Romans 8:23 "And not only this, but also we ourselves, having the first fruits of the Spirit, even we ourselves groan within ourselves, waiting eagerly for our adoption as sons, the redemption of our body." Galatians 5:5 "For we through the Spirit, by faith, are waiting for the hope of righteousness."

Thank you Lord Jesus for 2021, be thy will. I adore thy Name. You are In Control. My soul is subdued to thy mercy as I open a new book of my journey 2021! You never abondoned my soul and always visited me since I was formed to the end of days! Amen my Savior and Lord of hosts!

Ramsis Ghaly

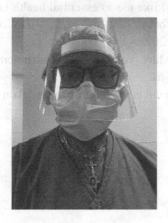

MR. Amen 🙏 God bless you

CA. So 2021 will be bad too?

TR. Thank you!! 🖤

SS. Amen!!

CB. Let's welcome 2021 with Love.....Peace..... And.......Joy.

KS. Happy new year to you doctor

FA, God bless you Dr Ghaly 🙏

AV. Amen! 💚🙏

SB. God bless you, Dr. Ghaly.

CR. I say amen to all you said!!! Thank you for your encouraging words from the Word of God.

BM. I really wish that people would take wearing a mask more seriously. I am not saying that it will cure it, but I believe it would slow it down. I am a mask wearer!

KC. Amen 🙏

CG. Welcoming 2021 with open eyes and open mind. Questioning things that need to be questioned and accepting the fact that only God knows what is in store for us in '21. Happy New Year! 💚🙏

NV. Amen 🙏 and God Bless you Doctor Ghaly! Wishing you Happy and Healthy 2021 🎆

DK. Keep our eyes on our Lord Jesus and don't be asleep or distracted for his return. It will happen...have faith....its just a question of when.

VG. Amin 🙏 i Bog Vas blagoslovio doktore.Veliko hvala na lepim rečima.Neka ova godina ode što pre, nanela nam je mnogo tuge i bola.Želim da vam Nova godina 2021 bude zdravija, uspešnija. 🌲💚💚 Amen 🙏 and God bless you doctors. Many thanks for the kind words. Let this year go as soon as possible, it has caused us a lot of sadness and pain. I wish that the New Year 2021 be healthier, more successful. 🌲💚💚💚💚

VM. Always stay safe bff like me as essential health care professionals. God is always blessings us for our best care to COVID victims.

AM. Praying for a better 2021! 🙏

DM. stay blessed and healthy. You are Gods instrument.my prayer that 2021 be a better one for all if us

CH. Continue to stay safe out there. You are an angel on earth to so many! Happy New Year to you.

Goodbye COVID19 and Welcome COVID20!

Ramsis Ghaly

With new year, let us say Goodbye China COVID-19 and Welcome UK COVID-20! But Regardless, Christmas remains so strong and so welcoming and spread hope and strengthen faith and renew God reconciliation to mankind and His promise for eternal salvation!

Four Thousands Lethal COVID Strains

COVID-19 —————— December 2019
COVID-20 —————— December 2020
COVID-21 —————— December 2021
COVID-22 —————— December 2022
COVID-23 —————— December 2023
COVID-24 —————— December 2024
COVID-25 —————— December 2025
COVID 4000 —————— December 6019

With new year, let us say Goodby China COVID-19 and Welcome UK COVID-20! Regardless, Christmas remains so strong and so welcoming and spread hope and strengthen faith and renew Hod reconciliation to mankind and His promise for eternal salvation

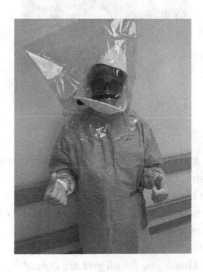

Just got called 1/17/2021 1130PM and I am going to help!

Here I go Mr COVID! Why did you enter to this man body and now they called me to help his breathing snd intubate him? Who send you to hurt us??

I put on my armor of faith and I drew the sign of my Lord Jesus Cross and in His Name I went and I did what was asked of me to do!

But I asked again that evil virus where did you come from??? The virus didn't reply!! But I wish I can send these viruses away and divert them from our human race!!

All I can do for now keep praying 🙏 to my Savior and keep my eyes 👀 open to His Holy visitation and my heart to His Love 🖤 and my ears to heaven to intercept the reply soon 🔜!

Thank you 🙏 Lord and speed recovery to the victims of COVID!!

Ramsis ghaly

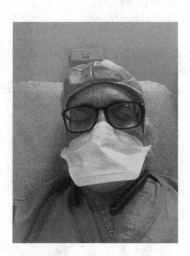

BL. You are awesome and God's blessing to so many, many, people.
MG. Prayers and blessing over u and your patient
ML. Much love to you Dr. Ghaly. 🖤🙏
FA. God bless you for helping Dr Ghaly you have a heart of 🤍
VL. I'm praying for you and with you 🙏🖤
TG. May Gd bless you and keep you safe!
KR. Please stay safe!! Thank you for all you are doing! 😇

ED. God bless you Doctor. May he continue to give you strength and mercy so that we can all follow in your path of spiritual healing and love 🙏❤️

BL. God bless you Dr Ghaly! ❤️🙏❤️🙏

YF. I pray that God keeps blessing your mind and those hands of yours & keeps working through you in Jesus name

AL. May God bless you, our prayers Will be heard

RV. 🙏🙏

BM. Praying for you and a hedge of protection around you and the other people. In the name of Jesus! Amen

BR., Stay safe.. 🙏🙏🙏

LM. Bless you and prayers for strength and peace

CP. May God keep you safe Ramsis so you may do what you do best.... Heal those around you....God Bless you 🙏🙏🙏

MP. Amén 💖😺

DC. God please bless and protect your servant Dr. Ramsis Ghaly! May he save lives today through your power and the gift of knowledge you have given him. May this virus be condemned and driven to the pit of hell!!! In Jesus name Amen! ✝️🙏🙏❤️

GK. May God give you strength to continue save the human race from this virus, may God bless you Doctor Ramsis Ghaly

RC. Spread recovery for all! Pray forma all

PR. much blessings to you

GS. Many blessings brother

KW. Be safe & be strong, my friend Dr Ghaly! You're blessed with many skills & we need you!

KE. Blessings Ramsis

BS. Be safe!!!

VG. Thank you so much for all that you do for your precious patients.

RF. God Bless you for helping.

VG. Amin 🙏

DT. Amen

AV. Thank you Dr. Ghaly for all u do! God continue to help & protect u! 🐱🙏

LT. May The Lord bless your hands and protect you from harm to keep helping and spreading Jesus's messages of hope

SK. Your patients are so blessed to have a Doctor like you!!

TG. May God help you give you strength to continue to safe the people on earth from this virus may God Bless you protect you. Many Blessings to you. 🙏🙏🙏🙏

The Year of 2021 Shall Give Birth to a New Brutal World!!

Written by Ramsis Ghaly

First day in 2021, it was so strange! I was dressed with a heavy cloth walking in the snow distancing away while masking up!

First I stopped by the church 🏛 to thank my Heavenly Father for the gift of life and let me live to 2021! However, the church was lockdown! No one was around. The gates were closed and the entire complex appeared abandoned! I could only hear the fallen ice mixed with snow drizzling down! I stood before the church doors in the freezing cold and looked up to My Father and I said Thank You 😊 Thank You 🙏 Thank You 🙏 Lord Jesus!

I continued my tour in the snow welcoming the New Year and taking few photos with what are remained from Christmas decoration before they are taken away! Again, there wasn't many around and the land looked abandoned with no evidence of cheer living!

With this strange beginning, I fell into deep reflection of 2021! I asked Miss 2021: "Who are you?? Miss 2021 replied: "I am glad you asked! I have been waiting for someone to ask me this questions but many had ignored me and continued to bury their heads in the sand! I am Miss 2021 and I shall give birth to the new world 🌑! This is my goal and I am determined! I will never go back and follow the years before me! COVID and much more shall keep me busy but it will help me to restructure the entire planet to a new world! Wait and see! Please go back and tell the world to expect much more!!!"

Immediately, I saw darkness fell as more clouds ☁☁ covered the sky. The sleet rain mixed with snow began to fall! The day signs continued to surprise my soul hinting for much of change is coming soon in the way! I prayed with tears to my Savior as I wondered in the words of Miss 2021 as I was waving goodbye at her! I couldn't take my eyes off Miss 2021 but she did rudely! He last words: "You won't see me again but you surely will here soon from me" She laughed and laughed as her laughs were fading away until she disappeared out of sight!!! I drew the sign of my Lord Jesus Cross! I knew this isn't a good sign! I screamed: "Lord have mercy please Lord don't leave me to 2021!"

I felt as if it was my end! I looked up to heaven and I asked my Father to take me back home! It wasn't the time to talk more but to reflect in these words and to be alone!

"Judge me, O God, and plead my cause against an ungodly nation: O deliver me from the deceitful and unjust man. [2] For thou art the God of my strength: why dost thou cast me off? why go I mourning because of the oppression of the enemy? [3] O send out thy light and thy truth: let them lead me; let them bring me unto thy holy hill, and to thy tabernacles. [4] Then will I go unto the altar of God, unto God my exceeding joy: yea, upon the harp will I praise thee, O God my God. [5] Why art thou cast down, O my soul? and why art thou disquieted within me? hope in God: for I shall yet praise him, who is the health of my countenance, and my God." Psalm 43

Ramsis Ghaly

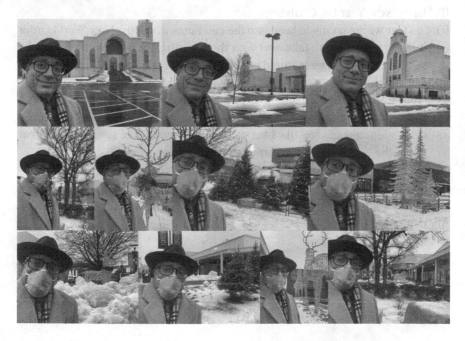

SM. Happy and blessed New Year Dr Ramsis Ghaly 🎆❤️🙏

SS. Tutte le forze ci portiamo dentro di noi stessi ...ognuno di noi che prega il Signore e una chiesa unità nella preghiera ... Preghiamo ..Dio di superare tutte le prove ..e uniamoci ...nella chiesa Di Dio ... tramite preghiera ...Gloria a Dio

ML. Happy New Year Dr. Ramsis Ghaly! Much love to you and many blessings for 2021 and beyond.

DCC. Quite profound and definitely prophetic.

JD. I believe you are correct Dr. Ghaly. Happy New Year. We must all pray! 🙏🙏🙏

BM. I believe that we must all pray for 2021.

If my people who are called by my name will Humble themself and pray and seek my face and turn from their wicked ways. Then I will hear from Heaven above, forgive their sins and Heal their Land! We must always put God First and PRAY! God Bless Everyone 💜🙏💜

JD. It's a strange world in which we live my friend

CD. Happy Blessed New Year!!

JB. 🙏🙏💜 Blessing in this New Year Dr.Ghaly.

TJ. Thank you Lord Jesus for bringing us through 2020; and into 2021. HIS grace is sufficient. God's continued blessings on you Dr. Ghaly.

ED. God's blessings Doctor. Let us pray that things will get better. Stay safe 🙏

PH. Oh my gosh, that is amazing and we all must pray every minute. You are so correct and many blessings to you.

CR. I couldn't agree with you more. Lord have mercy!

JP. Happy New Year Dr. Ghaly!

JO. I do fear we are trying to head into the end times where the New World Order is being structured to take over with the Antichrist at the helm. I do believe the Christians will be raptured prior to the 7 year tribulation. The microchip mark of the beast…

CG. Your words are like a painting. I see the vividness of what you see. Standing in front of an empty church feeling despair or looking at the Christmss decorations alone. I feel like I am standing there with you. Let us all pray that this is the beginning of a better year. Bless you! 🙏💜

Rc. Blesings in this strange world, ww can make a better 2021

Vg. Nek nam pomogne Blagoslov u ovoj Novoj godini. 🙏🙏💜

Dk. Happy 2021, Doctor Ghaly!

Ap. Happy New Year.

My First Monday of 2021 as COVID spread continues!

We pray! You all stay safe!

We pray for our Lord to crown this heat in His Name!

"Thou crownest the year with thy goodness; and thy paths drop fatness." Psalm 65:11 KJV

"Praise waiteth for thee, O God, in Sion: and unto thee shall the vow be performed. [2] O thou that hearest prayer, unto thee shall all flesh come. [3] Iniquities prevail against me: as for our transgressions, thou shalt purge them away. [4] Blessed is the man whom thou choosest, and causest to approach unto thee, that he may dwell in thy courts: we shall be satisfied with the goodness of thy house, even of thy holy temple. [5] By terrible things in righteousness wilt thou answer us, O God of our salvation; who art the confidence of all the ends of the earth, and of them that are afar off upon the sea: [6] Which by his strength setteth fast the mountains; being girded with power: [7] Which stilleth the noise of the seas, the noise of their waves, and the tumult of the people. [8] They also that dwell in the uttermost parts are afraid at thy tokens: thou makest the outgoings of the morning and evening to rejoice. [9] Thou visitest the earth, and waterest it: thou greatly enrichest it with the river of God, which is full of water: thou preparest them corn, when thou hast so provided for it. [10] Thou waterest the ridges thereof abundantly: thou settlest the furrows thereof: thou makest it soft with showers: thou blessest the springing thereof. [11] Thou crownest the year with thy goodness; and thy paths drop fatness. [12] They drop upon the pastures of the wilderness: and the little hills rejoice on every side. [13] The pastures are clothed with flocks; the valleys also are covered over with corn; they shout for joy, they also sing." Psalm 65

Ramsis Ghaly

705

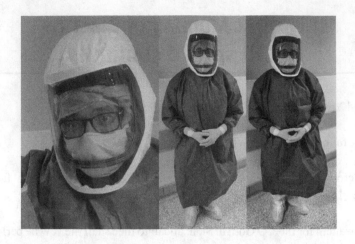

ED. Amen 🙏

MS. Amen.

KO. AMEN Dr Ghaly

PF. Amen 🙏 My you be healthy and safe 🖤

RA. God be with you Dr. Ghaly

AV. Amen! 😍🙏

JC. Stay safe Dr, you look like you are going to outer space 🙏🙏🙏

MS. You look like and astronaut 😷

AB. Amen

JM. Amen

CG. I pray for our Lord to stop this terrible virus. I look at you with all your PPE and I feel sad for you and all that are working with covid patients. I complain about wearing a little mask until I see you all in your many means of protection. I complain no more. Stay safe. 🖤🙏

KO. Few more I know are getting virus, young ones too, 🙏🙏 my heart goes out to them also

SJ. I do not know how you do it. I wear one mask and I get hot and my glasses fog up. You wear all of your protective gear and gloves and save people's lives. Praise to you and all the other front line workers. 😭🙏🖤

DM. Stay safe. Blood of Jesus cover you

COVID as a Shark Ready to Bite You and a Lion About to Kill You!

Every day more COVID Victims falling and needed intubations.

I urgently put on my PPE and ran to help. Every time I turn, Many around me are getting infected with COVID! Unbelievable!!!

Please you all stay away and stay safe!

COVID is a shark ready to bite you and a lion about to kill you!

Therefore run 🏃 away for now!

Ramsis Ghaly

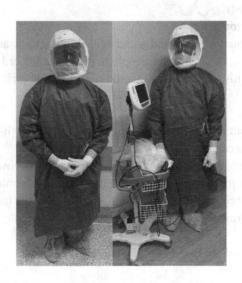

WG. Stay healthy Dr. Ghaly 👐
BB. Stay safe Dr. Ghaly
BS. Please stay safe! I can't understand why people Aren't still taking Covid seriously!
BS. I agree with you and the only thing that i can think of is that it hasn't effected their family or love one. God Bless!
PP. Stay safe Doc! It's an order 🖤

BM. Please stay safe as much as you can! God Bless you and all the other staff members. Dear Lord please put a Hedge of Protection around everyone who has to be on the front line on this virus. Please take this virus away. In the name of Jesus. Amen 🙏❤️🙏

JS. Stay Safe Ramsis! 🙏🙏🙏

PP. Message from my friend Doctor Ramsis Ghaly

Hay Bao Trong va Tranh xa COVID!

Message from my friend Doctor Ramsis Ghaly

How often in

BS. agree with you and the only thing that i can think of is that it hasn't effected their family or love one. God Bless!

LK. Yes, exactly!

PP. Stay safe Doc! It's an order ❤️

BM. Please stay safe as much as you can! God Bless you and all the other staff members. Dear Lord please put a Hedge of Protection around everyone who has to be on the front line on this virus. Please take this virus away. In the name of Jesus. Amen 🙏❤️🙏

JS. Stay Safe Ramsis! 🙏🙏🙏

JM. Blessings doctor

SS. May God break 🐍 head and stand with his strength above this enemy.. bringing life 🌸❤️🌸 and save people in the name of Lord Amen!!! Glory to God father to his son Jesus Christ and the Holy One Spirit through centuries Amen

JB. 🙏🙏🙏🙏😥

CG. Charlene Mentzer Glowaty Sending prayers for those with the Coronavirus and those who care for them. Stay safe doctor. ❤️🙏

LW. Everyone needs to get eight with Jesus because tomorrow is not promised. Fear is a killer just as well. Mismanagement is still a problem. Get treatment early, and chances are you will do well. I'm sorry foe the families and friends who are suffering. N...

TA. 🙏🙏

HW. Stay safe Dr. Ghaly!! God Bless you ❤️🙏

CP. 🙏

KG. Thank you for reminding us to do the right thing here, Dr. Ghaly 🙏

AL. Always be safe doc 🙏

RP. 🙏🙏

RR. Thank you!

JJ. May God bless you!!!

COVID Overpower Human Cells and Finally Crush Human Life to Dust!

Written by Ramsis Ghaly

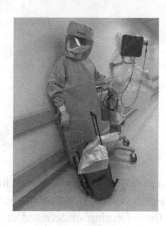

COVID fools many, finds a sneaky way to invade each human cell, makes human cell it's new home, paralyses the cell, massively replicate, mutate and reprogram, rapidly multiply within the entire human flesh forming undefeated army, overpower organ by organ and soon takeover, suffocate and exsanguinate the human cells and finally crush the human life to dust!

COVID TOOK OUR ANGEL AWAY! MIKE DID EVERYTHING TO STAY AWAY FROM COVID BUT COVID SOMEHOW GOT HIM!! COVID WENT TO HIS LUNGS AND AFTER HE WENT HOME, COVID WENT TO HIS HEART AND ENDED HIS LIFE!

YOU ALL PLEASE TAKE COVID SERIOUSLY, MIKE ONLY 49 YEARS OLD!

AFTER MY SURGERY TWO YEARS HE WAS GOLFING AND DOING GREAT UNTIL COVID. SO SAD. COVID IS AN EVIL ENEMY TO MANKIND!

Loss of smell!
Loss of taste!
Loss of appetite!
Loss of smile!
Loss of strength!

Loss of interest!
Loss of stamina!
Loss of weight!
Loss motivation!
Loss of feeling!
Loss of breathing!
Loss of immunity!
Loss of energy!
Loss of control!
Loss of hope!
Loss of defense!
Loss of blood!
Loss of heart!
Loss of fight!
Loss of life!

COVID fools many, finds a sneaky way to invade each human cell, makes human cell it's new home, massively replicate, mutate and reprogram, rapidly multiply within the entire human flesh forming undefeated army, overpower organ by organ and soon takeover, suffocate and exsanguinate the human cells and finally crush the human life to dust!

Ramsis Ghaly

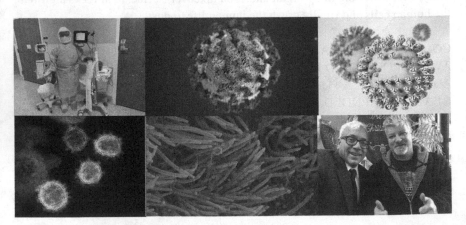

COVID TOOK OUR ANGEL MIKE AWAY!

MIKE DID EVERYTHING TO STAY AWAY FROM COVID BUT COVID SOMEHOW GOT HIM!!

COVID WENT TO HIS LUNGS AND AFTER HE WENT HOME, COVID WENT TO HIS HEART AND ENDED HIS LIFE!

YOU ALL PLEASE TAKE COVID SERIOUSLY, MIKE WAS ONLY 49 YEARS OLD!

AFTER MY SURGERY LAST YEAR M, HE WAS GOLFING AND DOING GREAT UNTIL COVID.

SO SAD! COVID IS AN EVIL ENEMY TO MANKIND!

<u>December 6, 2018</u> ·
Shared with Public

My patient ready to celebrate Christmas and New Year with no pain, back in his feet and soon ready to go back to work after a dead road full of miserable suffering.

Our Baby Jesus grant Michael a new lease in life with so much blessing

Merry Christmas and happy new year

<u>Ramsis Ghaly</u>

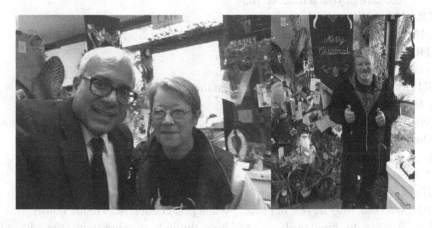

DS. Mary, so terribly sorry for your loss.
JM. Our Deepest Condolences
PU. Sending love 🖤
DA. I'm so sorry Mary. We all loved him so much.

JS. My heart goes out to all. Mike will be truly missed. We loved him so. You take care of yourself. Love you

DG. Mike will be dearly missed

MZ. my deepest condolences to you doctor and may God rest his soul in peace

TR. So very sorry for your loss. 🙏

TB. So very sorry to hear this 😢

KF. Mary many hugs n prayers for you n the family. 🖤🖤🙏🙏🙏🙏

EM. Strong prayers, so sad

MP. So so sorry How terrible

DI. I'm so sorry 😔

AP. So sorry for your loss

JD. So sorry to hear this! Prayers to all !!!JD. So so sad. May he rest in peace. My deepest condolences to his family

LS. Prayers to his family .. saw him through passing with the city of Wilmington 🙏🙏

DS. May he RIP 🙏 So sorry for your loss 🙏🖤

JS. So sorry for your loss 🙏🙏🙏

CG. This is very sad and so young. Sending healing prayers to his family.

CG. Unfortunately so true! Bless all the covid patients. 🖤🙏

DC, Mary, so terribly sorry for your loss.

PU. Sending love 🖤

DA. I'm so sorry Mary. We all loved him so much.

JS. My heart goes out to all. Mike will be truly missed. We loved him so. You take care of yourself. Love you

DG. Mike will be dearly missed

MR. my deepest condolences to you doctor and may God rest his soul in peace

TR. So very sorry for your loss. 🙏

TB. So very sorry to hear this 😢

KF. Mary many hugs n prayers for you n the family. 🖤🖤🙏🙏🙏🙏

EM. Strong prayers, so sad

MP. So so sorry

How terrible

DI. I'm so sorry 😔

AB. So sorry for your loss

JD. So sorry to hear this! Prayers to all !!!

JD. So so sad. May he rest in peace. My deepest condolences to his family 🖤

LS. Prayers to his family .. saw him through passing with the city of Wilmington 🙏🙏

DS. May he RIP 🙏 So sorry for your loss 🙏🖤

JS. So sorry for your loss 🙏🙏🙏

CG. This is very sad and so young. Sending healing prayers to his family.

TM. My condolences

PP. Sorry for your loss! ▲▲▲

BD. Prayers for you and his entire family ▲▲▲

BS. So sorry for your loss. He is with the angels.

TH. I am so sorry Dr Ghaly. We all must find a way to keep living yet keep our guard up against Covid.

DL. Sincere condolences to all his family/friends and also to you Dr. Ghaly.

IS. I'm praying for all who knew and loved him.

DM. Sorry for your loss...May he rest in peace

GS. Sorry for your loss Many blessings brother

GW. Oh my goodness Mary and family I am so so sorry to hear this love and prayers to all of you

DC. I'm so sorry Dr.Ghaly.

COVID the Darkest Evil Antihuman killer! Merciless Death

Written and Witnessed by
Ramsis Ghaly

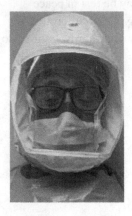

Coronavirus COVID-19 is so lethal and so evil. It does not leave the human body until it kills it!

I was called repeatedly in terminal cases and my eyes keep seeing! The army of viruses are eating the human fresh piece by piece as a starving roaring lions! Their bodies emanating screams of horrific pains experiencing hell gasping for air and oxygen which never enough, suffocation, terrors and imposed horrendous mutilations!!

The human tissues are converted to dark, hemorrhagic, necrotic, eaten up and unidentifiable tissues! The entire human body becomes toxic and totally destroyed!

After extreme suffering for two to three weeks, the blood 🩸 is turned to deep dark and no more viable human organs lifeless! The human flesh is disintegrated by the camp and nests full of lethal and evil viruses!

The entire person then get dumped in a heavy duty bag and wrapped in black bag and moved away in complete isolation since it is full of viruses 🦠!

These nests viruses 🦠 like an army ready jump to the next door victim another and eats him or her alive! These bodies are thrown one after another by the

714

morgues and trucks. The funeral homes and the land of death can't accommodate their burials!

Never in my life I have come across with daily dead and destroyed dark human bodies! No one could imagine not only what those patients are going through before they are wrapped in black bags but what healthcare workers are going through and witnessing non stop!

Sorry friends, mankind all over the world is defeated badly! Human bodies are just nothing and it turn out that in contrary, man is carrying a very weak human flesh can't stand these Nano invisible viruses!!!

Indeed these human bodies are formed from dust and the virus crushed them back to black bags full of dust! The world is only left with memories and photos of the past as soon the living nay become the virus casualties tomorrow. The inhabitants of the earth are racing for their death and it is just the beginning! Many believe man has control but in actuality man has nothing but just a big mouth with outspoken tongue ▼ with unsealed lips!!

In desperation having nothing to offer, you shed tears and cry 😿 in sadness and sorrows giving up!!! It reaches a time that indeed death is a blessing to the suffocated human body eaten up alive by a zoo of viruses!! Healthcare workers are melting away!!

This is the true picture I see every day! Isn't the good image I could present to you in the first day of the week but it has broken my heart and torn me and many apart knowing that I and we could do nothing but runaway!!!

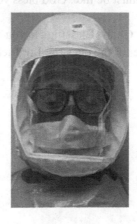

MU. Here and now and just for today: I share what is being lived in US hospitals this tremendous, revealing, sad, perhaps even horrendous, but it is the great message from Doctor Ghaly and if this happens there, imagine what happens here!!!, but let's accept the real thing and see clearly what can happen to our bodies in the face of this virus Read it carefully and reflect on the experience Dr Ghaly tells us. I wish you all Health and take care! 🙏🙏🙏💙

CR. This is a testimony from my doctor Ramsis Ghaly and it's what's really happening in hospitals where people continue to die horrific and uncontrollably. Let's not get tired of ending this virus because he hasn't tired of taking us down.

SR. mg!! How long will this all end? very strong Dr testimony Ghaly that looks like fiction. He is a very sensitive and compassionate person. She›s not having a good time. And that cove laying down?? It›s burned??

CR. I think that photo symbolizes the virus that by reproducing indiscriminately practically attacks the body until it leaves it lifeless.

SR. wow !!

And that's not even how people understand 😔

MF. My God have mercy on all humanity and forgive us all the evil we have done, bless all medical personnel, nurses, cleaning, police and maintenance, and Doctor Ghaly please do not give up the world needs Doctors and people like you Blessings to you and all around you!! 🙏🙏🙏

Am. How much master reality you also see in our hospitals fearing fall into despair but the will of our Lord embodies in us the virtue of not bending and seeking a better tomorrow. our faith will make us stronger. take care of yourself dr.

Ed. Many blessings to you brave Doctor 🙏🙏

CG. My heart aches for you and everyone who has to witness this on a daily basis. I can't imagine what it must be like. God bless you all and give you strength to carry on. 🖤🙏

RC. Thank you so much Dr. Ghaly. Blessings to you and new strength and grace for each day as you care for the ones the Lord sets in your way.

Even Late at Night COVID is Around!

Even Late at night, COVID is around! Busy busy!! The virus 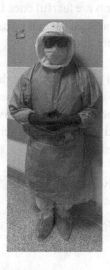 is keeping us wrapped and torn!!

Lord hear our prayers!

Ramsis Ghaly

KL. So sad! I pray for your safety
LK. Me too, Dr Ghaly. We need you!!
JB. Stay safe Dr. Ghaly!! 🙏❤️
FD. Please stay safe Dr Ghaly 🙏❤️
TH. Praying Dr. G!
KV. Prayers
VG. Praying 🙏🙏
MN. Prayers for you and all you do..thank you..
RN. Blessings Dr.Ghaly ❤️❤️🙏🙏
BV. In Jesus name amen
KO. Angels watch over all
CS. Stay safe Dr G!!
KG. Stay safe 🙏
DB. Keep safe!
SN. Praying for you and everyone else helping combat covid.
AV. MN. Just keep your self safe Dr .Ghaly

In hours, COVID patients' Oxygenation Get so Much Worse that We Run Racing to Intubate and Assist Them in Ventilators as a Life-saving!

In the early hours after midnight, our Lord with us to assist such a patient! As many, distressed COVID patients are fearful once intubated hearing next is death. So stressful and emotional facing such a lethal virus in a time of pandemic without treatment or expected cure—not knowing

It is neither flu nor traditional pneumonia, they look dry, dusky, pale and gray kissing the death! It is hard to explain as I approach those COVID victims with hard time breathing! I remember the very first patient back in March, I intubated and immediately I recognized that evil 🦠 when many others in the medical community denied and rejected me!

What a strong lethal and highly contagious virus 🦠

Coronavirus! Lord have mercy.

Psalm 46
God is our refuge and strength, a very present help in trouble. [2] Therefore will not we fear, though the earth be removed, and though the mountains be carried into the midst of the sea; [3] Though the waters thereof roar and be troubled, though the mountains shake with the swelling thereof. Selah. [4] There is a river, the streams whereof shall make glad the city of God, the holy place of the tabernacles of the most High. [5] God is in the midst of her; she shall not be moved: God shall help her, and that right early. [6] The heathen raged, the kingdoms were moved: he uttered his voice, the earth melted. [7] The Lord of hosts is with us; the God of Jacob is our refuge. Selah. [8] Come, behold the works of the Lord, what desolations he hath made in the earth. [9] He maketh wars to cease unto the end of the earth; he breaketh the bow, and cutteth the spear in sunder; he burneth the chariot in the fire. [10] Be still, and know that I am God: I will be exalted among the heathen, I will be exalted in the earth. [11] The Lord of hosts is with us; the God of Jacob is our refuge. Selah.

Psalm 31

In thee, O Lord, do I put my trust; let me never be ashamed: deliver me in thy righteousness. [2] Bow down thine ear to me; deliver me speedily: be thou my strong rock, for an house of defence to save me. [3] For thou art my rock and my fortress; therefore for thy name's sake lead me, and guide me. [4] Pull me out of the net that they have laid privily for me: for thou art my strength. [5] Into thine hand I commit my spirit: thou hast redeemed me, O Lord God of truth. [6] I have hated them that regard lying vanities: but I trust in the Lord. [7] I will be glad and rejoice in thy mercy: for thou hast considered my trouble; thou hast known my soul in adversities; [8] And hast not shut me up into the hand of the enemy: thou hast set my feet in a large room. [9] Have mercy upon me, O Lord, for I am in trouble: mine eye is consumed with grief, yea, my soul and my belly. [10] For my life is spent with grief, and my years with sighing: my strength faileth because of mine iniquity, and my bones are consumed. [11] I was a reproach among all mine enemies, but especially among my neighbours, and a fear to mine acquaintance: they that did see me without fled from me. [12] I am forgotten as a dead man out of mind: I am like a broken vessel. [13] For I have heard the slander of many: fear was on every side: while they took counsel together against me, they devised to take away my life. [14] But I trusted in thee, O Lord: I said, Thou art my God. [15] My times are in thy hand: deliver me from the hand of mine enemies, and from them that persecute me. [16] Make thy face to shine upon thy servant: save me for thy mercies' sake. [17] Let me not be ashamed, O Lord ; for I have called upon thee: let the wicked be ashamed, and let them be silent in the grave. [18] Let the lying lips be put to silence; which speak grievous things proudly and contemptuously against the righteous. [19] Oh how great is thy goodness, which thou hast laid up for them that fear thee; which thou hast wrought for them that trust in thee before the sons of men! [20] Thou shalt hide them in the secret of thy presence from the pride of man: thou shalt keep them secretly in a pavilion from the strife of tongues. [21] Blessed be the Lord: for he hath shewed me his marvellous kindness in a strong city. [22] For I said in my haste, I am cut off from before thine eyes: nevertheless thou heardest the voice of my supplications when I cried unto thee."

You all be safe. We pray Amen 🙏

Ramsis Ghaly

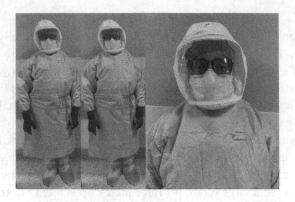

KP. Lord hear our prayers

DM. God have mercy on us

AC. May God continue to watch over you and cover you in His mantle of safety& protection, as you continue to save the lives of others in His Divine Mercy. 💜🙏🌷

JH. Prayers everyday. God Bless and keep you safe Dr. Thank you for all you do!

ML. Much love to you Dr. Ramsis Ghaly! You are my hero!

TH. Praying for you Dr. G!

MY. ربنا يرحم صنعه ايديه

JF. We thank our Lord for the dedicated, faithful servants as yourself. May He continue to bless you and keep you safe! 🙏

CB. Stay safe! 💜🙏

DR. Thank you 🙏
Stay safe & well 💜

LG. May the Lord shield you with His blue mantle of protection.

CR. Prayers for your strength and safety as well in Jesus name.

MG. Ramis !!
Stay safe and covered in Gods Grace & Protection!

JD. less you Dr. Ghaly. Heavenly Father wrap your healing and loving arms around everyone with this terrible virus and heal them and keep all of the front line workers safe. In Jesus name I pray! 🙏🙏🙏

CG. You are amazing! You never give up hope and you care so deeply for the covid patients. I join you in prayer for those patients
Bless you and stay safe. 💜🙏

AB. Amen

SC. I was hopeful that intubation was being replaced by therapeutics by this time. 🙏

JK. ربنا يقويك ويحميك دكتور رمسيس.

ML. Covid! Please be safe and wear your mask

JL. You forgot your N95

This what I do when I get emergency call to intubate a COVID patient. Put as much layers of PAPR & PPE So excited to help out and I run to save in my Lord Jesus Name!

What a blessing to serve our fellowmen and fellow women falling victims to COVID!

You aren't alone, we all here to serve you and care for you. It is our pleasure to do so! Be of good courage strong in faith and at peace and not to be in fears or terrorized by the media news. In Jesus our Savior Name. Amen 🙏

Ramsis Ghaly

Called today to help and there I went! I joined the caring team, honored and privileged to join and serve!

Bless you all and bless your hearts 💜 and your exceptional services!!

Ramsis Ghaly

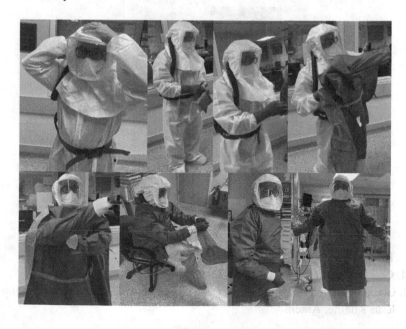

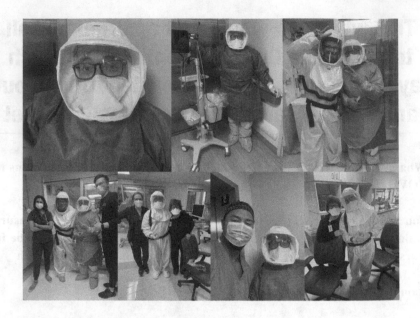

CS. Bless you! You are such an inspiration!

CG. Thank you all, stay safe and Bless you all. 🙏

FA. **Flor De Andocutin** Stay safe 🙏

JP. Your rewards will be great dear Facebook friend.

DL. My favorite doctor.

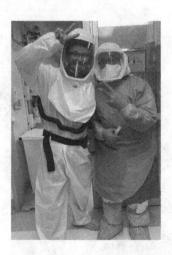

ML. Be safe Dr Ghaly!

LM. God Bless you for what you do 🙏🙏🙏💜

NE. God bless, strengthen and protect you as you continue to do this great job in Jesus's name, Amen!

BCD. You are Blessed sir. Amen

SK. Patients are so lucky to have a caring Dr., like you!!

KG. God Bless you, Stay safe and thank you for all you do for everybody. You are the angel for all of us! Xoxo

GV. God bless you for providing such wonderful and loving care to these sick, frightened people.

AR. God love you. Be safe Dr. Ghaly!

CR. Thank you Dr Ghaly

FL. God bless you 🙏

KC. Thank you for all you do, Dr. Ghaly

CG. I will never complain again about being hot and sweaty under a mask after I see what you have to wear. Bless you and all those helping the covid patients. They are so fortunate that you are there to help them. 😊💜

HH. God Bless You!

DE. Amen.

FA. God bless you 🙏 Dr Ghaly today and always ... THE DOCTOR WITH A HEART OF GOLD 🤍

JW. I commend you for your service Dr. Ghaly. By the way, all that stuff you put on kinda makes you look like an astronaut getting ready to walk on the moon!

AB. Amen praise God for His within you!

DL. Best doctor ever!

SN. Thank you for all you do, Dr. Ghaly. 🙏

CEE. Thank you for all you do! 💙

TJ. Dr. Ghaly, you are such a blessing to so many - thank God for giving you strength to be of service. God bless you always.

LB. What a blessing for your patients ✝️

BK. Thank you, thank you, thank you!!!

MH. God Bless you 🙏💜 and keep you safe during these trying times. Your an awesome Dr. With a Great Heart 💜

TW. God bless you, Dr. Ghaly, and all of your fellow health care workers for showing up and stepping up to care for these Covid patients. You are an amazing Dr. and PERSON! Thank you!

ZM. Dr.Ghaly on mission, May God bless you.

MMH. od Bless you 🙏💜 and keep you safe during these trying times. Your an awesome Dr. With a Great Heart 💜

TW. God bless you, Dr. Ghaly, and all of your fellow health care workers for showing up and stepping up to care for these Covid patients. You are an amazing Dr. and PERSON! Thank you!

CB. The Lord be with you.

JM. AMEN

JP. You are a angel of you he Lord.

BM. Praise God for DOCTORS like YOU!

Not again Getting called to intubate It isn't Deja vu but is real Friends be in the Watch!

MARCH 27, 2021
Ramsis Ghaly

Not again??? Getting called to intubate!! It isn't Deja vu but is real!! Friends be in the Watch!

COVID-19 is still around surging! Let Not your guard down!

Please be cautious! It is a strange virus 🦠 with no effective confirmed treatment!

Who knows why COVID-19 is still propagating?? And how that virus 🦠 is lasting behind worldwide??? It continues to create so much confusion and doubts as a result of lack of transparency in the land!

It certainly looks like mankind is under constant threat by highly smart and virulent virus 🦠 that is able to attack the human flesh day and night, in all seasons, all countries and involving all ethnicities and socioeconomic classes???

It shouldn't come to a surprise!! Science 🔬🧫🔬 didn't come yet with magic wand!! let us not forget poliomyelitis, HIV and Flue never left the land once imparted in the human land, flourished and found the world good home and the human flesh and an excellent host!!!

The ongoing prevalence of COVID-19 is indicative of failure of science to understand COVID-19 and failure of medicine to find a cure and not because the people aren't listening!! Understanding-ably, It took years to develop the universally effective and proven treatment and preventions of each! Why it shouldn't be any different for COVID-19??

Who is the mind master behind this so intelligent highly effective particle mastering the world 🌐 for the second year in the row shaking humanity conquering science and man manipulating human life and taking our serenity disturbing our peace and destroying our economy???

Ramsis Ghaly

724

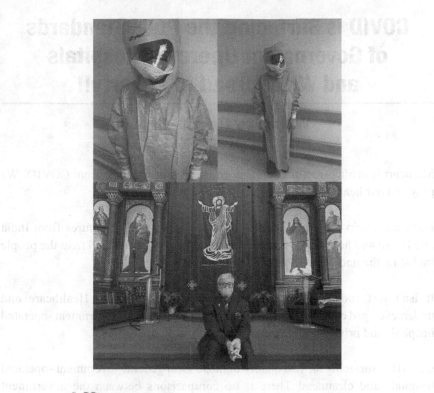

CP. Be safe 🙏❤️
VG, Čuvajte se, Bog Vas blagoslovio 🙏❤️
JB. Stay safe Dr. G. 💔💔💔🙏🙏
CR. Good questions!
Kg. Be safe and well. God Bless you!

COVID is Surfacing the Poor Standards of Government Operated Hospitals and Widespread of Poverty!!

Written by Ramsis Ghaly

My heart is aching from the so many causalities in India ⚑ from COVID! We pray and our hearts are with them!!

But I can't help it but comment in looking at the coming pictures from India and Brazil and hearing the news!! This isn't the way to care and treat the people including the underprivileged!!!

It isn't just India but all over especially under National Healthcare and underdeveloped countries. There is a huge gab between the Government -operated hospitals and private hospitals accepting only cash money!!!

COVID is surfacing the real quality of those local general government -operated hospitals and cleanness! There is no comparisons between the government operated hospitals serving the public the majority and the private serving the rich in these countries!

COVID is spreading in India and Brazil because of widespread low standard healthcare, extreme poverty and lack of cleanness!! It isn't all about the COVID vaccines but rather the poor health and healthcare, the extreme poverty, very dirty general hospitals and no supplies and no hygiene!

As usual, many are commenting that Indian and Brazilian people are not following the guidelines and they are to be blamed for the spread of COVID and not the government! Indeed the people are victims of the corrupted system!!

It isn't primarily the noncompliance of face-masks and lack of vaccines but rather the presence of slums and poor sanitations! Look at these pictures general hospitals no PPE—no medical coats —no uniforms, gloves—no clean stretcher!

COVID is sending a wake up! Look deep at the root of the problem and not just at the surface!! Reach out and help out——-etc

We cry for the public in India, Brazil and those have no money and no choice but to go to the so called "General Public Government Hospitals" and by no means they are any close to hospitals but slums!!

We pray for you!!

Ramsis Ghaly

Cg. So very sad for all the people. I pray for them. 🙏🙏🙏 My heart aches for them.

dl. Prayers for India.

727

Children And Unfolding COVID

COVID Lockdown Hurting Our Children Dreadfully
Written by Ramsis Ghaly

Hug your Children! Surround them with Love!
Reach Out and Open the Doors and gates!

And when we say: "Our children will never do this and they are big okay" Know we are at fault and furthermore, we don't know what deep inside their minds and hearts yet!

Be Vigilant! Protect 2.2 Billion Worldwide children!

There are more than 2.2 billion children in the world who constitute approximately 28% of the world's population. Those aged between 10 to 19 years make up 16 % of the world's population (UNICEF, 2019). COVID-19 has impacted the lives of people around the world including children and adolescents in an unprecedented manner.

For now, there is a dearth of hard research on how the pandemic is affecting children's mental health, mostly because the virus has been so fast-moving and studies take time. What data does exist is troubling.

Loneliness in lockdown is common for kids separated from their friends. But all children will not be emotionally rattled by the pandemic equally—or even at all; COVID-19 will affect them to different degrees and in different ways.

The country is on the verge of another health crisis, with daily doses of death, isolation and fear generating widespread psychological trauma.

Links to read
https://time.com/5870478/children-mental-health-coronavirus/
https://www.washingtonpost.com/.../mental-health.../
https://www.ncbi.nlm.nih.gov/pmc/articles/PMC7323662/
https://www.ncbi.nlm.nih.gov/pmc/articles/PMC7444649/
https://medicalxpress.com/.../2020-06-children-mental...
https://news.sky.com/.../coronavirus-lockdown...
https://www.cidrap.umn.edu/.../covid-19-tied-poorer...

Time.com

The Coronavirus seems to Spare Most kids From Illness, but Its Effect on Their Mental Health Is Developing. No Body is Immune to the Stress that comes with a Pandemic, but children may be at a particular!!!

CG. This is so true. I see this with my grandchildren. Some it doesn't effect but some it makes them anxious, depressed and withdrawn. Things have got to change. Children need to be in school.

WP. Totally agree with you Dr. Ghaly. Nobody leaves my house without an "I love yo

I am a Child in Agony! I am Lowly and Meek!
I am Love 💜 waiting to be Loved!

Written by Ramsis Ghaly

An Emotional Poem Dedicated to all our abandoned and abused children in agony worldwide; With Prayers, Love 💜 and Tears 😭 from my heart 💜

I am a child in agony!

+I am a child in agony! I am lowly and meek! Whosoever shall welcome me and give me to drink a cup of cold water does so to my Heavenly Father and receives my Lord Jesus!

I am a child in agony! I am a child 😊 of love 💜 searching for love 💜! Have you seen my mommy and daddy! My loss is so severe! I can't stop crying 😭 in tears! I am torn apart and I have no leg to stand! I am not ready for the dark days and nights! I am too young for them! I am running away from the evilness of man! Please, I beseech you in the Name of my Heavenly Father Jesus, come bring me to the shore and a safe haven to rest my soul!

I a child in agony! I miss my mommy and daddy! I have no place to go and shoulder to lean on! I am homeless sojourning among strangers and unmerciful people through many tortuous dry grounds! I am thrown in the corners and by the remote places! I am living in the dark and isolated from the world! I am shuffled by the basement and the doors and windows are sealed shut from the outside world! There is no water 💧 to drink 🍸 and no food 🍽 to eat! There is no bed 🛏 to sleep 💤 and no billow to rest my head! Please, I beseech you in the Name of my Heavenly Father Jesus, come bring me to the shore and a safe haven to rest my soul!

I am a child in agony! The days have been unbearable for me and my fellow children! I have been running away from the heat of the sun and the cold of the nights! All around me gloom, fears and terrors! My parents are no more and so are my people! There is no more home 🐿 for me! My heart is broken and I can't stop crying! Mom where are you? Dad where can I find you? Please, I beseech you in the Name of my Heavenly Father Jesus, come bring me to the shore and a safe haven to rest my soul!

I am a child in agony! To where I am going? What is above me? What is underneath me! What is in my side on the left? What is in my other side on the right? O what I left behind? What is today and what is for tomorrow? I lost my mind and I no longer could I think straight with my child 😊 brain 🧠! There is nothing left in me! I am a bruised reed and a smoking flax! Please, I beseech you in the Name of my Heavenly Father Jesus, come bring me to the shore and a safe haven to rest my soul! am a child in agony! I am sick 🤕! My heart is bleeding love 💜! My eyes are shedding tears! I am aching with broken soul and bones! My feet are weary and my legs can't support me any longer! There is no pasture or green around! There is no roads ir streets! There are no signs or marks! There are no phones 📱 or talks! There is no ears 👂 to hear me! There is no eyes 👀 to see me! I am lost in a strange land surrounded in danger and no place to rest my soul! Please, I beseech you in the Name of my Heavenly Father Jesus, come bring me to the shore and a safe haven to rest my soul!

I am a child in agony! My mouth is so dry and my stomach is so empty I am dying from hunger and cramping in pains! I am so thirst and my flesh dry as bone! There is life by me! I am all alone over the roof and under the curb! My mouth is shut and I can't speak! My ears are plugged and I can't hear 👂! My eyes 👀 are dim and no longer I can see! My clothes are old and dirty! My linen are weary and crusted with insects 🐛! If I am not bitten by man, I am bitten by bedbugs! There is no soap or shampoo! Skin lotions and perfumes are only in my dreams! I can only to look at them from far without touching them at my master bedroom! My shoes always with holes and my socks smell from far! Please, I beseech you in the Name of my Heavenly Father Jesus, come bring me to the shore and a safe haven to rest my soul!

I am a child in agony! I am bruised! My daily life is full of suffering! My eyes are usually red and swollen! My mouth is bleeding! My cheeks are wounded! My body is full of marks of the stripes! I am full of scars from being beaten up numerous daily! I am pushed around and around! As my parents get high in street drugs, it will be a torture night for me and memory of its own! It is just be the beginning of my scourging! When alcohol is spread around bottle after bottle shuffled from one to another, the night for me has no end! I will be mocked upon and spitted upon non stop! They will slab me left and right until nothing remained in my soul! I am a nightly sacrifice for their pleasure and lusts through the dawn until the sun rise! I am mocked day and night! I am always the center of their laughs and jocks! No one outside could hear since the rooms are sealed! By the time I go to my closet and through myself in the ground crying in tears to my Lord in secret, it will be the time for the school and O my gosh if I am a minute late! Please, I beseech you in the Name of my Heavenly Father Jesus, come bring me to the shore and a safe haven to rest my soul!

I am a child in agony! My school is my escape! No matter how much I wash and try to look clean, hiding my scars and bruises, it not always easy! My classmates are my fake friends! I am bullied all the time! My teachers are always harsh and rude! They are running away from me! It feels as if everyone is distancing themselves from me! It is lonely life in terror and fears with no peace! I am left with abused children like me! It is strange but it is true! I am attracted to those underprivileged and battered like me! Those are my friends! Perhaps one day we get courage and run away together! But we are living in fear and for now we are silent slaves for our household! Please, I beseech you in the Name of my Heavenly Father Jesus; come bring me to the shore and a safe haven to rest my soul!

I am a child in agony! I am a pleasure tool for many! I am a lust for adults! My own people starved me to death! My family deprived me from all things! They molusted me repeatedly! They have beaten me up day and night! My flesh was invaded violently so many times! I am forced to the corners of the house! I am smashed by the walls! I have been humiliated and mutilated! I became their food 🍞 everyday! My flesh is their destiny and their desire of lust! I can't take it anymore! I need you now! I need you by me now! Please harken and run fast to me! Please, I beseech you in the Name of my Heavenly Father Jesus, come bring me to the shore and a safe haven to rest my soul!

I am a child in agony! The love 🖤 in my heart! I am in dire need of motherly kisses! Please come and wipe my tears! May my Heavenly Father move your heart 🖤! I am praying to my Heavenly Father! I am bleeding for your mercy as my Lord of glory is patiently watching for your love 🖤! I can't take it anymore! I need you now! I need you by me now! Please harken and run fast to me! Please, I beseech you in the Name of my Heavenly Father Jesus, come bring me to the shore and a safe haven to rest my soul!

I am a Child in Agony! I am a Child of God born from Adam and Eve! I am a child and my years are only in the single digit! I am the fruit of my parents! I am the natives of our parents Adam and Eve! I am the new breath of my family tree ♠ ready to grow! I am at the beginning of my seed! Man made me with no cause unprivileged and unfortunate! There are tens of millions of me worldwide! I can't take it anymore! I need you now! I need you by me now! Please harken and run fast to me! Please, I beseech you in the Name of my Heavenly Father Jesus, come bring me to the shore and a safe haven to rest my soul!

I am a child in agony! I am your child in agony! Please rise up and rescue me! I have been walking barefooted looking for love! I don't know where I am going or where I am heading! I am searching for tender heart ♥ of love ♥, tender lips 👄 to kiss, tender chest to hug 🫂, tender hands 🤚 to thank and tender bosom to live! I can't take it anymore! I need you now! I need you by me now! Please harken and run fast to me! Please, I beseech you in the Name of my Heavenly Father Jesus, come bring me to the shore and a safe haven to rest my soul!

The children in Agony 😱 crying to the Lord! The children in agony! The cries of these children have reached the ears of the Almighty and the Divine Warrior the Lord of Just9 Now therefore, behold, the cry of the children of Israel is come unto me: and I have also seen the oppression wherewith the Egyptians oppress them." (Exodus 3:9)

Our Lord Jesus Christ said:

+" Then shall the King say unto them on his right hand, Come, ye blessed of my Father, inherit the kingdom prepared for you from the foundation of the world:35 For I was an hungred, and ye gave me meat: I was thirsty, and ye gave me drink: I was a stranger, and ye took me in:36 Naked, and ye clothed me: I was sick, and ye visited me: I was in prison, and ye came unto me.37 Then shall the righteous answer him, saying, Lord, when saw we thee an hungred, and fed thee? or thirsty, and gave thee drink?38 When saw we thee a stranger, and took thee in? or naked, and clothed thee?39 Or when saw we thee sick, or in prison, and came unto thee?40 And the King shall answer and say unto them, Verily I say unto you, Inasmuch as ye have done it unto one of the least of these my brethren, ye have done it unto me."(Matthew 25:34-40)

+" He that receiveth you receiveth me, and he that receiveth me receiveth him that sent me.—And whosoever shall give to drink unto one of these little ones a cup of cold water only in the name of a disciple, verily I say unto you, he shall in no wise los e his reward." (Matthew 10:40,42)

+"2 And Jesus called a little child unto him, and set him in the midst of them,3 And said, Verily I say unto you, Except ye be converted, and become as little children, ye shall not enter into the kingdom of heaven.4 Whosoever therefore shall humble himself as this little child, the same is greatest in the kingdom of heaven.5 And whoso shall receive one such little child in my name receiveth me.6 But whoso shall offend one of these little ones which believe in me, it were better for him that a millstone were hanged about his neck, and that he were drowned in the depth of the sea.7 Woe unto the world because of offences! for it must needs be that offences come; but woe to that man by whom the offence cometh!" (Matthew 18:2-7)

O The Great Wrath of God is come to those the Predators of the little children! The children in agony! Soon the great wrath of God shalll swallow the kings of earth unto pieces! great wrath of the Lamb has come to all those abusing the children of the Most High. As my Savior said: "16 And said to the mountains and rocks, Fall on us, and hide us from the face of him that sitteth on the throne, and from the wrath of the Lamb:17 For the great day of his wrath is come; and who shall be able to stand?" (Revelations 6:16-17)

The children in agony! Babylon the great is fallen, is fallen, and is become the habitation of devils, and the hold of every foul spirit, and a cage of every unclean and hateful bird. The wrath of God have burned the city of your predators! The day of your predators has come: "And he cried mightily with a strong voice, saying, Babylon the great is fallen, is fallen, and is become the habitation of devils, and the hold of every foul spirit, and a cage of every unclean and hateful bird. [3] For all nations have drunk of the wine of the wrath of her fornication, and the kings of the earth have committed fornication with her, and the merchants of the earth are waxed rich through the abundance of her delicacies. [5] For her sins have reached unto heaven, and God hath remembered her iniquities. [9] And the kings of the earth, who have committed fornication and lived deliciously with her, shall bewail her, and lament for her, when they shall see the smoke of her burning, [18] And cried when they saw the smoke of her burning, saying, What city is like unto this great city! [19] And they cast dust on their heads, and cried, weeping and wailing, saying, Alas, alas, that great city, wherein were made rich all that had ships in the sea by reason of her costliness! for in one hour is she made desolate." (Revelation 18:2-3,5,9,18-19)

The children in agony! Salivation is of the Lord O children in Agony: Be of Good Courage the Holy Lamb riding on the White Horse 🐎 is soon coming to rescue you all: "After this I beheld, and, lo, a great multitude, which no man could number, of all nations, and kindreds, and people, and tongues, stood before the throne, and before the Lamb, clothed with white robes, and palms in their hands; [10] And cried with a loud voice, saying, Salvation to our God which sitteth upon the throne, and unto the Lamb. [11] And all the angels stood round about the throne, and about the elders and the four beasts, and fell before the throne on their faces, and worshipped God, [12] Saying, Amen: Blessing, and glory, and wisdom, and thanksgiving, and honour, and power, and might, be unto our God for ever and ever. Amen. [13] And one of the elders answered, saying unto me, What are these which are arrayed in white robes? and whence came they"

The children in agony! O little angels soon our Savior shall dress you in white robes and sit you all by His throne: (Revelation 6:9-11) "[9] And when he had opened the fifth seal, I saw under the altar the souls of them that were slain for the word of God, and for the testimony which they held: [10] And they cried with a loud voice, saying, How long, O Lord, holy and true, dost thou not judge and avenge our blood on them that dwell on the earth? [11] And white robes were given unto every one of them; and it was said unto them, that they should rest yet for a little season, until their fellow servants also and their brethren, that should be killed as they were, should be fulfilled."

The children in Agony let us kneel and sing with the Psalmist to the Lord saying: Psalm 3; "LORD, how are they increased that trouble me! many are they that rise up against me.2 Many there be which say of my soul, There is no help for him in God. Selah.3 But thou, O LORD, art a shield for me; my glory, and the lifter up of mine head.4 I cried unto the LORD with my voice, and he heard me out of his holy hill. Selah.5 I laid me down and slept; I awaked; for the LORD sustained me.6 I will not be afraid of ten thousands of people, that have set themselves against me round about.7 Arise, O LORD; save me, O my God: for thou hast smitten all mine enemies upon the cheek bone; thou hast broken the teeth of the ungodly.8 Salvation belongeth unto the LORD: thy blessing is upon thy people. Selah."

A Cry 😭 to the World! A cry 😭 to the world! A plea to the Leaders! An appeal to man! A calling to all! Please rise and protect the children of the world 🌍! A cry 😭 to the world! A plea to the Leaders! An appeal to man! A calling to all! Please rise and protect the children of the world 🌍! Please come our Lord Jesus and protect our children from evil "He which testifieth these things saith, Surely I come quickly. Amen. Even so, come, Lord Jesus." (Revelations 22:20)

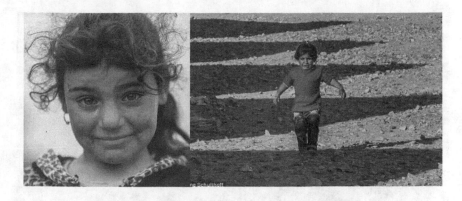

Bcd. this made my Soul tears stream down my face. We all are tortured children no matter what age we are. God Bless your kind 🖤🙏

ED. This breaks my heart.

SA. And we all say Amen and Amen!

CG. This is touching a poem. It is said with such compassion and emotion that touches my heart. Bless you 🖤

Diana Garcia

Our district has some children in person, hybrid and remote. Many want to come go in person but capacity limits restrict them. Today we received email that although rates below 1% we should anticipate there may be mandate for full remote. Makes me sad as they are working so hard to stay in. Today they had a drive by parade. As we circled around you could see beyond the masks for their eyes smiled as well. Made my day to see a COVID costume in the bunch 😊

CHILDREN DRAWING ARTS

Heather Mporokoso
Dameon's science project of the spine! Dr. Ramsis Ghaly

I think you would appreciate this project!! Dameon is learning so much about the brain and the human body. When my disk herniated into my nerve 3 years ago Dameon now understands what happened and can see where it happened so cool! #LoveHomeschooling

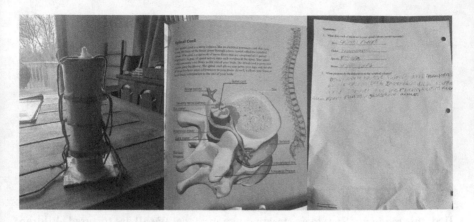

RG. It is outstanding work. Genius thank you 🙏

NM. Wow, so clever!!!! 😮😮😮

JL. Nice job Dameon!

The Coronavirus is sparing largely the babies children and pregnant mothers, in my Observation!

Whenever I get called to help out pregnant mothers, my heart aches but immediately I see the mercy of God on them!

But still very hard in a pregnant mom to go through the hardship of pregnancy and deliver and having COVID!!

I thank God for rescuing the backbone of mankind by protecting largely the newborns, babies, children and pregnant mothers??

May our Lord put an end to the pandemic of the century and lift up His wrath! We pray Amen 🙏 Amen 🙏

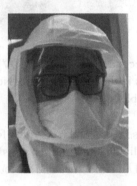

DM. i pray for your strength safety and health that you continue to be a blessing to humanity

CB. Amen 🙏🙏🙏

KG. Amen

BCD. Amen

VW. Amen

SS. Amen

CR. In Jesus name. Amen

MS. Amen 🙏

TA, 🙏 Amen

HD. Amen

CG. Prayers to end the pandemic. Blessings 🖤🙏

AV. Praying

Second Wave Is Here, Be in The Watch!!

11/18/2020

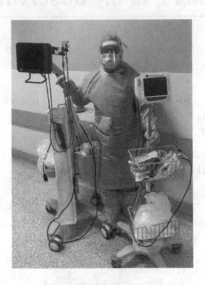

Not easy to be part of the second time round of COVID! More and more COVID cases to intubate and assess in the Intensive Care. Not only those vulnerable but also the so called invulnerable!!

Indeed, the Coronavirus is so lethal and tricky that found the weakest back door and easy access to each individual and human cells! It is engineered extremely well to target all people and all ethnicities and various climates and cultures!!

It is convenient to be virtual and away from such a contagious and stressful battlefield. But this where I find my Savior Jesus. He isn't as close in virtual remote areas but He always by me and each human soul in the depth of the battlefield, by the fire and by the mouth of lions, He is always protect and lift up His children and servants calling His Name.

So fatigued and can't believe it is back again nonstop since my very first case in March 2020. But I look up to heaven and to My Savior Lord Jesus and He gives me energy to keep going!

Very early at dawn, a COVID Victim is losing the battle to COVID and needed immediate help and to him I am going.

You all be safe

Ramsis Ghaly
Www.ghalyneurosurgeon.com

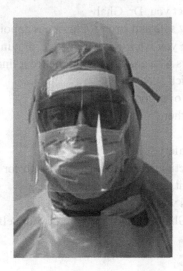

AS. Bless you be well

AK. God bless you and all of us who are suffering. Thank you, Dr Ghaly

BB. You are amazing 🙏

VD. Stay safe Dr Ghaly 🙏❤️

KC. Be safe Dr. Ghaly 🙏🙏🙏

CG. Please stay safe and Bless you. ❤️🙏

NM. Be safe 🙏🙏🙏

JV. Bless you with the strength, stamina and skill you need Dr. Ghaly, please be safe. ❤️

CY. Prayers that God will renew your strength and heal our nation from this Covid monster 🙏

VG. God Bless you 🙏🙏

KO. Lord keep you safe

HW. Thank you Dr. Ghaly for all that you do and God Bless you 🙏🙏

TJ. Thank you so much for your service. Praying for God to continue to give you strength to carry on.

AB. Praise God for your diligence to His will 🙏🙏🙏

PH. You are a true Blessing sent from GOD to care for all who need....Stay Safe!!

KG. Stay safe and well!

DS. God's Blessings 🙏 Be safe Doctor 🙏❤️🕊️

DR. Oh my bless your heart ❤️ and May God protect you 👋

SN, God Bless you Dr. Ghaly 🙏🙏❤️

JD. Take care of yourself too Dr. Ghaly !!!

RH. We can see that alarm and panic in your face. God bless you Dr. God bless all of the people that are trying to care and stop this virus.

SJ. God bless and protect you, Dr. Ghaly 🙏

JO. God Bless you! Stay safe and strong. Christ has appointed you to save many! Which hospital are you working now? 🙏❤️ praying for all the healthcare workers and doctors who are battling on the front lines. God Bless them and all those who are sick

VR. Please Lord watch over your son!

YR. Please be safe out there!

MB. Oh Lord!. 🙏🙏🙏

EM. Praying for your safety 🙏

KP. God give Dr protection from the virus, strength for every day, wisdom for treating each patient, and rest when he is weary.

KS. Stay safe God bless you for what you do

RN. God bless you Dr.Ghaly, please take care of your self!!

Please Consider My Advice During COVID Second Wave Surge!

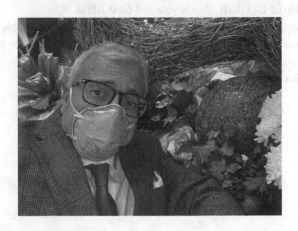

Think twice before you choose to have any elective surgery or attend any healthcare facility for non-urgent matters!

Healthcare is in crises and so is the care. No enough help, or resources, or back up or support or necessary reach out. And if something go wrong who will be around for you!!!

Hold your peace ✌️☮️ until the COVID storm 🌩️🌧️ passes by! Thank you. 🙏

Ramsis Ghaly

VF. Thank you, Dr. Ghaly!
CG. Sounds like good advice! 🖤🙏
CR. May God continue to bless and protect you 🙏
PH. Thank you for your amazing advice. 🙏😊
KO. Amen Dr Ghaly Lord bless all this world
ss. May God put under his hand ✋ and control this beast of the virus... with his own strength Amen.. and humanity that stays at peace... With all his brothers We pray.. for the whole world Amen
Sk. I agree!!
Tg. Thank you for good advice 🖤🙏
ED. I so agree with you Doctor 🙏
JP. My husband had lab work done. It turned out the best it's been in awhile. (my home-cooking instead of him going to McDonalds). He had an appointment

741

to see his GP and go over the results next week. I told him to cancel it. He goes every 3 months.

FA. Thank you Dr. Ghaly

CR. Thanks for the advice

RN. Totally agree Dr.Ghaly, thank you and God Bless. 🖤👀

JD. As you know Dr. Ghaly we are going through that very problem. It is very scary. You are the only doctor that I know that advocates for all ill people. Thank you from our whole family. 🙏

AP. Thanks for your advice

Be Ready to Put Your head and Face Sealed Inside Air Purifiers Connected to Filters and Air Tanks

Be Ready to Put Your head and Face Sealed Inside Air Purifiers Connected to Filters and Air Tanks After Double and Triple Face masks: Welcome to non-admitted Modern Incompetent Man-made Science and Robot Artificial Intelligence!!

Written by
Ramsis Ghaly

Caring for COVID patients and I now beat Fauci, I wear three face masks and soon I will put my head in an out-of-space air purifier container!!!

It my duty to serve those! They are my people, my own, my brothers and sisters and my cause!

Ramsis Ghaly

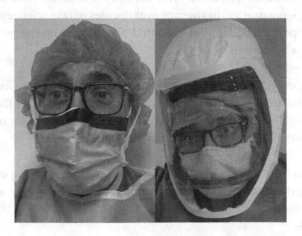

PF. Bless you please stay safe my friend 🖤
MS. Stay safe 💜
RH. Dearest doctor and friend..I look at you each picture and think how does he do it. I would feel claustrophobic. And my glasses always fog. But somehow you are still able to save lives and give the glory to God. I love you Dr.
BL. Can you breathe freely under all of that protection? 💕

CG. It's nice you still have a sense of humor. Bless you for all you do to care for the sick. ♥⚶

CM. Stay safe my friend. Did you get the vaccine??

FA. God bless you Dr Ghaly ⚶ please stay safe

AP. Be safe

KR. God Bless you

Science is stumbling!! The grandiose of man and artificial intelligence and so called "frontier science and modern robot and digital technology" brought to nothing!

Understandably, it is the Eleventh Pandemic in human history and science 🦠 does not know! It is simply above its head! There is nothing like this before and more are coming!!

To make things complicated, mankind decide to go global and to connect to the corners of earth for the first time. Son Now the pandemic had spread so fast in the speed of aircrafts and winds across the Sphere!

Furthermore, instead of the scientists, leaders, governments and politicians handle the pandemic with humility and admit their shortcoming, deficiencies, ignorance and negligence over decades of fake science and medicine and intense procrastination, they polluted and messed up the pandemic with politics and self-interest!!

Now you all expect Vaccine to be a miracle but indeed think twice and people will double and triple face masking and next generation is to place their faces and their heads totally inside an AIR PURIFIER and we all are going to walk as an astronauts with filters and tanks of clean airs and oxygen!!!

That minute virus 🦠 has a mind of its own and will be sweeping and sweeping out smarting the modern human minds and technology extremely well bringing them to nothing!!

Be Ready to Put Your head and Face Sealed Inside Air Purifiers Connected to Filters and Air Tanks After Double and Triple Face masks: Welcome to non-admitted Modern Incompetent Man-made Science and Robot Artificial Intelligence!!

This adverse progression and extensive Hand-Cuffed restrictions shall continue until God the Almighty find a down -to-earth humble loving heart ♥ non-politicians rejected by many viewed as weak and ignorant and from out of the establishment send and open his or her mind to discover the only way to stop ● and combat the virus 🦠 once and for all!

As man grandiose continues and his craziness, madness and self-interest and egocentricity and the non pure hearts and sorrowful spirits continue their own ways and take advantage, so shall the pandemic get more and more complex and sophisticated for human minds to find solutions!!

The traumatic scars will be difficult to handle in the years to come and the side effects in the new generations shall last for centuries to come. The causalities not just from COVID directly but related to COVID, shall increase more and more as collateral to the pandemic. The fragmentation of the societies and worldwide anti governmental riots, demonstrations and violence as the mistrust is in the rise!!

How much I wish that God had entrusted even if only one pure heart ♥ of a Spiritual Christian Leader to intervene and enter the heart of Heavenly Father and open His Divine Mercy!!!

Let us listen to the answer for the eleventh pandemic: "For it is written, I will destroy the wisdom of the wise, and will bring to nothing the understanding of the prudent. [20] Where is the wise? where is the scribe? where is the disputer of this world? hath not God made foolish the wisdom of this world? [21] For after that in the wisdom of God the world by wisdom knew not God, it pleased God by the foolishness of preaching to save them that believe. [25] Because the foolishness of God is wiser than men; and the weakness of God is stronger than men. [26] For ye see your calling, brethren, how that not many wise men after the flesh, not many mighty, not many noble, are called: [27] But God hath chosen the foolish things of the world to confound the wise; and God hath chosen the weak things of the world to confound the things which are mighty; [28] And base things of the world, and things which are despised, hath God chosen, yea, and things which are not, to bring to nought things that are: [29] That no flesh should glory in his presence. [30] But of him are ye in Christ Jesus, who of God is made unto us wisdom, and righteousness, and sanctification, and redemption: [31] That, according as it is written, He that glorieth, let him glory in the Lord."1 Corinthians 1:19-21,25-31 KJV

At that day let us utter Psalm 67: God be merciful unto us, and bless us; and cause his face to shine upon us; Selah. [2] That thy way may be known upon earth, thy saving health among all nations. [3] Let the people praise thee, O God; let all the people praise thee. [4] O let the nations be glad and sing for joy: for thou shalt judge the people righteously, and govern the nations upon earth. Selah. [5] Let the people praise thee, O God; let all the people praise thee. [6] Then shall the earth yield her increase; and God, even our own God, shall bless us. [7] God shall bless us; and all the ends of the earth shall fear him.

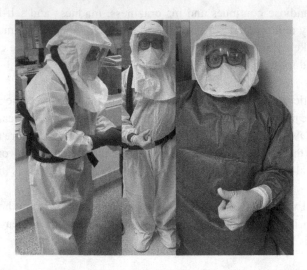

MN. Be careful Dr.Ghaly

CE. Please be safe Dr Ghaly!

RH. We love everything you do XOX

JM. Agree, The Pandemic Is "Polluted" With Politics and Self Interest!!

CG. Science and the politician's have failed America, you are correct. Who do we believe and who do we trust? ♥⅄

LA. "[God] wants men, so far as I can see, to ask very simple questions; is it righteous? is it prudent? is it possible? Now if we can keep men asking, "Is it in accordance with the general movement of our time? Is it progressive or reactionary? Is it the way that History is going?" they will neglect the relevant questions. And the questions they do ask are, of course, unanswerable; for they do not know the future, and what the future will be depends very largely on just those choices which they now invoke the future to help them to make." – Uncle Screwtape from C.S. Lewis - The Screwtape Letters

Persistent Fever in Early COVID Illness: Please listen to my advice!!

This is my advice to patients tested recently COVID-19 Positive and have persistent low grade fever: go to the hospital, get admitted and try to receive intravenous monoclonal antibody and dexamethasone as president Trump and other high hierarchy received!!!

My heart is saddened and feel sorrowful because one of my friends in Baltimore Maryland was tested positive from getting exposed to a positive person in a restaurant and John Hopkin rejected him and refused to admit him early as I advise him to do!

He started to suffer from only low grade fever otherwise he felt great. He continued to be quarantined at home. He texted me asking if I have done suggestions!

I called him. He told me he felt great no shortness of breath but he had a low grade temperature for a week. Everyone in the medical field told him to stay at home eat and drink and do not go to the hospital and no worries! They can only see him through Telemedicine. He found a Telemed doc who prescribed Ivermectin, prednisone and five-day supply of Zithromycin.

I took few moments and asked my Lord, Lord I am not his doctor and I don't practice in Baltimore !! I said to him: "Go to John Hopkins hospital Emergency Room where Dr Fauci practice and get admitted and try to receive intravenous monoclonal antibody and dexamethasone and perhaps remdesivir as president Trump and other high hierarchy received!!! He said, I am shocked from your advice especially everyone told me to stay at home and quarantine and you will be fine! My breathing is okay. I said with tearful eyes please go that hell virus can involve the heart and great vessels in no time causing strokes deadly heart attack. Once the virus started to cause persistent fever even if low grade it is unpredictable!!! I send him all medications available for treatment of COVID from Mayo clinic website!!

I was so hopeful that John Hopkins and Fauci have an aggressive early prevention from progression and early treatment from COVID 19. Bless his heart, he went and they send him away immediately without performing a single test and refuse to admit him or give him intravenous monoclonal antibody and dexamethasone and perhaps remdesivir! He insisted based in my advice but they refuse to listen!!

They just listen to his chest and heart and send him home! I wasn't happy at all and in my opinion sad especially he made a tripe and went to their doors!! What is the big deal to admit him and observe and give some intravenous dexamethasone and monoclonal antibodies and perhaps remdesivir and do some labs and xrays and send him home in few days!!!! There is a reason why fever is going on!! The man felt something in his health is going wrong and begged to be admitted, why you didn't listen to his heart especially he had a great health records shame on you hospitals and medical team!! You failed him and denied him!!

Four days later, my friend is suffering from severe decline with COVID pneumonia and hard to breath and talk getting admitted immediately to the intensive care unit!!

What is wrong of healthcare and common sense in Medicine!!! Shame on you John Hopkins and the ongoing medicine practice who reject such patients and common sense!! And only treat President Trump and other high hierarchy and whoever is connected and you know, differently than the regular public!!!

What about the regular hardworking Americans why they do not have access to president trump treatment and high hierarchy and get admitted for few days to monitor!! What is at home nothing but walls and TV and no medical care!!!! What is good in telemedicine and virtual other than some superficial pictures and carrying conversation with no hand s-on care!!!

Let us start prayer 🙏 chain for our beloved good hearted patient and all the sick like him in need for speed recovery, Amen 🙏

Ramsis Ghaly

JP. Prayers for your friend Dr. Ghaly. 🙏🙏🙏
DT. Very scary that hospitals and drs. Don't want to treat right away... don't understand why.... ?? Praying for your friend!!!!
WP. How the government, and by its extension the media, is handling this virus is sinful. TV commercials are now advertising the use of Regenerons monoclonal antibody. It's FDA approved now. Why would he be refused? He needs a lawyer to contact the hospital and add some pressure.
JZ. Prayers!
ML. It's such an unpredictable virus. I will pray for your friend. Although I have recovered from the virus, I am a long hauler and still feel the effects from this virus. Prayers for you my hero.

LR. Trump said this would work but he was blatantly belittled and made fun of by the asshat Steven Colbert and the rest of the jerks. The Pandemic was a political tool and now the vaccine is and the money that the powers that be are making from this virus. My heart goes out to your patients that have been treated like political pawns

DE. Thank you Dr.Ghaly 🙏

KB. Prayers for your friend!! 🙏

TD. What a sad situation, many prayers for your friend 🙏

SP. Prayers for your friend Dr. Ramsis Ghaly 🙏 When I hear things like this it upsets me that they have all the control and we are powerless over our own health care.

ED. Prayers 🙏🙏🙏🙏🙏🙏🙏

LN. We have commercials on TV (Arizona) in regards to people with high risk immune system and if they get covid to immediately call their health care for the monoclonal antibodies!

CG. My prayers go out to your friend. May our Lord bless him and protect him. 🙏🙏

JH. Will keep your friend in my prayers.

DL. Prayers for you dear friend. Can't imagine what India must be going through too. So sad. Prayers needed for everyone. Even other countries.

EH. Praying for your friend.

SS. 🙏 for a speedy recovery.

SL. So very sorry 😢 Sadly modern medicine, while having many caring and ethical individuals such as yourself, is also compromised by many corrupt people sworn to protect us and other outside evil influences my prayers are with you as always and for your dear friend 🙏❤️🙏

YF. I am so sorry to hear this 🙏🙏🙏🙏🙏 for all of us

MM. Praying for speedy recovery for your friend Dr.Ghaly, God is good

SM. Prayers for your friend doc!!

BS. My cousins daughter lives in Annapolis and is in her mid 40's
She was hospitalized and given that drug. She's home and doing good!
Is there a shortage of that drug ?

TA. Prayers 🙏🙏🙏 NV. Prayers for your friend Doctor Ghaly, 🙏

MD. I received monoclonal antibodies in January at Tampa General Hospital. They have a place called the Gedi Center (Global Emerging Diseases Institute) where they administer the infusion. Then they followed with you to see your progress.

MJ. Thank you Dr Ramsis Ghaly. For the stimulating post, we respect you sir

JD. Just wanted to share this with family & friends. This doctor who posted this did my back surgery and has quintuple certifications as a neurosurgeon. I trust him with my life. If his advice could help save one

life it is worth the share. Thank you Dr. Ramsis Ghaly for sharing your knowledge and advice!

JW. prayers to help Americans

DT. If you test positive go and get treatment ASAP .....

LA. Joining all others in praying for a full and speedy recovery for your friend and all those who are ill, and thanking the Lord in advance for hearing and answering our prayers.

KP. Prayers for you friend

AS. Sending my prayers! Behind all this is pharmaceutical mafia and we know very well that right now the most outspoken politicians making the biggest profit!

CR. This post brought me to tears. I couldn't agree more. We have such a broken system. Thank you for standing up for the ordinary person. Thank you for being my daughters doctor. Saving her life. I will be praying for this man.

EB. Prayers for your friend for fast recovery 🙏🙏🙏

SN. Sending prayers for your friend. 🙏

Ghaly Photos with PPE

Layers of protective clothing, gowns, gloves, circulating air with filters (PAPR)

Personal protective equipment is protective clothing, helmets, goggles, or other garments or equipment designed to protect the wearer's body from injury or infection. The hazards addressed by protective equipment include physical, electrical, heat, chemicals, biohazards, and airborne particulate matter.

What is personal protective equipment?

Personal protective equipment, commonly referred to as "PPE", is equipment worn to minimize exposure to hazards that cause serious workplace injuries and illnesses. These injuries and illnesses may result from contact with chemical, radiological, physical, electrical, mechanical, or other workplace hazards. Personal protective equipment may include items such as gloves, safety glasses and shoes, earplugs or muffs, hard hats, respirators, or coveralls, vests and full body suits.

What can be done to ensure proper use of personal protective equipment?

All personal protective equipment should be safely designed and constructed, and should be maintained in a clean and reliable fashion. It should fit comfortably, encouraging worker use. If the personal protective equipment does not fit properly, it can make the difference between being safely covered or dangerously exposed. When engineering, work practice, and administrative controls are not feasible or do not provide sufficient protection, employers must provide personal protective equipment to their workers and ensure its proper use. Employers are also required to train each worker required to use personal protective equipment to know.

Powered Air Purifying Respirator (PAPR)

- A PAPR (or tight-fitting goggles and an N-95 respirator) should be worn for high-risk aerosol-generating procedures. These respirators also meet CDC guidelines for protection against TB exposure. The equipment is battery operated, consists of a half or full facepiece, breathing tube, battery-operated blower, and particulate filters (HEPA only).
- PAPR uses a blower to pass contaminated air through a HEPA filter, which removes the contaminant and supplies purified air to a facepiece.
- PAPR is not a true positive-pressure device because it can be over-breathed when inhaling.

- A face shield may also be used in conjunction with a half-mask PAPR respirator for protection against body fluids.

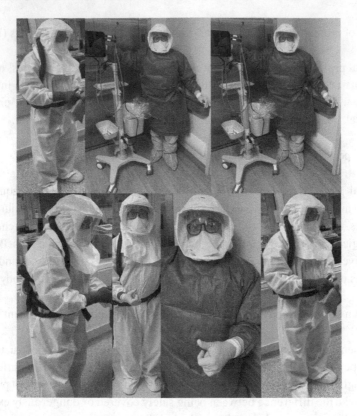

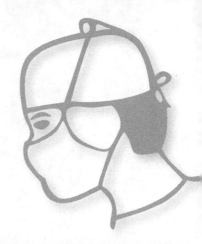

SECTION 13

Critical Look at COVID-19

COVID Pandemic My Critical Look!

A year had passed by with no single cure of COVID-19!! We must examine the Science and Medicine Failure immediately! We must hold senate meeting to surface the decades of corruption in science and medicine!! It is the time to reform Science and medicine and counter Bioweapon!

We must bring scientists and agents responsible to develop the medicine to protect mankind against viruses and pandemic to Justice! They all knew that it was a matter of time for such a pandemic to occur. They all were funded with federal money and tax money to defend our people and protect them against pandemics!! There were plentiful budgets and billions of dollars over decades were allocated and spent to recruit real scientists and to develop a countrywide plans and defense against the immediate threats of Bioterrorism!

The Nano Coronavirus proofed that man and science with their grandiosity are just nothing and fake!

The so called artificial Intelligence, the digital technology, computer electronics are all just a show.

All what they come out with lockdown and house arrest as our native mankind did 7000 years ago with their natural instinct and no so called fake science and fake degrees.

What a shame! What a massive corruption! It turns out there was never been a system in place or real scientists or genuine defense! Now they are depending on each state to lockdown people because there is no treatment and there is no enough hospitals. In fact, there was never been huge capacity hospital build to accommodate mass causalities! Look at Vegas, Montana, Dakotas,— and many others no enough hospital beds! So what medicine forced to do, let patients go and pull the plug early!!

What is the result of decades of corruption and darkness and dishonesty!!!!! The public pay the price, get locked down, arrested, penalized and die!!!

The COVID pandemic surfaced man corruption, dishonesty and fakeness! We all responsible since we all promoted such behavior!

Let us learn from this catastrophic pandemic, call for immediate reform, put the right people in the job, recruit real scientists, genuine gifted and skilled workers and put accountability and auditing in the progress!!

Respectfully
Ramsis Ghaly

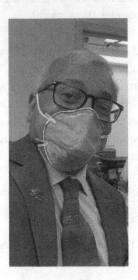

AS. When money (personal interest, and we know very well that pharmaceutical companies are like that) and politics are involved science cannot do much!

SC. Much respect, Dr. Ghaly.

DR. True - with the only caveat that AI is here and it will stay ....

JM. Yes I agree 😣

AV. Thank Dr Ghaly for this information! Truly we need people to turn to God for help & be accountable!! 🙏🙏

DR. yes so true and so wrong & sad 😔

PF. Yes Thank You! This is the truth we need to see it for what it is. Now it's time to leave the blame where lies and demand better for our survival. I can't say enough about you and the profession you are in. You all are our angeles trying to save who they can with no help. 😞

MB. Well said Dr.Ghaly. 🙏🙏🙏

MN. You are write there is no other way to explain that.

KO. Amen, be humble, be kind, to each other, this world needs to change 🙏🙏

RC. Right, unfortunately is general, in every ware!

Critical Look at the World Eleventh Pandemic!

Critical Look at the World 🌐 Eleventh Pandemic: The Entire World 🌐 lockdown because of a virus 🦠 causing only 0.028% Deaths!

Written by Ramsis Ghaly

My Weekend Critical Thesis

The world 🌐 nations is under man-made siege and surrendering to a virus 🦠 that killed only 0,03%!!! What about the lives of the 99.97% ?? Why are we ignoring the majority letting them die prematurely burying the 99.97% alive???

The world is still a good healthy and safe place to live! God is in control! The 99.97% of population are living and NO need to inflict unnecessary pains, suffering, hardships, losses, separation and deprivation that are leading to preventable causalities and social fragmentation, street and domestic violence, abuse and overdose!!!

The governments and so called scientists of the world are allowing the world to crash down because of a minute virus 🦠 causing less than 0.03% deaths and burying the entire God Grace and blessing on 99.97% of the world 🌐 populations!!

The entire economy down the drain and the world budget is directing to 1.3% of the population and taken away from the 98.7% of the world populations living dreadful in misery, darkness with little Hope!

The entire industry, production, social media, news and every day trading, transaction and move worldwide are concentrating on the 1.3% of the populations and nothing and ignoring the living giving just a little for 98.7% of populations and their needs, future, comfort, job and life security and peace of mind!!!

The 98.7% of the world 🌐 populations are starving out of jobs, not eating or working or living a life under house arrest and social isolation distancing away stopped-living because of a virus affecting 1.3%!! Is this fair or it is the

757

foolishness, ignorance and power to control and self interest of the rulers and so called scientists!!!

One day total world births are much more than the to-date total world COVID infected cases! TO-date total world COVID Deaths is almost nothing 4.3% of a single day world Deaths!

I wondered how the world leaders and so called political scientists justifying imprisonments of 98.7% of total world 🌍 population depriving them from living the life given to them by God and restraining the human souls of the growing new generations interrupting their development and taking their childhood and schooling away from them!!

Why those are looking at the little sip at the bottom of a cup ignoring the entire cup full of honey and passion fruit!!

The entire world is in standstill terrorized and forced in absolute Curfew because of virus 🦠 affecting only 1.3% of the population!

The so called wise rulers and scientists are imposing not just days or weeks or months but years of lifelessness ignoring the total population of Virus 🦠 free life living of 98.7%!

COVID is the ongoing man made world emergency and enslaving mankind all over the continents!!!

Did you know that Man and not virus 🦠 killed his own in World War I Deaths 20 million and total causalities 40 million
https://en.m.wikipedia.org/wiki/World_War_I_casualties

Did you know Man and not virus 🦠 killed his own in World War II Deaths 85 million
https://en.m.wikipedia.org/wiki/World_War_II_casualties

Stats and Facts
Total World Population 7,842,521,953
Total COVID Worldwide 102,546,473
Total COVID Recovered 74,450,404
Total COVID Deaths 2,214,076
Percentage of COVID to Total Population 1.3%
Percentage of COVID Deaths to Total Population 0.028%

123,539 Daily Births
51,865 daily Deaths
https://www.worldometers.info/world-population/
https://www.worldometers.info/coronavirus/

There is a belief that either way with or without treatment, the virus has to infect and kill certain numbers before fades away!

The world 🌑 is at loss with the Eleventh pandemic of humanity over thousands of years and don't know what to do. Everything is "Emergency" and every tip is a "Breaking News"— The Ten Previous Worst Pandemics

First Pandemic 541
The Plague of Justinian arrived in Constantinople, the capital of the Byzantine Empire, in 541 CE. It was carried over the Mediterranean Sea from Egypt, a recently conquered land paying tribute to Emperor Justinian in grain. Plague-ridden fleas hitched a ride on the black rats that snacked on the grain. The plague decimated Constantinople and spread like wildfire across Europe, Asia, North Africa and Arabia killing an estimated 30 to 50 million people, perhaps half of the world's population.

Second Pandemic 1347
The plague never really went away, and when it returned 800 years later, it killed with reckless abandon. The Black Death, which hit Europe in 1347, claimed an astonishing 200 million lives in just four years.

Third pandemic 1348-1665
London never really caught a break after the Black Death. The plague resurfaced roughly every 10 years from 1348 to 1665—40 outbreaks in just over 300 years. And with each new plague epidemic, 20 percent of the men, women and children living in the British capital were killed. The Great Plague of 1665 was the last and one of the worst of the centuries-long outbreaks, killing 100,000 Londoners in just seven months.

Fourth Pandemic 15th century
Smallpox was endemic to Europe, Asia and Arabia for centuries, a persistent menace that killed three out of ten people it infected and left the rest with pockmarked scars. But the death rate in the Old World paled in comparison to the devastation wrought on native populations in the New World when the smallpox virus arrived in the 15th century with the first European explorers.

759

Fifth Pandemic 19ᵗʰ century
In the early- to mid-19ᵗʰ century, cholera tore through England, killing tens of thousands. The prevailing scientific theory of the day said that the disease was spread by foul air known as a "miasma."

Sixth Pandemic 19ᵗʰ century
H1N1 virus 🦠 pandemic infected 500 million and killed 50 million worldwide! The 1918 influenza pandemic was the most severe pandemic in recent history. It was caused by an H1N1 virus with genes of avian origin. Although there is not universal consensus regarding where the virus originated, it spread worldwide during 1918-1919. In the United States, it was first identified in military personnel in spring 1918. It is estimated that about 500 million people or one-third of the world's population became infected with this virus. The number of deaths was estimated to be at least 50 million worldwide with about 675,000 occurring in the United States.
https://www.cdc.gov/.../pandemic.../1918-pandemic-h1n1.html

Seventh Asian Flu
According to the CDC, the "Asian Flu" began in East Asia in 1957. The influenza virus was an H2N2 strain, first discovered in Singapore. From there, the virus made its way to Hong Kong and to the coastal cities in the United States. Of the 1.1 million people who died of the Asian flu worldwide, 116,000 of them were in the United States

Eighth Pandemic Hong Kong Flu
The Hong Kong flu pandemic of 1968 originated in China. Caused by an influenza A virus (H3N2), it was the third pandemic flu outbreak to occur in the 20ᵗʰ century, killing one million people worldwide, 100,000 in the United States.

Ninth Pandemic Swine Flu
The "swine flu" occurred in 2009 with a novel influenza virus, H1N1. According to the CDC, the virus was actually first detected in the US, and spread quickly across the US and the world. Between April 12, 2009 and April 10, 2010, there were 60.8 million cases reported, 274,304 hospitalizations, and 12,469 deaths due to the virus. The CDC estimates 575,400 people died worldwide.

Tenth Pandemic HIV/AIDS
Human immunodeficiency virus, HIV, and acquired immunodeficiency syndrome, AIDS, were first discovered in the early 1980s. AIDS was first detected in American gay communities but it's thought to have developed from a chimpanzee virus from Africa in the 1920s. According to the World Health Organization, 75

million people have been infected with the virus since it was discovered, resulting in 32 million deaths worldwide. An estimated 38,000 new HIV infections still happen in the U.S. each year.

https://www.history.com/.../pandemics-end-plague-cholera...

https://abc7news.com/.../pandemic-epidemic.../5974174

The people run away to hide, in terrors and fears and all the news around full of threats, intimidation, rules, and regulations with penalties and humiliation! While the politicians are exercising their powers while life in the Brave land is restrained by force!

For a year now, the world 🌐 is under continuous attacks made by man unrelenting and no stop! What is wrong of the world! Where is the emergency? What kind of emergency ⚓ that is lasting for a year? I understand for a day or two or a week or two for a month or two but not for a year and is still going!!!

Why those are looking at the little sip at the bottom of a cup ignoring the entire cup full of honey and passion fruit!!

Let us be thankful to our Lord for the 99.97% living of all people! Our Savior is in control Colossians 3:15-17 KJV 15] And let the peace of God rule in your hearts, to the which also ye are called in one body; and be ye thankful. [16] Let the word of Christ dwell in you richly in all wisdom; teaching and admonishing one another in psalms and hymns and spiritual songs, singing with grace in your hearts to the Lord. [17] And whatsoever ye do in word or deed, do all in the name of the Lord Jesus, giving thanks to God and the Father by him. Psalm 107:1,8-9 KJV 1] O give thanks unto the Lord, for he is good: for his mercy endureth forever. [8] Oh that men would praise the Lord for his goodness, and for his wonderful works to the children of men! [9] For he satisfieth the longing soul, and filleth the hungry soul with goodness.

Let us praise our Savior for His abundance of grace and plentiful of blessing wirjdeude saving 99.97% of all people! Jesus is in Control: Psalm 150:1-6 KJV 1] Praise ye the Lord. Praise God in his sanctuary: praise him in the firmament of his power. [2] Praise him for his mighty acts: praise him according to his excellent greatness. [3] Praise him with the sound of the trumpet: praise him with the psaltery and harp. [4] Praise him with the timbrel and dance: praise him with stringed instruments and organs. [5] Praise him upon the loud cymbals: praise him upon the high sounding cymbals. [6] Let every thing that hath breath praise the Lord. Praise ye the Lord.

I thought I may be missing something as I went through facts s as d statistics!!! I looked from my windows may be the cause of ongoing emergency 🔔 are the falling billions of rockets and explosive bombs bombarding every corner upon the face of earth but I couldn't see any!! I searched more and more and I continue to see God Grace and blessing in abundance! I thought may be Ramsis and Moses time came back with the pestilences! But o my gosh nothing like those days!!!

The world 🌍 is still a good healthy and safe place to live! God is still with us shining the sun ☀ at day time and the moon 🌑 at nighttime, the millions of stars ⭐ covering the sky, the fresh air flowing around the planet 🌍, the ground is giving plentiful of grass trees 🌿🌲 and fruits 🍌🍎🍊, the creeping animals in the fields, the birds 🦅 and towels are flying high and the whales 🐋 and fish 🐟🐠 are filling the seas and oceans and the waters erupting in the wills for the billions and billions of the living to drink!!! What is wrong of this world! God is in control and why call it crises when there isn't one since our Heavenly Father is alive and working!! Let us be thankful and give thanksgiving and joyful in the Lord!

Let us follow Jesus and let the dead bury their dead as it is written: "And he said unto another, Follow me. But he said, Lord, suffer me first to go and bury my father. [60] Jesus said unto him, Let the dead bury their dead: but go thou and preach the kingdom of God. [61] And another also said, Lord, I will follow thee; but let me first go bid them farewell, which are at home at my house. [62] And Jesus said unto him, No man, having put his hand to the plough, and looking back, is fit for the kingdom of God." Luke 9:59-62 KJV

Our Lord is with us who can be against us! COVID and rumors of pandemics and fears and terrors of pestilences shall never take over our lives and take our hears away from the love and prosperity of living day and night with our living Savior forever and ever more as it is written: "What shall we then say to these things? If God be for us, who can be against us? [32] He that spared not his own Son, but delivered him up for us all, how shall he not with him also freely give us all things? [35] Who shall separate us from the love of Christ? shall tribulation, or distress, or persecution, or famine, or nakedness, or peril, or sword? [36] As it is written, For thy sake we are killed all the day long; we are accounted as sheep for the slaughter. [37] Nay, in all these things we are more than conquerors through him that loved us. [38] For I am persuaded, that neither death, nor life, nor angels, nor principalities, nor powers, nor things present, nor things to come, [39] Nor height, nor depth, nor any other creature, shall be able to separate us from the love of God, which is in Christ Jesus our Lord."

Romans 8:31-32,35-39 KJV
Be in good comfort knowing billions of people are healthy living and not touched by so called COVID!

Be of good cheer, the world 🌍 is our Savior land and a beautiful place to live! Don't live in fear! Don't let the days go by in hide: "Be strong and of a good courage, fear not, nor be afraid of them: for the Lord thy God, he it is that doth go with thee; he will not fail thee, nor forsake thee." Deuteronomy 31:6 KJV

"Cast your burden on the Lord, and He shall sustain you; He shall never permit the righteous to be moved" (Psalms 55:22)

Be in peace and give thanksgiving to the Lord in Jesus name! He is alive and our Savior and our Father! "Peace I leave with you, my peace I give unto you: not as the world giveth, give I unto you. Let not your heart be troubled, neither let it be afraid." John 14:27

Numbers 6:24-26 NKJV "The LORD bless you and keep you; The LORD make His face shine upon you, And be gracious to you; The LORD lift up His countenance upon you, And give you peace."

Emergency 🚑 and isn't Emergency! The world 🌍 is still a good healthy and safe place to live and God in Control!

Written by Ramsis Ghaly

"Be anxious for nothing, but in everything by prayer and supplication, with (B) thanksgiving, let your requests be made known to God; 7 and (C)the peace of God, which surpasses all understanding, will guard your hearts and minds through Christ Jesus." Philippians 4:6-8

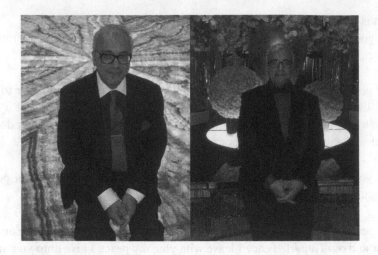

LW. Thank you Ramsis!

AV. Thank you Dr Ghaly! Stay safe! 🌸🙏

KG. How informative and beautiful are your thoughts, Dr. Ghaly! You give us hope 🙏

FA. Yes Dr Ghaly you give us hope 🙏

VW. Thank you, Dr. Ghaly!

AP. You give us hope

CG. Doctor you are always so positive and reassuring. God bless you! 💜🙏

JM. There's always hope when the Lord is involved. Too much Fear in the world your post hit the nail on the head! 🙏

JM. Facts about Pandemic.

SB. Very interesting and informative. Surprised Zucker Book hasn't removed this article that goes against their agenda. Maybe because it's sunday...

LA. Words of wisdom from Dr. Ramsis Ghaly ~

LG. More wise words from a Neurosurgeon in Chicago who has been working on the front lines since the beginning....

LM. Thanks, Lisa. Dr. Ghaly's advice is appreciated.

BS. This is how Fake News on a Daily basis causes Fear, And I am truly sorry for those we have lost, But Ruining the other 97 % of the country.

Looking Back at COVID Pandemic!! Deep Reflections

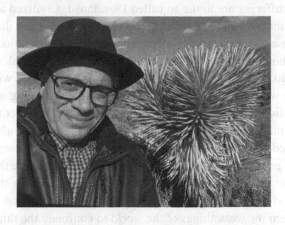

"It is of the Lord's mercies that we are not consumed (by COVID19 viruses 🦠🦠🦠), because his compassions fail not." Lamentations 3:22 KJV

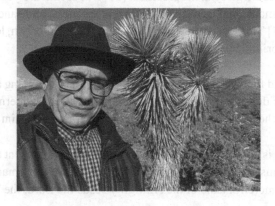

+ COVID is in its way out because of inherited natural immunity created by the Almighty and to God is all the credit!!!

+ COVID showed the world a little Nano-virus can defeat the heaviest army of men overnight and wipe out countries in no time!

+ COVID showed that the builders of Babylon tower and modern sky high rise can be conquered and brought down to the ground in a matter of seconds from a little particles of the invisible despite the sophistication of intelligence, cameras and satellites!!

+ The worst countries got hit hard in regarding to numbers of casualties, death, sickness and suffering are in the so called Developed, Civilized and Advanced countries and the poor and under developed and not as civilized did much better and still living as the virus never wiped them out!!! So proud nations think twice of what you should be proud of and return to your roots!! Think for a moment and reflect unto these words as it is written: "For it is written, I will destroy the wisdom of the wise, and will bring to nothing the understanding of the prudent. [20] Where is the wise? where is the scribe? where is the disputer of this world? hath not God made foolish the wisdom of this world? [21] For after that in the wisdom of God the world by wisdom knew not God, it pleased God by the foolishness of preaching to save them that believe. [25] Because the foolishness of God is wiser than men; and the weakness of God is stronger than men. [27] But God hath chosen the foolish things of the world to confound the wise; and God hath chosen the weak things of the world to confound the things which are mighty; [28] And base things of the world, and things which are despised, hath God chosen, yea, and things which are not, to bring to nought things that are: [29] That no flesh should glory in his presence. [30] But of him are ye in Christ Jesus, who of God is made unto us wisdom, and righteousness, and sanctification, and redemption: [31] That, according as it is written, He that glorieth, let him glory in the Lord." 1 Corinthians 1:19-21,25,27-31 KJV

+ No one should fool you or take credit for the Coronavirus going away!!! This is what pandemic does for thousands of years and this what modern medicine and science fooled the world when they are incompetent and proclaim false claim!!

+ COVID soon is going away NOT because of previous or present administration and NOT because of the vaccine or CDC or WHO or pharmaceuticals BUT because of the merciful hand of the Almighty Jesus the Lord, the True Healing!

+ COVID taught us that modern medicine and so called artificial intelligence and science 🖋️ is untrustworthy and so limited and irresponsible and the people shouldn't depend on blindly and never take things for granted!!

+ COVID exposed science, modern medicine and technology and alerted them of having a long way to go and never ever think for a moment that artificial computerized robots will replace the mighty human brain created by God the Lord!!

+ COVID brought the human race to their knees and showed mankind how weak, how vulnerable and how vanishing is human life in earth!!

+ COVID brought people together in suffering, loss and difficult times! In these times we have one another!

+ COVID also surfaced the Corporate corruption and selfishness of mankind and greediness of humanity and manipulative politicians!!

+ Covid awaken man to go back to his routes and return to God's creation! COVID made us explore the nature more and more and run away from the cities and industrial pollution and crowding and noisy electronics looking up to God the Almighty as our eternal destiny!!

+ COVID called for humanity to wake up from the fake dreams and lengthy naps and examine the truth about mankind and whom to depend on but God Almighty and not the fiction of science!

+ COVID made us appreciate the gift of life more and more and the health and made us to be much appreciative and content to what we have and more than ever give thanks to the Lord and Thanksgiving!

+ COVID demonstrated to many how they fell victims to the untruth and must examine the sources of the spirits!! And God Almighty provided His children with the armor of faith and what it take to conquer the enemies!!

Psalm 70 Make haste, O God, to deliver me; make haste to help me, O Lord. [2] Let them be ashamed and confounded that seek after my soul: let them be turned backward, and put to confusion, that desire my hurt. [3] Let them be turned back for a reward of their shame that say, Aha, aha. [4] Let all those that seek thee rejoice and be glad in thee: and let such as love thy salvation say continually, Let God be magnified. [5] But I am poor and needy: make haste unto me, O God: thou art my help and my deliverer; O Lord, make no tarrying.

+ This generation is given nothing better than Lamentations 3: "It is of the Lord's mercies that we are not consumed, because his compassions fail not. [24] The Lord   is my portion, saith my soul; therefore will I hope in him. [25] The Lord is good unto them that wait for him, to the soul that seeketh him. [40] Let us search and try our ways, and turn again to the Lord. [41] Let us lift up our heart with our hands unto God in the heavens. [42] We have transgressed and have rebelled: thou hast not pardoned. [43] Thou hast covered with anger, and persecuted us: thou hast slain, thou hast not pitied. [44] Thou hast covered thyself with a cloud, that our prayer should not pass through. [46] All our enemies have opened their mouths against us. [47] Fear and a snare is come upon us, desolation and destruction. [48] Mine eye runneth down with rivers of water for the destruction of the daughter of my people. [49] Mine eye trickleth down, and ceaseth not, without any intermission, [50] Till the Lord look down, and behold from heaven. [51] Mine eye affecteth mine heart because of all the daughters of my city. [52] Mine enemies chased me sore, like a bird, without cause. [53] They have cut off my life in the dungeon, and cast a stone upon me. [54] Waters flowed over mine head; then I said, I am cut off. [55] I called upon thy name, O Lord, out of the low dungeon. [56] Thou hast heard my voice: hide not thine ear at my breathing, at my cry. [57] Thou drewest near in the day that I called upon thee: thou saidst, Fear not. [58] O Lord, thou hast pleaded the causes of my soul; thou hast redeemed my life. [59] O Lord, thou hast seen my wrong: judge thou my cause. [60] Thou hast seen all their vengeance and all their imaginations against me. [61] Thou hast heard their reproach, O Lord, and all their imaginations against me; [62] The lips of those that rose up against me, and their device against me all the day. [63] Behold their sitting down, and their rising up; I am their musick. [64] Render unto them a recompence, O Lord, according to the work of their hands. [65] Give them sorrow of heart, thy curse unto them. [66] Persecute and destroy them in anger from under the heavens of the Lord."

"It is of the Lord's mercies that we are not consumed (by COVID19 viruses), because his compassions fail not." Lamentations 3:22 KJV

Amen

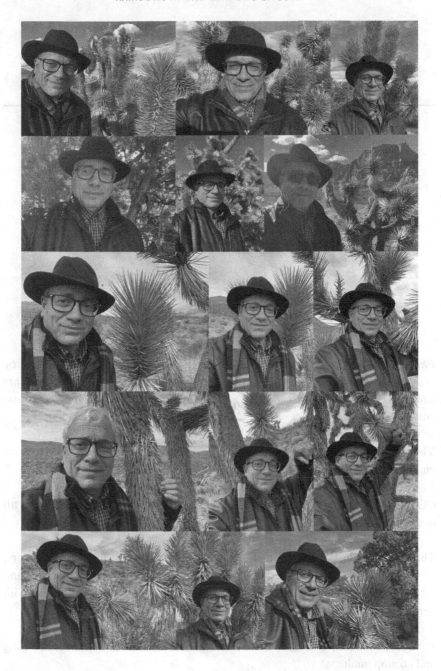

Cg. Yes, covid has done many things this past year.

It has brought families closer together and also closer to God. Thank you for sharing. 🖤🙏

Emergency and isn't Emergency! The world is still A Good Place to Live and God is in Control!

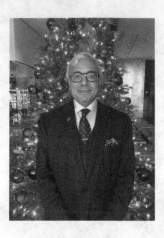

Philippians 4:6-7 Do not be anxious about anything, but in every situation, by prayer and petition, with thanksgiving, present your requests to God. And the peace of God, which transcends all understanding, will guard your hearts and your minds in Christ Jesus.

Thessalonians 5:16-18 Rejoice always, pray continually, give thanks in all circumstances; for this is God's will for you in Christ Jesus.

COVID is the ongoing man-made world emergency and enslaving mankind all over the continents!!!

Those few made the people in the entire world run away to hide, in terrors, paralyzed minds and brain washed, and day and night fears and night mares and all the news around are full of threats, intimidation, rules, and regulations with penalties and humiliation!

For a year now, the world 🌑 is under continuous attacks made by man unrelenting and no stop madness!

I kept looking from my windows watching for what the world was told of the emergency because of those billions of invisible rockets and explosive bombs bombarding every corner upon the face of earth but I couldn't find any!! Where are those enemies or ghosts causing the year of ongoing emergency upon the face of the earth!!

I said what is wrong of the world! Where is the emergency? What kind of emergency ⬛ that is lasting for a year? I understand for a day or two or a week or two for a month or two but not for a year and is still going!!!

There is no transparency what so ever and every minute there is a change, no consistency as mother and father used to tell their kids when they behave like angry cats yelling and screaming and running around trying to get attention with no purpose: O son don't act immature and irrational as a chicken rambling around chaotic with no head?

Guess what the people aren't taking it anymore, riots, demonstrations and antigovernment are in the rise and just building up!!

What those rulers are doing instead of being truthful and wise? They are tightening the people freedom and the people they serve aren't able to breath and angry and mad like hell and yet the rulers and regulators are imposing more and more social isolations and curfews!!

As if this not enough, Marshall law and military guards are in the streets and cities and in front of buildings! As if they never learned from history that this isn't the way to lead the people!!!

Ghaly cascade of man destruction: When there is no transparency, there is conspiracy and when there is conspiracy, there is no truth and when there is no truth, there is no trust and when there is no trust, there is anger, unrest and uprise and when there are unrest, uprise and anger, there is revolution and when there is revolution, there is destruction and when there is destruction, there is no peace and when there is no peace, there is ongoing bloodshed and when there is bloodshed, there is mass casualties! What is the treatment? Love, truth and transparency!!!

There is sufficient time passes by to examine the facts and screen the data and do follow ups. What was emergency yesterday isn't today! Really the world is still good place to live, the rockets of fires and explosive bombs aren't in any existence and nothing of that source could be found. In contrary of what we are being told, there is nothing invisble or UFO shooting down at every part of earth nonstop to keep calling emergency!

Be ready for life post COVID!! Don't kid yourself!! Life forever changed, those behind the scene made this way and new global beneficiaries are in full blown!!

The opportunistic and capitalists found a new heaven with land full of world honey! They kept the world under a continuous terror for more than year and forcing the billions to run away and hide!

Those are telling us it is so called "emergency rules", yet I have never once heard of Marshall law emergency when there wasn't emergency 🔔 rather than man-made emergency!

Emergency 🔔 lasts minutes and seconds and few hours but not weeks, months and year! Emergency a sudden serious, unexpected, and often dangerous situation requiring immediate action "your quick response in an emergency could be a lifesaver"

Brethren worldwide:

God is in control and is providing all the people good and bad and the entire earth with His grace, blessing and peace! Let us be thankful to the Lord of the creation. God is overshadowing 24/7 our world and sending the world with the free blessing and gifts. The sun is shining during the day, the moon is lightening at the nights, the air is fresh and filling the earth, the ground gives the life full of greens, grass, trees, planets and fruits, the earth is full of abundance of drinking waters, the wells, seas and oceans are quiet and the living whales and fishes and under the seas animals are multiplying in billions in joy and the creeping animals in variety and numbered in millions creeping over the face of earth, the fowels and birds are filling our skies. Few are sick and billions are healthy kicking and seeing, hearing and touching all of these God blessing upon the face of earth. Emergency and there isn't emergency but man-mad madness!

Be Thankful and give to the lord thanksgiving: **Ephesians 5:18-20** *Do not get drunk on wine, which leads to debauchery. Instead, be filled with the Spirit, speaking to one another with psalms, hymns, and songs from the Spirit. Sing and make music from your heart to the Lord, always giving thanks to God the Father for everything, in the name of our Lord Jesus Christ.* **Colossians 2:6-7***So then, just as you received Christ Jesus as Lord, continue to live your lives in him, rooted and built up in him, strengthened in the faith as you were taught, and overflowing with thankfulness.* **Colossians 3:15-17***Let the peace of Christ rule in your hearts, since as members of one body you were called to peace. And be thankful. Let the* *message of Christ dwell among you richly as you teach and admonish one another with all wisdom through psalms, hymns, and songs from the Spirit, singing to God with gratitude in your hearts. And whatever you do, whether in word or deed, do it all in the name of the Lord Jesus, giving thanks to God the Father through him.* "Giving thanks always and for everything to God the Father in the name of our Lord Jesus Christ," Eph. 5:20 "The Lord is my strength and my shield; My heart trusts in Him, and I am helped; Therefore my heart exults, And with my song I shall thank Him." Ps. 28:7 **Ezra 3:11***With praise and thanksgiving they sang to the Lord: "He is good; his love toward Israel endures forever." And all the people gave a great shout of praise to the Lord, because the foundation of the house of the Lord was laid.* **Psalm 7:17***I will give thanks to the Lord because of his righteousness; I will sing the praises of the name of the Lord Most High.* **Psalm9:1** *I will give thanks to you, Lord, with all my heart; I will tell of all your wonderful deeds.* **Psalm 35:18** *I will give you thanks in the great assembly; among the throngs I will praise you.* **5. Psalm 69:30***I will praise God's name in song and glorify him with thanksgiving.* **Psalm 95:1-3** *Come, let us sing for joy to the Lord; let us shout aloud to the Rock of our salvation. Let us come before him with thanksgiving and extol him with music and song. For the Lord is the great God, the great King above all gods.* **Psalm 100:4-***Enter his gates with thanksgiving and his courts with praise; give thanks to him and praise his name.*

For the Lord is good and his love endures forever; his faithfulness continues through all generations. **Psalm 106:1***Praise the Lord. Give thanks to the Lord, for he is good; his love endures forever.*

Be in good comfort knowing billions of people are healthy living and not touched by so called COVID!

Be of good cheer, the world 🌐 is our Savior land and a beautiful place to live! **Deuteronomy 31:6** Be strong and of good courage, do not fear nor be afraid of them; for the LORD your God, He is the One who goes with you. He will not leave you nor forsake you. (NKJV) **Joshua 1:9** "This is my command—be strong and courageous! Do not be afraid or discouraged. For the Lord your God is with you wherever you go." (NLT) **1 Chronicles 28:20** also said to Solomon his son, «Be strong and courageous, and do the work. Do not be afraid or discouraged, for the LORD God, my God, is with you. He will not fail you or forsake you until all the work for the service of the temple of the LORD is finished.» (NIV) **1 Corinthians 16:13** Be on your guard; stand firm in the faith; be men of courage; be strong. (NIV) **Psalm 27:1** The LORD is my light and my salvation; Whom shall I fear? The LORD is the strength of my life; Of whom shall I be afraid? (NKJV) **Psalm 56:3-4** When I am afraid, I will trust in you. In God, whose word I praise, in God

I trust; I will not be afraid. What can mortal man do to me? (NIV) **Isaiah 41:10** So do not fear, for I am with you; do not be dismayed, for I am your God. I will strengthen you and help you; I will uphold you with my righteous right hand. (NIV) **Isaiah 41:13** For I am the LORD, your God, who takes hold of your right hand and says to you, Do not fear; I will help you. (NIV) **Isaiah 54:4** Do not fear, for you will not be ashamed; Neither be disgraced, for you will not be put to shame; For you will forget the shame of your youth, And will not remember the reproach of your widowhood anymore. (NKJV) **Matthew 10:26–28** "But don't be afraid of those who threaten you. For the time is coming when everything that is covered will be revealed, and all that is secret will be made known to all ... Don't be afraid of those who want to kill your body; they cannot touch your soul. Fear only God, who can destroy both soul and body in hell." (NLT) **Romans 8:15** For ye have not received the spirit of bondage again to fear; but ye have received the Spirit of adoption, whereby we cry, Abba, Father. (KJV) **2 Corinthians 4:8-11** We are hard-pressed on every side, but not crushed; perplexed, but not in despair; persecuted, but not abandoned; struck down, but not destroyed. We always carry around in our body the death of Jesus, so that the life of Jesus may also be revealed in our body. For we who are alive are always being given over to death for Jesus' sake, so that his life may be revealed in our mortal body. (NIV)

Emergency 🪓 and isn't Emergency! The world 🌍 is still good place to live and God in Control! Man-made Crises when there is no crises!

Ghaly cascade of man destruction: When there is no transparency, there is conspiracy and when there is conspiracy, there is no truth and when there is no truth, there is no trust and when there is no trust, there is anger, unrest and uprise and when there are unrest, uprise and anger, there is revolution and when there is revolution, there is destruction and when there is destruction, there is no peace and when there is no peace, there is ongoing bloodshed and when there is bloodshed, there is mass casualties! What is the treatment? Love, truth and transparency!!!

God is in control and is providing all the people good and bad and the entire earth with His grace, blessing and peace! Let us be thankful to the Lord of the creation. God is overshadowing 24/7 our world and sending the world with the free blessing and gifts. The sun is shining during the day, the moon is lightening at the nights, the air is fresh and filling the earth, the ground gives the life full of greens, grass, trees, planets and fruits, the earth is full of abundance of drinking waters, the wells, seas and oceans are quiet and the living whales and fishes and under the seas animals are multiplying in billions in joy and the creeping animals in variety and numbered in millions

creeping over the face of earth, the fowels and birds are filling our skies. Few are sick and billions are healthy kicking and seeing, hearing and touching all of these God blessing upon the face of earth. Emergency and there isn't emergency but man-mad madness!

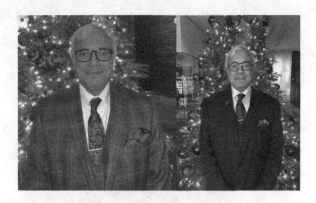

LM. Well said.....

MS. Nice pictures, beautiful flowers.

CB. Happy to see you without the mask.

AK. What an inspirational man you are, I'm so glad I had the pleasure of meeting you a few times. ❤️🙏

JM. Agree!

LG. This man is a well known Neurosurgeon who practices in Chicago and has been working on the front lines since the beginning of the pandemic:

AM. Very well said 👍👍

SA. Thank you, Dr. Ghaly, Director Ghaly Neuroscience Neurosurgery

CG. You're correct that the world is a good place to live as long as God is part of it. ❤️🙏

BL. "Love truth, and transparency." Those are now my words of daily use and inspiration. Thank you Dr Ghaly. I often. think of my (now deceased) brother, Larry Swarens, and then my thoughts turn to you and how much he, and our family, admire you.

Numbers 6:24-26 NKJV "The LORD bless you and keep you; The LORD make His face shine upon you, And be gracious to you; The LORD lift up His countenance upon you, And give you peace."

LR. Well said, and it provides comfort amongst all the havoc, conspiracy theories, etc going on today. What a true gift it was to meet you onboard my flight that day. I continue to follow, and take advise from one so wise. Thank you for sharing your wisdom...you are truly gifted in so many ways. 🙏😊😃

Eccentricity of Science and Researchers and lack of Realism!

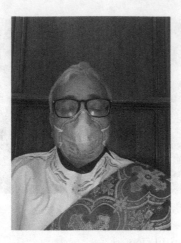

Science and Researchers were spending billions of tax dollars and years of researching so called "Global Warming"

Yet, Science and Researchers were spending pennies and nil time to proactively prevent and treat the imminent and known worldwide biologic weapons such as Coronavirus!

Science and Researchers were and are so eccentric and they love to play "God" lacking realism!

More than 100 million infected and rising while Science and Researchers of human intelligence are standstill don't know what to do stumbling and crushed! They are Unable to control and unable to treat and just pointing fingers to the innocent people as if the problem is not wearing the mask tight enough and not separating themselves far enough!

Ramsis Ghaly

CG. You are absolutely correct. Is this vaccine really going to cure covid? From what I have been reading, no. 🖤🙏

Show me a Worldwide COVID Hotspot Map that Matches Poverty Hotspot Map!!

Written by Ramsis Ghaly

Why America is still Hotspot Despite all the Unbelievable Restriction the Governments Imposing unto their People!!

If what we reporting is true and what science advocate is true, then COVID WORLDWIDE HOT SPOT SHOULD MATCH POVERTY HOTSPOT and THE SEVERITY OF COVID SPREAD SHOULD BR LINEAR RELATIONSHIP TO THE DEGREE OF POVERTY HOTSPOT!

So Why America is still Hotspot Despite all the Unbelievable Restriction the Governments Imposing unto their People!!

https://www.npr.org/.../new-federal-covid-19-data-release...

It does not make any sense or match any truth.

I came from Egypt 🇪🇬 and I know poverty! I lived it and so my countrymen and women! I lived at times of epidemics!! Over 6 feet, three families with 25 members are literally sleeping over each other with absolutely no hygiene, no clean waters, dirt and filth and waste and sewage—no masks, no barriers, no cloth, no distance away- no nutrition - no clinics no hospital no beds no couches no furniture no streets no clean food, no fresh sir, starvation, flies and cockroaches are all over instincts crawling eating their human flesh, no toilets, no spray, no papers, no soap, no transportations, no pharmacy, walking naked with no shoes—-NO NOTHING!

In other words, COVID should flourish and multiply and mutate in seconds, like no tomorrow, in these areas among 1 billion people instantly worldwide. In 24 hours we should see villages and cities full of dead bodies with COVID! It has nothing to do with accurate testing in these regions since the mass causalities will be in the millions and certainly it will make the news! Think for a second, we should hear daily not thousands but million of victims dying in these extreme poor countries! If science, USA and government tight regulations are true then 22% of the world populations should have been already dead 💀!

777

If I am mindless, I will still not believing what is being presented of statistics!! If it is true show me a Map of COVID Hotspots world wide matches very well the Extreme poverty worldwide Map and distribute linearly!! Last time I checked USA are leading country in wealth and we already having vaccines, houses, beaches, furniture, luxury of 6 feet distancing, masks, fresh air, parks, land, cloths, hygiene, food, clean waters, cars,—-and much money!!!

Here is the fact: "Total of a billion people are living in poverty. 689 million people live in extreme poverty, surviving on less than $1.90 a day. ... 1.3 billion people in 107 developing countries, which account for 22% of the world's population, live in multidimensional poverty. 644 million children are experiencing multidimensional poverty."

https://ourworldindata.org/.../world-population-in...
https://lifewater.org/.../9-world-poverty-statistics-to.../
https://howmuch.net/.../people-living-in-extreme-poverty...

Why America is still hotspot despite all the unbelievable restriction the governments imposing unto their people?

https://www.dailymail.co.uk/.../Almost-county-America...
https://www.nytimes.com/.../us/coronavirus-us-cases.html

Why not other parts of the world that theoretically should millions and millions not wearing masks or distancing away not using spray snd hand sanitizers be dead by now since they all aren't following USA and SCIENCE restrictions guidelines and are packed together with no Walls, masks, PPE living in extreme poverty!

I am talking millions should have been dead daily if the COVID data and spread are matching correctly!! I mean millions. Do you know the extreme poverty in the third world, COVID should have wiped them out of the map if things match!!

In fact, COVID WORLDWIDE HOT SPOT SHOULD MATCH POVERTY HOTSPOT and THE SEVERITY OF COVID SPREAD SHOULD BR LINEAR RELATIONSHIP TO THE DEGREE OF POVERTY HOTSPOT

I am at loss and hope you too!!!

JD. I absolutely agree Dr. Ghaly. 💯
MK. Yes, agreed. This cannot continue! People are dying from suicide, alcohol, drugs, abuse!

DC. I thought this was a excellent way to put some perspective and truth to all of the misinformation.

ESSENTIAL FACTS

JS. I love your investigative work.

JU. Excellent work Dr Ghaly

BCD. I do not know either

CG. I really am frustrated with all these lies that are being fed to the American people. Doesn't anybody but you, question what's going on?

JC. A must read... Thank you Ramsis.

NP. VERY TRUE READ THIS AND SHARE TRUTH!!! Thank you Dr. Ramsis Ghaly for sharing Factual Knowledge and Truth. 🙏

Ramsis Ghaly Cascade for Man Destructions!

COVID and Events during COVID made me look at the root cause analysis and I came with Cascade:

When there is no transparency, there is conspiracy and when there is conspiracy, there is no truth and when there is no truth, there is no trust and when there is no trust, there is anger, unrest and uprise and when there is unrest, uprise and anger, there is revolution and when there is revolution, there is destruction and when there is destruction, there is no peace and when there is no peace, there is ongoing bloodshed and when there is ongoing bloodshed madness, there is mass casualties!

What is the treatment? Love, truth and transparency!!!
Written by Ramsis Ghaly

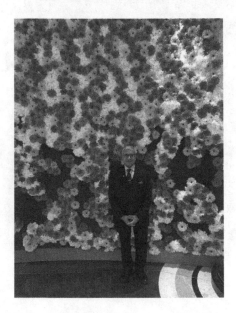

RH. Amen
JM. Amen

My Deep Reflection on Face Mask!!

Written by Ramsis Ghaly

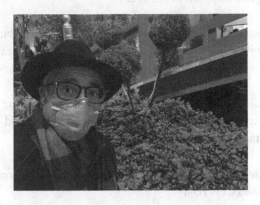

2021 is the year of Face Mask! Facemask should become our human logo and in every country flag! China may need to replace the snake 🐍 with face mask!! Facemask is an essential part of 2021 look and dress as well as center for 2021 fashion design!

It never been in human life since the beginning of creation Adam and Eve until 2020 that one item never existed before imposed and is so essential and talked about it millions and million times worldwide as that of facemask!

Face mask is a federal law and disobedient can get you into jail federal offense and felony charges! And wearing a facemask is a sign of being a good citizen and patriot obeying the law in 2021! And not wearing facemask is considered a crime and inhuman! It is the utmost political topic and hot subject going until the second year and rank high at any list!

What was considered a punishment now is considered mandatory! What was odd and extremely offensive, now is imposed as normal! In fact, facemask was a way to chastise outspoken children in my country and a disciplinary action to ask the undisciplined school children with profane words to shut up and limit their freedom!

Face mask is the only item made it to the constitution debate and all government branches and highly endorsed and personally enforced by all the officials from the highest rank the president to Fauci and CDC to WHO, UN,——to the local police 👮 !

Face mask is a touchy word in every day debate and a cause to instant termination! Facemask is the most common topic of the day! It came with no warning, with no clear understanding, from no where all of a sudden and dominate human life as an unwelcoming parasite ✿ invading unto our homes and mandated in every outdoor clothing and imposed to our faces!

Face mask is essential item in the White House, federal building, schools, classrooms, hospitals, Restaurants, bars, shops, malls. jails, trains, air shuttles, buses, cars and ——much more!

Facemask is considered as essential as drinking water and eating food! Facemask is being introduced as aspirin for stroke and heart attack and as Excedrin for migraine and antacids for stomach upset!

In fact, worldwide myth is that face mask is the only effective treatment available for Coronavirus and COVID-19!

What is so fascinating and puzzling human minds that PhD doctors are describing the facemask as if it is a premier revolution in science and medicine and not just a piece of cloth!

Face mask is a sharp two edged sword in the political debate that made Trump lost the reelection! Facemask discussion is a center of hostility and firing and a ground to kick you out of a plane!

Face mask super pass anything else in human daily living for the last two years in a row! The first thing to do in the morning is to find a mask and put it on as fast and the last thing to do is to take off or ripe off the facemask and go to sleep!

Billions of face masks 🦋 are distributed worldwide at any given day!

Face mask should never be forgotten or left behind as the underwear and other essentials of the daily attire!

Facemask is viewed as a tool to control, a power to intimidate, a way to terrorize and a cause to freak out! The number of face masks superseded the numbers of the hoky books, the shoes and utensils worldwide!

In fact, any household can convert his or her home to be a manufacturer of face masks with no necessary schools or preparations or regulations! It is as easy as just cut a piece of cloth and wrapped around the lower half of the face and give it a shape. And indeed it is a quality legal facemask to wear according to the federal regulations!

It is the easiest task to please and to mark the box of the day and push the button in your smart phone! It is the easiest item to make and to put it on! Face mask is in every home, every unit, every room!

Facemask is worn by every household including all ages children and elders!

If you look from far, face mask is a show converting a gorgeous human face to a face with a small nub as a little elephant nose!

Facemask is becoming an excuse for people to cover their faces, hide their looks, not to come close to each other, or flatter one another, or kiss or hug or change lips ● or put make up or brush teeth or care about mouth smell or wash the face!

Recently, Face mask is becoming a part of fashionable show matching the dress, suit and uniform!

Look out!! Face mask is becoming a sexy item with pink color and fantasy drawing! And the closet is full of various types and forms!

Revealing the Truth

Modern science and medicine were supposed to be equipped to provide immediate vaccine before the virus spread as both were funded to do so as part of combating bioterrorism since 1973! But medicine and science failed the people! Modern medicine and science after years of federal funding should have been able to instantly produce the correct vaccine!! Frontier medicine and science in the hands of the good people should have been an easy task to do especially with the era of artificial intelligence, electronics, computers, nanotechnology and digitalization! Medicine and science should have be better than this!! They missed the boat and they were napping for years and only treatment they offer is wrapping the lower face!!!

So really what is facemask and it's relationship of Coronavirus?? It is a simple barrier to cover the mouth and nose until medicine and science catch up to find a cure or the pandemic take its course and victims and leave as other previous pandemic had done! In fact, the Pandemic is in its way out as in the ancient days of Adam and Eve prior to civilization, because the natural human immunity weakened the virus and not because of science!

Therefore facemask is just a mask to bridge until the virus 🌑 goes away while covering for the incompetent science and medicine in the modern artificial intelligence era! In other hand, it should never been that way with facemask dominance if medicine and science had done what they promised thy people to do early on!

So what do we do best other than pointing fingers at the innocent people as if the problem is the people are not listening to facemasking and distancing rather than pointing fingers at themselves for not doing their job and eradicating the virus from time zero! With all the millions of dollars of tax money spend over decades on virology laboratories and institutes, especially at the intelligence federal kevel where bioterrorism has been real threat, a real scientist should have come with creating vaccine on the spot to combat any virus and treatment Drug regimen!

2021 is the year of Face Mask! Facemask should become our human logo and in every country flag! China may need to replace the snake 🐍 with face mask!! Facemask is an essential part of 2021 look and dress as well as center for 2021 fashion design!

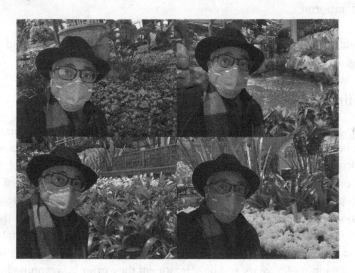

TH.. So much truth! I laughed, realizing how people are replacing simple hygiene with a mask! Brush those teeth!! Lol!

MN. See Dr.Ghaly you look good dressed up with a mask on its the way of life or death stay Safe

JG. Very well written 😄😄

CG. Good reflection. Hopefully we can all bear our faces soon, give a hug and a kiss and say goodbye to the virus. Be safe and blessings to you. 🖤🙏

JM. Thank You Dr. Ghaly about FACE MASKS!!

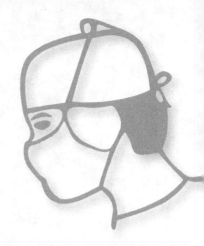

SECTION 14

VACCINATION CONTROVERSY

Is COVID Vaccine is a "True" or a "False" Security for Immunity?

Ramsis Ghaly

Any new post vaccine data from the Americans already received the vaccine other than those data we were told by the initial pharmaceutical trial!! If you know documented antibodies as a result of the vaccine please share!!

Why Now articles are showing up that those received the vaccine must continue the strict restriction of face masking, distancing away and social separation!

If the vaccine is that effective 95% why now articles coming up! Why the pharmaceuticals and politicians aren't demanding testing to all the millions of Americans receiving the vaccine for antibodies! Is COVID Vaccine is just a Cover Up as an Opioid to "Feel Good" and to Provide a "False Security for Immunity or Real Vaccine! Are you spending billions of dollars to support the populations to become a huge laboratory for industry!

Everyone received the Vaccine I talked to or read about, repeating what the Social Media promotes: "I feel great, in fact I ran 3 miles after receiving the vaccine. I just had a little discomfort, minor fever but I went back to work and I feel great" I replied: "Vaccine never been given for feeling good but for immunity? How do you know the vaccine made you immune and you have antibodies?" Their reply is again similar to social media news: "Because the trial was effective and mRNA is safe and effective!!!"

O smart minds, the COVID vaccine was administered as an emergency basis not to test its safety but to provide Immediate immunity! And yet, now articles as attached started to come up! No grantee of immunity against COVID, keep wearing the masks, distance yourself 6 feet, social and physical separations —-all the same!

And by the way, there is no testing prior or after vaccination for effectiveness of the vaccine and developing of antibodies!!! Are we spending billions of dollars to give false sense of relief and "feeling good"

Is this a hint that Now the Vaccine might not do what promised to do!!! By the way you must sign a legally defensive consent before receiving the vaccine to release all the liabilities and in addition, No grantee for immunity and we aren't

787

paying for any testing prior or after vaccination to ensure effective vaccine!!! And regulatory government agents aren't enforcing nationwide testing for antibodies!!

Reasons why you should keep wearing the masks and distancing away after vaccination!!

No one thus far and no reports of those US healthcare workers replied to my question: "Is anyone American, not in the trial by pharmaceutical, received Vaccine recently and developed effective immunity and antibodies when he or she was tested compared to prior vaccination?"

We owed to the world, in particular to the American people and to the scientific community, to get the fact straight!!! We must demand testing prior and after COVID vaccination to proof antibodies developed as a result of the vaccine indicative of effective immunity of those more than millions of American healthcare workers just received Vaccine the emergency release against FDA standard approval guidelines!

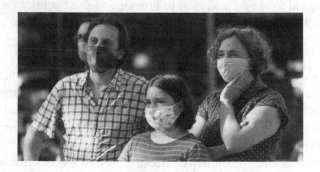

APPLE.NEWS
Why you still need to mask up after getting COVID-19 vaccine — ABC News
Getting the vaccine does not mean you can ignore precautions.

LR. Thank you!!!!
CG. My question exactly. Why get vaccinated if there is no guarantee you will not get covid?
LN. 🫤 makes one wonder?!
TH. I'm so confused 🤦‍♀️

Any US Recently Vaccinated Volunteers Was Tested Positive for Antibodies as a Result of receiving the COVID Pfizer vaccine and was not Positive Prior Vaccination!!!! No Information Available Yet!!

More than a Million US received vaccine!

We are looking for any information directly!

If any of the US healthcare workers whom never had COVID prior vaccination and was tested after being vaccinated recently and demonstrated had antibodies against COVID, please let us know!

https://www.cnbc.com/.../covid-vaccine-us-has-vaccinated...

Ramsis Ghaly

CNBC.COM

The U.S. has vaccinated just 1 million people out of a goal of 20 million for December

The total number of vaccines administered is still a long way off from the federal government's goal to inoculate 20 million Americans by the end of the year.

MO. I had the antibody test a few months ago but not directly prior to receiving the vaccine. I have not had any exposures since other than at work with proper PPE. I had not considered getting the antibody test after but I wonder if others will

KM. Shokran Khteer! Xoxo Blessings from Egypt. Stay safe, Be well and God Bless you as you continue to help us all in these tragic times. Xoxo

Hard talk to so called "Science" of vaccine! Thoughts for the day!!
Written by ramsis ghaly ON 1/28/2021

Why it is so difficult for vaccine pharmaceuticals, CDC, WHO and free standing independent academic researchers, institutes and journals to share, demand and release actual results of immunity success in the millions worldwide people have already received vaccines since September of 2020 including the study group.

There is so sufficient time passes by to examine the facts and screen the data and do follow ups. What was emergency yesterday isn't today! Really the world is still good place to live, the rockets of fires and explosive bombs aren't shooting every part of earth nonstop to keep calling emergency!

Where are the thousands and thousands of independent academic centers and their results of actual immunity yes or no after these teens if vaccines being introduced??? It is not just about safety but these billions of dollars and subjected close to billions for mass injections should be about effectiveness?? The better government business bureau and better science bureau should do their own investigations on the vaccine effectiveness as any other standard treatment or product!

When we are going to treat COVID and vaccines with the standard science and not with political science!!

What happen to the thousands of volunteers that received initial doses of vaccines 8 months ago?? Are they immune??? Anyone knows? Those that pharmaceuticals used their results to get emergency FDA approvals are they still well and virus free and developed immunity???

It is a simple question: do the millions of people received vaccines are already immune and no need to restriction and go back to normal life???

What is wrong?? Why the results of vaccines are so secretive and we have to listen to daily to Fauci gut feeling!!! They keep talking about we must listen to science??? Where is the science if no transparency of the actual follow up and results???

I am really sick of so calked the MRNA is safe!! Do these vaccines actual work in the mass vaccination stage in the public?? Do we know the NS deer yet?? It has been 6 months follow up??

This what I know about political science recommendations:

1) March 2020 political science said face mask and distancing away 6 feet and curfew for two weeks which should have completed by April 2020! The curfew is still going on for a year!!
2) December 2020, political science said vaccine should make people celebrate Christmas normally with no restrictions! February 2021, complete restriction continues the same as those received no vaccine!

Now, they are hanging their excuses on mutations! Are you serious, so is flu virus and do all the viruses ????

Respectfully

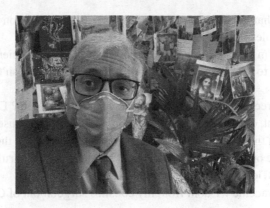

BCD. Thank you for your comments. I feel the same. This is a control and conquer political tactic.

JC. 100 per cent agree with you 👍👍 well said!

PS. I am so grateful for your voice!!!!! Please keep sharing! So many need to hear this! I always knew you were one of the smartest people I knew. I only hope. People will listen to you

KG. I applaud your knowledge and expertise. Yet, I like you, await the release of the Science and Data and only seeing more of the same. I'm not rushing to take some injection I've heard and seen people actually become hospitalized from just the first one.

I'm starting to question this whole entire thing with no data or Science and only a handful of "Experts" spouting the same mess we heard at the beginning with no better results. I am questioning are we soon to be relying on a China Vaccine? When TOP Pharmaceuticals suddenly get a conscience and back out of their contract for vaccines indeed makes one pause and wonder. Just what are we doing?

People die from the Influenza/ Flu and Pneumonia every year. With symptoms so like These I am starting to wonder. WHY aren't we hearing about the Flu anymore or Pneumonia even? Sounds like a profiteering racket entirely to me. While we all suffer.

Stay safe, well and Be Blessed. Thank you for all that you do! God Bless you!

BP. Scientific consensus does nothing but hold back actual science.
Remember, we have a political class that says men can give birth!

CS. Thanks Dr G!!! I agree show us the data!!!

CG. Thank you for your insightfulness. I agree with you as do many who have not gotten the vaccine. I need to see data that this vaccine has no lasting side affects or that it truly works. I will always trust your opinion before political opinions. Bless you. 🖤🙏

JT. 💯 agree! I'm shocked at the number of people "trusting science"!

HW. Yes! Glad to hear from a healthcare professional that doesn't just follow the masses! 👀

CH. Totally agree with you. Why aren't they sharing the data? Everything is so inconsistent, even going to multiple doctors. Some let a spouse in, some make you wait in the waiting room, some even make you wait in the car. Everyone needs to be on the same path instead of so many different rules. It's g

JM. So very difficult, I AGREE show us the DATA!!!

KS. Excellent vaccine wisdom from my cousin's surgeon out of Chicago Illinois

What about this conspiracy theory???

Spread a virus that cause worldwide loss of TASTE, SMELL & LIBIDO

Imagine life living without TASTE, SMELL & LIBIDO!!!

What kind of life would be!??? Perhaps the society be transformed to submissive ordered by socialism a communist!!! The end result as follows: Weight loss, cost saving, no complaints or demonstrations, no sexual harassment or rape, low maintenance, no enjoyment, followers with low demands, loss of self-esteem and submission to the authoritarianism!!!!

Ramsis Ghaly

Cg. Sounds like communism!

Jd. We just went to a wake tonight to say goodbye to a good friend who died from covid. Infuriates me with the stupid people in this country who still think it's just like the flu or worse yet that it is a hoax! 🤢

Bcd. No future babies. All will be AI robots at the control of China

The way COVID is going around out of control, I decided to call my parent in Heaven thinking that Coronavirus flew also out of space???

My father and mother told me, the angels made mass testing and everyone in the paradise including themselves were tested positive! But they are doing well!!

I asked mom and dad why everyone nowadays on earth and paradise is positive for COVID?? They replied: "Son it is just a test!

I asked how did you know that you might have COVID? They replied the first thing we noticed was loss of taste and smell toward all evil dialogues and Gossips!

They also heard from the archangel Michael that every soul in hell weren't tested and when they complained, archangel Michael told them: "For what!!! What difference does it make. The judgment and the destiny are already determined" They are already living in terrors and fears. They are struggling horribly with or without COVID-19!!"

I asked my dad and mom about facemask, distancing away and getting the vaccine! They replied: "No need for us to do so but for you go back down from where you came from!!!

Thank you 🙏 mom and dad

Ramsis Ghaly

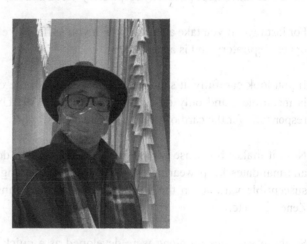

Lr. Great advice!
Kg. Love this
Jm. AGREE!!
Nv. Love it, God bless you Doctor Ghaly 🙏😊
Cg. This is delightful. 🖤🙏
Mh. I'm impressed 🤍😎
Cr. Thank you for painting such beautiful pictures for us as a magnificent truth from the Word of God.

COVID VACCINE

Any good viral immunologist can explain why the only consistent worldwide major complication of the current COVID vaccines is VASCULAR (Causing hyper-coagulable state—) and not Respiratory knowing that Coronavirus is a respiratory virus and not cardiac or vascular????

It is interesting to see whatever the vaccine kind, the number one side effect is vascular complications and not any respiratory complications!!! It is very strange since Coronavirus is primarily respiratory virus and not vascular!!

For instance, if you take a flu vaccine, if you suffer Sid effects, it is a form of flu upper respiratory and is acceptable!!

If you look carefully, it should tell a human mind, the current COVID vaccine is incomplete and only target not the CORONAVIRUS itself but the protein responsible for the cardiovascular complications!

Now, it makes big sense why taking COVID vaccine doesn't prevent infection and mandates keep wearing the facemasks, distancing away, not open, more susceptible variants in the way, much fear, hold Johnson and Johnson, hold Zeneca, —etc.

So these vaccines all along were developed as a quick fix against the protein responsible for vascular complication and not against the virus itself! Majority were left in the dark to guess and few weren't????

If my analogy is true, it surfaces a bigger issue which is the vaccine wasn't developed carefully and examined thoroughly and it is just a temporary proposal to learn the results. And the coronaviruses are still flying free and mutating in any shape or form because yet no effective precise vaccine against them!!! And the watch dogs are terrified and establishing the grounds to further fourth mutation to the reason behind spread and lack of COVID control!!

Furthermore, the war against COVID isn't over awaiting more surprises as the world is becoming a laboratory 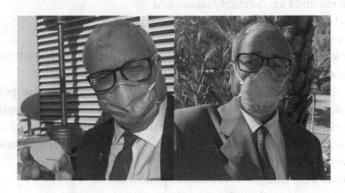 to find out!!!!!!

Now I wonder what it takes develop the correct vaccine and establish the correct treatment for life to return to normal again????

Transparency is lacking and we are left to guess!!!

Ramsis Ghaly

DL. Amén!

AK. 💯 agree

JB. Thank you for speaking up, I really appreciate your input. This is so important for people to hear and understand.

SH. Very considering opinion.

CR. Thank you for being a truth teller.

SA. 💯!!! Thank you for speaking up!!

ED. Thank you Dr Ghaly 🙏

SC. Thanks Dr

ML. You are brilliant! 🖤🙏

SK. Yes, I worry we'll be seeing a tv commercial in a few years asking if we had Covid injection and suffered side effects to call Lawyers. 😌

CL. Thank you Dr Ghaly! You are so Godly. We all need to listen to you as I feel God has you representing us! I will NOT get this shot! 🖤🙏

SL. The pharma companies are saying they recommend a booster every year so that falls within your thoughts that future versions would target differently. Thank you for your thoughts on this as I was wondering same things -

KE. I always value and respect your insight!

DC. Thank you Dr. Ghaly. I haven't wanted the vaccine all along!! I don't intend to get it. As a man of God what's your opinion on how can we ever get around their restrictions on traveling?

LW. Thank you my friend for being so honest. I truly believe in everything you are saying but reluctanctly took the J&J vaccine since it will be required to travel. We are all in a limbo....

LH. Couldn't agree more!

BCD. Thank you Sir. I agree 💯 percent.

YR. Thank you for reminding me to use my brain 🧠 again and not fall victim to the pressures of media to put something in my body that had not been proven. I wish everyone could read your truth! God 🙏 you, Dr Ghaly!

LM. Oh gosh I was wondering this also as I did just get my second vaccine of the moderna and I am definitely concerned 😖

mh. Wow! Glad I didn't get the shot. Thank you for posting this!

Sp. I haven't done it.....

Ka. Thank you Dr Ramsis Ghaly I have not gotten my shot....and will not

Jg. Had both my Mederma shots.

Mp. My thought: is the effect of COVID virus on lung is on the pulmonary vascular system, not the lung tissue per se? Which would explain why "standard of care" treatment of respiratory failure (PEEP, high FiO2) isn't always successful. And might explain why those with HTN/abnl vasculature are disproportionately affected.

Bl. Thank you Dr. Ghaly; I have much to ponder. 🤯

Jm. I just hope it is the Right Decision!!

Lk. No vaccine for me period or any other family member either. Will will need to rely on hydroxychloriquine or ivermectin with vitamin C, D and zinc. Have FAITH and not Fear.

YV. Words from a very wise man, Dr

KG. Thank YOU, Dr Ghaly

Well Renowned Neuro Surgeon and Author of Multiple books
Front line Covid worker
And
Beloved Man of God!
Leave it to Dr Ghaly to put this all into the simplest perspective even a child can understand.
WHY are we so afraid from a Respiratory
Breathing VIRUS
And
Taking the Vaccines is causing Vascular problems?
We take the Influenza vaccine and we get the Flu and that's acceptable
We take these Covid Vaccines and we get Blood clots and a Memo goes out
Oh it's normal!
These are side effects

Only 16 people out of 6 million died.
Yes really?
WHY is a Virus that causes Respiratory distress
Being treated with incomplete Vaccines that cause Vascular Blood Clot issues
That can very well worsen in time?
Still rushing off to get the vaccines
The world is the experimental lab rat
God Bless you, Dr Ramsis Ghaly!

Thank you so much!

LH. Have respect for Dr Ghaly. Excellent Dr. man of faith.

IO. Good points

AL. Just something to think about!

LS. 💯 focused on my immune resilience

SS. Very important esp. If you have vascular and cardiac disease.

EM. A neurosurgeon explains his theory of why you can still become infected after (Ovid va((inaction, and why blood clots are the. most prevalent side effect.

SQ. Beware! Not for me!

KG. Thanks for posting this. Dr Ghaly Is The Very Best!

OB. Dr Ghaly is an amazing Dr who holds 4 board certificatios. When he speaks you should listen...

JS. Thank you Ramsis Ghaly Very important information ...

CH. It's all so confusing! Who do you believe?

CM. Take the I-MASK+ set of supplements with the ivermectin! True destruction of the virus, prevention of infection and reversal of long-Covid. We have seen it work. The media is not allowed to let you know about it. The only prescription needed is for the ivermectin.

JU. Thank you doctor Ghaly for speaking out.

MH. Wow! Glad I didn't get the shot. Thank you for posting this!

SP. I haven't done it.....

KA. Thank you Dr Ramsis Ghaly. I have not gotten my shot....and will not

JU. Today life was claimed in my cousin family one week after 2nd Pfizer job.
Massive blood clotting.
Doesn't matter if you are young or old it is serious issue.
How many more people have to die of this madness?

BA. thank you. So sad that we can't be on same page. Even some friends did get 1st one.

BL. Thank you Dr. Ghaly; I have much to ponder. 🤦

JM. I just hope it is the Right Decision!!

LK. No vaccine for me period or any other family member either. Will will need to rely on hydroxychloriquine or ivermectin with vitamin C, D and zinc. Have FAITH and not Fear.

MH. Wow! Glad I didn't get the shot. Thank you for posting this!

SP. I haven't done it.....

KA. Thank you Dr Ramsis Ghaly. I have not gotten my shot....and will not

JG. Had both my Mederma shots.

MP. My thought: is the effect of COVID virus on lung is on the pulmonary vascular system, not the lung tissue per se? Which would explain why "standard of care" treatment of respiratory failure (PEEP, high FiO2) isn't always successful. And might explain why those with HTN/abnl vasculature are disproportionately affected.

My residents graduation 🎓 is at Sears Towers (Wills Tower)

Tight restriction for those didn't take the vaccine as follow:

1) Must have negative COVID test!
2) Must sit in a remote table and isolated from other tables!
3) Cannot mix with other people!
4) Will have a separate waiters and waitress!

Therefore, I am not going!!! I will zoom in virtual. It is very hard to feel discriminated and excluded and restricted just because!!

Every one of them not only forcing the vaccines per so called CDC guideline but also forcing to sign a consent releasing them from any responsibilities and Sid effects !!

Look at Wills sky deck:

Important Notice Regarding COVID-19
Willis Tower and Skydeck Chicago have implemented measures consistent with CDC and local and federal guidance to try to reduce the spread of COVID-19 on the premises, including enhanced cleaning protocols. Even with these procedures in place, PLEASE BE ADVISED that building occupants, building and Skydeck visitors, or others currently or previously present upon this property and/or the Skydeck MAY HAVE CONTRACTED OR BEEN EXPOSED TO COVID-19 or other infectious diseases, and may expose you. By accessing and using building common areas, the Skydeck, and their associated amenities, you and your party voluntarily assume all risks of your use—INCLUDING THE RISK OF

EXPOSURE TO INFECTIOUS DISEASE—and you waive all claims, including claims for negligence, against Willis Tower, Skydeck Chicago, and their respective owners, managers, affiliates, agents and representatives, arising out of such use. The above parties hereby disclaim all liability for any injuries arising out of your use of this property and the Skydeck, including exposure to infectious disease.

Accept and ContinueAccept and Continue

SL. I'm very concerned the discrimination will continue to get much worse at least here in IL and especially Chicago. 😢
JS. I totally agree with you Dr Ghaly.

The man took the vaccine and he assumed as he was told that he should receive some protection!

He is a business man and wants to go out and meet people and that is the reason he took the vaccine to give him some protection!!!

Unfortunately, he didn't know that it despite it made sense, it was a false protection!

What CDC response, it is his underlying condition!!!! They always have a response for their failures!!

NBCCHICAGO.COM
After Fully-Vaccinated Father Dies of COVID-19, Family Hopes Story Raises Awareness

Report of COVID Vaccines Danger of introducing Toxin Spike protein into human body and blood stream unexpectedly and be stored in various essential organs affecting the normal human host cells with short and long term consequences!

"Editor's Note: This article has been amended to note that 11 of 13 vaccinated subjects in a recent Ogata study had detectable protein from SARS coronavirus in their bloodstream including three people who had measurable spike protein. Whereas the article referenced a statement from Professor Bridle's group stating that spike protein was present for 29 days in one person, the study in question states that spike protein was found in the person on Day 29, one day after a second vaccine injection and was undetectable two days later. May 31, 2021 (LifeSiteNews) — New research shows that the coronavirus spike protein from COVID-19 vaccination unexpectedly enters the bloodstream, which is a plausible explanation for thousands of reported side-effects from blood clots and heart disease to brain damage and reproductive issues, a Canadian cancer vaccine researcher said last week. "We made a big mistake. We didn't realize it until now," said Byram Bridle, a viral immunologist and associate professor at University of Guelph, Ontario, in an interview with Alex Pierson last Thursday, in which he warned listeners that his message was "scary."

Another link:
SARS-CoV-2 Spike Protein Elicits Cell Signaling in Human Host Cells: Implications for Possible Consequences of COVID-19 Vaccines

Abstract
The world is suffering from the coronavirus disease 2019 (COVID-19) pandemic caused by severe acute respiratory syndrome coronavirus 2 (SARS-CoV-2). SARS-CoV-2 uses its spike protein to enter the host cells. Vaccines that introduce the spike protein into our body to elicit virus-neutralizing antibodies are currently being developed. In this article, we note that human host cells sensitively respond to the spike protein to elicit cell signaling. Thus, it is important to be aware that the spike protein produced by the new COVID-19 vaccines may also affect the host cells. We should monitor the long-term consequences of these vaccines carefully, especially when they are administered to otherwise healthy individuals. Further investigations on the effects of the SARS-CoV-2 spike protein on human cells and appropriate experimental animal models are warranted.

https://www.mdpi.com/2076-393X/9/1/36/htm
WWW-LIFESITENEWS-COM.CDN.AMPPROJECT.ORG
Vaccine researcher admits 'big mistake,' says spike protein is dangerous 'toxin' | News | LifeSite

'Terrifying' new research finds vaccine spike protein unexpectedly in bloodstream. The protein is linked to blood clots, heart and brain damage, and potential risks to nursing babies and fertility.

KB. As of May 28, 2021, there have been 259,308 confirmed cases of SARS-CoV-2 infections in Canadians 19 years and under. Of these, 0.048% were hospitalized, but only 0.004% died, according to the CCCA statement. "Seasonal influenza is associated with more severe illness than COVID-19." Given the small number of young research subjects in Pfizer's vaccine trials and the limited duration of clinical trials, the CCCA said questions about the spike protein and another vaccine protein must be answered before children and teens are vaccinated, including whether the vaccine spike protein crosses the blood-brain barrier, whether the vaccine spike protein interferes with semen production or ovulation, and whether the vaccine spike protein crosses the placenta and impacts a developing baby or is in breast milk.

DT. Soooo scary!!

DB. Thank you, Ramsis.

COVID Vaccine and Toxin Spike Protein in Blood stream!

Report of COVID Vaccines Danger of introducing Toxin Spike protein into human body and blood stream unexpectedly and be stored in various essential organs affecting the normal human host cells with short and long term consequences!

"Editor's Note: This article has been amended to note that 11 of 13 vaccinated subjects in a recent Ogata study had detectable protein from SARS coronavirus in their bloodstream including three people who had measurable spike protein. Whereas the article referenced a statement from Professor Bridle's group stating that spike protein was present for 29 days in one person, the study in question states that spike protein was found in the person on Day 29, one day after a second vaccine injection and was undetectable two days later. May 31, 2021 (LifeSiteNews) — New research shows that the coronavirus spike protein from COVID-19 vaccination unexpectedly enters the bloodstream, which is a plausible explanation for thousands of reported side-effects from blood clots and heart disease to brain damage and reproductive issues, a Canadian cancer vaccine researcher said last week. "We made a big mistake. We didn't realize it until now," said Byram Bridle, a viral immunologist and associate professor at University of Guelph, Ontario, in an interview with Alex Pierson last Thursday, in which he warned listeners that his message was "scary."

Another link:
SARS-CoV-2 Spike Protein Elicits Cell Signaling in Human Host Cells: Implications for Possible Consequences of COVID-19 Vaccines

Abstract
The world is suffering from the coronavirus disease 2019 (COVID-19) pandemic caused by severe acute respiratory syndrome coronavirus 2 (SARS-CoV-2). SARS-CoV-2 uses its spike protein to enter the host cells. Vaccines that introduce the spike protein into our body to elicit virus-neutralizing antibodies are currently being developed. In this article, we note that human host cells sensitively respond to the spike protein to elicit cell signaling. Thus, it is important to be aware that the spike protein produced by the new COVID-19 vaccines may also affect the host cells. We should monitor the long-term consequences of these vaccines carefully, especially when they are administered to otherwise healthy individuals. Further investigations on the effects of the SARS-CoV-2 spike protein on human cells and appropriate experimental animal models are warranted.

Vaccine researcher admits 'big mistake,' says spike protein is dangerous 'toxin' | News | LifeSite

'Terrifying' new research finds vaccine spike protein unexpectedly in bloodstream. The protein is linked to blood clots, heart and brain damage, and potential risks to nursing babies and fertility.

Partly False Information. Checked by independent fact-checkers.

See Why

Dt. Soooo scary!!

Db. Thank you, Ramsis.

Kp. As of May 28, 2021, there have been 259,308 confirmed cases of SARS-CoV-2 infections in Canadians 19 years and under. Of these, 0.048% were hospitalized, but only 0.004% died, according to the CCCA statement. "Seasonal influenza is associated with more severe illness than COVID-19."

Given the small number of young research subjects in Pfizer's vaccine trials and the limited duration of clinical trials, the CCCA said questions about the spike protein and another vaccine protein must be answered before children and teens are vaccinated, including whether the vaccine spike protein crosses the blood-brain barrier, whether the vaccine spike protein interferes with semen production or ovulation, and whether the vaccine spike protein crosses the placenta and impacts a developing baby or is in breast milk.

803

The Man took the COVID Vaccine and Died of COVID!

The man took the vaccine and he assumed as he was told that he should receive some protection!

He is a business man and wants to go out and meet people and that is the reason he took the vaccine to give him some protection!!!

Unfortunately, he didn't know that it despite it made sense, it was a false protection!

What CDC response, it is his underlying condition!!!! They always have a response for their failures!!

NBCCHICAGO.COM
After Fully-Vaccinated Father Dies of COVID-19, Family Hopes Story Raises Awareness

A suburban Chicago family who lost their fully vaccinated father to COVID-19 said they hope his story can help others with certain pre-existing conditions and immune deficiencies as they say his unexpected passing left them with a major "what if."

Jo. Sadly the Vaccine is causing Autoimmune symptoms and horrible side effects... he had no chance to fight Covid. I believe, from the numerous people's stories on developing serious complications from the vaccines, that the spike protein is doing more harm than good. If you want to see all of the horror stories go to Telegram.

rr. unfortunately, no enough follow up data on the effectiveness of the vaccine other than the early reports, some insurance doesn't approve to test the antibodies titer. and when the vaccines will be approved properly with enough studies and data) instead of emergency approval . it is always the underlying conditions to blame. but this should be avoided if we have good screening parameters!! 😠😠😠

mm. Is not the efficacy of the vaccine 95%? This means that every 100 vaccinated persons 5 may be infected. In our church out of 500 individual who got vaccinate, 25 may get infected. Yet we did not see this number getting sick, thank God. It is very sad that we lose a beloved one. But let us not create a scare that discourages people from getting the vaccine. It still does more good than harm.

cg. Very sad! Prayers for him and his family 🙏🙏🙏

lv. lv. I know folks who got the shot and got covid.

Mandatory Vaccine Consent

December 16, 2020

When you receive the vaccine NOW you consent that you understand fully that the vaccine has only been tested for NEARLY 44,000 participants for ONLY two months follow up! And immunity tested post injection is over ONLY two months!!

You are also consenting and understand and agree that the vaccine was not subjected to regular FDA. The vaccine has received FDA emergency use authorization 12/11/2020 due to the COVID pandemic, but this is different than full FDA approval and follow up safety data are limited to only at least two months of observation.

The results in NEARLY 44,000 participants for ONLY two months follow up appears to be 95% effective at preventing COVID-19 disease. The most common vaccination side effects include mild to moderate injection site pain, along with fatigue, headache, and muscle pain. Fever, chills, and joint pains occurred in some trial participants, but were less common.

Have the vaccine showed 95% effectiveness when tested in the vulnerable groups such as nursing homes and above 65 years ok'd with coexisting medical problems?????????

Who is liable?? Who is taking full responsibility of serious side effect even if it is 1:45,00??? They washed their hands by the signed consent!! If the vaccine is so perfect why such a well design consent prepared by experts, is showing up at the last minute and must be signed??

Certainly, COVID Pandemic continues to push the world to an edge! Mankind is stumbling and despair! Can you really trust the Science and Politics behind the vaccine?? It appears the world is becoming a huge Experimental laboratory and the people are the participants and the animals are spared!

The true results are indeed when the vaccine is administered over ample time to much larger numbers over many centers and regions! Only then shall be known the trustworthy short term and long term results!!

The vaccine market is highly politicized and very biased with unimaginable secondary gains extremely high in demand, so profitable targeting 8 billion customers worldwide!!!
https://www.globenewswire.com/.../Vaccine-Market-Size...

As America, Germany and United Kingdom leading the vaccine market in the West!!!
https://www.globaldata.com/us-uk-germany-top.../

China is leading vaccine distribution in Latin America and Africa!!!
https://www.nytimes.com/.../coronavirus-southern-command...
https://www.theafricareport.com/.../china-africa-to.../amp/
https://www.nature.com/articles/d41586-020-02807-2

Ramsis Ghaly

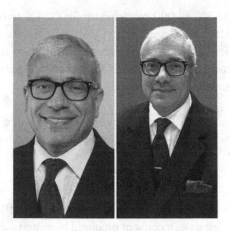

JD. Thank you Dr Ghaly!

DH. Thanks for the informed update, Doc BCD. Great photo of you

RH. It doesn't that we are the guinea pigs. I would rather stay in my house by myself and be one of the first ones.

SS. Thank you so much for your insight
The question is did you or will you take the vaccine?

VA. I trust in the greatness of God. I do believe he has allowed this vaccine to be created. God sees his suffering people.

N. Thank you Dr.Ghaly! ♥🙏🙏

CB. Thank you so much Dr. Ghaly 🙏♥🙏

JD. So are you getting it?

CH. Thank you Dr. Ghaly

CS, Very interesting. I appreciate the information. Thank you.

SL. Thanks Dr Ghaly for sharing this!!! I too have serious concerns about taking this because I have had anaphylaxis several times in my life and my allergist told me I can't even have anymore allergy shots because even if they have a crash cart on standby he said once anaphylaxis starts there is no guarantee it can be stopped

DI. Thanks for the info Dr!

M. Thank you dr. Ghaly! 😂

AV. Thank you Dr. Ghaly for your thoughts on this vaccine! 🙏🇺🇸

LL. Thank you

MS. Thanks for the info.

FL. I am not consenting to this!

BH. Really great photos of you. It made me smile and is a welcome break from the horrors associated with this pandemic. Thank you for sharing your brilliant insights on this inoculation that is getting shoved down our throats. It's almost terrifying. So glad to see you looking so well. Happiest of holidays dear Man, and Happy New Year to you!! 🖤🎄🖤🎄🖤

JT. Very Well Where the hell do we stand Now could Somebody explain this thing to me as if I was 5yrs old, is the damn thing safe or not??? 👀

AL. OMGVG.

VG. Very interesting!! Thank you Dr Ghaly. 🙏🙏🖤

CG. I have read enough to know that the vaccine will not be put in my body. Your info confirms what I have tread. Thank you! 🖤🙏

JL. 👀 wide open

BV. A local neurosurgeon, speaks out about the cov)d vax. Please do your research!!

DI. Great Neurosurgeon 👆

CS. 'm sharing the post because I trust the doctor who wrote this. I know him & his character, personally. It's just something to consider; a bit of information to think over.

JO. My Neurosurgeon is extremely smart. 🙏

MO. It will be a while before the general public would have the opportunity to get the vaccine. Everyone can see what happens to us healthcare workers. Personally I weighed risk versus benefit and to me the risk is worth not infecting my elderly parents who may not do so well with it. I am getting my shot Friday. This is probably the only way to move beyond this limbo we are living in.

AM. God Bless the Lord for people like him! 🙏😊🖤

AB. Read and weep, snowflakes

DH. This Just In...From the Neurology Department: For those seeking information, and wishing to make informed decisions...

JS. Thank you Ramsis for explaining this ....

JU. Thank you Dr. Ghaly!

JO. praying there's no bad side effects. 🙏🙏🙏 Personally I think Congress and Senators should be the first ones. 😜

CM. i don't see this as privilege, I see it as an experiment. One with zero culpability. I have a 99.8 percent of chance of surviving this virus. 90 percent of the people I know do, as well. The other 10 percent, over 70, are taking precautions much safer by being extra hygienic and avoiding crowds. I hope your dose works and has zero side effects! best of of luck.

CH. "Sometimes you must cut off a finger, to save a hand." Chinese proverb

RR. Thank you for the info!

JD. Thank you for the information and insight and No thank you to the vaccine. I will take my chances with my body's own immune system.

BS. Thank you for sharing this

js. This is why I say "No!" to the vaccine.

RM. Know before you go

MI. Thank you for sharing this with us Dr. Ramsis! Good pics btw.

AJ. I have so many friends who are excited to take this. I can early next week but I just can't bring myself to do that yet. People say follow the science. Yep that is what I am doing. Pfizer is the most unethical drug company its common knowledge, they have never had a vaccine before yet were the first ones to distribute and they have studied Sars for years yet never have they given a vaccine like this to humans?. 😧 They don't know the long-term because that's impossible to know. The future isn't here yet. Oh People say well Americans eat McDonald's cheeseburgers. Yep and you are correct i don't know what is in that Nasty little cheeseburger but I do know its been consumed over 50 years and know the outcome.

DJ. To many unknowns...

Like nearly all things new - improvements will be needed and unforeseen issues/ problems to be fixed. I'm going to wait...

FYI:
I do have a strong belief in getting PROVEN vaccinations.

JR. This is really crazy. mRNA is very sensitive and we contain it in our body. I think it's comparable to hyaluronic acid. We also have that in our body and we also put it on our face in our face creams.

Because it disintegrates and is so fragile it would be unexpected to have any long term side effects. Studies also show that some of the people that developed side effects were in the placebo group and also didn't fall out of the standard number or cases of Bell's palsy for a given population so it wasn't rectified by the data.

The vaccine was given to all ethnicities. Race and ages and they did have comorbidities. the most important piece of this to me is that unlike the flu shot it did not lose efficacy over the last 2-3 months. The flu shot drops it's efficacy 10% each month. This is why the elderly have to take a higher dose.

VA. I trust in the greatness of God. I do believe he has allowed this vaccine to be created. God sees his suffering people.

RB. and what about all the suffering people with cancers and other illnesses?!! God sees all who are suffering in so many ways, even worse than COVID symptoms. Many are suffering way beyond this virus. I do not trust this rushed vaccine!!!!

TS. This sounds like a typical liability waver. All side effects are typical or actually less. They are way oversensatonalizing allergies. No one has died and they happen with every vaccine and medication, including Tylenol.

Now, that being said, the testing numbers are low and so was the testing period. Those are fair reasons to be a little nervous. However, we are in a complete state of emergency and our health system is overrun. I have friends and family that have died, been severely ill and left with chronic conditions, and in the medical field begging for this. It's way worse than the flu. I have essentially had to quarantine since March, I'm so high risk. I don't have options. I have only seen one friend because of extreme circumstances. The bonfire was going to be a risk, but I'm sick of my own 4 walls and outside is safer.

Anyhow, it's people's lives and we're getting sensationalized reports of 3 people with non lethal allergic reactions which are always expected. In truth, because of the low number of people tested, I'm happy that it has to go through health care workers, essential high risk workers then high risk me...then it will have essentially had enough testing for me to feel safe. However, it's still going to take a 1 1/2 to 2 years for us to come anywhere close to herd immunity even with the vaccine. It would be virtually impossible without. I will continue to wear a mask and social distance like a responsible citizen of the world. And we'll still be learning about this new disease and the vaccine, but we'll be at a better place. And hopefully, the worse viruses will still be way off in the future.

Lastly, you essentially sign a waiver of liability when you buy and open any over the counter medication from the store. Herbs don't even have FDA approval although that's by design by the pharmaceutical companies and it pisses me off. Anyway...it's a basic liability waiver...and I'm not sure why it's scary.

I just want the news to stop sensationalizing allergic reactions, so that if anything real happens their story will have real merit.

CR. Thank you for sharing such an important point of view. God bless you always. Stay safe. We love you.
BL. Dear Dr Ghaly, I am grateful for your article. I believe it is needed and should be shared as much as possible. You have treated my Brother, Larry Swarens and my niece Wendy Swarens. I am in awe of your work and your passions; thank you for sharing your talents and compassion. I hope to get to see you some day for your medical opinion concerning my physical challenges.
ER. Thank you for your insight.
Dg. Insight from Dr who has been risking himself-sometimes working alone-from day 1. So I'm not too upset my facility not priority for health department. We will continue our procedures and hope and pray cases are minimal for patients and staff.

I think in general the expected trust but the decreased testing pool but definitely the extreme short duration for study. He isn't extreme. He wears a mask and does encourage being safe. In the early months when some were too scared of exposure. He suited up and had to intubate and modify care because he was doing it solo. He wants a solution but proper and safe guidelines. The "emergency" protocols can curb routine safety. I did same with H1N1. Pass on 1st round- I was nursing an infant. I waited for following seasons for it to be incorporated into annual that's fair, I'll probably take it whenever it gets to my area since I work with the public, but I do plan to wait for the kids until it's been out longer. It came off as "if it's safe why do we need to sign a consent?" and I was immediately skeptical of him lol

jr. This is really crazy. mRNA is very sensitive and we contain it in our body. I think it's comparable to hyaluronic acid. We also have that in our body and we also put it on our face in our face creams.

Because it disintegrates and is so fragile it would be unexpected to have any long term side effects. Studies also show that some of the people that developed side effects were in the placebo group and also didn't fall out of the standard number or cases of Bell's palsy for a given population so it wasn't rectified by the data.

The vaccine was given to all ethnicities. Race and ages and they did have comorbidities. the most important piece of this to me is that unlike the flu shot it did not lose efficacy over the last 2-3 months. The flu shot drops it's efficacy 10% each month. This is why the elderly have to take a higher dose.

Antibody Testing Prior and After Vaccination Is Not Being Mandated or Part of the Requirements! Why???

Written by Ramsis Ghaly

It is already well established mandatory guidelines, except for unknown reasons in COVID vaccination, if someone receiving hepatitis vaccine or tuberculosis TB, to be tested prior vaccination to see if he or she ever got infected before and has antibodies already. And also must be tested after vaccination to confirm the effectiveness of vaccine and development of the antibodies in that particular subject!

It is the right thing to do. It is patient safety. It is for better industry pharmaceutical oversight control. It is part of keeping them honest! It is for accurate data collection! It won't delay the process at all! So why isn't done or implemented ASAP! After all you are authorizing use of vaccine to the entire world that is not even completely studied, might as well follow the quantitative accurate results for free to audit and to ensure what are you giving the public that the vaccine is safe and is doing what supposed to do!!

For COVID vaccine prior and after, obligatory testing has been waived and been told we must assume that 95% effectiveness! A company study results does not mean the public is indeed harmonious group with the previous pharmaceutical operated study!! In addition, certainly recipients would like to know if vaccination is really needed especially if already antibodies in the system from previous sub clinical infection! And also recipients would like to know if the vaccine was effective or he or she is of the 5% non-responders! Why the recipient must pay to be tested if it should be part of the CDC mandatory on experimental vaccine conducted by the pharmaceutical?

Isn't considered violation of patients Safety in support of Industry Regulation Rules!

So far volunteers are receiving vaccine without being tested before and after! And if any of them interested, they must pay for it! In the same time no steps have been taken to examine accuracy of the vaccine to the recipients!

As the experimental vaccination continues, the pharmaceuticals should schedule the volunteers for free antibody Titer test prior and after vaccination! And they must keep the books straight and clean? CDC and public safety shouldn't allow short cuts when it comes to patients safety facing industry involvement!

Otherwise how you test the effectiveness of the experimental vaccine you are giving to the public in an emergency basis? How are you studying the vaccine? What data you are collecting to keep the records straight and examine the results??? Are we giving the pharmaceuticals free path here and taking advantage of the imposed public emotional vulnerability fear and terrors!

Nowadays, people are getting vaccinated rushing without being tested prior to see if they already had COVID antibodies and therefore vaccination is needed to start with or after to see if the vaccine was effective! They decided if isn't required and it us individual preference and must pay for it (average $500) Each vaccine recipient must also be tested after vaccination to confirm effectiveness of vaccine and development of adequate antibodies!

Ideally each one should demand to be tested for free prior to receiving the vaccine and after receiving the vaccine for antibody title as all other historic vaccine guidelines!

Respectfully
Thank You 🙏

VS. Hm, retrospective analysis of blood samples collected for other reasons than Covid showed that about 29-25 prcent already had antibody.
AP. Yes!!!
DI. It sure should be.
RP. I would certainly have my antibodies checked prior. The newest test available is a quantitative test and Mt. Sinai in NYC is performing this blood test. My husband just had it done.
LR. THANK YOU!!!!!
SL. God Bless you for speaking the truth and advocating for all healthcare workers as well as patients!!!

We need more brave and honest doctors like you

RC. Seems a lot more about the $$, not the science.
FA. Thank you Dr Ghaly

JS. I thought it was because people seem to not carry antibodies for long after having the virus ? (Either because they loose them or because we can't properly test for it)

DD. Antibodies should be routinely tested on all patient that have recovered from covid and to those who are receiving the vaccine. This data is very important!

LA. for sharing your expertise with us!! May God's protection be with you as you fight the good fight. Much love and blessings to you! 🖤

VG. I am not a doctor, but this sounds right to me!

MG. Dr Ghaly if we test positive for antibodies do we still need vaccine? how long do you think i might be immune ?

DI. no one knows yet except it is short two months or less. For that reason antibodies testing is so important and keep testing

DG. I have a brother out of town who had in spring and then living in household of family who had in October and didn't get. He didn't get antibodies but was tested for active virus and negative. No quarantine precautions aside staying home with others. My family(no contact with this household) tested in August no antibodies. None for all except 11 y.o.-0.37 but not considered til over 1. We tested positive early November. She was only one who was not sick. Rest of us all symptoms down for weeks.

SP. These are facts !!!! The nurse died who msm downplayed earlier today on the news. Even if she had prexisting conditions, even more of a reason of research before vaccinating people. Any fact checkers disclaiming this issue, at this point, should be sued as individuals outside of their employers like Soros, the social media owners etc. etc

JS. More good information about Covid-19...

Thank you
Ramsis

... You are in our prayers on the front line. Thank you! 🙏🙏🙏

Out of millions of the people, Is any any any Anyone worldwide who received the COVID vaccine had a blood test confirming that he or she now immune by that vaccine??????

All I am getting is the news of millions are getting the vaccine but there is no single report yet that the newly administered vaccine worldwide is successful through a follow up blood test of providing immunity?? Unless you know??

Ramsis Ghaly

813

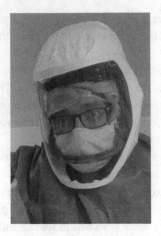

RC. I've wondered that too!

HC. No. This v does not give u immunity they already know that

HC. It's just to reduce symptoms like the whooping cough one

VA. I think it is too early. But i trust God is leading us.

TH. Good question!

GH From what I understand, you can still get covid after vaccines and spread it. They said to continue wearing masks and social distancing. If one does contract covid after receiving vaccine, the symptoms shouldn't be as bad???? Now I've also heard, it's only good for 6 months.

AM. Hmm now that is really something to be considered!

AL. Order me a test and We will find out!

GR. I was told that the vaccine is an immune booster shot that will help you blood cells fight viruses and combat Covid19, if contracted.

BK. I think many still have to get the second shot

LM. Good question

CG. That's what I want to know. I hope someone answers this. 🖤🙏

HM. Is this not how they determined efficacy in the clinical trials?

NP. Canceled my appointment today. During Q&A with our leadership I asked a question if after Covid infection antibodies disappear from the blood within 90 days what about after covid vaccination? Do we have to get vaccine every three months? They couldn't answer to my question.

SZ. Did you here about the doctor in Florida who died after receiving the vaccine??? Scary

My apologies for accidentally misspelling the correct form! Glad you were "here" to correct me. 💜

AV. Good question! 🦠🙏🇺🇸

814

AL. Great Question Doctor.

ED. I agree, I really don't want to be a Guinea pig.

AK. Yes, you can ask for the spike protein ab test.

The nucleoside ab test is post infx.

So yes. Available

RP. Question? Since the vaccine is a 2 part administration how long do you need to wait for it to start working? I know the flu vaccine starts kicking in about 2 weeks after injection. Any idea?

Compensation for the Victims of COVID Vaccine Complications!!

Ramsis Ghaly

Whenever I see patients with complications related to COVID vaccine and or/ occurred after receiving the vaccine, I feel helpless and disturbed in the same time!! The complications I have seen are neurological and vascular related. And the immediate response of the officials: "They are related to the coexisting diseases and not to the vaccine".

Dr Fauci and CDC said "I do not understand those people refuse the COVID Vaccine." If Dr. Fauci and his team feel strongly that the COVID Vaccine is absolutely safe and effective and risk free, why the patients have to sign a well written Legal consent that provides unlimited immunity to be sued to all the vaccine manufacturers and officials??

It is only fair to compensate those participants of taking the vaccine and developed complications.

Ramsis Ghaly

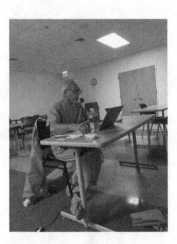

JC. Strongly agree Dr. 😌
ND. Yes!!!!
JR. Please share details about type of vaccine that caused complications. Number of patients you saw. How morbid are the complications. Are you reporting

these to CDC.. still anecdotal experience is not reliable enough to share and discourage the public to take the vaccine.

DST. My ex husband Jills Dad had a stroke after first shot five days later.... he is fine now and lucky with no problems from stroke which was a clot in his brain..... he would have died if not gotten to hospital under 5 minutes...... they live close to hospital in Palm Springs CA..... so scary

DP. Agree with you Dr. I'm not doing the shot because it has not been vetted to the point where they don't require signing such an agreement. you sign for most vaccines...Ever since my kids were small. I will not be taking this one tho. I understand. However, the difference is this consent exempts the manufacture from being sued for any reason because it's being issued during a pandemic.

SL. In 1986 Regan signed into law that all vaccine manufacturers are liability free for all vaccine injuries for every type of vaccine given Agree with you Dr. I'm not doing the shot because it has not been vetted to the point where they don't require signing such an agreement. you sign for most vaccines...Ever since my kids were small. I will not be taking this one tho.

SL. In 1986 Regan signed into law that all vaccine manufacturers are liability free for all vaccine injuries for every type of vaccine given

BCD. YES, AND THANKS!

DL. Totally agree with you. However, it will eventually become mandatory for all large gatherings and travel

JU. no it will not we the people have power to stop them.

SD. agreed. Making something like this mandatory, taking away freedoms is not why we originally settled in this country

SD. plus that 💩doesn't even works.

DL. absolutely not. I'll be getting a religious exemption if that EVER happens.

SH. I took the vaccine because I was told the reason I developed AFIB was due to having COVID. Now I have to have an ablation in May, I'm not sure if getting the vaccine was the right decision. 🙍

LA. My cousin was diagnosed with Bell's palsy the day after she got her second Pfizer vaccine last week

DL. Thank you doc for speaking out

RH. Absolutely

SB. My EP Cardio @ Rush said their seeing an increase of POTS after people get Covid!

I have POTS and its brutal

JK. Yep, that's why I decided not to get the so called vaccine!!! To many unknowns!!! GOD WILL DELIVER ND. I have to agree, Dr. Ramsis Ghaly I also just learned about COVID psychosis. What are your thoughts on that?

DG. A co worker mentioned fatigue to me. Not a normal fatigue but what she had imagined when I told her I had with covid. Also continue to have. Have seen a few patients with new elevation in blood pressure. And one mentioned he noticed it started after vaccine. Also a symptom I have had post covid but for me only diastolic. His is both. I know of few others with no other previous medical conditions who have had blood pressure issues post covid so with the vaccine I think the patient may be on to something. Seems they are getting same long hauler issues. Also have had some getting virus after taking vaccine. I am taking note of who gets and which vaccine they had.

JB. Thank you, I appreciate your advice, concerns and information.

SL. God Bless you for speaking truth!!! We need more courageous doctors to do the same 🙏❤️🙏

SC. im not reciving it i do not belive its safe just me

AC. Thank you for speaking up.

MM. Amen! God bless you for being honest with us! 🖤

BCD. I agree 💯 percent. Way too many lies

SD. My surgeon who helped me walk upright again. Christian man, author, and the man you will always have, and always want to have on your side. So proud of you Dr Ghaly for all you do to help so many!

DH. Amen

JW. Kind of interesting ... coming from a Doctor.

SF. There's not much that can be done once a adverse reaction happens from the vaccine. Uncharted Territory for everyone in the medical profession

MK. 🙏🙏 totally agree.!!!

YR. I share your information and none of my friends even try to look at the truth. Shameful agree, they've all been brainwashed and scared to death. it is really sad. I get more views on a random picture of a cat than important info about your health

GG. Have you seen anybody with neurological and vascular complications from getting the Covid virus? The complications from the disease are 30 times more frequently seen than the ones from the vaccine. Who will you sue then? Trump? China? God?

JB. Where is the research that backs up what you are saying? What complications and are you and other doctors reporting them? I have heard about complications from covid but very few compared to complications from the number of people vaccinated.

LC. Im not taking this shot...First they dont know enough about it,,,,It was tested for 9 months,,Something that should take years..Now they say its safe even hearing people getting side effects,,Well i dont take chances in life,,my luck something happens,,I have a friend who family member is a doctor..This doctor said DONT TAKE THE SHOT,,Not everyone is on agreement with this,,,Take it you can still get the virus and get a booster,,Now there talking about a 3 rd booster,,Keep the muzzles on..come on now Get real..Not to mention of side effects down the road for years to come ..

Anti- COVID Coat!!

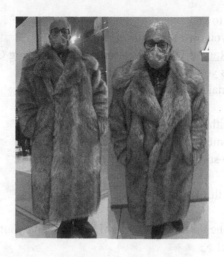

I won't take the vaccine!
But instead I found this coat that will instantly swallow COVID-19 and kill any coronavirus come close!!

Ramsis Ghaly

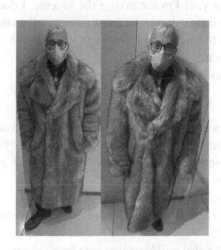

CG. I love it!
ND. You make me laugh 😄
JO. You're cracking me up! But seriously don't take the vaccine! Lol
TH. Dr. G!! Lol!
MK. Thank God dooooooo not take it!

MS. I love the coat, it looks it can take a
30 below temperature 🐻

DI. Love it!

PR. Good weekend to you.

CR, Please tell me you own this coat 😆

KG. Blessings, Dr <u>Ramsis Ghaly.</u> We arent either! Looking Great! Stay safe and
   well. God Bless you and Merry Christmas!

DR, 🖤 it and you make my days brighter 👏

KC. Love it!!

FL. I won't take it either!

BV. Thats an awesome coat!!

DH. You look like a surgical teddy bear!

JW. Awesome Doc!

EH. Why don't you think it is safe

JT. Love
That coat! No vaccine for me and my family!! No thank you!

VG. Thats awesome! 😊

GP. Love that coat!

RF. Dr. Ramsis Ghaly,, that's a beautiful coat 🖤

JJ. COVID-19 is definitely scared of that!!!! Is it wolf? 🐺😄

JC. Love it!

CT. Doc Da Fashionister ✨🎩✨

DC. A warm coat for you! I'm not taking the vaccine. I doubt they will tell us
   what's in it, and if they do can we trust them to tell us the truth? Americans
   don't know who to trust when it comes to vaccines. 😔

AS. Hilarious.. I love it !! 😅😅

CW. You are hilarious! Don is cracking up too

TR. I love it!!Grrrrrr

WP. Lol

JP. You may be attacked by animal rights activists if you wear it in public 😄

LR. Love love love the "Covid Coat" 😅

KW. Looking handsomely safe from any virus! Have a great Christmas 🎄
   season! Miss you out here!

ML. Where did you get that fur? I love it! 😅

BS. I have a shorter mink look jacket. I don't want the vaccine either, if I don't
   need it!

AP. I don't know if the coat will keep you safe from the virus but it is a beautiful
   coat be safe and healthy have a Merry Christmas

TJ. I will not be taking the vaccine either. Guess I better get me one of those
   coats too.

GG. Best advice as always! Wear with pride!

JJ. That will keep you warm Dr.

SP. I'm not taking the vaccine either. However, I may need to borrow that coat to remain safe!!! 😇😳😊😳😊😊❤️😊🙏🙏🙏

PC. Legendary

JF. I love it! I want a matching one so we can be twins!!! #PastorJeff90210

RH. Now your taking a action 👋👆😭

LG. FABULOUSLY SAFE AND SHIELDED.

EG. No to mandated vaccines.

PS. Can I ask you why you're not taking the vaccine? I'm a 60 year diabetic with heart issues and I'm not sure what to do about taking the vaccine.

DH. Seriously?

BCD. Good idea

CP. That will keep you warm ‼️

DL. Lol. Love it

NE. I love it! Get me one 😂😂

VG. Divni ste legendo. Najbolji savet. Nosite sa ponosam i ja se pridružujem. Ponosim se sa Vama dr.Ramis Ghali! 🙏🙏🖤🖤 You are a wonderful legend. The best advice ever. Wear with pride and I join. I am proud of you Dr. Ramis Ghali! 🙏🙏🖤🖤🖤🖤

NV. I won't take the vaccine either! and thank goodness I don't have the coat 😭 God Bless you Doctor Ghaly and stay safe 🙏😸

RF. Need a Hat to match.

DS. I love my COVID coats as well!!! Safety can be luxurious!

GS. You wont take the vaccine? Why not Dr?

LP. Wondering why you will not take the vaccine? No comment on the coat. I hope you will explain.

NV. You are looking for the doctor to tell you what to do, so later if there are side effects you can say well I followed what this doctor did! I can tell you why I am not taking the vaccine ✒️! It takes 5-12 years to develope and test the vaccines before being available. This coronavirus vaccine was developed to fast and for me there was not enough sufficient testing time to see what if any long term side effects will have. Everyone should decide for themselves if they want to get the vaccine or not!

AR. Your are rocking that coat! Keep on shining ✨🤍

ED. Loving the coat Doctor! Not sure I'll take the vaccine either. Will wait and see.

KC. Love it

BM. Love it! It looks my size, hint, hint 🤍😭🤍

TN. Looks VW. That statement you made about not taking the vaccine has really got me thinking? Can you please explain? I'll buy your fur 😊

NA. It's beautiful and looks cozy!!

SC. the kids and i have no desire for the vaccine

MN. Awesome covid coat...I'm not taking the vaccine either..not enough research or tests behind it...and if there is...that means they already had the vaccine ready....?!?! And for what????

SL. Looking sharp brother love your fur 😃

MP. You look Russian comrade 😉

AP. 🖤🖤🖤 me either!

AP. I'm with you, Doctor. I will not take it neither 🙏

KM. Only you can pull this off! Looks great.

JC. Would you take the vaccine?

ED. To cute!

LM. Love the coat.

HG. YES to the vaccine, NO to the Fur-coat

TL. Loving the coat!!

JM. Looking Good Dr. Ghaly 💕 Covid Will never get you in that coat 💕

LH. Looking good, stay well and safe 🖤

LM. Love the coat.

JM. King Good Dr. Ghaly 💕 Covid Will never get you in that coat 💕

LH. Looking good, stay well and safe 🖤

BB. How will you refuse ? I heard county employees have to take it 😔

BS. This may be the best post ever. We love you dr Ghaly

JM. Love it Doc, and I say YES to the coat, and no to the Vaccine

SP. Happy to see you have manage to maintain your sense of humor 😊 Thank you for risking your health to care for Covid patients. You are a hero.

NP. I'm with Dr. Ghaly, No Vaccination for me and mine 💯 God has us 🙏🖤

AP. I won't get vaccinated no way, no how. My Heavenly Father is my only Healer and He is all I need. 🙏🖤

LP. That's a beautiful fur coats yeah I agree with you it'll kill covid-19and everything else.

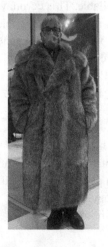

Discriminatory Treatment Based on Vaccinated and Unvaccinated!!

My residents graduation 🎓 is at Sears Towers (Wills Tower)
Tight restriction for those didn't take the vaccine as follow:
1) Must have negative COVID test!
2) Must sit in a remote table and isolated from other tables!
3) Cannot mix with other people!
4) Will have a separate waiters and waitress!

Therefore, I am not going!!! I will zoom in virtual. It is very hard to feel discriminated and excluded and restricted just because!!

Every one of them not only forcing the vaccines per so called CDC guideline but also forcing to sign a consent releasing them from any responsibilities and Sid effects!!

Look at Wills sky deck:

Important Notice Regarding COVID-19
Willis Tower and Skydeck Chicago have implemented measures consistent with CDC and local and federal guidance to try to reduce the spread of COVID-19 on the premises, including enhanced cleaning protocols. Even with these procedures in place, PLEASE BE ADVISED that building occupants, building and Skydeck visitors, or others currently or previously present upon this property and/or the Skydeck MAY HAVE CONTRACTED OR BEEN EXPOSED TO COVID-19 or other infectious diseases, and may expose you. By accessing and using building common areas, the Skydeck, and their associated amenities, you and your party voluntarily assume all risks of your use—INCLUDING THE RISK OF EXPOSURE TO INFECTIOUS DISEASE—and you waive all claims, including claims for negligence, against Willis Tower, Skydeck Chicago, and their respective owners, managers, affiliates, agents and representatives, arising out of such use. The above parties hereby disclaim all liability for any injuries arising out of your use of this property and the Skydeck, including exposure to infectious disease.

Accept and Continue Accept and Continue

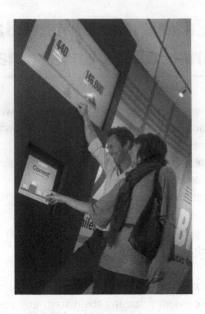

THESKYDECK.COM

Plan Your Visit to Skydeck Chicago | Hours, Wait Times, Accessibility
Skydeck can personalize your visit to the highest observation deck in the US! Plan you visit with inside tips, hours, wait times, prices, and more.

Visit the COVID-19 Information Center for vaccine resources.

Get Vaccine Info

Sl. I'm very concerned the discrimination will continue to get much worse at least here in IL and especially Chicago 😨
Js. I totally agree with you Dr Ghaly.
Rw. Totally agree
Cg. YOU are so correct. We are being forced to get the vaccine if we want to do the things we love to do and live the life we had. I am one of those who said I would never get the vaccine BUT I love traveling and the European countries are only allowing th...
Sc. my dad use to take me& my siblings there when it was sears tower hated it scared of heights

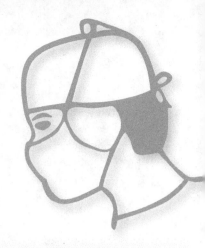

SECTION 15

Medical Issues during COVID-19

COVID Should Never be an Excuse to Let our Beloved Old People Go Prematurely!

Written by Ramsis Ghaly

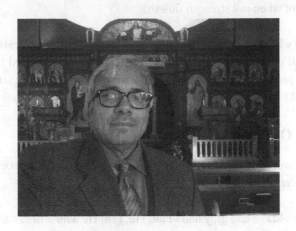

COVID should never be an excuse to let our beloved old people go prematurely! COVID is not an excuse to pull the plug in our dearest elders, the blessed! COVID is not a reason to turn your back in the senior loved ones!

covid should never be used as an excuse to withdrawal life short from our elders that otherwise could be saved!

We all should fight for the lives of all the sick regardless of age, sex, demographic, ethnicity and socioeconomic status!

The entire planet and each household is loaded with the blessing of our senior citizens! Please do not take them away! Why should we do that to them?? They have the same rights if not even more to deserve the best Medical care!

Our elders are living in fears and terrors because the youngsters are not fighting for their health and existence and they won't defend them!

Elders' lives should be cherished and we the siblings should stand by them and be their advocate and their voice! Please don't put your loved ones in hospice if they do not belong there not just because they are old!

827

We should take it as an opportunity to do more and appreciate them more and more and stand by them all the way and not to leave them half way!! If we do God prolong our lives and make them well as He promised! Don't bring a curse upon yourself!!!

God hears their outcry: Psalms 71:9 - Cast me not off in the time of old age; forsake me not when my strength faileth.

God Almighty love them so much as He said in day one in the creation: "Honour thy father and thy mother, as the Lord thy God hath commanded thee; that thy days may be prolonged, and that it may go well with thee, in the land which the Lord thy God giveth thee." Deuteronomy 5:16 KJV

Honor the Old Age:

Look to kind words of God to care for our loved elders and do the best we can we shall never ever cut their life short:

"Even to your old age and gray hairs I am He, I am He who will sustain you. I have made you and I will carry you; I will sustain you and I will rescue you." Isiah 46:4

"Stand up in the presence of the aged, show respect for the elderly and revere your God. I am the Lord." Leviticus 19:32

"Do not cast me away when I am old; do not forsake me when my strength is gone." Psalm 71:9

"To the elders among you, I appeal as a fellow elder and a witness of Christ's sufferings who also will share in the glory to be revealed." 1Peter 5:1

"Do not rebuke an older man harshly, but exhort him as if he were your father. Treat younger men as brothers; 2. older women as mothers, and younger women as sisters, with absolute purity." 1 Timothy 5:1-2

Acts 20:35 - I have shewed you all things, how that so labouring ye ought to support the weak, and to remember the words of the Lord Jesus, how he said, It is more blessed to give than to receive.

1 Timothy 5:8 - But if any provide not for his own, and especially for those of his own house, he hath denied the faith, and is worse than an infidel.

828

1 Timothy 5:1 - Rebuke not an elder, but intreat [him] as a father; [and] the younger men as brethren;

Leviticus 19:32 - Thou shalt rise up before the hoary head, and honour the face of the old man, and fear thy God: I [am] the LORD.

Ephesians 6:2 - Honour thy father and mother; (which is the first commandment with promise;)

1 Timothy 5:4 - But if any widow have children or nephews, let them learn first to shew piety at home, and to requite their parents: for that is good and acceptable before God.

James 1:27 - Pure religion and undefiled before God and the Father is this, To visit the fatherless and widows in their affliction, [and] to keep himself unspotted from the world.

Psalms 71:9 - Cast me not off in the time of old age; forsake me not when my strength faileth.

1 Timothy 5:3-4 - Honour widows that are widows indeed. (Read More...)

1 Timothy 5:17 - Let the elders that rule well be counted worthy of double honour, especially they who labour in the word and doctrine.

Isaiah 46:4 - And [even] to [your] old age I [am] he; and [even] to hoar hairs will I carry [you]: I have made, and I will bear; even I will carry, and will deliver [you].

Exodus 20:12 - Honour thy father and thy mother: that thy days may be long upon the land which the LORD thy God giveth thee.

Matthew 15:4-6 - For God commanded, saying, Honour thy father and mother: and, He that curseth father or mother, let him die the death. (Read More...)

1 Timothy 5:16 - If any man or woman that believeth have widows, let them relieve them, and let not the church be charged; that it may relieve them that are widows indeed.

https://www.nature.com/articles/d41586-020-02483-2
https://www.nbcnews.com/news/amp/ncna1244853
Ramsis Ghaly

PP. Well said Dr. Ramsis Ghaly

KO. Thank You Dr Ghaly from all us elderly folks 💜

AK. Very true 💜

Dr. Are you Coptic Orthodox. You probably said before, but do not remember

CG. What you say is so true. The elder deserve all the care, respect and love we can give them. 💜🙏

JD. Happy New Year Dr. Ghaly !!! You are a blessing to us all !!!

SJ. The U.S. is a throw away society - even our elders. We do not value their histories, wisdom, dedication, love or age. They are not beautiful. Thank you for speaking out on this often overlooked group. It would be such a blessing if the U.S. valued its elders like the native Americans, Japanese, etc. It would provide great value to all if we Lived in multigenerational homes.

CB. I'm so touch with you post regarding the elderly. In my country we take care of our elders until the last breathe of their life. That's how we respect and love them.

VG. Well said doctor!!! 💜💜💜

Virtual Medical Management in Modern Post COVID Medicine

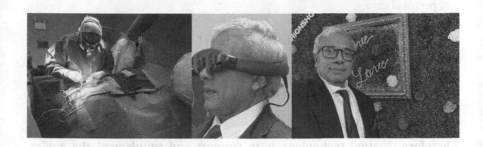

Technology made for Man and NOT Man for Technology!!
As Our Teacher and Master Jesus Taught us: "The sabbath was
made for man, and not man for the sabbath:" Mark 2:27

Virtual Medical Management (VMM) is on the rise, rightly so during COVID-19 to comply with social isolation and physical distancing. The fear that VMM is replacing the standard in person care and in remote counties is offered as the only method to provide care.

VMM has its place in providing care but not all care. For instance, VMM is acceptable for established patients, medication refill, initial evaluation especially in remote areas. But VMM cannot replace the gold standard of care, In Person, and Hands On. The physical touch, in person interaction, the various human intuition, perceiving signals through in person examination cannot be replaced by robotic arms and cameras. Medical management relies on not only boxes to mark but full input and comprehensive in-person data collection to interpret and come up with correct diagnosis and sound faultless medical management plans. This is what patients wants and what quality healthcare demand of us.

Through my career, I cannot make any medical and surgical diagnosis, decisions and come up with the best plans for that particular patient without hands-on In person care leaving all things outside the room and interact fully with the patient one-to-one without any barriers. Medicine is an High hierarchy Art and demand the best of in person care that can offer!!

In Person Medical Management (IPMM) and In Person Medical Team (IPMT) use all the unlimited Godly gifted senses and skills first hand without the need of additional barriers through wiring, video cameras, teleconferencing.

Furthermore, the technology is in infantile stage lacking many sensitive medical sensors and devices to examine patients fully from far. Technology is not there yet for virtual reality and bring remote virtual care to become similar to hands-on care. Not only in person provide superb hands-on care but also, warmth, tender, and personal care.

IPMM provides care to all ages and to all kind of diseases especially challenging patients, disabled, uncooperative, not savvy in technology –etc. Confronting patients with serious illness and life changing health events cannot be handled by remote virtual robots but best handled by in person, private, attentive, hands on close IPMM.

Therefore, Virtual technology is to support and supplement the golden standard of In-person Hands-on Care! VMM and VMT is for IPMM and IPMT.

Technology made for Man and NOT Man for Technology!!

As Our Teacher and Master Jesus Taught us: "The sabbath was made for man, and not man for the sabbath:" Mark 2:27

The sabbath was made for man, and not man for the sabbath
Technology made for Man and NOT Man for Technology!!
VMM and VMT is for IPMM and IPMT and NOT
IPMM and IPMT for VMM and VMT!
Virtual technology is to support and supplement the
golden standard of In-person Hands-on Care!

An example of VMM went bad:
Virtual Medical Team (VMT) received a Medical Emergency!
VMT get the message but VMT can't download!!
Every time doctor try to download the message, it doesn't download!
VMT calls IT (Informatics) person, the IT voice mail has 9 options to select one!
VMT couldn't get hold of alive IT, VMT select wrong options, and finally hang up!
VMT decided the best way was to turn off the VMT system and allowed to Reboot!
VMT gets panic yell and scream for emergency help, call the police but there is no police already defunded, call 911 but no more dispatchers, they are only available for murders by GSW!

Finally the VMT rebooted the system but the message was deleted and emergency message was gone!

Another new message comes to VMT and the message was do not bother the patients are dead call the funeral to take the bodies! died!

Finally a patterned in VMT get hold to IT person and was able to retrieve the message but it was too late!

The IT said no worries it was just a computer glitch and a night hacker hacked our system but we are running antivirus program and will fix all computer problems!

What is the lesson? Patient care should never be under the mercy of technology and must continue to be Hands-on care! Technology for Medical Care and NOT Medical Care for Technology! Technology for Medical Doctors and NOT Medical Doctors and Staff for Technology

Let us remember Technology made for Man and NOT Man for Technology!!

As Our Teacher and Master Jesus Taught us: "The sabbath was made for man, and not man for the sabbath:" Mark 2:27

In Conclusion

The sabbath was made for man, and not man for the sabbath
Technology made for Man and NOT Man for Technology!!
VMM and VMT is for IPMM and IPMT and NOT IPMM and IPMT for VMM and VMT!
Virtual technology is to support and supplement the golden standard of In-person Hands-on Care!

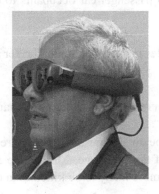

Motorcycle Riders, during COVID: Did You Know!!!

Ramsis Ghaly

Many Riders drive out during COVID escaping from the imposed curfews. I wish Motorcyclists know that despite full protection gear, leather clothes and helmet, they aren't protected against fatal and semi fatal accidents by no fault of the motorcyclists.

Two patients within a week suffered almost fatal accidents and lifelong permanent non fixable injuries and it wasn't their faults: one case because a flat tire and the second accident, a car cut across and he tried to avoid it!!

Both patients said they will never ever ride a motorcycle again and they advise others to do the same!

Unfortunately, in the industry, motorcycle dealerships and manufactures may not make it clear that full gear protection isn't grantee of self-protection even if the motorcyclist is an expert one!

Traveling on a motorcycle carries a much higher risk of death or injury than driving the same distance in a car. In 2006 US motorcyclists had a risk of a fatal crash that was 35 times greater than that of passenger cars, based on 390 motorcyclist deaths per billion vehicle miles and 11.1 car fatalities for that distance. In 2016 this rate was 28 times that for automobiles. In 2018, 4,985 motorcyclists died in motorcycle crashes, down 5 percent from 5,229 in 2017, according to the National Highway Traffic Safety Administration (NHTSA). In 2018, motorcyclists were 27 times more likely than passenger car occupants to die in a crash per vehicle miles traveled.

Motorcycle rider death rates increased among all rider age groups between 1998 and 2000

Motorcycle rider deaths were nearly 30 times more than drivers of other vehicles

Motorcycle riders aged below 40 are 36 times more likely to be killed than other vehicle operators of the same age. Motorcycle riders aged 40 years and over are around 20 times more likely to be killed than other drivers of that same age. Since about 2004 over 4,000 people have died every year up to 2014 in motorcycle accidents, and in 2007 and 2008 deaths exceeded 5,000 per year.[4] At the same time occupant deaths of other types of vehicles have decreased in the 21st century, so motorcycle accident deaths have become an increased share of all deaths and noted for being 26 times more deadly than cars.[4] Operators of sport motorcycle models had a higher rate of death compared to other motorcycle types, and speeding was noted in roughly half of fatal sport and super sport accidents compared to about a fifth for fatal accidents of other types.[6] Sport and super sport riders were also likely to be younger among those involved in a fatal accident, with an average age of 27 (for the year 2005).[6] The number of fatalities of those under 30 has gone from 80% percent in 1975 to 30% in 2014.

https://en.m.wikipedia.org/.../Motorcycle_fatality_rate...
https://en.m.wikipedia.org/wiki/Motorcycle_safety

My Chicago Thanksgiving Between COVID and Gun Victims

But neither COVID nor guns shall separate us from the love of Christ!
Look at the days what brought us to!!
Who ever imagine 2020 Thanksgiving will be like this????

My thanksgiving is between COVID victims and the Wild West of Chicago guns and stabs

Yet nothing will separate us from the Love 🖤 of our Savior and Redeemer Jesus our God, Amen 🙏

Neither COVID nor Pandemic nor tribulations nor guns nor distress nor social isolation nor physical distancing nor rules nor regulation—-Nothing nothing shall separate us from our Love 🖤 to our Savior Jesus

"Who shall separate us from the love of Christ? shall tribulation, or distress, or persecution, or famine, or nakedness, or peril, or sword? [36] As it is written, For thy sake we are killed all the day long; we are accounted as sheep for the slaughter. [37] Nay, in all these things we are more than conquerors through him that loved us. [38] For I am persuaded, that neither death, nor life, nor angels, nor principalities, nor powers, nor things present, nor things to come, [39] Nor height, nor depth, nor any other creature, shall be able to separate us from the love of God, which is in Christ Jesus our Lord." Romans 8:35-39 KJV

Happy Thanksgiving 🍁🦃🍽 and Be Safe!
Ramsis Ghaly

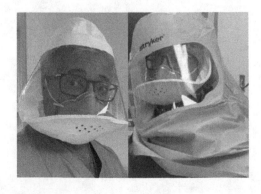

KM. Happy Thanksgiving Dr. SJ. Happy Thanksgiving, Dr. Ghaly

TP. Happy Thanksgiving Dr. Ghaly! Thank you for service and care. May God bless you.

RZ. Happy Thanksgiving!

DC. Happy Thanksgiving Dr. Ghaly. God bless you for the care you give to those in need. ✝🙏❤️

SS. GLORIA A Dio

HD. Blessing to you this Thanksgiving 2020

JB. Happy Thanksgiving Dr.G. Please be safe!!

AB. Praise God!

MY. مع المسيح ذاك افضل جدا الرب يعنا ونصل اليه بلا عيب ولا دنس لأنه هو رجائنا آمين ثم آمين
يارب العالمين ونشكرك يارب ونحمد فضلك يا ابن الله اللحى 🖤🖤🖤🖤🖤

ER. Agreed Dr. Ghaly 🖤. Stay safe and Happy Thanksgiving 🦃

CY. Happy Thanksgiving Dr Ghaly

ER. Stay safe Doctor!

Bless you and Happy Thanksgiving 🦃

MM. Happy Thanksgiving! Good luck! 🍀

CB. Happy Thanksgiving! 🍁🦃

DC. Happy thanksgiving 🍁🍗🦃

CP. Happy Thanksgiving. ☺️

AF. Thank you!! Wishing you a happy and healthy Thanksgiving

AV. Thankful for you & your coworkers! God Bless you! 🖤🙏 and Happy Thanksgiving!

NM. Happy Thanksgiving!!

CR. Amen

CE. Happy Thanksgiving to you, Doctor!

RH. You are on my mind often.

So grateful for your love of Jesus and your my church 🙏😷😋😷🙏

My Chicago Thanksgiving Between COVID and Gun Victims

High from Chicago Highway!!! Express from Chicago Expressway!!! Bullets are flying in Chicago Freeways!!

The more COVID sad News floating around, the more highway shooting!!

The more of viruses news are spreading, the more causalities of intoxicated and Overdose victims!

837

Chicago in particular and other major cities in America are in dire need of structural and moral help!!

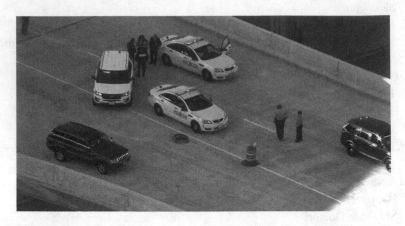

NBCCHICAGO.COM

Chicago Area Sees Daily Expressway Shootings For Last 8 Days

The Chicago area has reported shootings on expressways in the past eight days, including one in which a man was fatally shot Friday on the Eisenhower Expressway.

RF. Week in Progress (11/29 – 12/5)
Shot & Killed: 9
Shot & Wounded: 54
Total Shot: 63
Total Homicides: 11
Chicago Crime 2020

RF. The new norm.
RF. So now the Loop, North Michigan Avenue, and the Expressways are unsafe.... What's next?
GH. Stay safe Dr. I had a round trip ticket I didn't use to visit my sister a s family in Chicago! Very sad...

Patient Empowerment with Faith

A Real Story

Always remember my quote especially nowadays in healthcare: "Patient empowerment: trust yourself, advocate for your health and settle for no less"

God blessed me to help a patient came desperately to my clinic with horrific pain in the face. Her doctors thought it was coming from a rare disease called Idiopathic Trigeminal Neuralgia. It was getting worse and worse. Although her doctors missed to make the correct diagnosis, God made her aware in her heart that it was the bad tooth!

However, she couldn't go anywhere, because no one doctor yet was making the correct diagnosis. So the merciful God intervened and didn't allow the shortcoming of man to worsen her condition and endanger her life and deteriorate into life threatening infection, she was guided by one of her friend to come and see me for evaluation to treat the trigeminal neuralgia.

As she was describing to me: she said "The pain started as horrible toothache—". I examined her and I said: "You are absolutely correct and medicine has failed you. You Do Not have Idiopathic Trigeminal Neuralgia but you have a serious dental infection resulted from a tooth abscess that wasn't treated early and aggressively. So sorry, you must go right away to the hospital to drain the abscess before it spreads to the head and neck and you will not be able to breath and then it became life threatening —Do not leave the hospital, the tooth must come out and start intravenous antibiotics and drain the abscess—-and settle for no less—-".

Understandably, It wasn't easy to convince her and her husband since they already seen the doctors and they told her: "No by big N and this is "Idiopathic Trigeminal Neuralgia" and she was treated accordingly and get more medications for the pains! To make it easy and convince her, I took a picture and text it to her to show it to her and to take it to the emergency room so that she can be helped and not be turned away!!

Next day, I called, I was so happy and proud of her! She did exactly that and today she is back home with no pain and very happy. Praise our Lord Jesus. Thank you Lord for using me to help this patient, a mother of big family, despite the fact I am neither an oral surgeon nor a dentist!!

Always remember my quote especially nowadays in healthcare: "Patient empowerment: trust yourself, advocate for your health and settle for no less"

Respectfully
Ramsis Ghaly
GHALYNEUROSURGEON.COM
Neurosurgeon | Brain surgery, spine surgery | Treating carpal tunnel symptoms, spinal stenosis, sciatica in Auruora, Il

LW. Thank you once again Dr Ghaly for taking good care of my friend! So glad she got to you in time!!

Ghaly Novel Checklist in Anesthesia and Neurological Surgery: Editorial Publication

I wish to share with you an exciting news!! My Novel Checklist for Anesthesia and Surgery/ neurosurgery just got published as an Editorial in a prestigious international Journal to help safe anesthesia and surgery/ Neuro worldwide. It is much more comprehensive and specific compared to the current Surgery safety checklist

Link to article
https://surgicalneurologyint.com/.../a-novel-checklist.../

Ramsis Ghaly

Ghaly Checklist for General and Neuro-Anesthesia

A) Preoperative
1. Anesthesia machine checked, self-test passed
2. Preoperative Assessment completed, medical/surgical history and laboratory values reviewed
3. Patient consent signed, surgical site marked
4. Preoperative medications and choice of regional blockade

B) Monitors (Connected and functioning)
1. O_2 Saturation. 2.Blood pressure. 3. EKG 4. $etCO_2$

   Anesthesia setup completed

C) Airway
1. ETT/LMA checked and available (need for specialty ETT?)
2. Head positioning optimized for intubation, preoxygenation adequate ($etO_2 > 80\%$)
3. Intubating device functioning (direct laryngoscopy, video laryngoscopy, fiberoptic awake/asleep), difficult airway backup plans
4. Suction available and working

D) Induction and Lines
1. IV access adequate and functioning
2. Need for Arterial line and/or Central venous line placement
3. Induction agents available, drawn and labelled

E) Intraoperative

1. Patient positioning and operating room setup (prone, lateral decubitus, supine), pressure points protected
2. Anesthetic maintenance regimen selected (volatile anesthetic, TIVA, balanced)
3. Antibiotic of choice administered, perioperative subcutaneous heparin requested
4. ERAS protocols indicated?
5. Invasive and noninvasive cardiac/hemodynamic monitoring
6. Warming: forced air blanket, fluid warmer
7. Blood pressure parameters, pressor/antihypertensive drips
8. Anticipated blood loss and management plans (TXA, cell saver, blood/FFP/ platelet transfusion)
9. Prophylaxis for postop nausea/vomiting
10. Intraop and postop pain management plan selected/discussed (prn IV medications, PCA, regional blocks, neuraxial)

F) Emergence

1. Awake or deep extubation vs keep patient intubated
2. Need for postoperative ventilatory support (mechanical ventilation, BiPAP, High flow, nasal cannula, room air)
3. Postoperative Patient disposition (Phase I PACU, Phase II, medical/surgical floor, telemetry, Stepdown, ICU)
4. Post-operative blood pressure and pain control

G) Specific for Neuroanesthesia

1. Specific neurosurgery positioning requirements (head of bed, head pins, horseshoe, sitting, Jackson table)
2. Cervical spine stability/airway management (video laryngoscopy, awake/ asleep fiberoptic intubation, in-line stabilization) and post-intubation neuro assessment
3. Anesthetic Regimen (Awake, TIVA, volatile agents) and neuromuscular blockade use (can non-depolarizing paralytics be used for induction?)
4. Intraoperative fluoroscopy, IR Angiography, Navigation and other imaging modalities
5. Neuromonitoring (Awake, TCD, SSEP, MEP, EEG, EMG)
6. Air Emboli Risk (Transthoracic doppler, TEE)
7. ICP concerns and EVD management (drainage level and rate, max allowable drainage per hour)
8. Recommended $PaCO_2$ and $etCO_2$ level

9. Perioperative blood pressure parameters (systolic/mean), pressor/antihypertensive drips
10. IV crystalloids/colloid choice, fluid restriction indicated?
11. Specific medications and neuroprotective agents (Steroids, antiepileptics, osmodiuretics, burst suppression, hypothermia, etc.)
12. Pre-extubation neuroassement, awake vs deep extubation
13. Postop infusion drips (Nicardipine, pressors, propofol)
14. Postoperative imaging (CT, interventional neuroradiology)

H) Any Additional Requests and Concerns from the Team
Abbreviations: EKG, electrocardiogram; etCO2, end-tidal carbon dioxide; ETT, endotracheal tube; LMA, laryngeal mask airway; etO2, end-tidal oxygen; IV, intravenous; TIVA, total intravenous anesthesia; ERAS: Enhanced Recovery After Surgery; TXA, tranexamic acid; FFP, fresh frozen plasma; PCA, patient-controlled analgesia; BiPAP, bilevel positive airway pressure; PACU, post-anesthesia care unit; ICU, intensive care unit; IR, interventional radiology; TCD, transcranial doppler; SSEP, somatosensory evoked potentials; MEP, motor evoked potentials; EEG, electroencephalogram; EMG, electromyogram; TEE, transesophageal echocardiography, ICP, intracranial pressure; EVD, external ventricular drain; $PaCO_2$, arterial pressure of carbon dioxide; CT, computed tomography

COMMENTS

ML. Well deserved Dr. Ramsis Ghaly. Way to go! 🙏❤️
LL. Great job Dr Ghaly!
DL. Yay. Bravo!
JB. Congratulations Dr. Ghaly!!
Another wonderful accolade!!! 💜
MM. Congratulations
CG. How wonderful that you are able to share your knowledge worldwide.
Congratulations on another great accomplishment! ❤️🙏
MK. Excellent piece of work

Worse Days Ahead for Chicago Violence!!

Ramsis Ghaly

My Father's Day is aching while with my residents caring for young adults dying from the extreme violence and insanity in Chicago Land!! Chicago isn't proud from their betrayals for taking its peace and prosperity away inflicting suffering across the city and taking away human lives spreading terrors and fears in our nation! It is the words in the street nowadays of lacking morality and degrading humanity! To get some sanity from the senseless acts of evil, I went solo to church of God in sadness with all my burden sitting by the Alter of our Lord Jesus in tears with broken heart 💔 praying 🙏 "Lord Have Mercy in thy People".

I have been involved in Chicago Trauma Resuscitation and caring for Chicago trauma victims since 1987 and never seen the horrific causalities in a daily basis in Chicago. It is worse than the battlefield between real the enemies!

The love of Christ is dissipating—! Chicagoans are no longer in love with themselves and with each other! The price of life is trivial in recent days and the disrespect to each other is shocking! The people are fed-up!!!

The Chicago Violence nowadays is Unreal and the number of Trauma Victims unbearable. All colors of young adults are being shot, stabled and murdered. The brutality among the people are unimaginable as we are running out of space and resources to try save what we can!

So many of us healthcare workers are 24/7 round the clock working and doing our best. In the same time, we are crying and our hearts are torn seeing our fellow women and men getting brutally killed.

It is no longer certain group of people, but all kinds! For instance, tonight in June 2021, most of the victims are young women and not colored??? Go figure!!!

People had it with the extreme hardship since March 2020!! Many are suicidal and are in the edge!! The purpose of further living isn't strong anymore after the hell they had seen from the politics and the news and the uprise!!

The reasons are obvious including Rising cost, unemployment, nuances of politics, fake news, racial unrest, coming out of COVID Curfews—/

Never 👎 we saw Chicago going down!! All day and night long trying to keep sanity in our once before a beloved city!! Regardless of what side you belong in politics, No one should over joy in the disastrous Chicago violence and the killing that goes around nowadays in early days of the summer!!

For how long Chicago will be in the dark and the nation news of top city of Chicago violence and murders??? We pray? 🙏

Live a life of love to each other listening to these biblical words: Ephesians 5:1-2 KJV "1] Be ye therefore followers of God, as dear children; [2] And walk in love, as Christ also hath loved us, and hath given himself for us an offering and a sacrifice to God for a sweet-smelling savour."

Ephesians 4:1-6 KJV "1] I therefore, the prisoner of the Lord, beseech you that ye walk worthy of the vocation wherewith ye are called, [2] With all lowliness and meekness, with longsuffering, forbearing one another in love; [3] Endeavoring to keep the unity of the Spirit in the bond of peace. [4] There is one body, and one Spirit, even as ye are called in one hope of your calling; [5] One Lord, one faith, one baptism, [6] One God and Father of all, who is above all, and through all, and in you all."

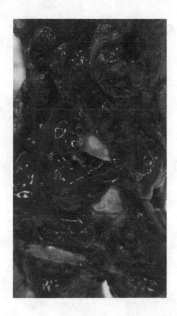

LM. It's not just Chicago, it's all over the country! that's so true, all over this world needs prayers 🙏💜😥🖤

TJ. So sad!

NC. So true it's heartbreaking 🙏🙏🙏

ED. Prayers for Chicago and our Country. God please help us. 🙏🙏

CG. What has happened to our country? The fighting, racism, and destruction of our cities and its people. This is so hard to comprehend. Prayers for all healthcare workers that have to deal with this daily. Be safe! ❤️🙏🙏🙏

DK. As long as politicians work against police and tie their hands from stopping crime the worse it will get. Chicago needs people willing to get dirty working for clean money and not abiding by laws to get more dirty money. All violence is a hate crime and people need to be put away in prison for murder and mayhem. It's so sad and so senseless. This is what happens as Jesus and God are forced out of our country and schools etc.

HAIR SAMPLES

Corporate Health Systems are now requiring hair samples to replace urine samples for toxi screen!

Is it only for criminal background check and 3month worth of drug screening? But I don't think so, Perhaps to take more personal data without consent such as DNA,—-

So between social media and smart phones and hair samples the government and corporate have all the personal information in details. Now if it is hacked by conspirators and foreign agencies how much damage will result?

I looked up why hair samples replacing urine toxi screen, I came with much information about forensic and FBI labs and DNA

We never had hair samples. This is my first time ever to have my hair cut!!

I wonder What are the reasons for corporates other than toxi screen to take actual hair samples and what other information the corporate and government collect behind the scene?

DT. Dr Ghaly what reasons do they need DNA? What will they do with it…..? I'm not schooled in this like you are……. 🤩
GG. Big Brother
SP. I love it when you get political, I feel like we have a connection 😝.

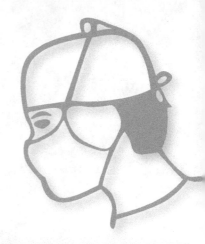

SECTION 16

Future COVID

Coronavirus a Powerful Bioterrorism Please Stay Away!

Please don't blame God! Our Almighty will never ever do something like that! But blame those Sodom and Gomorrah among you! At James said: "Do not err, my beloved brethren. [17] Every good gift and every perfect gift is from above, and cometh down from the Father of lights, with whom is no variableness, neither shadow of turning." James 1:16-17 KJV and he also wrote: "Let no man say when he is tempted, I am tempted of God: for God cannot be tempted with evil, neither tempteth he any man: [14] But every man is tempted, when he is drawn away of his own lust, and enticed. [15] Then when lust hath conceived, it bringeth forth sin: and sin, when it is finished, bringeth forth death." James 1:13-15 KJV

It is a spiritual ware by Satan and satanic people against humanity and human race living!! COVID neither care nor target animals or plants. The target is only Mankind and no other creation with extreme anti-Godly selfishness and animosity against the children of God controlling the freedom of man and the way of living thrown in jail cells and curfews with extreme restrictions drooling through face masks limiting the natural fresh air! Look at the world 🌐 is being destroyed, churches closed, minds are full of godly doubts and hate and no love and people are distancing from each other, families and friends bring separated, all running in terrors and fears and being isolated and arrested and their forms and all what man about have been shut down before our eyes!

Please do as the angel of the Lord told Lot's wife "Escape for thy life; look not behind thee, neither stay thou in all the plain; escape to the mountain, lest thou be consumed" lest be consumed as a COVID Pillar dead 💀 like her became a pillar made of salt: "And it came to pass, when they had brought them forth abroad, that he said, Escape for thy life; look not behind thee, neither stay thou in all the plain; escape to the mountain, lest thou be consumed. [20] Behold now, this city is near to flee unto, and it is a little one: Oh, let me escape thither, (is it not a little one?) and my soul shall live. [26] But his wife looked back from behind him, and she became a pillar of salt." Genesis 19:17,20,26 KJV

If you aren't a Frontliner sacrificing your life to care for COVID patients run away and stay away from them!

The entire COVID pandemic is highly suspicious for satanic people behind the scene and hence much more evil 🦹 mutated particles will continue to be released

851

to our atmosphere! It won't stop ⬤, until Satan sees more and more human tragedies! This isn't a typical natural pandemic or do novo natural disaster! This is series of handmade satanic disasters!!

Please O people do as the angel of God advised

Please stay away until better government highly intelligent federal agents get to the bottom of COVID-19 and who is behind the Hunan mass destruction!

Coronavirus is known to be a powerful Bioweapon for centuries and it was expected to used by 1973!

Coronavirus bioweapon is known to be replicated and mutated frequently!

Coronavirus is an invisible billions of particles spreads globally without borders operated by invisible behind the scene enemies that cannot be traced!

The entire world economy is crumbled!
The world populations are terrorized and fearful!
The world structure and the global Powers are being reformed!

Billions of dollars are being spent on VOVID Vaccines and new ways of living dependent on technology 100%!

What a Supernatural highly intelligent well thought off satanic Bioterrorism perfectly engineered to invade all human cells and has unlimited power to replicate, calculable innumerable ways to mutate, infect, invade and kill without fingerprints!

"How long wilt thou forget me, O Lord ? for ever? how long wilt thou hide thy face from me? [2] How long shall I take counsel in my soul, having sorrow in my heart daily? how long shall mine enemy be exalted over me? [3] Consider and hear me, O Lord my God: lighten mine eyes, lest I sleep the sleep of death; [4] Lest mine enemy say, I have prevailed against him; and those that trouble me rejoice when I am moved. [5] But I have trusted in thy mercy; my heart shall rejoice in thy salvation. [6] I will sing unto the Lord, because he hath dealt bountifully with me." Psalm 13

"In the Lord put I my trust: how say ye to my soul, Flee as a bird to your mountain? [2] For, lo, the wicked bend their bow, they make ready their arrow upon the string, that they may privily shoot at the upright in heart. [3] If the foundations be destroyed, what can the righteous do? [4] The Lord is in his holy temple, the Lord's throne is in heaven: his eyes behold, his eyelids try, the children of men. [5] The Lord trieth the righteous: but the wicked and him that loveth violence his soul hateth. [6] Upon the wicked he shall rain snares, fire and brimstone, and an horrible tempest: this shall be the portion of their cup. [7] For the righteous Lord loveth righteousness; his countenance doth behold the upright." Psalm 11

Ramsis Ghaly

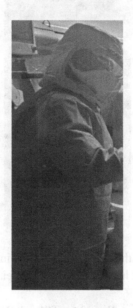

HH. Happy Thanksgiving My Dr. Ramsis Ghaly.!!
CG. I don't believe and can't believe that people believe God is at fault for covid. It's difficult to understand why a country would develop such a bioweapon that would destroy thousands of lives including their own people. 💜🙏
JM. Amen
CP. I remember some of the "Elites" talking about "trimming" the world population in interviews and how this virus has a patent.

Look Beyond the Surface of COVID Pandemic!

Written by Ramsis Ghaly

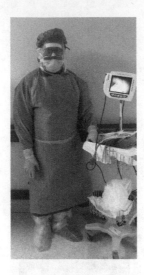

I was called in the middle of the night to assess and intubate a COVID patient and I prayed and my Lord didn't leave me! It was challenging!

Later on my mind fell into deep thoughts of "Look Beyond the Surface of COVID Pandemic"

Who are Behind the scene Beneficiaries of the COVID Pandemic!!

Although there are so much loses from COVID Pandemic not only human lives but also much of tourism and traditional workforce. In fact, the COVID Pandemic is like 9/11 will leave everlasting finger prints and forever will change how we live and earn living! As if all of a sudden a huge stone descended down from out of space upon the shinning predictable world with bright future and put an immediate stop ⬤ and the inhabitants of earth are still in shock and not seeing the entire picture and "Look 👀 Beyond the Surface of COVID Pandemic"

Those highly skilled team of highly intellectual modern evil 🦹 Gangs didn't like the current world power and the way of people living and decided in highly sophisticated and calculable tactic to put a stop ⬤ and immediate change the world to their benefits!!! They took the powers away from those in power and retained to themselves!! It is no longer the power comes from the well-equipped Army or swords or weapons but rather the invisible anti human enemies manufactured by nanotechnology scientists of bioweapons. In the past it was nuclear weapons but currently worked invisible mass destructive overpowering militants!

The COVID PANDEMIC is giving unlimited powers for those behind the smart wireless and digital technology. In fact, the movers and shakers are no longer the White House or kings, or queens, or leaders, or military commanders or selfish human servants but the wild industrial minds hiding in remote placed and operate overseas millions of mikes away unrecognized and unnoticed by the world! It is almost look like a Net of Team Globally well Coordinating secrecy flipping the world upside down to their benefits and believes!

But one of the most serious impact is destabilizing the world powers and redistribute the global beneficiaries!

China 🏴 and Canada 🇨🇦 least affected
China signed agreement with 2 billion people contract
Turkey is moving undercover to take over Armenia and Cyprus
Iran is expanding—
America and Europe are falling
Churches are closing
Computer and digital Industry and technology are taking over the world—-

Digital wireless technology—Computers—Mobile smart phones-Team Microsoft—Zoom—On-line services such as shopping—Amazon —-social Media such as Facebook, LinkedIn, Twitter—search engine such as googles—

Certainly COVID Pandemic is not good for poor low class and even middle class—-

It is like that Net Team formed over internet is looking to control the world and have the absolute power of the future of the world.

It also includes Global warming and out of space industries. Those Net Team is acting as if they are gods of the entire Universe surpassing the True God!!

"The earth is the Lord's, and the fullness thereof; the world, and they that dwell therein. [2] For he hath founded it upon the seas, and established it upon the floods. [3] Who shall ascend into the hill of the Lord? or who shall stand in his holy place?

[4] He that hath clean hands, and a pure heart; who hath not lifted up his soul unto vanity, nor sworn deceitfully. [5] He shall receive the blessing from the Lord, and righteousness from the God of his salvation. [6] This is the generation of them that seek him, that seek thy face, O Jacob. Selah. [7] Lift up your heads, O ye gates; and be ye lift up, ye everlasting doors; and the King of glory shall come in. [8] Who is this King of glory? The Lord strong and mighty, the Lord mighty in battle. [9] Lift up your heads, O ye gates; even lift them up, ye everlasting doors; and the King of glory shall come in. [10] Who is this King of glory? The Lord of hosts, he is the King of glory. Selah." Psalm 24:1-10 KJV

"God be merciful unto us, and bless us; and cause his face to shine upon us; Selah. [2] That thy way may be known upon earth, thy saving health among all nations. [3] Let the people praise thee, O God; let all the people praise thee. [4] O let the nations be glad and sing for joy: for thou shalt judge the people righteously, and govern the nations upon earth. Selah. [5] Let the people praise thee, O God; let all the people praise thee. [6] Then shall the earth yield her increase; and God, even our own God, shall bless us. [7] God shall bless us; and all the ends of the earth shall fear him." Psalm 67:1-7 KJV "Make haste, O God, to deliver me; make haste to help me, O Lord. [2] Let them be ashamed and confounded that seek after my soul: let them be turned backward, and put to confusion, that desire my hurt. [3] Let them be turned back for a reward of their shame that say, Aha, aha. [4] Let all those that seek thee rejoice and be glad in thee: and let such as love thy salvation say continually, Let God be magnified. [5] But I am poor and needy: make haste unto me, O God: thou art my help and my deliverer; O Lord, make no tarrying." Psalm 70:1-5 KJV

Respectfully

IS. You read my mind this morning 😔

SC. I think you speak with understanding.

RH. Love to you

MB. Take care of yourself dear Dr. Ghaly, please! 🙏🙏🙏

KB. Stay safe Dr. Ghaly Have happy Thanksgiving.

CG. Thank you for sharing your look beyond the pandemic. I guess I never thought about it before. What you say makes perfect sense. Thank you for sharing your thoughts once again. 💙🙏

HV, From your mouth to GODS ears!! 🙏 I pray 🖤🖤🖤

SD. Thanks to all of health care worker For your unconditional commitment to all of us. God bless you

VG. Thank you for sharing your thoughts. Speak with understanding. I owe you thanks for this. Beware of dr. Galia god bless you 💚🙏

Two years later no Treatment for COVID 19!!

I just recently have two gentlemen where they had done everything were told to do to prevent and to treat COVID-19 and didn't help or prevent them from getting the worse form of COVID-19, one died yesterday and the other is still in ventilator!!

Putting politics on the side and no sugar coating, the fact is, there is no cure or magic treatment yet for COVID-19!

Science, medicine and artificial intelligence and all the wisdom of man failed to find a cure against COVID 19! The data are shaky, misleading and surrounded with much doubts! The officials are wishy washy and flip flop!

O Science and O man: Are you aware In few months, it will be two years since COVID-19 invaded our planet and targeted the human race in entirely with no exception of racial m, socioeconomic class or demographic variables!

Millions after millions and it keeps going as COVID-19 victims from every corner of the earth are falling down!!

In fact, there is no household that didn't get infected or it's loved ones weren't infected!

And whoever standing strong be in the watch because more variants are in the way! The people are in constant fears and terrors, awaiting their day!!

Where all the science, modern medicine and technology to find a cure?? Finally, man grandiose and science corruption are surfaced and demand is high for immediate structural Reformation!!

What we left with facemask, distancing away and pray to the Lord of hosts to have mercy upon mankind and the world!!!

The people need no lip service and nothing but a cure and transparency! Please be honest and find a cure!!

Ramsis Ghaly

857

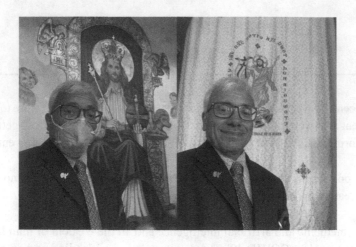

EG. What a summary!
DL. True facts.
AB. Amen

Why Demonstrations and wars do not result in highly expected Hot Spots For COVID-19??

If what we were told is true, we should by now seeing so many hot spots in America across the violent states????

Why wars and frequent huge demonstrations spread COVID-19???

We never heard over two years this far a "hot spot" for COVID during or following wars and demonstrations and crowd???

By now I thought for sure DC and Minneapolis will be hot spots for COVID especially after the huge crowd and weeks of demonstrations?

We know very well that COVID-19 loves people talk, shout and crowd and these what occurs during American demonstrations and general wars????

Ramsis Ghaly

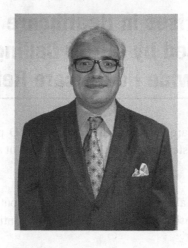

DT. Very interesting and true...... maybe we are being fooled.... maybe? It took you so long to figure it out?

LV. Nice photo!

CP. Very nice picture. ☺

CG. We have been deceived about a lot of things especially covid.

AP. Very nice picture

MH. Nice suite, you take a good picture.

MH. I think Covid 19 was all about population control otherwise we would be seeing a lot more of covid-19 out brakes and we haven't yet?

RW, It's about fear and panic. A universal social experiment

SC. fabulous

SC. We were lied to from day 1! Fear played a great deal, people die every day of different causes, even flu complications. Yes, this virus was different, so it was swine flu...I don't even remember what I was doing that year. "What we resist persists"

VM. Hello genius BFF. You're the best Neurosurgeon. Always be safe.

The Crises in Healthcare is not Caused by COVID Calling for Worldwide Healthcare Reform!!

The Crises in Healthcare isn't caused by the COVID pandemic! It is in the healthcare corporate system itself not only worldwide but also US State level and Federal levels!!

Perhaps if we are honest about it, we can do something about it for the future instead of beating around the bush and confuse the public and continue to cover the truth!!

A lesson each country Worldwide has learned from the ongoing uncontrolled numbers of patients! You must have hospital capacity and resources to accommodate mass causalities!! You shouldn't wait to the last minute! You must have an active and reserve similar to the army ready to take care of all thy people at any given time!!! It shouldn't never have happened! Every country knew it is coming soon, instead, the officials turn their backs against what is imminent!

Now the care of COVID and Non COVID patients are crumbling! The hospitals including in America are dangerous places to be! Not just no enough man power and resources but also no RESERVE and no back up plans in place! Much of the working force not enough personnel to start with, because the hospitals and medical facilities were cutting costs but also the active staff currently are pushed around, fatigued and tired! The environment is chaotic toxic and the system is no longer sustainable! We tried to do a change when doctors and nurses were pushed away! These sound ideas and plans were pushed away because in the business mentality and corporate organizational development, it did not make sense! I wrote much in my books since 2007 and it turn out that Healthcare corporate is full of red tap, bureaucracy and corruption!

The federal and states knew Mass causalities ought to occur at any time, yet the business class and the corporates didn't do other than "cost effective" and "evidence base practice" medicine and narrowed the service to almost nothing close to accommodate few hundreds of patients! In fact, if a city gunshot victims exceeded few, the hospital will go to bypass since each patient may require up to 30 staff to resuscitate and provide the life-saving measures!!

The problem is in each hospital, each city, each state and the entire country at the State level and Federal level!

No one paid attention! No one cared enough to think ahead, no future plans nothing that shall ever make sense of how they were thinking!

Does this ever make sense! Las Vegas has close to million hotel rooms but only three hospitals and less than a thousand beds!! Or big cities such as Chicago and New York have so many high rise buildings and yet have no enough hospital beds for the living patients and their hardworking tax payers' patients!

Thank God we only dealing with one pandemic not even close to the historic flu or plague pandemics!

Have modern civilized highly developed countries never downloaded a simulated computer predictable map for such a catastrophic event as they always do daily to justify future projects! I find it hard to believe!!

Ramsis Ghaly
Www.ghalyneurosurgeon.com

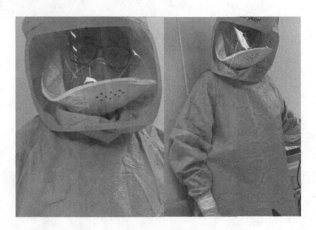

AV. So true! Praying for our country!! 😳🌸🙏🇺🇸
JJ. Truth bomb!!!!! God bless you, Ramsis.
DM. As long as big pharma and insurance company lobbyists have unlimited, uncontrolled access to our elected officials and hospital CEO's- nothing is going to change. It has taken less than a year to put us on a pathway to becoming another 3rd world country. This virus may kill some but just wait as our healthcare continues to crumble.
CG. It is a shame that our country and healthcare system is in a shambles. Praying that someday our country and healthcare will be the quality we all deserve. 🖤🙏

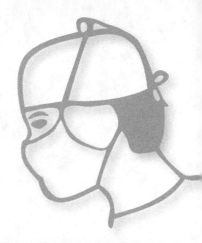

SECTION 17

Spiritual Philosophy

Two Secrets of Life Where Lord Visitation to Earth Full of Holiness and Blessing: Giving Birth to a Newborn and Taking a Faithful Human Soul! Looking Deeper to Theological Aspect!

Written by Ramsis Ghalyl

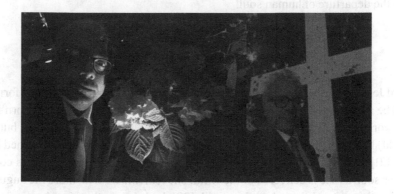

Let me share with you all the two secrets full of mystery, holiness and blessing to those taking part of both!

Indeed the Lord actually remembers His people and descends down to visit the earth and bringing with Him tremendous blessing and grace to all those are taking part of the two heavenly celebration and memorial events!

Standing By And Be part of the Moments of a Mother Giving Birth to Her Newborn and the Departing Soul are the Two Moments are the Most Holy and Full of Blessing

Two Moments, the heavens open to earth with the Lord visit where the most blessed and glorious times: the birth of a newborn and the death!

It is in the daily Spiritual calendar since the creation of mankind after the descend of our parent Adam and Eve and it shall continue until the end of the world!

The two moments where the heavens open to earth and the Divine decision be made and announced! The joy of the heaven of the new born and saved departed human souls are beard all over and shared by many especially those present and taking active part of the two events!

Although externally, the naked human senses may not see what transpired spiritually but indeed it was shielded from their carnal senses as ordered by the Creator! In addition, the spiritual sceneries aren't tolerated by the limited mortal body and its senses!

So O human souls be part of those two heavenly events: the birth of a newborn and the departure of human soul!

1) Moment of Giving Birth to a Newborn

Lord Jesus describe the heavenly joy for each newborn as a new a child is formed and be a celebrated addition to the Lord flock "—for joy that a man is born into the world." "Verily, verily, I say unto you, That ye shall weep and lament, but the world shall rejoice: and ye shall be sorrowful, but your sorrow shall be turned into joy. [21] A woman when she is in travail hath sorrow, because her hour is come: but as soon as she is delivered of the child, she remembereth no more the anguish, for joy that a man is born into the world. [22] And ye now therefore have sorrow: but I will see you again, and your heart shall rejoice, and your joy no man taketh from you." (John 16:20-22 KJV)

On the other hand, a mother carries a newborn and the moment of giving birth, is a glorious and sacred time. So many examples of the feasts and celebrations at the time of giving birth as in our fathers Isaac, Samuel and Samson. The Lord visits the womb and overshadow the conception since a child is born fur His flock. For the birth of Isaac is well described: "And the Lord visited Sarah as he had said, and the Lord did unto Sarah as he had spoken. [2] For Sarah conceived, and bare Abraham a son in his old age, at the set time of which God had spoken to him. [3] And Abraham called the name of his son that was born unto him, whom Sarah bare to him, Isaac." Genesis 21:1-3 KJV

And in Samuel birth, God remember his mom Hannah as it is written: "Then Eli answered and said, Go in peace: and the God of Israel grant thee thy petition that thou hast asked of him. [18] And she said, Let thine handmaid find grace in thy sight. So the woman went her way, and did eat, and her countenance was no more sad. [19] And they rose up in the morning early, and worshipped before the Lord, and returned, and came to their house to Ramah: and Elkanah knew Hannah his wife; and the Lord remembered her. [20] Wherefore it came to pass, when the time was come about after Hannah had conceived, that she bare a son, and called his name Samuel, saying, Because I have asked him of the Lord. [21] And the man Elkanah, and all his house, went up to offer unto the Lord the yearly sacrifice, and his vow." 1 Samuel 1:17-21 KJV

And in Samson birth not only the conception is a glorious time between heaven and earth for a newborn is formed to be a child of God and a new addition to the Lord' flock but also a sacred time and the mother must watch what she puts in from food and drink and protect that development of tgat innocent soul as it is written: "She may not eat of any thing that cometh of the vine, neither let her drink wine or strong drink, nor eat any unclean thing: all that I commanded her let her observe." "And the angel of the Lord appeared unto the woman, and said unto her, Behold now, thou art barren, and bearest not: but thou shalt conceive, and bear a son. [4] Now therefore beware, I pray thee, and drink not wine nor strong drink, and eat not any unclean thing: [5] For, lo, thou shalt conceive, and bear a son; and no razor shall come on his head: for the child shall be a Nazarite unto God from the womb: and he shall begin to deliver Israel out of the hand of the Philistines. [14] She may not eat of any thing that cometh of the vine, neither let her drink wine or strong drink, nor eat any unclean thing: all that I commanded her let her observe. [24] And the woman bare a son, and called his name Samson: and the child grew, and the Lord blessed him. [25] And the Spirit of the Lord began to move him at times in the camp of Dan between Zorah and Eshtaol." Judges 13:3-5,14,24-25 KJV

Perhaps, the best ever celebration and blessing was the birth of the Savior of the world, the heavens and heaven opened their doors and the Son of Bod from heaven was incarnated and born and so the heavenly hosts came down and sang the praises and so are the stars and the entire universe worshipping the New Born. Not only those at that time but the entire world since tbe beginning of ages until the end of ages are so blessed and honored with the birth of the Most Holy Newborn Baby Jesus! As it is well described: "And so it was, that, while they were there, the days were accomplished that she should be delivered. [7] And she brought forth her firstborn son, and wrapped him in swaddling clothes, and laid him in a manger; because there was no room for them in the inn. [9] And, lo, the angel of the Lord came upon them, and the glory of the Lord shone round about them: and they were sore afraid. [10] And the angel said unto them, Fear not: for, behold, I bring you good tidings of great joy, which shall be to all people. [11] For unto you is born this day in the city of David a Saviour, which is Christ the Lord. [12] And this shall be a sign unto you; Ye shall find the babe wrapped in swaddling clothes, lying in a manger. [13] And suddenly there was with the angel a multitude of the heavenly host praising God, and saying, [14] Glory to God in the highest, and on earth peace, good will toward men. [15] And it came to pass, as the angels were gone away from them into heaven, the shepherds said one to another, Let us now go even unto Bethlehem, and see this thing which is come to pass, which the Lord hath made known unto us. [16] And they came with haste, and found Mary, and Joseph, and the babe lying in a manger. [20] And the shepherds returned, glorifying and praising God for all the things that they had heard and seen, as it was told unto them." Luke 2:6-7,9-16,20 KJV

2) Moment of Departure

At the moment of death, the liberating Christian soul joins heaven and the world loses a person. The flesh disintegrates back to dust and the spirit fly up high to where belongs! The moment of death journey dying soul at the Moment of Departure is the Most Holy full of Blessing!

The moment of death is mystery hidden and shielded from the eyes and ears and senses of mankind throughout the generations until the end of the world

It is that time where the Righteousness and darkness present the books and the sum of the person's life journey good and bad and the taker of the spirit according to the Divine Justice to the Paradise or Hades!

Living the final days with the loved ones is blessing since it is the most sacred time where the Holy Spirit with heavenly hosts prepare to descend down and wish to take the Hunan soul away from Satan as long as the account of person's life checked by the Divine Just and Mercy to be in favor with God, the Almighty!

It is indeed a huge Spiritual war between the Righteous Spirit and evil spirits. Although the human naked senses aren't perceiving that war! The Almighty is hidden it away from the world!

Yet the dying person usually begin to sense his and her actual destiny as the very final moments where there is no further return, almost all done, the final check point!

Although externally quiet, but yet spiritually is the most heated moments in the entire life journey of the dying person. It is almost as a spiritual war fighting for whom receiving the newly departed human soul, the heavenly hosts to the paradise or the demons to Hades!

It is the daily spiritual calendar and meeting of spiritual powers since the descend of Adam and Eve to the world condemned with the death sentence!

The only time that the Spiritual war revealed to the naked eyes and ears at the moment of Jesus departure at the Cross as it is written: "And, behold, the veil of the temple was rent in twain from the top to the bottom; and the earth did quake, and the rocks rent; [52] And the graves were opened; and many bodies of the saints which slept arose, [53] And came out of the graves after his resurrection, and went into the holy city, and appeared unto many." Matthew 27:51-53 KJV

Elijah, disciple Elisha, took the spiritual blessing of his master Elijah, through his mantle at the moment of Elijah was taken up by the whirlwind as it is written: "And it came to pass, when they were gone over, that Elijah said unto Elisha, Ask what I shall do for thee, before I be taken away from thee. And Elisha said, I pray thee, let a double portion of thy spirit be upon me. [10] And he said, Thou hast asked a hard thing: nevertheless, if thou see me when I am taken from thee, it shall be so unto thee; but if not, it shall not be so. [11] And it came to pass, as they still went on, and talked, that, behold, there appeared a chariot of fire, and horses of fire, and parted them both asunder; and Elijah went up by a whirlwind into heaven. [12] And Elisha saw it, and he cried, My father, my father, the chariot of Israel, and the horsemen thereof. And he saw him no more: and he took hold of his own clothes, and rent them in two pieces. [13] He took up also the mantle of Elijah that fell from him, and went back, and stood by the bank of Jordan; [14] And he took the mantle of Elijah that fell from him, and smote the waters, and said, Where is the Lord God of Elijah? and when he also had smitten the waters, they parted hither and thither: and Elisha went over." 2 Kings 2:9-14 KJV

The moment of death for God's children is that time where the Heavens open its gate to earth and come down to earth where the previous soul is and takes up to the glory of Jesus the King. A spectacular example is at the time of St Stephen death, he saw the glory of God, and Jesus standing on the right hand of God, and St Stephen said: "Behold, I see the heavens opened, and the Son of man standing on the right hand of God.": "But he, being full of the Holy Ghost, looked up stedfastly into heaven, and saw the glory of God, and Jesus standing on the right hand of God, [56] And said, Behold, I see the heavens opened, and the Son of man standing on the right hand of God. [57] Then they cried out with a loud voice, and stopped their ears, and ran upon him with one accord, [58] And cast him out of the city, and stoned him: and the witnesses laid down their clothes at a young man's feet, whose name was Saul. [59] And they stoned Stephen, calling upon God, and saying, Lord Jesus, receive my spirit. [60] And he kneeled down, and cried with a loud voice, Lord, lay not this sin to their charge. And when he had said this, he fell asleep." Acts 7:55-60 KJV

Rest assure that there is no death to the faithful Christian! Spending the last hours with the loved ones are fruitful with high measure of blessing emanate from the departed soul especially at the time of death

I will tell you a secret, touching the soul of a Christian believer while departing and the spirit is getting separated from the body, you shall receive multitudes of blessing in Jesus Name!

At the moment of death is where the maximal Spiritual visitation come down from heaven to pick up the soul and protect the Christian believer from the evil spirits!

In fact, it is that time the Divine cast out the evil by the blood of Jesus Cross and by justice throughout Satan of that spirit!

This spiritual interaction occurs quietly as all the Lord works yet it is a celebration of heaven that one more person joined the heavenly hosts and becomes the pride of the Bridegroom!

While you are crying and your heart ♥ is grieving, put your Spiritual glasses so that our Savior open your eyes to see the Spiritual victory as archangel Michael is kicking Satan far away from your lived one in Jesus Name!

Our Heavenly Father chose to keep it out of physical sight until His Day of Coming back where all secrets shall be revealed and the physical barriers be melted away!

So rush and touch the departed soul and say Our Heavenly Father's Prayer, you shall receive the person's life blessing and the Spiritual grace at that moment in faith!

Conclusions

Although God is present all the time and the heavenly host descends and ascends all the time since His Holy Conception, these two moments are so special and where the Holy Spirit supervise and guide the entire events and fill the surrounding with His infinite and spectacular blessing grace! Our Lord promised of His kingdom at hand: "And saying, The time is fulfilled, and the kingdom of God is at hand: repent ye, and believe the gospel." Mark 1:15 KJV

With the two events, there are much happening as well exchange between heaven and earth with participations of all parties! A heaven giving birth to a new human soul welcoming and release him or here to grow and be tested on earth and bring him or her back to home as a winner! In both events the heaven is fully participating and the world subdued by Satan is envy of each! A woman given birth to a future child of God and Satan is forever forbidden to be God child! And a saved human soul departed from the world and going unto her seat by the kingdom of God and Satan is!

With the newborn, the heaven welcome a new addition to the Lord army and with death, heaven also welcome a new addition with a faithful Christian soul. Both incidents the Divine hope is more and more of His children get born to fill the heavens and save each soul so that it won't any empty seats and empty mansions in heaven that don't host His people everyone by his and her name! For that reason our Lord Jesus said Satan is falling as lightening from heaven and the names of Hid children are written in His Kingdom: "And he said unto them, I beheld Satan as lightning fall from heaven. [19] Behold, I give unto you power to tread on serpents and scorpions, and over all the power of the enemy: and nothing shall by any means hurt you. [20] Notwithstanding in this rejoice not, that the spirits are subject unto you; but rather rejoice, because your names are written in heaven. [23] And he turned him unto his disciples, and said privately, Blessed are the eyes which see the things that ye see:" Luke 10:18-20,23 KJV

As the heavenly God descended and incarnated and lived with us as a man in the flesh, the cleavage between heaven and earth was removed and the heavenly angels come down and go up all the time between earth and heaven. Jesus the Lord said: "And he saith unto him, Verily, verily, I say unto you, Hereafter ye shall see heaven open, and the angels of God ascending and descending upon the Son of man." John 1:51 KJV

And the moment of Jesus departure, the entire was between earth and heaven was rented and no more in existence: "And, behold, the veil of the temple was rent in twain from the top to the bottom; and the earth did quake, and the rocks rent; [52] And the graves were opened; and many bodies of the saints which slept arose," Matthew 27:51-52 KJV

Giving birth to a Newborn and departure of a human soul are events take place only once in each living soul. As each human soul means so much to our Savior and His purpose is that human soul salvation by all means as it is written: "Either what woman having ten pieces of silver, if she lose one piece, doth not light a candle, and sweep the house, and seek diligently till she find it ? [9] And when she hath found it, she calleth her friends and her neighbours together, saying, Rejoice with me; for I have found the piece which I had lost. [10] Likewise, I say unto you, there is joy in the presence of the angels of God over one sinner that repenteth." Luke 15:8-10 KJV

As our Lord ascended, He opened the gate for 24/7 all year around heavenly visitations as He said: "And he said unto them, Go ye into all the world, and preach the gospel to every creature. [16] He that believeth and is baptized shall be saved; but he that believeth not shall be damned. [17] And these signs shall follow them that believe; In my name shall they cast out devils; they shall speak with new tongues; [18] They shall take up serpents; and if they drink any deadly thing, it shall not hurt them; they shall lay hands on the sick, and they shall recover." Mark 16:15-18 KJV

In both moments of the conception and birth of newborn and the dying human flesh and departure if the soul, gracious is the Lord and holy is His Name and good will to man: "Gracious is the Lord, and righteous; yea, our God is merciful. [6] The Lord preserveth the simple: I was brought low, and he helped me. [7] Return unto thy rest, O my soul; for the Lord hath dealt bountifully with thee. [8] For thou hast delivered my soul from death, mine eyes from tears, and my feet from falling. [9] I will walk before the Lord in the land of the living. [10] I believed, therefore have I spoken: I was greatly afflicted:" Psalm 116:5-10 KJV

Standing by and bd part of the Moments of a Mother Giving Birth to Her Newborn and the Departing Soul are the Two Moments Most Holy and Full of Blessing Two Secrets of Life Where Lord Visitation to Earth Full of Holiness and Blessing: Giving Birth to a Newborn and Taking a Faithful Human Soul! So O human souls be part of those two heavenly events: the birth of a newborn and the departure of human soul!

Both are living wonders full of mystery and holiness and proof of God Love, mercy and grace and both have times of beginning and end: a conception with giving birth to a newborn and a departure of human soul after a life journey on earth! What a remarkable two events externally visible in the surface but their depth are invisible to naked human senses, yet Spirituality revealed in depth manifested in heaven!

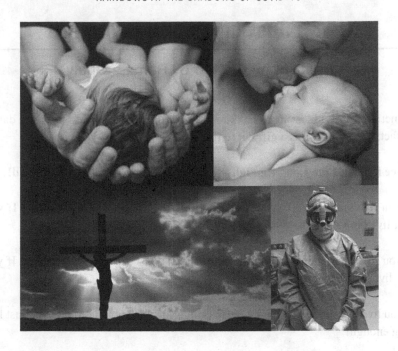

BCD. Very beautiful

AB. Wonderful, Brother!

CG. I truly enjoyed reading this. Both birth and death are described as they are perceived by me. Thank you! 🖤🙏

BL. Thank you for your insightful and enriching writings. I look forward to them. 💜🖤💜

LA. Gloria Gaither expresses precisely what Dr. Ramsis Ghaly

refers to as the two secrets full of mystery, holiness and blessings to those taking part in both! For a moment - just for a moment the door flap between here and eternity opens and the angel dust of eternity gets on you and for a moment life gets real, and you are transformed, and you're never the same again.

JP. My sweet grandson was delivered on Feb 5, only 32 weeks gestation. He was born with a club foot, but other than that, through the power of many prayer warriors, he's perfect and thriving. He's appropriately named Kendric (champion) and Gabriel (God is my strength); indeed He is.

BL. Thank you for your insightful and enriching writings. I look forward to them. 💜🖤💜

JM. AMEN!!

VG. Beautifully described birth and death!

RH. What a wonderful message in order 👍 Amen

873

If You Just Live Long Enough!!!

Philosophy Written by Ramsis Ghaly

Sometimes, it is a blessing to not know! Sometimes, it is good to be in the dark!! In fact, sometimes, it is a gift not to live long enough!

Since if "You Live Long Enough——", you may wish you hadn't, indeed!

If you live long enough, you may see things you wish you hadn't see! If you just live long enough!

If you live long enough, you may hear things you wish you hadn't hear! If you just live long enough!

If you live long enough, you may read things you wish you hadn't! If you just live long enough!

If you live long enough, you may come across things you wish you hadn't! If you just live long enough!

If you live long enough, you may witness things you wish you hadn't witness! If you just live long enough!

If you live long enough, you may do things you wish you hadn't done! If you just live long enough!

If you live long enough, you may fall you wish you didn't! If you just live long enough!

If you live long enough, you may get that senile you wish you hadn't! If you just live long enough!

If you live long enough, you may become so frail you wish you hadn't hear! If you just live long enough!

If you live long enough, you may get so ill you wish you hadn't hear! If you just live long enough!

If you live long enough, you may loose much you wish you hadn't! If you just live long enough!

If you live long enough, you may commit evil things you wish you didn't! If you just live long enough!

If you live long enough, you may reveal things you wish you didn't! If you just live long enough!

If you live long enough, you may figure things you wish you didn't! If you just live long enough!

If you live long enough, you may discover things you wish you didn't! If you just live long enough!

If you live long enough, you may find things you wish you didn't! If you just live long enough!

If you live long enough, you may know things you wish you didn't! If you just live long enough!

If you live long enough, you may stand before the facts you wish you hadn't! If you just live long enough!

If you live long enough, you may come to face the truth you wish you hadn't! If you just live long enough!

If you just live long enough! If you just live long enough! If you just live long enough! Therefore, sometimes, it is a blessing to not know! Sometimes, it is good to be in the dark!! In fact, sometimes, it is a gift not to live long enough!

Therefore give thanks to the Lord in all circumstances: 1 Thessalonians 5:18 ESV "Give thanks in all circumstances; for this is the will of God in Christ Jesus for you"

And whatever you do, work heartily: Colossians 3:23 ESV "Whatever you do, work heartily, as for the Lord and not for men" Remembering: Job 14:1 ESV: "Man who is born of a woman is few of days and full of trouble"

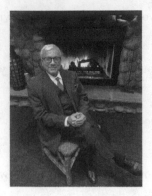

LK. Really wonderful photo!

CG. This is so splendid. I am sure a lot of us have thought "If I just live long enough..." Love the picture! Stay safe. 🖤🙏

RC. Good reflections

MH. What a lovely picture Dr. Ghaly. Very elegant! 🙏

LC. Looking good

BS. Yes, and love the writing! I shared.

GS. Always quite the dashing dapper gentleman! Many blessings brother

CP. Bless you always Dr. G 🙏

HH. Good Morning my Dr..I wish YOU good health a long Live. ! !

SC. very nice picture dr lovin it!

ML. I enjoy reading your beautiful words. They always seem to bring me up when things look down. Thank you for inspiring me to look at life in a different shade. 🙏🖤

CP. Very nice. 😊

FA. Great pic Dr Ghaly, I love seeing your posts every morning 🔽

RH. Very true

DC. Nice picture Dr. Ghaly..Gods Blessings and be safe. 🙏🖤😌

JD. I wish I would have read this a year ago. 🙏🙏🙏

KJ. Unbelievable during these times how compromised we all are. The greatest blessing from God is to be born with Health. Too much for us to comprehend as technology and submissiveness in the Dark ages coming. Never give in or give up. Reasoning and intelligence should never be challenged. Adding the DNA of an Animal is against the principle and laws of Nature. This is dead wrong to be forced into taking inoculations against our will.

CE. The world sure needs a great doctor like you. Stay safe! You look so good, by the way! 💜

MN. Amen Dr. Ghaly stay safe.

EM. Love reading your posts. Great picture!

KE. Precious

TM. Thank you for your post!

Friends This How Days Pass By Quickly!!!

Written by Ramsis Ghaly

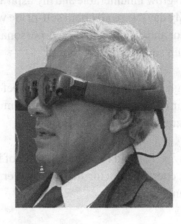

This is my life story!!!

I wanted to start to live but I am afraid it is almost over!

I thought the time is near for me to start living, I never realized it flew so fast!

I asked myself; "Soul when I am going to enjoy life and do what I always wanted to do?" I found myself looking at the mirror! My mouth 👄 whispered it is done and gone!!

I always thought tomorrow shall come, and then I will begin my life but never acknowledged that I might be wrong!

I kept waiting for better tomorrow and I didn't know the old days were the good days for me to live!

There were so much going on and I was much absorbed in facing the daily challenges! And I kept waiting when those would clear up so I could start living!

I found myself entangled in so many projects and jobs pulled in so many directions and the hours of the days were never sufficient! My soul was burdened in all kind of countless commitments. And I kept waiting when those would clear up so I could start living!

My life was a marshal following the military clock 🕰 and my schedule was always overbooked as I was engaged unto everyday countless world businesses! And I kept waiting when those would clear up so I could start living!

My ambition continued to grow innumerable and my aspiration never ceased as my passion never got cold! My days were all about self-pride with over achievements, always grade A with honor and disciplined type A personality! And I kept waiting when those would clear up so I could start living!

Nothing was good enough for me! I let my life slide before me day by day and month by month and year by year expecting more and more are coming with no end! I woke up one day and it was that end already!

Indeed, my days swept by so fast and I reached the end of life unnoticeably! I had that image of me young energetic doctor that will never age and perhaps those passed away wee them and never me!

A surprise arrived as a shock one day, when my eyes opened wide looking at myself in mirror 🪞 saying who am I? What have I done all these years!

I was running 🏃 in a race and that race consumed my entire life and now it is over! I looked age fragile and senility took hold of me! My mind isn't as Sharpe and i can hardly walk! I no longer count in myself! it isn't me any longer! but perhaps it wasn't ever me since I didn't get chance to know me that well! is this the so called "life" of an ambition man meant well!!

My last days are full of regrets and guilts! I wish I could re-live those days again! the clouds are covering my sight and my ears are hardwearing, my apatite is gone and so is my energy! i am a frail man, I must accept and acknowledge my all my failures since I was never serious to come to grip unto the reality of humanity and so called "Facts of Life"! My brain center for desires is shut down and that of ambition is no longer around!

Indeed, what my father Job once said: Job 14:1 ESV "Man who is born of a woman is few of days and full of trouble." And the wisdom of my father Solomon: Ecclesiastes 1:4 ESV "A generation goes, and a generation comes, but the earth remains forever" Ecclesiastes 6:12 ESV "For who knows what is good for man while he lives the few days of his vain life, which he passes like a shadow? For who can tell man what will be after him under the sun."

My life was just a show and vapor disappeared the minute it was started and the blossom of my youth withered away! My name vanished away and all me was buried under the ground!! When the death came to my door, I wasn't ready! I tried to fight it but I lost the fight! In seconds I was gone! No one claimed my body so I was buried with the unknowns of the world ⬤! My already disintegrated flesh was thrown away and mixed with the corps of the neglect! As it is written in James 4:14 KJV "Whereas ye know not what shall be on the morrow. For what is your life? It is even a vapour, that appeareth for a little time, and then vanisheth away." Psalm 144:4 ESV "Man is like a breath; his days are like a passing shadow." 1 Peter 1:24 ESV "For "All flesh is like grass and all its glory like the flower of grass. The grass withers, and the flower falls," Psalm 102:11 ESV "My days are like an evening shadow; I wither away like grass." Psalm 102:3 ESV "For my days pass away like smoke, and my bones burn like a furnace."

If I can just rewind the clock back and bring the pendulum all the way to the beginning of my days, I will have lived each day to its fullest and never counted on tomorrow! Perhaps, I would attend a crash course in reality of life and facts of living so I will never be distant in a remote fantasy of my own!! I would have listened to these biblical words: James 4:13 KJV "Go to now, ye that say, Today or tomorrow we will go into such a city, and continue there a year, and buy and sell, and get gain:" Psalm 90:12 ESV "So teach us to number our days that we may get a heart of wisdom."

Listen to me, my little soul, although my days are almost over, let us then look forward to the life to come after my departure! No more time to waste and don't this final chance slide by!!

O my soul, It is never too late even if I got few minutes to live! Turn thy back in those old days! Learn from the past, stand up and gird thyself and be steadfast! Let thy loin be girded about, and thy light be burning and wait on the Lord! Sell that I have, and give alms; provide myself bags which wax not old, a treasure in the heavens that faileth not, where no thief approacheth, neither moth corrupteth. Wait on the Lord, the second watch, the third watch fear ⌞OBJ⌟ not be ready and Watch!

At the end of life, O soul you only have Jesus your only Savior and loving of mankind that never ever left thy sight even when you were in the dungeon pit. He wasn't seen when you got lost but He was within you carrying you around protecting you from the darkness of the world rescuing your soul. Your Savior words to you tonight in the beginning and at the end and in between: "Fear not, little flock; for it is your Father's good pleasure to give you the kingdom. [33] Sell that ye have, and give alms; provide yourselves bags which wax not old, a treasure in the heavens that faileth not, where no thief approacheth, neither moth corrupteth. [35] Let your loins be girded about, and your lights burning; [36] And ye yourselves like unto men that wait for their lord, when he will return from the wedding; that when he cometh and knocketh, they may open unto him immediately. [37] Blessed are those servants, whom the lord when he cometh shall find watching: verily I say unto you, that he shall gird himself, and make them to sit down to meat, and will come forth and serve them. [38] And if he shall come in the second watch, or come in the third watch, and find them so, blessed are those servants. [40] Be ye therefore ready also: for the Son of man cometh at an hour when ye think not." Luke 12:32-33,35-38,40 KJV

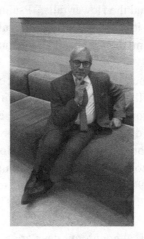

KE. Bless You Ramsis
Loving Prayers
NE. Beautiful!
KG. Be well and be ready 🙏
SA. God bless you Dr. Ghaly 🙏
FA. God bless you Dr Ghaly 🙏
MW. 💜 Beautiful 💜
JP. If I could rewind my life; I would want you as my teacher. Keep speaking the truth Doctor; we need your wisdom.
JB. Sending blessings Dr. Ghaly. Let us remember, it is not only the destination, but what we do with the journey. 💜
CB. May the good Lord bless and keep you Dr. Ghaly.
CM. My Dear Dr. Ghaly you are far from "unnoticeably". You have touched so many. You've helped so many and no doubt that it's all been through your love of and through God. You are truly a gift straight from God. Larry left 12yrs ago Sunday and today is his birthday. You made such a difference in our lives and will always be in my heart. God Bless 🤗

Please Do Not Look Down at My Age!!

Written by Ramsis Ghaly

Please, don't look down at my age!! The days had done so with my form!

Please, don't look down at my wrinkles!! The struggles I went through and triumphed had done so to my body!

Please, don't look down at my skin!! The heat of the sun during the day and that of the moon at night had done so to my flesh!

"Look not upon me, because I am black, because the sun hath looked upon me: my mother's children were angry with me; they made me the keeper of the vineyards; but mine own vineyard have I not kept." Song of Songs 1:6 KJV

Judge not at my appearance but listen to my inner soul; *"I am black, but comely, O ye daughters of Jerusalem, as the tents of Kedar, as the curtains of Solomon."* Song of Songs 1:5 KJV

God look not at the outward appearance but the inward heart 💜 as He said to Samuel when He chose David the least of Jesse's children to be the king of Israel and become the descendent of Jesus: *"But the Lord said unto Samuel, Look not on his countenance, or on the height of his stature; because I have refused him: for the Lord seeth not as man seeth; for man looketh on the outward appearance, but the Lord looketh on the heart."* 1 Samuel 16:7 KJV

Jesus said: *"Judge not according to the appearance, but judge righteous judgment."* John 7:24 KJV

As Paul advice his disciple the young Timothy saying: *"Remember them which have the rule over you, who have spoken unto you the word of God: whose faith follow, considering the end of their conversation. [8] Jesus Christ the same yesterday, and today, and forever."* Hebrews 13:7-8 KJV

Every stage of human life isn't the same!

There are pluses and minuses in everything as there are gains and loses!

There are the pros and cons as there are the good and not so good! !

As a man or a woman ages, the external physic may be limited but the internal heart ♥ is exceptional!

I am advance in age but yet I am walking in my own feet!

Perhaps I am no longer youngster but I am moving around in pride!

I may not be racing or flying but my foundation is well established and my shadow speaks volumes!

I might have that appearance because my wealth is within and my treasurers are countless!

I may not look as sharp but I made it through the tough days and I pulled through against the giant waves before me!

I am quiet and you may think I have no youth within me! But isn't the case but rather youth is in my mind and thoughts!

You may think I am ancient and I may not caught up with what is new and recent! It is rather my way of picking thoroughly beyond the surface of things!

I may not have your energy but certainly I got the wisdom, experience and the mind to analyze the impossible!

Therefore, what a man does during his early years shall bring him to the top in his late years as he had accomplished unprecedented achievements and shall gain unwavering support in his old age!

Therefore, what a woman does during her early years shall bring her to unparalleled achievement and towering intellect to the top in here late years as she had accomplished sterling credentials and shall gain unyielding support in here old age!

At Paul said in his late years: *"I have fought a good fight, I have finished my course, I have kept the faith: [8] Henceforth there is laid up for me a crown of righteousness, which the Lord, the righteous judge, shall give me at that day: and not to me only, but unto all them also that love his appearing."* 2 Timothy 4:7-8 KJV

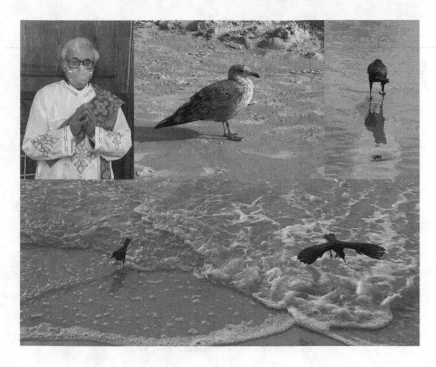

TJ. BEAUTIFUL!

AV. God continue to Bless you Dr. Ghaly!! 🐾🙏

MA. Amen

MN. Amen Dr. Ghaly you have accompanied more than anyone young or old you have a huge heart of Gold you are the best man I know Dr. Ghaly the only man other than you is my father.

CG. This is beautifully written. Many of us can relate to this. Although you dear doctor are like the Energizer bunny. You are young at heart and just keep on going no matter what you are doing. God bless you! 🖤🙏

Minority A Philosophical View

Written by Ramsis Ghaly

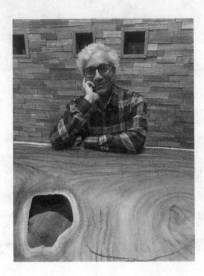

Minority is not only about race or religion although both are most common!

Minority is Standing alone in whatever condition among the majority at a particular place and at a given time!

Minority in rare inherited or acquired situation isn't a choice but most of the time is a choice mostly and it is a part of humanity and globalism!

Minority is not a static situation but it is dynamic and always changing!

In certain condition, minority can be lifetime such as colored race in a no colored majority or a Christian among majority non-Christians, a woman among men majority, a naturalized citizen among born citizen —!

But in many circumstances, minority is temporary at a particular time and region and situation!

For instance I was a minority persecuted Christian in my hometown Egypt 🇪🇬 in the past but now I am in America no longer Christian minority!

For instance, I was a minority foreigner in Neurosurgery when I entered in neurosurgery 1980's but now 30 years later, foreigners are no longer minority!

I continue to be minority as a determined patient advocate and not a corporate advocate hated by the majority admired by few!

I continue to be minority in my belief to save lives regardless of the underlying dire condition and have God to pull the plug and not a man!

I used to be among the majority back in 1970's and 1980's when I committed my life to church and medicine and no life style or much of extracurricular activities, but now I am minority among the majority which is not as committal with much of extracurricular enthusiasm!

Heroism is commonly in Minority and not majority! They are numbered!

Minority is those entering into strait gate and majority is those entering into the wide gate!

Minority is those walking into narrow way and majority is those walking into the broad way!

As our Lord Jesus said: "Enter ye in at the strait gate: for wide is the gate, and broad is the way, that leadeth to destruction, and many there be which go in thereat: [14] Because strait is the gate, and narrow is the way, which leadeth unto life, and few there be that find it." Matthew 7:13-14 KJV

The elect saved human souls that chose Jesus their Savior and followed Him to the end are minority compared to the billions majority didn't follow Jesus and drank from His blood and ate from His bread!

Jesus our Lord said: "For many are called, but few are chosen." Matthew 22:14 KJV

In fact a minority is those not conforming with the majority in the world: "And be not conformed to this world: but be ye transformed by the renewing of your mind, that ye may prove what is that good, and acceptable, and perfect, will of God." Romans 12:2 KJV

Biblical Verses

Matthew 7:14 For the gate is small and the way is narrow that leads to life, and there are few who find it.

Luke 13:23 And someone said to Him, "Lord, are there just a few who are being saved?" And He said to them,

Revelation 3:4 But you have a few people in Sardis who have not soiled their garments; and they will walk with Me in white, for they are worthy.

1 Peter 3:20 who once were disobedient, when the patience of God kept waiting in the days of Noah, during the construction of the ark, in which a few, that is, eight persons, were brought safely through the water.

Mark 6:5 And He could do no miracle there except that He laid His hands on a few sick people and healed them.

Isaiah 24:6 Therefore, a curse devours the earth, and those who live in it are held guilty. Therefore, the inhabitants of the earth are burned, and few men are left.

Matthew 9:37 Then He *said to His disciples, "The harvest is plentiful, but the workers are few.

Daniel 11:23 After an alliance is made with him he will practice deception, and he will go up and gain power with a small force of people.

Proverbs 14:28 In a multitude of people is a king's glory, But in the dearth of people is a prince's ruin.

Numbers 26:54 To the larger group you shall increase their inheritance, and to the smaller group you shall diminish their inheritance; each shall be given their inheritance according to those who were numbered of them.

Numbers 33:54 You shall inherit the land by lot according to your families; to the larger you shall give more inheritance, and to the smaller you shall give less inheritance. Wherever the lot falls to anyone, that shall be his. You shall inherit according to the tribes of your fathers.

Numbers 35:8 As for the cities which you shall give from the possession of the sons of Israel, you shall take more from the larger and you shall take less from the smaller; each shall give some of his cities to the Levites in proportion to his possession which he inherits."

Genesis 34:30 Then Jacob said to Simeon and Levi, "You have brought trouble on me by making me odious among the inhabitants of the land, among the Canaanites and the Perizzites; and my men being few in number, they will gather together against me and attack me and I will be destroyed, I and my household."

1 Kings 20:27 The sons of Israel were mustered and were provisioned and went to meet them; and the sons of Israel camped before them like two little flocks of goats, but the Arameans filled the country.

Deuteronomy 7:7 The Lord did not set His love on you nor choose you because you were more in number than any of the peoples, for you were the fewest of all peoples,

Deuteronomy 26:5 You shall answer and say before the Lord your God, 'My father was a wandering Aramean, and he went down to Egypt and sojourned there, few in number; but there he became a great, mighty and populous nation.

Psalm 105:12 When they were only a few men in number, Very few, and strangers in it.

Ecclesiastes 9:14 There was a small city with few men in it and a great king came to it, surrounded it and constructed large siegeworks against it.

Deuteronomy 4:27 The Lord will scatter you among the peoples, and you will be left few in number among the nations where the Lord drives you.

Deuteronomy 28:62 Then you shall be left few in number, whereas you were as numerous as the stars of heaven, because you did not obey the Lord your God.

Nehemiah 7:4 Now the city was large and spacious, but the people in it were few and the houses were not built.

Jeremiah 42:2 and said to Jeremiah the prophet, "Please let our petition come before you, and pray for us to the Lord your God, that is for all this remnant; because we are left but a few out of many, as your own eyes now see us,

Ezekiel 12:16 But I will spare a few of them from the sword, the famine and the pestilence that they may tell all their abominations among the nations where they go, and may know that I am the Lord."

1 Samuel 14:6 Then Jonathan said to the young man who was carrying his armor, "Come and let us cross over to the garrison of these uncircumcised; perhaps the Lord will work for us, for the Lord is not restrained to save by many or by few."

Jeremiah 44:28 Those who escape the sword will return out of the land of Egypt to the land of Judah few in number. Then all the remnant of Judah who have gone to the land of Egypt to reside there will know whose word will stand, Mine or theirs.

Isaiah 21:17 and the remainder of the number of bowmen, the mighty men of the sons of Kedar, will be few; for the Lord God of Israel has spoken."

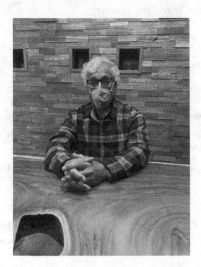

KO. Wow, such a awesome person you are Dr Ghaly.

KJ. Beautiful 💜💜💜 I agree 100% with you. Let God pull the plug.

JM. I love your thinking

CG. There is no doubt about it that you are definitely in the minority. There is no other doctor that I know of who cares about his patients like you do. Another great picture. Bless you 💜🙏

MA. Amen in Jesus name

JF. Beautiful words. I love Dr.

LK. Yes, this doctor is so awesome. I will never forget he called me personally when I was in so much pain on a Friday evening. He is one of a kind.

MG. Thank You Shin M

MH. Wow! Never knew persecuted minority Christian in your own hometown. So glad you're in America now, and using your healing hands to heal others. As the Lord wants you too.

Diversity in life!

Sometimes, someone might wonder if life is fair!

Written by Ramsis Ghaly

One born and one unborn!
One is alive and one is dead!
One is Christian and one is unchristian!
One is saved and one us unsaved!
One is royal and one is lowborn!
One is crowned and one is crownless!
One is privileged and one is unprivileged!
One is fortunate and one is unfortunate!
One is lucky and one is unlucky!
One is of minority and one of majority!
One is colorful and one is colorless!
One is supported and one is unsupported!
One is obedient and one is rebellious!
One is gentle and one is hostile!
One is polite and one impolite!
One is covered and one is naked!
One loses and one wins!
One dies and one lives!
One succeeds and one fails!
One swims and one drowns!
One climbs and one stumbles!
One scores high and one scores low!
One is free and one is captive!
One is agreeable and one is stubborn!
One says yes and one says no!
One is strong and one is weak!
One is fertile and one is infertile!
One is barren and one is productive!
One is impotent and one is potent!
One in love and one in hate!
One is angry and one is meek!
One is tall and one is short!
One is intelligent and one is stupid!

One is straight "A" and one us straight "Z"!
One is above average and one is below average!
One is lucky and one is unlike!
One is healthy and one is sick!
One is skilled and one is unskilled!
One is talented and one is not!
One is gifted and one is ungifted!
One is rich and one is poor!
One is affluent and one is impoverished!
One full and one is hungry!
One is handsome and one is not!
One is pretty and one is not!
One is tall and one is short!
One is fair and one is unfair!
One is colored and one is uncolored!
One is accepted and one is rejected!
One is male and one is female!
One is sad and one is happy!
One is laughing and one is crying!

It is really heartbreaking to live through those extreme diversity and what it appears as unfairness! It was a night of silence and slowly replies started to rain !!

Are you forgetting that the life in the world is temporary and not the life eternity! Do not worry son and not to be in doubt, the life to come shall all be about fairness, wholeness and holiness!

Let us examine the books:

While I was sad and feeling sorrow for many, I heard a voice perhaps the most joyful and least accountable are those ignored by the world and looked down by the people? Have you ever thought about the poor Lazerus is now much happier than the rich? Luke 16:19-31 KJV There was a certain rich man, which was clothed in purple and fine linen, and fared sumptuously every day: [20] And there was a certain beggar named Lazarus, which was laid at his gate, full of sores, [21] And desiring to be fed with the crumbs which fell from the rich man's table: moreover the dogs came and licked his sores. [22] And it came to pass, that the beggar died, and was carried by the angels into Abraham's bosom: the rich man also died, and was buried; [23] And in hell he lift up his eyes, being in torments, and seeth Abraham afar off, and Lazarus in his bosom. [24] And he cried and said, Father Abraham, have mercy on me, and send Lazarus, that he may dip the tip of his finger in water, and cool my tongue; for I am tormented in this flame. [25] But Abraham said, Son, remember that thou in thy lifetime receivedst thy good things, and likewise Lazarus evil things: but now he is comforted, and thou art tormented. [26] And beside all this, between us and you there is a great gulf fixed: so that they which would pass from hence to you cannot; neither can they pass to us, that would come from thence. [27] Then he said, I pray thee therefore, father, that thou wouldest send him to my father's house: [28] For I have five brethren; that he may testify unto them, lest they also come into this place of torment. [29] Abraham saith unto him, They have Moses and the prophets; let them hear them. [30] And he said, Nay, father Abraham: but if one went unto them from the dead, they will repent. [31] And he said unto him, If they hear not Moses and the prophets, neither will they be persuaded, though one rose from the dead."

+Perhaps those born blind and in infirmity are much fortunate than those born with eye sight and limbs yet they are buried in their sins??? Let us read the parable of the Talents:

Matthew 25:14-46 KJV For the kingdom of heaven is as a man travelling into a far country, who called his own servants, and delivered unto them his goods. [15] And unto one he gave five talents, to another two, and to another one; to every man according to his several ability; and straightway took his journey. [16] Then he that had received the five talents went and traded with the same, and made them other five talents. [17] And likewise he that had received two, he also gained other two. [18] But he that had received one went and digged in the earth, and hid his lord's money. [19] After a long time the lord of those servants cometh, and reckoneth with them. [20] And so he that had received five talents came and brought other five talents, saying, Lord, thou deliveredst unto me five talents: behold, I have gained beside them five talents more. [21] His lord said unto him, Well done, thou good and faithful servant: thou hast been faithful over a few things, I will make thee ruler over many things: enter thou into the joy of thy lord. [22] He also that had received two talents came and said, Lord, thou deliveredst unto me two talents: behold, I have gained two other talents beside them. [23] His lord said unto him, Well done, good and faithful servant; thou hast been faithful over a few things, I will make thee ruler over many things: enter thou into the joy of thy lord. [24] Then he which had received the one talent came and said, Lord, I knew thee that thou art an hard man, reaping where thou hast not sown, and gathering where thou hast not strawed: [25] And I was afraid, and went and hid thy talent in the earth: lo, there thou hast that is thine. [26] His lord answered and said unto him, Thou wicked and slothful servant, thou knewest that I reap where I sowed not, and gather where I have not strawed: [27] Thou oughtest therefore to have put my money to the exchangers, and then at my coming I should have received mine own with usury. [28] Take therefore the talent from him, and give it unto him which hath ten talents. [29] For unto every one that hath shall be given, and he shall have abundance: but from him that hath not shall be taken away even that which he hath. [30] And cast ye the unprofitable servant into outer darkness: there shall be weeping and gnashing of teeth. [31] When the Son of man shall come in his glory, and all the holy angels with him, then shall he sit upon the throne of his glory: [32] And before him shall be gathered all nations: and he shall separate them one from another, as a shepherd divideth his sheep from the goats: [33] And he shall set the sheep on his right hand, but the goats on the left. [34] Then shall the King say unto them on his right hand, Come, ye blessed of my Father, inherit the kingdom prepared for you from the foundation of the world: [35] For I was an hungred, and ye gave me meat: I was thirsty, and ye gave me drink: I was a stranger, and ye took me in: [36] Naked, and ye clothed me: I was sick, and ye visited me: I was in prison, and ye came unto me. [37] Then shall the righteous answer him, saying, Lord, when saw we thee an hungred, and fed thee ? or thirsty, and gave thee drink? [38] When saw we thee a stranger, and took thee in? or naked, and clothed thee ? [39] Or when saw we thee sick, or in prison, and came unto thee? [40] And the King shall answer and say unto them, Verily I say unto you, Inasmuch as ye have done it unto one of the least of these my brethren, ye have done it unto me. [41] Then shall he say also unto them on the left hand, Depart from me, ye cursed, into everlasting fire, prepared for the devil and his angels: [42] For I was an hungred, and ye gave me no meat: I was thirsty, and ye gave me no drink: [43] I was a stranger, and ye took me not in: naked, and ye clothed me not: sick, and in prison, and ye visited me not. [44] Then shall they also answer him, saying, Lord, when saw we thee an hungred, or athirst, or a stranger, or naked, or sick, or in prison, and did not minister unto thee? [45] Then shall he answer them, saying, Verily I say unto you, Inasmuch as ye did it not to one of the least of these, ye did it not to me. [46] And these shall go away into everlasting punishment: but the righteous into life eternal.

In my deep thoughts and dilemmas of what is fair and unfair, I was referred to some of the biblical verses: Everyone is according to his gifts and talents:

Romans 12:4-8 For as we have many members in one body, and all members have not the same office: [5] So we, being many, are one body in Christ, and every one members one of another. [6] Having then gifts differing according to the grace that is given to us, whether prophecy, let us prophesy according to the proportion of faith; [7] Or ministry, let us wait on our ministering: or he that teacheth, on teaching; [8] Or he that exhorteth, on exhortation: he that giveth, let him do it with simplicity; he that ruleth, with diligence; he that sheweth mercy, with cheerfulness.

1 Peter 4:10-11 KJV As every man hath received the gift, even so minister the same one to another, as good stewards of the manifold grace of God. [11] If any man speak, let him speak as the oracles of God; if any man minister, let him do it as of the ability which God giveth: that God in all things may be glorified through Jesus Christ, to whom be praise and dominion for ever and ever. Amen.

C- Those with talents will ask more of than those with least talents According to the Deeds:

Romans 2:1-6 Therefore thou art inexcusable, O man, whosoever thou art that judgest: for wherein thou judgest another, thou condemnest thyself; for thou that judgest doest the same things. [2] But we are sure that the judgment of God is according to truth against them which commit such things. [3] And thinkest thou this, O man, that judgest them which do such things, and doest the same, that thou shalt escape the judgment of God? [4] Or despisest thou the riches of his goodness and forbearance and longsuffering; not knowing that the goodness of God leadeth thee to repentance? [5] But after thy hardness and impenitent heart treasurest up unto thyself wrath against the day of wrath and revelation of the righteous judgment of God; [6] Who will render to every man according to his deeds:

Biblical verses according to gifts:

2 Corinthians 9:15 Thanks be to God for His indescribable gift!

1 Peter 4:10 As each one has received a special gift, employ it in serving one another as good stewards of the manifold grace of God.

Romans 11:29 for the gifts and the calling of God are irrevocable.

Romans 12:6 Since we have gifts that differ according to the grace given to us, each of us is to exercise them accordingly: if prophecy, according to the proportion of his faith;

1 Corinthians 12:4 Now there are varieties of gifts, but the same Spirit.

Ephesians 2:8 For by grace you have been saved through faith; and that not of yourselves, it is the gift of God

2 Timothy 1:6 For this reason I remind you to kindle afresh the gift of God which is in you through the laying on of my hands.

Ephesians 4:7 But to each one of us grace was given according to the measure of Christ's gift.

1 Corinthians 12:7 But to each one is given the manifestation of the Spirit for the common good.

Romans 6:23 For the wages of sin is death, but the free gift of God is eternal life in Christ Jesus our Lord.

James 1:17 Every good thing given and every perfect gift is from above, coming down from the Father of lights, with whom there is no variation or shifting shadow.

1 Timothy 4:14 Do not neglect the spiritual gift within you, which was bestowed on you through prophetic utterance with the laying on of hands by the presbytery.

John 4:10 Jesus answered and said to her, "If you knew the gift of God, and who it is who says to you, 'Give Me a drink,' you would have asked Him, and He would have given you living water."

1 Peter 4:11 Whoever speaks, is to do so as one who is speaking the utterances of God; whoever serves is to do so as one who is serving by the strength which God supplies; so that in all things God may be glorified through Jesus Christ, to whom belongs the glory and dominion forever and ever. Amen.

1 Corinthians 12:28 And God has appointed in the church, first apostles, second prophets, third teachers, then miracles, then gifts of healings, helps, administrations, various kinds of tongues.

Ephesians 3:7 of which I was made a minister, according to the gift of God's grace which was given to me according to the working of His power.

Ecclesiastes 5:19 Furthermore, as for every man to whom God has given riches and wealth, He has also empowered him to eat from them and to receive his reward and rejoice in his labor; this is the gift of God.

Psalm 127:3 Behold, children are a gift of the Lord,
The fruit of the womb is a reward.

1 Corinthians 12:31 But earnestly desire the greater gifts. And I show you a still more excellent way.

2 Timothy 1:7 For God has not given us a spirit of timidity, but of power and love and discipline.

Ephesians 4:8 Therefore it says,
"When He ascended on high,
He led captive a host of captives,
And He gave gifts to men."

1 Corinthians 7:7 Yet I wish that all men were even as I myself am. However, each man has his own gift from God, one in this manner, and another in that.

Biblical verses According to the deeds

Matthew 16:27 For the Son of Man is going to come in the glory of His Father with His angels, and will then repay every man according to his deeds.

Jeremiah 17:10 I, the Lord, search the heart, I test the mind, Even to give to each man according to his ways, According to the results of his deeds.

Lamentations 3:64 You will recompense them, O Lord, According to the work of their hands.

Proverbs 24:12 If you say, "See, we did not know this," Does He not consider it who weighs the hearts?
And does He not know it who keeps your soul?
And will He not render to man according to his work?

Romans 2:6 who will render to each person according to his deeds:

Revelation 22:12 "Behold, I am coming quickly, and My reward is with Me, to render to every man according to what he has done.

Jeremiah 25:14 For many nations and great kings will make slaves of them, even them; and I will recompense them according to their deeds and according to the work of their hands.)'"

Jeremiah 32:19 great in counsel and mighty in deed, whose eyes are open to all the ways of the sons of men, giving to everyone according to his ways and according to the fruit of his deeds;

Job 34:11 For He pays a man according to his work And makes him find it according to his way.

2 Corinthians 5:10 For we must all appear before the judgment seat of Christ, so that each one may be recompensed for his deeds in the body, according to what he has done, whether good or bad.

Isaiah 3:10 Say to the righteous that it will go well with them, For they will eat the fruit of their actions.

Jeremiah 21:14 But I will punish you according to the results of your deeds," declares the Lord,
"And I will kindle a fire in its forest
That it may devour all its environs."'"

Ezekiel 24:14 I, the Lord, have spoken; it is coming and I will act. I will not relent, and I will not pity and I will not be sorry; according to your ways and according to your deeds I will judge you," declares the Lord God.'"

Ezekiel 36:19 Also I scattered them among the nations and they were dispersed throughout the lands. According to their ways and their deeds I judged them.

Ezekiel 33:20 Yet you say, 'The way of the Lord is not right.' O house of Israel, I will judge each of you according to his ways."

Hosea 12:2 The Lord also has a dispute with Judah,
And will punish Jacob according to his ways;
He will repay him according to his deeds.

Micah 7:13 And the earth will become desolate because of her inhabitants, On account of the fruit of their deeds.

Zechariah 1:6 But did not My words and My statutes, which I commanded My servants the prophets, overtake your fathers? Then they repented and said, 'As the Lord of hosts purposed to do to us in accordance with our ways and our deeds, so He has dealt with us.'"'"

John 5:29 and will come forth; those who did the good deeds to a resurrection of life, those who committed the evil deeds to a resurrection of judgment.

1 Corinthians 3:8 Now he who plants and he who waters are one; but each will receive his own reward according to his own labor.

2 Corinthians 11:15 Therefore it is not surprising if his servants also disguise themselves as servants of righteousness, whose end will be according to their deeds.

2 Timothy 4:14 Alexander the coppersmith did me much harm; the Lord will repay him according to his deeds.

Hebrews 6:10 For God is not unjust so as to forget your work and the love which you have shown toward His name, in having ministered and in still ministering to the saints.

1 Peter 1:17 If you address as Father the One who impartially judges according to each one's work, conduct yourselves in fear during the time of your stay on earth;

Revelation 2:23 And I will kill her children with pestilence, and all the churches will know that I am He who searches the minds and hearts; and I will give to each one of you according to your deeds.

Revelation 20:12 And I saw the dead, the great and the small, standing before the throne, and books were opened; and another book was opened, which is the book of life; and the dead were judged from the things which were written in the books, according to their deeds.

Revelation 20:13 And the sea gave up the dead which were in it, and death and Hades gave up the dead which were in them; and they were judged, every one of them according to their deeds.

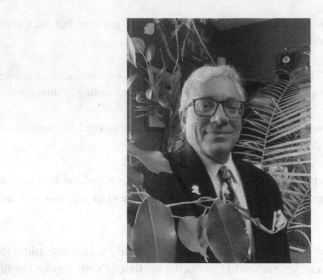

JM. Wow Thank You Dr. Ghaly 💕 Quite a Read.........beautiful

CG. Your writings are beautiful. I always look forward to reading them. Bless you! 🖤🙏

JH. Excellent picture a meaning in each sentence of expression

Quality Before Quantity

Written Ramsis Ghaly

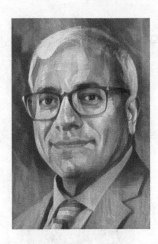

What is good to have Health insurance for everyone and having no quality healthcare but corporate books!

What is good to have a very good health insurance and yet having no quality healthcare system!

What is good to have very good health insurance and yet having no quality doctors, surgeons and nurses!

What is good to have the best healthcare insurance but the laborites are with no autonomy, limited experience and skill, restrained, constrained and pushed around and fatigued!!

Healthcare is in crises! It is becoming more and more a computerized medical cook book and many of the good medical care providers are running away, quieting and retiring! My heart is aching from keep losing my very good friends of physicians, surgeons and nurses!!

In the meantime, litigations, trial attorney and malpractice going after doctors and staff is sky rocketing while the hospital system and healthcare industry is getting restrictive, punitive and less rewarding!

What is so sad many of doctors and nurses leaving their jobs, talents and skills are going in less stressful jobs working from homes, working through computers, —- any job distancing themselves far away from stress, liabilities and punitive systems!

Ramsis Ghaly
www.ghalyneurosurgeon.com

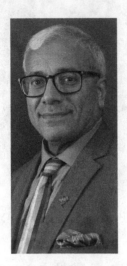

AV. Praying that our Heavenly Father will continue to watch over you & keep u safe! 💝🧎😊
HH. My Dream Friend of America,. I WISH YOU GOOD HEALTH AND A LONG LIVE! !
MS. Good portrait 😊🌷
CG. It is sad that today's doctors can't just be doctors they also have to know the correct coding for procedures. It is very stressful for the doctors I know. Especially for their patients that are medicare. I often wondered when the insurance companies took over medicine. 🙏
AA/ Handsome Dude!
AB. Thank you, Brother!
KE. Gallant Brilliant Doctor*

"Quality Builds Team And That Team Enforces Quality"

Written by Ramsis Ghaly

Quality Builds Team and Team Builds quality!

It is factual and true! Quality first! Who stay with you and not fall off is your team who will embrace core values and your vision!

Some Corporates of America believes: "Building a Team First and then "Quality" Comes Second"!!

I believe the Opposite: "Building Quality First and Subsequently Team Comes by itself"

I care so much about Quality, Dedication and Pure Commitment and everything else follows!!!

Life has taught us if you care about the deep of things and not the surface of things! Build on solid grounds and the rains won't blew what established of quality and team!

Jesus our Lord pointed to us his important is the depth and the heart of things: Matthew 15:17-20 KJV 17] Do not ye yet understand, that whatsoever entereth in at the mouth goeth into the belly, and is cast out into the draught? [18] But those things which proceed out of the mouth come forth from the heart; and they defile the man. [19] For out of the heart proceed evil thoughts, murders, adulteries, fornications, thefts, false witness, blasphemies: [20] These are the things which defile a man: but to eat with unwashen hands defileth not a man."

And also said: Matthew 7:24-27 KJV 24] Therefore whosoever heareth these sayings of mine, and doeth them, I will liken him unto a wise man, which built his house upon a rock: [25] And the rain descended, and the floods came, and the winds blew, and beat upon that house; and it fell not: for it was founded upon a rock. [26] And every one that heareth these sayings of mine, and doeth them not, shall be likened unto a foolish man, which built his house upon the sand: [27] And the rain descended, and the floods came, and the winds blew, and beat upon that house; and it fell: and great was the fall of it."

Therefore, "Quality Builds Team And That Team Enforces Quality"

Ramsis Ghaly

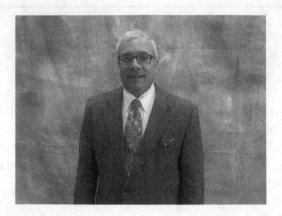

CG. I agree with you 100%
SP. Well said ♥
KP. Great message
CP. Very nice picture. ☺
KP. Great message
DK. Thank you, doctor!
RC. Quality is very important because is the truth of everything.

Reforming Modern Definition of Corporate Professionalism!

Written by Ramsis Ghaly

How much I pray to reform the ongoing understanding of "Corporate Professionalism" to be equal to the traditional old time "Professionalism" and return to the original form of "Professionalism" as my parents and forefathers understood it!!

Professionalism is NOT:

The pass to make more money 💰 and quick cash! Be smarter by making more while working less!

Professionalism is judged not base in quality, dedication and full commitment but rather Life style, work shifts, and extracurricular activities!

After Emotional satisfaction!
Empty words that are lacking Substance!
Trading Ethics, values and morals for cheating and earning the team!
Untruth, unreal and fake and never be upfront!
Preoccupied to make up stories and dinged and nothing but lies and be smart!
Cover up and be in hide and work under the table and never be known!
Unrevealing much and not straightforward!
Numbing the facts and ignoring the roots!
Busy in the surface and patching the core!
Priority is to be nice, team player and go along with peers in the cost of defending the truth!
Eager to not rock the boat and go along with mainstream and never stand alone!
Not after permanent cure but quick fix and temporary solutions!
Staying away from the narrow gate and run far from the straight gate!
Being liked is essential but not Skills, Talents and experiences!

Manipulation is the name of the game! No need to sweat 😓 just climb in the shoulders of others and enter into the others' labors!

Take advantage of the hard laborers and be opportunistic!!
Lip service rather than doer of good!

Laziness and do the least always taking the easy way out!
Do not believe in the Extra mile spirit to help out and reach out!
Miles away from Sacrifice!
Playing smart yet Fools and laughable!

Make clean the outside of the cup and the platter; but your inward part is full of ravening and wickedness!

Ye tithe mint and rue and all manner of herbs, and pass over judgment and the love love

Ye love the uppermost seats in the synagogues, and greetings in the markets.

Ye are as graves which appear not, and the men that walk over them are not aware of them.

Ye lade men with burdens grievous to be borne, and ye yourselves touch not the burdens with one of your fingers! Luke 11:39-44,46-50 KJV

Our Master also said!

"Enter ye in at the strait gate: for wide is the gate, and broad is the way, that leadeth to destruction, and many there be which go in thereat: [14] Because strait is the gate, and narrow is the way, which leadeth unto life, and few there be that find it. [15] Beware of false prophets, which come to you in sheep's clothing, but inwardly they are ravening wolves. [16] Ye shall know them by their fruits. Do men gather grapes of thorns, or figs of thistles? [17] Even so every good tree bringeth forth good fruit; but a corrupt tree bringeth forth evil fruit. [18] A good tree cannot bring forth evil fruit, neither can a corrupt tree bring forth good fruit. [19] Every tree that bringeth not forth good fruit is hewn down, and cast into the fire. [20] Wherefore by their fruits ye shall know them. [21] Not every one that saith unto me, Lord, Lord, shall enter into the kingdom of heaven; but he that doeth the will of my Father which is in heaven. [22] Many will say to me in that day, Lord, Lord, have we not prophesied in thy name? and in thy name have cast out devils? and in thy name done many wonderful works? [23] And then will I profess unto them, I never knew you: depart from me, ye that work iniquity. [24] Therefore whosoever heareth these sayings of mine, and doeth them, I will liken him unto a wise man, which built his house upon a rock:" Matthew 7:13-24 KJV

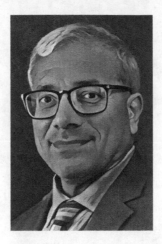

KG. Your words ever so wise, resonate with all. Thank you so much for these words of yours that lift my spirit in the darkest of times. Thank God for you! Were that the world a better place. A place where the hearts were pure. Thank God for you, Dr Ghaly. God Bless you! Blessings from Egypt

MW. Beautiful photo

BCD. I like the picture

CG. You truly are a professional in the true sense of the word. You care about your appearance, you're reliable and you have ethics. You are a blessing to us all. Great photo! 🖤🙏

GS. Many blessings brother

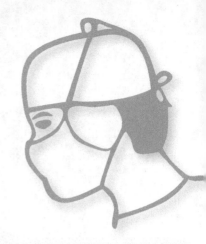

SECTION 18

Political Events During COVID Decline

Where was the Wise? Where was the Scribe? Where was the Disputer of this world?

Written by Ramsis Ghaly

TWO decisions if both have been taken, they would have changed the entire course and prevented much of harm! If there was enough pure Love, humility and egoless!

1) **A declaration of postponing all kind of USA elections for a year once the COVID virus Pandemic is controlled. Not only for safety of American people to avoid spread of virus but also to concentrate the effort to combat imminent lethal threat! While leaving the elections to go through when the American people under no more threat of virus and restrictions with uplifting spirit!**

2) **President Donald Trump instead of keep fighting the repeated battles and lately asking his supporters to defend his policies, he should have stepped back and even resign! There isn't any reason for 70 years old man to keep fighting the impossible and neither healthy nor productive for US Capitol under so much divisions! And he could return should the Capitol politics change and the American people want him!**

Indeed, where was the Wise? Where was the Scribe? Where was the Disputer of this world? Bible said about the foolishness and weakness of man: "For it is written, I will destroy the wisdom of the wise, and will bring to nothing the understanding of the prudent. [20] Where is the wise? where is the scribe? where is the disputer of this world? hath not God made foolish the wisdom of this world? [21] For after that in the wisdom of God the world by wisdom knew not God, it pleased God by the foolishness of preaching to save them that believe. [25] Because the foolishness of God is wiser than men; and the weakness of God is stronger than men. [26] For ye see your calling, brethren, how that not many wise men after the flesh, not many mighty, not many noble, are called: [27] But God hath chosen the foolish things of the world to confound the wise; and God hath chosen the weak things of the world to confound the things which are mighty; [28] And base things of the world, and things which are despised, hath God chosen, yea, and things which are not, to bring to nought things that are: [29] That no flesh should glory in his presence. [30] But of him are ye in Christ Jesus, who of God is made unto us wisdom, and righteousness, and sanctification, and redemption:

[31] That, according as it is written, He that glorieth, let him glory in the Lord." 1 Corinthians 1:19-21,25-31 KJV

To us wisdom, and righteousness, and sanctification, and redemption: [31] That, according as it is written, He that glorieth, let him glory in the Lord." 1 Corinthians 1:19-21,25-31 KJV

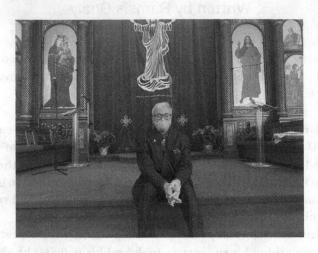

AC. Just need to believe ... Life is beautiful 🙈

MG. I think it was gods will that removed Trump from office right now... I know I have prayed for it for four years

BCD. President Trump knew many of the men/women in congress were doing illegal things. His tactics were used to get them to show their true agenda.

All evidence from all sources is in and the Deep State is going Down quickly. We will see all of it as it unfolds. The UGLY TRUTH OF IT ALL. It might take a few weeks for all information to be given to us citizens and the world. God is Good, we are Blessed to see a new world and peace coming for all of us.

ED Amen Amen Amen

Voting During COVID Unfolding

America 🇺🇸 Let us Pray for God Annointee!
Let us Pray for Peace!
Written by Ramsis Ghaly 11/7/2020

"And there was much murmuring among the people concerning him: for some said, He is a good man: others said, Nay; but he deceiveth the people." John 7:12 KJV 🙏

"And the Lord said unto Samuel, Hearken unto the voice of the people in all that they say unto thee: for they have not rejected thee, but they have rejected me, that I should not reign over them." 1 Samuel 8:7 KJV

"Judge not according to the appearance, but judge righteous judgment." John 7:24 KJV

Lord Jesus Elect for America 🇺🇸 Your Anointed! Let us Pray for Peace!

"The Lord shall fight for you, and ye shall hold your peace." Exodus 14:14 KJV

Our father Moses says: "And Moses said unto the people, Fear ye not, stand still, and see the salvation of the Lord, which he will shew to you today: for the Egyptians whom ye have seen today, ye shall see them again no more forever." Exodus 14:13 KJV

America 🇺🇸, Let us lift our heart 💙 to the Lord to elect a President to lead His people and our Beloved country America!

America 🇺🇸, Let us rise early Sunday morning to pray to our Savior to nominate the president of our nation in His Name!

America 🇺🇸, Let us look up high calling His Name lifting our arms and hands up to heaven appealing to the Most High to intervene for His Name sake!

America 🇺🇸, Let us pray in faith, love and humility to Lord God of our land and ask Him to announce the chosen Shephard for our land!

911

America 🇺🇸, Let us subdue to the results and pray it won't be our choice king Saul but His choice king David!

America 🇺🇸, Let us pray for Peace! Our Lord Jesus says: "Peace I leave with you, my peace I give unto you: not as the world giveth, give I unto you. Let not your heart be troubled, neither let it be afraid." John 14:27 KJV

Since God look deep in the heart as He said when He chose king David: "But the Lord said unto Samuel, Look not on his countenance, or on the height of his stature; because I have refused him: for the Lord seeth not as man seeth; for man looketh on the outward appearance, but the Lord looketh on the heart." 1 Samuel 16:7 KJV

"As ye have therefore received Christ Jesus the Lord, so walk ye in him: [7] Rooted and built up in him, and stablished in the faith, as ye have been taught, abounding therein with thanksgiving. [8] Beware lest any man spoil you through philosophy and vain deceit, after the tradition of men, after the rudiments of the world, and not after Christ. [9] For in him dwelleth all the fulness of the Godhead bodily. [10] And ye are complete in him, which is the head of all principality and power:" Colossians 2:6-10 KJV Amen

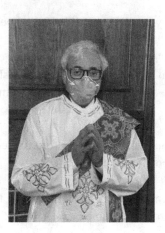

MA. Amen
HD. Amen
AK. Amen!
AM. Amém... Deus conosco sempre...
MM. Amen
CG. Bless us and give us wisdom to be able tp accept the outcome of the election. Amen! 🖤🙏

MA. Amen

BCD. Thank you for these prayers. I'm sharing this.

Today I Went to Vote for My Lord Jesus!

Today early morning I put on my Deacon cloth and went to meet whom my soul love 💜 most!

Today I went to the church of my Lord Jesus and cast my Vote 🗳 to my Savior!

Today I went to cast my voting ballot. I voted for One and only One Jesus. I elected One and only one my Savior Jesus Christ!

Today I Voted 🗳 for my Beloved who had loved 💜 me from the time I was formed in the womb of my mother and to all the way to the end of ages and never changed once, Jesus Christ who gave His life for me and many, Jesus who shed His blood for me, and many, the Son of God who was crucified for me and many, Jesus who give His Holy Body and Blood to me and many, Christ who died for me and many, who rescued my soul and many from eternal damnation, my Redeemer who granted me and many life eternity, my King who open His kingdom to me and many, my Light who brighten my soul and illuminate my darkness, my Bread, my Way, my Truth, my Salvation, my God and Good Samaritan Who covered my nakedness, soaked my wounds and put me at the Inn and visited me soul, my Savior, my Lord and God, my Heavenly Father, my Creator who formed me out of nothing, my Father who forgive my sins and give me free Amnesty, my Good Father who made me His son and granted me citizenship and build me a mansion in His kingdom, my Bridegroom who accepted me the way I am and never once was ashamed of me, my Lord who let me sit in his table and dine with me, my Savior who knocks in my door and bring me the good news and enter in my heart, my Beloved who kiss me with kisses the Rose of Sharon, the Great Pearl, the only Silver Coin I have, my Shield in the wars, my Refuge, my Rock, my Love, the Morning Star, the Living Fountain, the Spring of Waters, the living Tree, my Healer who raise me up from death even after four days, my Father who reach out to me all the time and the time in need and who I reach out all the time with no prior screening or appointments, my Lord who picked me up from my infirmity and broken bones and made me walk again, my Almighty who is full of mercy and grace, my God who wipe my tears and comfort my soul and ease my sorrows, my God who bring me joy and happiness, my Beloved who give me His richness and holiness, my Master who is fair and just forever, my Teacher who teaches me and many one to One, my physician who heals me and many for free, my Ruler who never tax me or take anything from me or in return, my Good Shepherd who made an existence for my soul and my people out of no existence, God the Lord who came down and degraded from His glory to live with me and take me up high with Him—This who I voted for the Lord of hosts and The King of Glory, Amen ⚞

Today I Voted 🗳 for my Beloved who had loved 💜 me from the time I was formed in the womb of my mother and to all the way to the end of ages and never changed once, Jesus Christ who gave His life for me and many, Jesus who shed His blood for me, and many, the Son of God who was crucified for me and many, Jesus who give His Holy Body and Blood to me and many, Christ who died for me and many, who rescued my soul and many from eternal damnation, my Redeemer who granted me and many life eternity, my King who open His kingdom to me and many, my Light who brighten my soul and illuminate my darkness, my Bread, my Way, my Truth, my Salvation, my God and Good Samaritan Who covered my nakedness, soaked my wounds and put me at the Inn and visited me soul, my Savior, my Lord and God, my Heavenly Father, my Creator who formed me out of nothing, my Father who forgive my sins and give me free Amnesty, my Good Father who made me His son and granted me citizenship and build me a mansion in His kingdom, the Son of God who is eternal never dies and the first fruit who conquer death, my Bridegroom who accepted me the way I am and never once was ashamed of me, my Lord who let me sit in his table and dine with me, my Savior who knocks in my door and bring me the good news and enter in my heart, my Beloved who kiss me with kisses the Rose of Sharon, the Great Pearl, the only Silver Coin I have, my Shield in the wars, my Refuge, my Rock, my Love, the Morning Star, the Living Fountain, the Spring of Waters, the living Tree, my Healer who raise me up from death even after four days, my Fortress, my Deliverer, my Father who reach out to me all the time and the time in need and who I reach out all the time with no prior screening or appointments, my Lord who picked me up from my infirmity and broken bones and made me walk again, my Almighty who is full of mercy and grace, my God who wipe my tears and comfort my soul and ease my sorrows, my God who bring me joy and happiness, my Beloved who give me His richness and holiness, my Master who is fair and just forever, my Teacher who teaches me and many one to One, my physician who heals me and many for free, my Ruler who never tax me or take anything from me or in return, my Good Shepherd who made an existence for my soul and my people out of no existence, God the Lord who came down and degraded from His glory to live with me and take me up high with Him—This who I voted for the Lord of hosts and The King of Glory, Amen ⚞

"The earth is the Lord's, and the fulness thereof; the world, and they that dwell therein. [2] For he hath founded it upon the seas, and established it upon the

floods. [3] Who shall ascend into the hill of the Lord ? or who shall stand in his holy place? [4] He that hath clean hands, and a pure heart; who hath not lifted up his soul unto vanity, nor sworn deceitfully. [5] He shall receive the blessing from the Lord, and righteousness from the God of his salvation. [6] This is the generation of them that seek him, that seek thy face, O Jacob. Selah. [7] Lift up your heads, O ye gates; and be ye lift up, ye everlasting doors; and the King of glory shall come in. [8] Who is this King of glory? The Lord strong and mighty, the Lord mighty in battle. [9] Lift up your heads, O ye gates; even lift them up, ye everlasting doors; and the King of glory shall come in. [10] Who is this King of glory? The Lord of hosts, he is the King of glory. Selah." Psalm 24:1-10 KJV

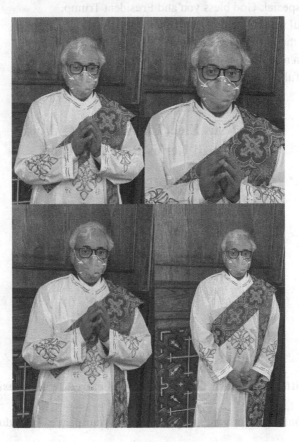

TM/. Thank you Dr. Ghally 🙏

HB. Thanks Dr Ghaly

FA God bless you Doctor

MA. God bless Dr

SS. Gloria a Dio a suo figlio Gesù e allo Spirito Santo ...speriamo che Dio ci protegge tutti noi e ci salva di tutti malvagi Amen nei secoli

MY. يباركك الرب ويحرسك مع محبهَ رب المجد يسوع المسيح ابن الله اللحى آمين ثم آمين يارب
JC. العالمين God bless you Dr Ghaly 💜💜

MA. Amen alleluia the power of God

MP. Absolutely love the sentiment, cast your vote for Jesus. I participate in elections for politicians but I already have a King. Rock on

KB. Amen

SL. Amen, God Bless You

AF. تعيش وتصلى د. رمسيس الشماس والخادم الأمين الرب يبارك حياتك ويفرح قلبك دايما .

AB. Amen !!

MH. I pray for our safety & good health for all.

EH. That is special. God bless you and President Trump.

CG. Beautiful words from a beautiful mind. Bless you! 🖤🙏

MN. i know the Lord will be with you forever Dr.Ghaly Amen

JJ. We need a real Pope, not the false profit we have now.

JD. Wonderful

Lord Jesus Elect for America 🇺🇸 Your Anointed! Let us Pray for Peace!

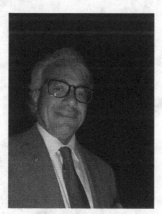

Written by Ramsis Ghaly 11/1/2020 before Election results

"The Lord shall fight for you, and ye shall hold your peace: " Exodus 14:14 KJV

Our father Moses says: "And Moses said unto the people, Fear ye not, stand still, and see the salvation of the Lord, which he will shew to you today: for the Egyptians whom ye have seen today, ye shall see them again no more forever." Exodus 14:13 KJV

America 🏴, Let us lift our heart 💜 to the Lord to elect a President to lead His people and our Beloved country America!

America 🏴, Let us rise early Sunday morning to pray to our Savior to nominate the president of our nation in His Name!

America 🏴, Let us look up high calling His Name lifting our arms and hands up to heaven appealing to the Most High to intervene for His Name sake!

America 🏴, Let us pray in faith, love and humility to Lord God of our land and ask Him to announce the chosen Shephard for our land!

America 🏴, Let us subdue to the results and pray it won't be our choice king Saul but His choice king David!

America 🏴, Let us pray for Peace! Our Lord Jesus says: "Peace I leave with you, my peace I give unto you: not as the world giveth, give I unto you. Let not your heart be troubled, neither let it be afraid." John 14:27 KJV

Since God look deep in the heart as He said when He chose king David: "But the Lord said unto Samuel, Look not on his countenance, or on the height of his stature; because I have refused him: for the Lord seeth not as man seeth; for man looketh on the outward appearance, but the Lord looketh on the heart." 1 Samuel 16:7 KJV

America 🏴, Who will be the president the chosen Vessel unto Lord Jesus?? "The Lord said to the president elect: "But the Lord said unto him, Go thy way: for he is a chosen vessel unto me, to bear my name before the Gentiles, and kings, and the children of Israel: [16] For I will shew him how great things he must suffer for my name's sake." Acts 9:15-16 KJV

And for the President elect saint Paul says: "I charge you in the presence of God, who gives life to all things, and of Christ Jesus, who in his testimony before Pontius Pilate made the good confession, to keep the commandment unstained and free from reproach until the appearing of our Lord Jesus Christ, which he will display at the proper time—he who is the blessed and only Sovereign, the King of kings and Lord of lords, who alone has immortality, who dwells in unapproachable light, whom no one has ever seen or can see. To him be honor and eternal dominion. Amen." (1 Timothy 6:15, ESV)

2 Thessalonians 2:13 "But we should always give thanks to God for you, brethren beloved by the Lord, because God has chosen you from the beginning for salvation through sanctification by the Spirit and faith in the truth."

Psalm 20
The Lord hear thee in the day of trouble; the name of the God of Jacob defend thee; [2] Send thee help from the sanctuary, and strengthen thee out of Zion; [3] Remember all thy offerings, and accept thy burnt sacrifice; Selah. [4] Grant thee according to thine own heart, and fulfil all thy counsel. [5] We will rejoice in thy salvation, and in the name of our God we will set up our banners: the Lord fulfil all thy petitions. [6] Now know I that the Lord saveth his anointed; he will hear him from his holy heaven with the saving strength of his right hand. [7] Some trust in chariots, and some in horses: but we will remember the name of the Lord our God. [8] They are brought down and fallen: but we are risen, and stand upright. [9] Save, Lord: let the king hear us when we call.

Psalm 91
[1] He that dwelleth in the secret place of the most High shall abide under the shadow of the Almighty. [2] I will say of the Lord, He is my refuge and my fortress: my God; in him will I trust. [3] Surely he shall deliver thee from the snare of the fowler, and from the noisome pestilence. [4] He shall cover thee with his feathers, and under his wings shalt thou trust: his truth shall be thy shield and buckler. [5] Thou shalt not be afraid for the terror by night; nor for the arrow that flieth by day; [6] Nor for the pestilence that walketh in darkness; nor for the destruction that wasteth at noonday. [7] A thousand shall fall at thy side, and ten thousand at thy right hand; but it shall not come nigh thee. [8] Only with thine eyes shalt thou behold and see the reward of the wicked. [9] Because thou hast made the Lord, which is my refuge, even the most High, thy habitation; [10] There shall no evil befall thee, neither shall any plague come nigh thy dwelling. [11] For he shall give his angels charge over thee, to keep thee in all thy ways. [12] They shall bear thee up in their hands, lest thou dash thy foot against a stone. [13] Thou shalt tread upon the lion and adder: the young lion and the dragon shalt thou trample under feet. [14] Because he hath set his love upon me, therefore will I deliver him: I will set him on high, because he hath known my name. [15] He shall call upon me, and I will answer him: I will be with him in trouble; I will deliver him, and honour him. [16] With long life will I satisfy him, and shew him my salvation. Amen let us pray

DS. God Bless you.. Dr. Ghaly 🙏❤️
MH. Amen
HD. Aen

CG. Let's pray that America makes the best choice for President. Great picture! 🖤🙏

RH. 🙏🙏🙏🙏🙏 on our knees. Amen

KJ. I LOVE WHEN YOU TAKE YOUR PRESCIOUS TIME TO ENRICH OUR LIVES WITH WISDOM. AMEN.

AB. AMEN!

JH. I love to read the anointing words the lord shares to your heart which allows you to share the words to the followers of God a true gift 📖

Civil Unrest America 🇺🇸 My Posts on October 22 and October 31!

https://www.facebook.com/1150861349/posts/10223631214505682/?d=n
https://www.facebook.com/1150861349/posts/10224181091052252/?d=n

Nation shall Mourn!!
Written by Ramsis Ghaly on October 22, 2020

Isaiah 24:4 "The earth mourns and withers, the world fades and withers, the exalted of the people of the earth fade away."

Isaiah 33:9 "The land mourns and pines away,
Lebanon is shamed and withers;
Sharon is like a desert plain,
And Bashan and Carmel lose their foliage."

Jeremiah 4:28 "For this the earth shall mourn
And the heavens above be dark,
Because I have spoken, I have purposed,
And I will not change My mind, nor will I turn from it."

Lamentations 1:4 "The roads of Zion are in mourning
Because no one comes to the appointed feasts.
All her gates are desolate;
Her priests are groaning,
Her virgins are afflicted,
And she herself is bitter."

Isaiah 3:26 "And her gates will lament and mourn,
And deserted she will sit on the ground."

Lamentations 2:8 "The Lord determined to destroy
The wall of the daughter of Zion.
He has stretched out a line,
He has not restrained His hand from destroying,
And He has caused rampart and wall to lament;
They have languished together."

Joel 1:10 "The field is ruined,
The land mourns;
For the grain is ruined,
The new wine dries up,
Fresh oil fails."

Amos 1:2 "He said,
"The Lord roars from Zion
And from Jerusalem He utters His voice;
And the shepherds' pasture grounds mourn,
And the summit of Carmel dries up."

Isaiah 24:7 "The new wine mourns,
The vine decays,
All the merry-hearted sigh."

Isaiah 29:2 "I will bring distress to Ariel,
And she will be a city of lamenting and mourning;
And she will be like an Ariel to me."

Ezekiel 32:16 "This is a lamentation and they shall chant it. The daughters of the
nations shall chant it. Over Egypt and over all her hordes they shall chant it,"
declares the Lord God."

Zechariah 12:11 "In that day there will be great mourning in Jerusalem, like the
mourning of Hadadrimmon in the plain of Megiddo."

Matthew 13:42
Verse Concepts
and will throw them into the furnace of fire; in that place there will be weeping
and gnashing of teeth.

Revelation 18:8 "For this reason in one day her plagues will come, pestilence and mourning and famine, and she will be burned up with fire; for the Lord God who judges her is strong."

Amos 8:10 "Then I will turn your festivals into mourning
And all your songs into lamentation;
And I will bring sackcloth on everyone's loins
And baldness on every head.
And I will make it like a time of mourning for an only son,
And the end of it will be like a bitter day."

Amos 5:16-17 "Therefore thus says the Lord God of hosts, the Lord,
"There is wailing in all the plazas,
And in all the streets they say, 'Alas! Alas!'
They also call the farmer to mourning
And professional mourners to lamentation.
"And in all the vineyards there is wailing,
Because I will pass through the midst of you," says the Lord."

Joel 1:8-13 "Wail like a virgin girded with sackcloth
For the bridegroom of her youth.
The grain offering and the drink offering are cut off
From the house of the Lord.
The priests mourn,
The ministers of the Lord.
The field is ruined,
The land mourns;
For the grain is ruined,
The new wine dries up,
Fresh oil fails.

read more."

Amos 5:17 "And in all the vineyards there is wailing,
Because I will pass through the midst of you," says the Lord."

"Therefore humble yourselves under the mighty hand of God, that He may exalt you at the proper time, casting all your anxiety on Him, because He cares for you." 1 Peter 5:6-7

Lord Jesus Elect for America 🇺🇸 Your Anointed! Let us Pray for Peace!

Written by Ramsis Ghaly on October 31

"The Lord shall fight for you, and ye shall hold your peace." Exodus 14:14 KJV

Our father Moses says: "And Moses said unto the people, Fear ye not, stand still, and see the salvation of the Lord, which he will shew to you to day: for the Egyptians whom ye have seen to day, ye shall see them again no more for ever." Exodus 14:13 KJV

America 🏳, Let us lift our heart 💜 to the Lord to elect a President to lead His people and our Beloved country America 🏳!

America 🏳, Let us rise early Sunday morning to pray to our Savior to nominate the president of our nation in His Name!

America 🏳, Let us look up high calling His Name lifting our arms and hands up to heaven appealing to the Most High to intervene for His Name sake!

America 🏳, Let us pray in faith, love and humility to Lord God of our land and ask Him to announce the chosen Shephard for our land!

America 🏳, Let us subdue to the results and pray it won't be our choice king Saul but His choice king David!

America 🏳, Let us pray for Peace! Our Lord Jesus says: "Peace I leave with you, my peace I give unto you: not as the world giveth, give I unto you. Let not your heart be troubled, neither let it be afraid." John 14:27 KJV

Since God look deep in the heart as He said when He chose king David: "But the Lord said unto Samuel, Look not on his countenance, or on the height of his stature; because I have refused him: for the Lord seeth not as man seeth; for man looketh on the outward appearance, but the Lord looketh on the heart." 1 Samuel 16:7 KJV

America 🏳, Who will be the president the chosen Vessel unto Lord Jesus?? "The Lord said to tge president elect: "But the Lord said unto him, Go thy way: for he is a chosen vessel unto me, to bear my name before the Gentiles, and kings, and the children of Israel: [16] For I will shew him how great things he must suffer for my name's sake." Acts 9:15-16 KJV

And for the President elect saint Paul says: "I charge you in the presence of God, who gives life to all things, and of Christ Jesus, who in his testimony before

Pontius Pilate made the good confession, to keep the commandment unstained and free from reproach until the appearing of our Lord Jesus Christ, which he will display at the proper time—he who is the blessed and only Sovereign, the King of kings and Lord of lords, who alone has immortality, who dwells in unapproachable light, whom no one has ever seen or can see. To him be honor and eternal dominion. Amen." (1 Timothy 6:15, ESV)

2 Thessalonians 2:13 "But we should always give thanks to God for you, brethren beloved by the Lord, because God has chosen you from the beginning for salvation through sanctification by the Spirit and faith in the truth."

Psalm 20
The Lord hear thee in the day of trouble; the name of the God of Jacob defend thee; [2] Send thee help from the sanctuary, and strengthen thee out of Zion; [3] Remember all thy offerings, and accept thy burnt sacrifice; Selah. [4] Grant thee according to thine own heart, and fulfil all thy counsel. [5] We will rejoice in thy salvation, and in the name of our God we will set up our banners: the Lord fulfil all thy petitions. [6] Now know I that the Lord saveth his anointed; he will hear him from his holy heaven with the saving strength of his right hand. [7] Some trust in chariots, and some in horses: but we will remember the name of the Lord our God. [8] They are brought down and fallen: but we are risen, and stand upright. [9] Save, Lord: let the king hear us when we call.

Psalm 91
[1] He that dwelleth in the secret place of the most High shall abide under the shadow of the Almighty. [2] I will say of the Lord, He is my refuge and my fortress: my God; in him will I trust. [3] Surely he shall deliver thee from the snare of the fowler, and from the noisome pestilence. [4] He shall cover thee with his feathers, and under his wings shalt thou trust: his truth shall be thy shield and buckler. [5] Thou shalt not be afraid for the terror by night; nor for the arrow that flieth by day; [6] Nor for the pestilence that walketh in darkness; nor for the destruction that wasteth at noonday. [7] A thousand shall fall at thy side, and ten thousand at thy right hand; but it shall not come nigh thee. [8] Only with thine eyes shalt thou behold and see the reward of the wicked. [9] Because thou hast made the Lord, which is my refuge, even the most High, thy habitation; [10] There shall no evil befall thee, neither shall any plague come nigh thy dwelling. [11] For he shall give his angels charge over thee, to keep thee in all thy ways. [12] They shall bear thee up in their hands, lest thou dash thy foot against a stone. [13] Thou shalt tread upon the lion and adder: the young lion and the dragon shalt thou trample under feet. [14] Because he hath set his love upon me, therefore will I deliver him: I will set him on high, because he hath known my name. [15] He shall call upon

me, and I will answer him: I will be with him in trouble; I will deliver him, and honour him. [16] With long life will I satisfy him, and shew him my salvation.

Amen 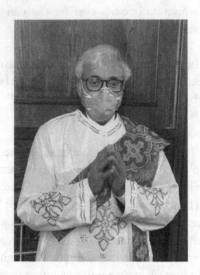 let us pray

Let us get some debate about the similarities of the mysterious exit for both Pope Benedict 16th and President Trump other than holiness!!
Your thoughts of the week

JD. Well Dr. Ghaly, never in the history of the Catholic Church has a Pope ever stepped down. Correct me if I am wrong please. They usually stay until they pass on. My gut told me that there was something fishy going on there. This has never been a fight between Democrats and Republicans. It has been and continues to be a battle between Good and evil. Now regarding President Trump, we know for CERTAIN that there are illegalities going on. More and more proof every day is coming out. So, I would say after much prayer, that there is a lot of evil going on in this world. If we lose President Trump and they make the USA a Communist Country, there is no where else for us to flee to. I am right with God and I hope everyone else that believes in him is too. God help us all! 🙏🙏🙏

Let us Not Forget!!

Through the unrest, let us not forget! Thank you President Trump and Thank you American 🇺🇸 troops and president Puten and Russian military for saving

the Coptic and Middle East native ancient Christians against the genocide and the brutality of centuries of the evil NON CHRISTIAN sword!

Ramsis Ghaly

NC. Women, children, men continually mass slaughtered throughout the Middle East. Because they are Christians. Syria, Iraq, Jordan, Armenia, Egypt, Lebanon (my George is a survivor). Many have fled, spent huge sums of money, emigrated legally, taking years.....to South America, to Canada, to the US. They do not get "special help" or "special assistance" from the governments. They are not awarded "refugee" status. Many have watched the mass slaughter of their town, their village, their families. But they emigrate legally. They go to school and learn their new home country's language. They go to more school and become legal citizens. They pay taxes. They educate their children. They contribute to their new communities. Las Vegas is an example of many, many Christian Lebanese, Iraqis, Jordanians, Armenians, Egyptians, who became contributors to our community. They lost everything. They came with nothing. They re-built from scratch, and many successful professionals and business owners emerged here. They have drive, honesty, loyalty, a sense of community. You do not see roving gangs of Christian Middle Eastern kids preying upon neighborhoods here. In fact, these are the kids who will have your back when you cry for help. There is a difference in immigrants, and we need to start paying attention.

Let America Abd the World know that the Christians of Egypt and Middle East appreciate so much president Trump whom immediately put a stop to the brutality and bloodshed of Christians by Islamic sword as soon as he got in the Office 2016. The Islamic brutality used to be in the rise in the Christmas time and many of us used to mourn in the Christmas for those who brutality murdered! Let us never forget! Thank you Mr. President Trump, Thank you.

The Christians of the Middle East are left behind: inside view
A Christmas message written by
Ramsis Ghaly

I hear a crying voice from very far, I see the hidden tears from miles away: I screamed and said with so many with one voice you are not alone. Who can reach my brother and my sister? Who can feed my child and my parents? This all because they are Christians from the Middle East. One day the real story will be told and we all will be ashamed from what we have not done. Let us put our shoes and go and do. It is not too late friends!!

My brothers and sisters, Christians of Egypt, Syria, Iraq and neighbor countries are left behind.

It was not long ago when so many Middle East christians came to America and Europe leaving the persecution behind. It was during my time back then in 1970's and 1980's.

I hear a crying voice from very far, I see the hidden tears from miles away: I screamed and said with so many with one voice you are not alone. Who can reach my brother and my sister? Who can feed my child and my parents? This all because they are Christians from the Middle East. One day the real story will be told and we all will be ashamed from what we have not done.

Since the beginning of this century, no much of Christians are allowed or able to leave their countries. They all are left behind waiting to be tortured or killed.

They are suppressed, oppressed and speechless. There is no hand to reach.

In fact, they have no money and no resources, it was all taken away from them.

Every day, a Middle East Christian is in the death row waiting for his or her time to depart.

Otherwise, they either threatened or slaved or become cheap labors.

I hear a crying voice from very far, I see the hidden tears from miles away: I screamed and said with so many with one voice you are not alone. One day the real story will be told and we all will be ashamed from what we have not done.

They were denied from going by to Europe and join the refugee.

After waiting the days and the nights to get into a boat from the Syrian shore, they were thrown away to the streets.

I hear a crying voice from very far, I see the hidden tears from miles away: I screamed and said with so many with one voice you are not alone. Who can reach my brother and my sister? Who can feed my child and my parents? This all because they are Christians from the Middle East. One day the real story will be told and we all will be ashamed from what we have not done. Let us put our shoes and go and do. It is not too late friends!!

The media ignored them, the politicians turned their backs on them and the truth is buried and many stories were turned around and covered up.

They have no help or assistance from any human right groups worldwide

In Christ they put their lives and their destiny in full

I hear a crying voice from very far, I see the hidden tears from miles away: I screamed and said with so many with one voice you are not alone. One day the real story will be told and we all will be ashamed from what we have not done.

The access was blocked. The telephones were disconnected. The electricity was no longer. The water supply was stopped. There was no enough food left behind. Who can reach my brother and my sister? Who can feed my child and my parents? This all because they are Christians from the Middle East.

There is no advocate and the society alienated them and took their name off one by one.

They learn not to talk or express their rights otherwise more will be tortured and killed.

A Christian brother went to the American Embassy and found the staff are all non-Christians and he was asked to leave immediately.

He went ahead and mailed the embassy and his request was denied and thrown away.

I hear a crying voice from very far, I see the hidden tears from miles away: I screamed and said with so many with one voice you are not alone. Who can reach my brother and my sister? Who can feed my child and my parents? This all because they are Christians from the Middle East. One day the real story will be told and we all will be ashamed from what we have not done. Let us put our shoes and go and do. It is not too late friends!!

A Christian sister went to a travel agency looking for s cheaper flight and was told what equal to 10,000.0 American dollars for a two flight ticket.

I wonder if someone can reach My brothers and sisters, ancient Christians of Middle East Egypt, Syria, Iraq and neighbor countries.

I wonder if there is a Good Samaritan that will heal their wounds and help them. In this Christmas season, I join so many speaking up and sharing saying you are not alone our beloved souls.

I hear a crying voice from very far, I see the hidden tears from miles away: I screamed and said with so many with one voice you are not alone. Who can reach my brother and my sister? Who can feed my child and my parents? This all because they are Christians from the Middle East. One day the real story will be told and we all will be ashamed from what we have not done. Let us put our shoes and go and do. It is not too late friends!!

Thank you
Ramsis Ghaly

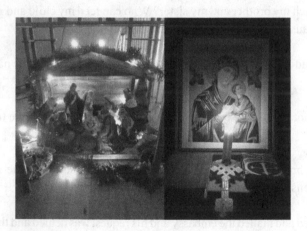

Pay Attention to the Unfolding Truth about Turkey and its Followers and the Christians of the West!! The ongoing slain in Austria and France!

It goes back to little under thousand years of Islamic Turks and Ottoman against the Christians of the west and east, south and north!

On the other hand, Jesus Who they persecuted teaches His followers Neither open their mouth nor get any revenge but in return pray, forgive and love 💜. Our Lord Jesus was blasphemed against and His followers were brutally killed, murdered and mass raped and molested and saying all the kind of vulgar words against Jesus the Incarnated Son of God and denied by the Ottoman empire under the leadership of the Islamic leaders including Mehmet with sword declaring wars against all the Christians for 500 years?

O my gosh about the brutal murders of the Christians in the West and Middle east by the Ottoman leaders?? How can we forget?? The Ottoman Empire is also known as the Turkish Empire and was founded by Turkish tribes around 1299. The Empire expanded and gained a lot of power after it took control of Constantinople in 1453. It persecuted and murdered the Christians throughout--.

https://www.independent.co.uk/.../genocide-christian...
https://study.com/.../the-long-war-christians-vs-turks-by....

America wake Up!! It isn't about Democrats or Republicans. It is about America and protecting America against the wolves dressed in sheep cloths antichrists!!!

As President Emmanuel Macron has promised to intensify a clampdown on Islamist radicalism in France, days after Paty was murdered in broad daylight in a quiet Paris suburb for having shown and discussed caricatures of the Prophet Mohammad in a civics class. An escalating crackdown on groups suspected of aiding or abetting Islamist extremists has prompted accusations that the French government is riding roughshood over legal protections in the wake of the gruesome murder of 47-year-old teacher Samuel Paty last week. Samuel Paty, 47, was targeted for showing cartoons of the Prophet Muhammad to his students.

His killer, 18-year-old Abdullakh Anzorov, was shot dead by police shortly after last Friday's attack. But seven people, including two students and a parent of one of Mr Paty's pupils, were detained in the days following the killing.

https://www.npr.org/.../france-turkey-and-the-charlie...
https://www.nbcnews.com/.../offensive-charlie-hebdo...
https://www.bbc.com/news/world-europe-54632353
https://www.france24.com/.../20201022-anger-at-beheading...

CG. It almost mirrors what is happening in some of our cities.

The Latest Events Both Parties Are To Be Blamed While Not Excusing the President Trump!!

Written by Ramsis Ghaly

Goodbye Mr. President! The Latest Events both parties are
to be blamed while not excusing President Trump!!
Written by Ramsis Ghaly

While we all pointing fingers at President trump, we should also point fingers at ourselves and the system. We all failed as one country! Where were all the past four years?? Just now waking up and taking serious decisions?? It isn't any more working-together US Capitol for America!! It is the time to reform and start a New Formed Unified US Capitol of America!

A mother with a disturbed son that always make trouble and many just point fingers at him! Yet the mother and good people around him are always blame themselves for not doing enough for the son to success! America, the system and we all to be blamed for president Trump failure. Always ridiculing the president actions and words, yet We never did enough to make him successful!

Let me start by acknowledging out loudly and tell the world and president Trump thank you for doing the best to protect the ancient helpless Christians of Egypt and Middle East from the brutality of the Islamic sword! Those Christians were left to die and tortured heavily before president Trump became president. Forever grateful!!

I do feel for president Trump! He meant well to the country and for the people! And his failures and latest event could have been avoided if the adversaries stopped the absolute hatred!

Although ultimately his fault and he is fully responsible for his behavior! He was placed for a position with No enough guidance and a trusted shoulder he can lean on except his supporters! He was consistently has been provoked and many enabled him to continue his rhetoric's!

However, the other party has also blame to take because they couldn't work with him and earn his trust other than make a fool out of him for everything he did!

Fallen in hands of God but much better than fallen in hands of man as king David said: "And David said to Gad, "I am in great distress. Please let us fall into the hand of the LORD, for His mercies are great; but do not let me fall into the hand of man." 2 Samuel 24:14

I can't imagine that there was no single person existing in his family and the Oval office that could not help, filter, vent and guide the president against wrongdoing?? If those around him cared so much and determined to work out!!

And if there wasn't anyone among the people around him and in the US Capitol, then those should have searched externally for a talented mentor and professional Coaches!!

The dark events and uncontrolled rhetoric's should have been prevented and cared for by professional Coaches and those who are talented enough to earn the trust of president Trump!

Because of those around him didn't work hard enough, they joined the president in the ultimate America failure! The end result is that no one won but we're all America's lost! In addition, the entire world is laughing at America!!!

America is full of talented people professional and spiritual coaches such as Billy Graham and many others doing the impossible and we choose not to extend our hands too hard enough! Pure love with no agenda or secondary gains does the impossible and faith bridges for all miracles! As it is written: "Love never fails. But whether there are prophecies, they will fail; whether there are tongues, they will cease; whether there is knowledge, it will vanish away" 1 Corinthians 13:8

While we are saying goodbye to president Trump, we must thank him for all the good things he had done for the country and people and acknowledge the failures of all those around him!

Before pointing our fingers at president Trump, let us look at our failures to do enough to support him and truly love him and coach him and let him flourish to do the best for our country other than belittle him and keep berating him more and more! Let us look at ourselves the mote and beam out as it is written; Matthew 7:1-5 KJV "Judge not, that ye be not judged. [2] For with what judgment ye judge, ye shall be judged: and with what measure ye mete, it shall be measured to you again. [3] And why beholdest thou the mote that is in thy brother's eye, but considerest not the beam that is in thine own eye? [4] Or how wilt thou say to thy brother, Let me pull out the mote out of thine eye; and, behold, a beam is in thine

931

own eye? [5] Thou hypocrite, first cast out the beam out of thine own eye; and then shalt thou see clearly to cast out the mote out of thy brother's eye."

America is about not making fool of ourselves but unity, helping each other and reach out hard enough to compliment the shortcomings among us! As he is a Patriot American!

St Paul said; "4Love suffers long and is kind; love does not envy; love does not parade itself, is not [b]puffed up; 5does not behave rudely, does not seek its own, is not provoked, [c]thinks no evil; 6does not rejoice in iniquity, but rejoices in the truth; 7bears all things, believes all things, hopes all things, endures all things. 8Love never fails. But whether there are prophecies, they will fail; whether there are tongues, they will cease; whether there is knowledge, it will vanish away. 9For we know in part and we prophesy in part. 10But when that which is [d]perfect has come, then that which is in part will be done away." 1 Corinthians 23:4-10

Last president Trump
speech https://fb.watch/2UGEX8nXnD/

Please use professional language and tell us your thoughts????

Goodbye President Trump! Thank you 🙏 and may the remaining years to be guided by our Lord Jesus to lead you to safety according to His promise and your family to His kingdom. Ours Lord is the ultimate Judge and knows all things. I am not worthy to judge and we all sinful and all fell short as it is written: Romans 3:22-24 KJV "Even the righteousness of God which is by faith of Jesus Christ unto all and upon all them that believe: for there is no difference: [23] For all have sinned, and come short of the glory of God; [24] Being justified freely by his grace through the redemption that is in Christ Jesus:" And "8If we say that we have no sin, we deceive ourselves, and the truth is not in us. 9If we confess our sins, he is faithful and just to forgive us our sins, and to cleanse us from all unrighteousness. 10If we say that we have not sinned, we make him a liar, and his word is not in us." 1 John 1:7-9)

Thank you 🙏 and Goodbye Mr President Donald Trump!

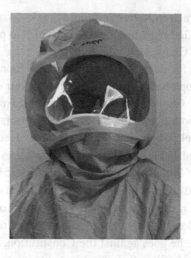

JP. Thank you Doctor for your words of encouragement. We have a God that's greater than all that's happening. My hope is in Him and Him alone.

Thank you Doctor for all you do.

GB. Thank you.

CR. Do not agree with you this time. Stay safe. We love you.

VA. Well said.

NV. Very well said! God Bless you Doctor Ghaly 🙏

TJ. Dr. Ghaly, I always love & respect your opinion, but have to disagree. My nephew was part of President Trumps CIA security detail. So he had firsthand experience that there were very capable people there to advise & council the President, except he chose not to listen to anyone. Furthermore, he is a racist, a criminal, and an overall horrible human being. I have never seen a president be as unpresidential as he has been. He DELIBERATELY incited a riot where people were seriously injured and lost their lives. What kind of President does that. All because he's too small of a person to except defeat and move on. I agree that those who provoked and enabled him are to blame as well. But I believe in Father God just as you do. Therefore, I have to forgive & trust my faith that God can change even somebody as EVIL as Donald Trump.

SC. very well stated my good friend love it

MG. Strongly disagree

RP. Thank you 🙏

RP. Thank you 🙏

CR. Thank you so much for always putting yourself out there with an open heart. This was extremely well said. May the Lord continue to bless you and keep you in all that you do.

MA. Thank you doc Amen in Jesus Christ and thanks to our president of United states of America God bless him God is with him to protect him amen

DC. Thank you Doctor Ghaly, well said.

CC. Please don't blame President Trump for the breech on the Capital. Antifa or the American gestopo was behind it. God now is our only salvation

BS. Very well said, Dr. Ghaly. I am thankful for President Trumps 4 yrs. I also believe fault is on both sides and social media is absolutely no help to anyone. This election, I feel is bringing us all closer to Jesus. I have friends and relatives who turned on me due to politics. It hurts, yes. I pray for our country all day every day. If President Trump is having erratic behavior, he was under pressure and turned on from the time he threw his hat in the ring. Perhaps the stress is causing a crack under pressure. I know the Lord was with him, or he wouldn't have held up as long as he has. I am going to give Biden a chance, but if at ANY time he goes against the Constitution, and brings a socialist/communist agenda, I will definitely object.

CH. Beautifully said! I was a Trump supporter all the way and felt the same, nobody ever gave him a chance to prove himself. If everyone worked together I think the world would have been a better place.

JS. The thing is, both parties have issues. They ridicule him for his actions and words (and sometimes they are correct); however, they themselves act and do things like ripping up speeches on national TV and attempt a coup and waste time, money and energy on fictitious claims. Both sides need to behave like adults and do the right things for our country and not special interest groups that grease their palms.

JP. Perfectly said Doctor Ghaly!

TG. Thanks you to our President Trump of United states of America. He do the best he can for American trying to keep American great again All the Congress in white house no one is standing by him and support him, this is sadness time for us who love President Trump and thanks for everything he has done, joe Biden and his son going to sell American to China because Joe Biden son corrupt take billions Dollars from china. One say anything and do anything about. This is wakeup call for America. I Prayers for President Trump i pray for God help America. Not to become the china communist. 🙏🙏

AL. Amen 🙏

RM. God bless 🙏 Amen

MN. Well stated Dr. Ghaly. The intense hatred that so many had towards Trump blinded them from ANY positive contributions he made to the country. So very sad indeed.

SA, Well said Dr. Ghaly. Can I share? Thanks

CG. There is nothing left to say. You doctor said it all. Bless you and our President Trump. 💜🙏

TR. Well said, Dr. Ghaly! I admire, your choice of words and deep devotion to our faith! Yes! Everything you said, is true. He is subjected to many, challenges by the left but overall he did more for the country than other presidents.. in the last 4 years. More, than his promises. Thanks, President Trump, My heart breaks & hope the fraudulent election be rectified & truth be restored. God Bless.

ML. Amen Dr **Ramsis Ghaly**

KG. Very well said. 🙏

VW. This is absolutely amazing. Thank you for giving the Godly truth

VL. The lickspittles in congress are determined to destroy our country.

KK. I like this it's not one sided. Thank you!

JJ. May God bless America! 🇺🇸 I am concerned with the future ahead; our rights must be protected. Thankfully, I know God is in control.

DR. Socialism will prevail. We didn't do enough but social media giants have taken over. It's already here, shutting down businesses and now taking a business down. Parler have been shut down by big tech. We must not have another view. These are scary times, but as you well know, God is so much bigger.

DK. Well said. Look at all he accomplished with all the hatred and lies from trying to rid the white house etc of corruption and people who are paid off by special interest groups etc. Just imagine how good it COULD have been for the citizens of the U.S. if all the.ones against him had just once tried to work with him and hear him out and looked at the bigger picture and saw the good he was doing. I doubt anyone after him will be looking to protect Israel and with that not happening God will no longer protect anyone who doesn't. Hopefully and prayerfully people will focus on the king of kings and the Lord of Lords because the biggest part of history(besides Jesus birth) hasn't happened yet...but it will!! **#TheKingIsComing**

Sadness over the land and gloominess all around! Post During Riots Before Washington DC Capitol 1/5/2021

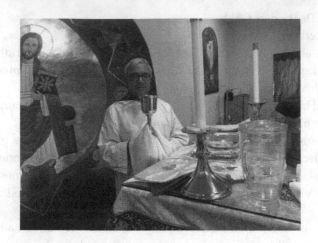

Sadness over the land and gloominess all around!
Love of power is a killer and competition to control is an evil!
Man ambition is blind and the ways are tedious!
The divisions are in the rise! Man is at standstill and many victims are becoming hostage!
The enemy made fool out of the nation!
The conspirators are planning the wars!
Their tactics are deceiving and their aiming is bloodshed!
They are going after the Messiahs!
The screams are coming out of the cages!
I see the bruised faces shattered by the laughing spirits!
The dead bodies can no longer be resuscitated!
The spread of suffocated souls is about to get unreal!
I see Satan ignites the fire!
I hear the devil 😈 spiraling the crowd!
I feel the dark spirits lined up outside!
I witness much more demons are in the way!
The hearts are pierced by the arrows!
The inwards are empty of goodness!
The godliness is running short!
The Divine lodging is rare!
The visitations are cut short!

The evil is dominating and the enemy of mankind is overpowering!
Go home everyone! Let us pray!
Please don't let them in!
Drew the sign of Jesus Cross in our souls and homes!

In unity and obedience with spiritual humility and broken hearts in one voice: "After this manner therefore pray ye: Our Father which art in heaven, Hallowed be thy name. [10] Thy kingdom come. Thy will be done in earth, as it is in heaven. [11] Give us this day our daily bread. [12] And forgive us our debts, as we forgive our debtors. [13] And lead us not into temptation, but deliver us from evil: For thine is the kingdom, and the power, and the glory, forever. Amen." Matthew 6:9-13 KJV

Amen 🙏

GB. Wisdom. Thank you.
BCD, Keep the Faith, Trump is on it. They cheated on Georgia. Votes were changed with Dominion system again. There is proof.
JC. Amen! Hope this ends soon 😨
JP. Thank you for shining your light on this darkness we are living in. Praying for peace to take over our land. God is God and we know how this story will end.
AS. So true God bless you
ED. Amen 🙏. Bless you Doctor.
CG. Such a sad time in our country. I have to ask is all this a test of our faith? What has God got planned for us?
RL. Amen
CR. Getting nearer to the end of this age. Satan knows his time is short.
KO. AMEN CHAR, GOD'S IN CONTROL ALWAYS, PRAYING FOR THIS WORLD 🙏🙏
BL. Thank you and God bless you.
MH. Praying for an end to the virus, peace & joy to return once again.
TG. It sadness time in our country. I praying for peace to take over our land. God got planned for us this is wake up call for all of us. Prayers 🙏🙏
VA. So much hate now. Satan is rejoicing.

Jesus Name During 2021 Presidential Inauguration!

Written by Ramsis Ghaly

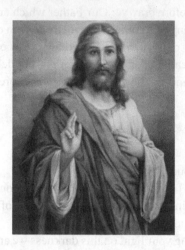

Does placing the one's hand on the Bible is considered an oath of using the Bible for a way of life and in every decision made in the White House leading the nation! Or it is just a ceremonial???? Who is worthy to touch the Bible giving oath and proclaiming Jesus the Lord and Word of God! Let us examine ourselves before placing our hand on the Holy Book of the Word of God and the Wisdom of God otherwise For he that eateth and drinketh unworthily, eateth and drinketh damnation to himself, not discerning the Lord's body—as it is written: 1 Corinthians 11:26-30 KJV "For as often as ye eat this bread, and drink this cup, ye do shew the Lord's death till he come. [27] Wherefore whosoever shall eat this bread, and drink this cup of the Lord, unworthily, shall be guilty of the body and blood of the Lord. [28] But let a man examine himself, and so let him eat of that bread, and drink of that cup. [29] For he that eateth and drinketh unworthily, eateth and drinketh damnation to himself, not discerning the Lord's body. [30] For this cause many are weak and sickly among you, and many sleep."

Therefore, placing the one's hand on the Bible is indeed the most sacred to declare an oath before the Lord and the nation. It is a lifetime Vow subjected to the Judgment day as it is written: Numbers 30:2 "If a man makes a vow to the Lord, or takes an oath to bind himself with a binding obligation, he shall not violate his word; he shall do according to all that proceeds out of his mouth." And: Deuteronomy 23:21-23 "When you make a vow to the Lord your God, you shall not delay to pay it, for it would be sin in you, and the Lord your God will surely require it of you. However, if you refrain from vowing, it would not be sin in you. You shall be careful to perform what goes out from your lips, just as you have voluntarily vowed to the Lord your God, what you have promised."

I thought the leaders of United States of America will draw Jesus Cross sign upon themselves and say in the beginning and at the end: "The love and peace of our Father, His Son Jesus Christ and the Holy Spirit One God Amen" Perhaps I should consider it isn't the church of Christ but I thought the White House is!! Perhaps America is no longer the land of Christ but I thought it is!!

I wish the opening of Inauguration especially the President of United States and Vice President and Chief Commander, to be with our Heavenly Father's prayers "Our Father which art in heaven, Hallowed be thy name—" and to be concluded in Lord Jesus Name "for thine kingdom, glory and power for every and ever Amen 🙏" This is especially true in difficult times! While the administration is calling for healing and unity, the true healing and the true unity is in truth and not without the truth and in Jesus and not without Jesus! Perhaps the nation knows more than one God and no longer Jesus is its Only God for America?

The fact is the Lord God is the True Healer and His Name is Jesus: "Come to me, all you who are weary and burdened, and I will give you rest. Take my yoke upon you and learn from me, for I am gentle and humble in heart, and you will find rest for your souls. For my yoke is easy and my burden is light." ~ Matthew 11:28-30 "Peace I leave with you; my peace I give you. I do not give to you as the world gives. Do not let your hearts be troubled and do not be afraid." ~ John 14:27 "Heal me, O Lord, and I will be healed; save me and I will be saved, for you are the one I praise." ~ Jeremiah 17:14 Is anyone among you sick? Let them call the elders of the church to pray over them and anoint them with oil in the name of the Lord. And the prayer offered in faith will make the sick person well; the Lord will raise them up. If they have sinned, they will be forgiven." ~ James 5:14-15

Where were all the gorgeous chains and earrings and neckless carrying Jesus icons and St Mary and Jesus Cross!!! Where were all the signs of Jesus and Christianity ✝ !!!!! Where were the beautiful blessed faces of Christ's at the Inauguration! Perhaps I should know in 2021, America is for all non-domination and all the Christians signs and words should taken away from our public!! Christmas 🙏 is no longer Christmas but Happy Holiday and there is no "Under God" and God shouldn't be in the constitution or the school or government or politics!!!!

The fact is we should be proud of Jesus Cross: Galatians 6:14,18 KJV 14] But God forbid that I should glory, save in the cross of our Lord Jesus Christ, by whom the world is crucified unto me, and I unto the world. [18] Brethren, the grace of our Lord Jesus Christ be with your spirit. Amen." 1 Corinthians 1:18,23-24 KJV 18] For the preaching of the cross is to them that perish foolishness; but unto us which are saved it is the power of God. [23] But we preach Christ crucified, unto the Jews a stumbling block, and unto the Greeks foolishness; [24] But unto them which are called, both Jews and Greeks, Christ the power of God, and the wisdom of God.

It isn't putting the hand over the Bible is what count but rather doers of what is written in the Bible!! Only God knows the hearts of people and tomorrow the books shall be open!! Three different bibles are used during inauguration! It should never be anything over the Bible but a clean holy and sincere hand of a faithful servant well heartedly standing before God Almighty Jesus the Lord! Perhaps, it is all just routine and the knowledge of what is in the heart is within?

But the fact is the Lord Name should never be used in vain! 1. Deuteronomy 5:10-11 "But I lavish unfailing love for a thousand generations on those who love me and obey my commands. "You must not misuse the name of the LORD your God. The LORD will not let you go unpunished if you misuse his name." 2. Exodus 20:7 "You shall not take the name of the LORD your God in vain, for the LORD will not hold guiltless anyone who takes his name in vain."3. Leviticus 19:12 "Do not bring shame on the name of your God by using it to swear falsely. I am the LORD."

The fact is Jesus taught us how to pray saying Our Father in Matthew 6:9-15 KJV "After this manner therefore pray ye: Our Father which art in heaven, Hallowed be thy name. [10] Thy kingdom come. Thy will be done in earth, as it is in heaven. [11] Give us this day our daily bread. [12] And forgive us our debts, as we forgive our debtors. [13] And lead us not into temptation, but deliver us from evil: For thine is the kingdom, and the power, and the glory, for ever. Amen. [14] For if ye forgive men their trespasses, your heavenly Father will also forgive you: [15] But if ye forgive not men their trespasses, neither will your Father forgive your trespasses."

The fact is we should never be ashamed of mentioning Jesus name in public if we are indeed sincere and believe in Him and His Commandments! Jesus said; Matthew 10:32-33 KJV 32] Whosoever therefore shall confess me before men, him will I confess also before my Father which is in heaven. [33] But whosoever shall deny me before men, him will I also deny before my Father which is in heaven. Amen 🙏

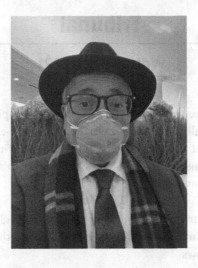

AP. Those who love and value the Bible know how to demonstrate that conviction when making a vow.

CC. Agreed!

JF. Amen and amen!!! #PastorJeff90210

jf. Well said. It was ceremonial use of the Bible only.

Kb. Will said Dr.

Mh. Hopefully they will do what is right & up hold their vowls. Also give the people the much needed money & cheaper rent here in AZ. They need to put a cap on what they are charging. Hopefully he will help us 🇺🇸 & make us proud to call him our president 🙏

ds. Swearing on a million bibles doesn't mean they will keep America free, safe, abide by our constitution and protect us from socialism. Honor our men in blue, support our troops, protect the unborn, freedom of speech, right to bare arms and worship. The swamp is beyond bigger than we knew. Praying for our country.

jm. That particular bible had a hidden message deeper than many realize. Biden is not a Christian leader.

Sa. ربنا يبارك حياتك د. رمسيس فأنت دكتور ومبشر للسيد المسيح ايضا . ربنا يبارك خدمتك الرائعه الحقيقيه 🙏🙏

Gb. I appreciate your words, Dr. Ghaly. Using the Bible to place one's hand for the purpose of ceremony, (regardless if it's a family heirloom), is way different than using the Bible for a way of life. I surely am praying...

941

Tribunal

Written 1/21/2021

Within three Days, three months and three years!!! My spirit today directed my soul to watch and recall the Knesset Court that condemned Jesus! Indeed I saw the High Priests, Chief Priests, lawyers, Scribes and officers as the Council of Old, Conspirators, Conspiracy ———-! It is unbearable to see injustice and what men can do to his fellowmen!!!

Interestingly, as I searched the biblical words during Jesus trial with chief priests and Pilates, I came across Two words mentioned the Bible "Tumult" and "Insurrection" as follows

"When the morning was come, all the chief priests and elders of the people took counsel against Jesus to put him to death: [2] And when they had bound him, they led him away, and delivered him to Pontius Pilate the governor. [17] Therefore when they were gathered together, Pilate said unto them, Whom will ye that I release unto you? Barabbas, or Jesus which is called Christ? [18] For he knew that for envy they had delivered him. [19] When he was set down on the judgment seat, his wife sent unto him, saying, Have thou nothing to do with that just man: for I have suffered many things this day in a dream because of him. [20] But the chief priests and elders persuaded the multitude that they should ask Barabbas, and destroy Jesus. [21] The governor answered and said unto them, Whether of the twain will ye that I release unto you? They said, Barabbas. [22] Pilate saith unto them, What shall I do then with Jesus which is called Christ? They all say unto him, Let him be crucified. [23] And the governor said, Why, what evil hath he done? But they cried out the more, saying, Let him be crucified. [24] When Pilate saw that he could prevail nothing, but that rather a tumult was made, he took water, and washed his hands before the multitude, saying, I am innocent of the blood of this just person: see ye to it. [25] Then answered all the people, and said, His blood be on us, and on our children. [26] Then released he Barabbas unto them: and when he had scourged Jesus, he delivered him to be crucified." Matthew 27:1-2,17-26 KJV

"And straightway in the morning the chief priests held a consultation with the elders and scribes and the whole council, and bound Jesus, and carried him away, and delivered him to Pilate. [2] And Pilate asked him, Art thou the King of the Jews? And he answering said unto him, Thou sayest it. [3] And the chief priests accused him of many things: but he answered nothing. [4] And Pilate asked him again, saying, Answerest thou nothing? behold how many things they witness against thee. [5] But Jesus yet answered nothing; so that Pilate marvelled. [6] Now at that feast he released unto them one prisoner, whomsoever they desired. [7] And there was one named Barabbas, which lay bound with them that had made insurrection with him, who had committed murder in the insurrection. [8] And the multitude crying aloud began to desire him to do as he had ever done unto them. [9] But Pilate answered them, saying, Will ye that I release unto you the King of the Jews? [10] For he knew that the chief priests had delivered him for envy. [11] But the chief priests moved the people, that he should rather release Barabbas unto them. [12] And Pilate answered and said again unto them, What will ye then that I shall do unto him whom ye call the King of the Jews? [13] And they cried out again, Crucify him. [14] Then Pilate said unto them, Why, what evil hath he done? And they cried out the more exceedingly, Crucify him. [15] And so Pilate, willing to content the people, released Barabbas unto them, and delivered Jesus, when he had scourged him, to be crucified." Mark 15:1-15 KJV

"And they began to accuse him, saying, We found this fellow perverting the nation, and forbidding to give tribute to Caesar, saying that he himself is Christ a King. [3] And Pilate asked him, saying, Art thou the King of the Jews? And he answered him and said, Thou sayest it. [4] Then said Pilate to the chief priests and to the people, I find no fault in this man. [5] And they were the more fierce, saying, He stirreth up the people, teaching throughout all Jewry, beginning from Galilee to this place. [10] And the chief priests and scribes stood and vehemently accused him. [18] And they cried out all at once, saying, Away with this man, and release unto us Barabbas: [19] (Who for a certain sedition made in the city, and for murder, was cast into prison.) [20] Pilate therefore, willing to release Jesus, spake again to them. [21] But they cried, saying, Crucify him, crucify him. [22] And he said unto them the third time, Why, what evil hath he done? I have found no cause of death in him: I will therefore chastise him, and let him go. [23] And they were instant with loud voices, requiring that he might be crucified. And the voices of them and of the chief priests prevailed. [24] And Pilate gave sentence that it should be as they required. [25] And he released unto them him that for sedition and murder was cast into prison, whom they had desired; but he delivered Jesus to their will." Luke 23:2-5,10,18-25 KJV

"Then Pilate therefore took Jesus, and scourged him. [2] And the soldiers platted a crown of thorns, and put it on his head, and they put on him a purple robe, [3] And said, Hail, King of the Jews! and they smote him with their hands. [4] Pilate therefore went forth again, and saith unto them, Behold, I bring him forth to you, that ye may know that I find no fault in him. [5] Then came Jesus forth, wearing the crown of thorns, and the purple robe. And Pilate saith unto them, Behold the man! [6] When the chief priests therefore and officers saw him, they cried out, saying, Crucify him, crucify him. Pilate saith unto them, Take ye him, and crucify him: for I find no fault in him. [7] The Jews answered him, We have a law, and by our law he ought to die, because he made himself the Son of God. [8] When Pilate therefore heard that saying, he was the more afraid; [9] And went again into the judgment hall, and saith unto Jesus, Whence art thou? But Jesus gave him no answer. [12] And from thenceforth Pilate sought to release him: but the Jews cried out, saying, If thou let this man go, thou art not Caesar's friend: whosoever maketh himself a king speaketh against Caesar. [13] When Pilate therefore heard that saying, he brought Jesus forth, and sat down in the judgment seat in a place that is called the Pavement, but in the Hebrew, Gabbatha. [15] But they cried out, Away with him, away with him, crucify him. Pilate saith unto them, Shall I crucify your King? The chief priests answered, We have no king but Caesar. [16] Then delivered he him therefore unto them to be crucified. And they took Jesus, and led him away." John 19:1-9,12-13,15-16 KJV

Authoritarian "Brain Wash and further away from the truth" Society!!

"The further a society drifts from truth the more it will hate those who speak it." George Orwell

1984 Novel An authoritarian Society of totalitarianism, mass surveillance, and repressive regimentation of persons and behaviours within society while deprograming those speak out the truth Thematically, Nineteen Eighty-Four centres on the consequences of totalitarianism, mass surveillance, and repressive regimentation of persons and behaviours within society. The novel examines the role of truth and facts within politics and the ways in which they are manipulated. This is the idea that the world would divide into three totalitarian superstates that were rigidly hierarchical, in complete control of information and expression, and engaged in perpetual and unwinnable wars for world domination. Capitalism and liberal democracy seemed moribund; centralized economies and authoritarian regimes looked like the only way modern mass societies could be governed.

I wondered about 3 days, 3 months and 3 years?? I heard no reply back!!

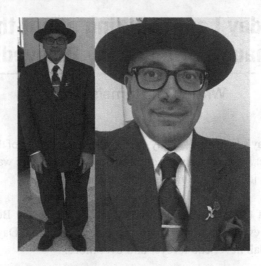

BL. Wonderful gentleman! 💕 Thank you for sharing he message!

CG. Never realized how this has a close similarity to what happened to our last President. Thanks for sharing. You look wonderful as usual, dressed to perfection. 🖤🙏

TM. Yes, I see now the tribunal clearly. Three months....... 🖤

JM. "Fascinating" but True!!

Today I am Thinking about the Inauguration of my Beloved!

Written by Ramsis Ghaly

As I watched today's Inauguration, my eyes shed tears thinking of the Inauguration of my Only Love: Jesus Christ my Lord and Savior! His Name wasn't mentioned once! He is to be inaugurated and celebrated worldwide!

I joined many of the unpopular and have reached out to my Beloved: O Lord waiting for Your everlasting Inauguration and no another that Day of victory and salivation that shall never end forever and ever more!

When are You coming my Lord and Savior! I am ready to take the oath and to return to You my Heavenly Father as the prodigal son had taken and run toward You to be worthy at that Day of thou Inauguration!

The Inauguration shall be for our Lord Jesus! The Son of God, the Only Begotten Son Risen from the death as it is written: "I am Alpha and Omega, the beginning and the ending, saith the Lord, which is, and which was, and which is to come, the Almighty. [13] And in the midst of the seven candlesticks one like unto the Son of man, clothed with a garment down to the foot, and girt about the paps with a golden girdle. [14] His head and his hairs were white like wool, as white as snow; and his eyes were as a flame of fire; [15] And his feet like unto fine brass, as if they burned in a furnace; and his voice as the sound of many waters. [16] And he had in his right hand seven stars: and out of his mouth went a sharp twoedged sword: and his countenance was as the sun shineth in his strength." Revelation 1:8,13-16 KJV

My Beloved inauguration shall not be in the Capitol made of man but it shall be in the Holy City: New Jerusalem coming down from God out of heaven, prepared as a bride adorned for her husband, God shall be with His people as it is written: "And I John saw the holy city, new Jerusalem, coming down from God out of heaven, prepared as a bride adorned for her husband. [3] And I heard a great voice out of heaven saying, Behold, the tabernacle of God is with men, and he will dwell with them, and they shall be his people, and God himself shall be with them, and be their God. [4] And God shall wipe away all tears from their eyes; and there shall be no more death, neither sorrow, nor crying, neither shall there be any more pain: for the former things are passed away." Revelation 21:2-4 KJV

I looked at the ancient Bibles in today's inauguration as they put their hands swearing the solemn oath to fulfill the Constitution promise! My heart ♥ cried to my Lord and Savior saying O DC His Name Jesus and with His Holy Spirit these bibles were written: don't be ashamed to mention His Glorious Name in public!

My heart ♥ is sick love ♥ for my Beloved! He is our True Healer and the Healer of all nations!

At the Inauguration, My Beloved shall restore Justice, holiness and wholeness! Please Come Soon my Lord God!

My Beloved's servants not love in word or in tongue but in deed and in truth: "17 But whoever has this world's goods, and sees his brother in need, and shuts up his heart from him, how does the love of God abide in him? 18 My little children, let us not love in word or in tongue, but in deed and in truth" (1 John 3:17-18)

My Beloved gives no speech but gives Life eternity! My Beloved is the True King of Kings and Lord of Lords Who's Kingdom has no end!

My soul is waiting for the Inauguration of my Heavenly King!

I bought my special uniform and rehearsed my the words of my songs to my Lord at His Inauguration Day!

I am preparing my best ever written poem for my Savior Jesus Christ!

My Beloved knows each one by name and He knows what is in the heart ♥! The constituents are His own children! He created them out of nothing! In His Coming Inauguration He shall sit them by Hus side and dine with Him in His table at His Inauguration Day!

O my Lord when are You coming? Thy people waiting for You!

There is neither a day or night whereas my soul is not thinking of You my Beloved!

You never came to give a talk or to be with a special party!! But You died for all people and shed Your Own Precious blood ◐ for the least before the rich and for the uncommon before the common and for the defame before the fame!

My Beloved is Mighty and coming soon riding over a white horse 🐎 full of Grace and Glory!

My Beloved is so sweet like honey and awesome God! He is indeed shall heal thy people and wipe their tears! He shall lift us up to heaven and manifest Himself to His followers and faithful servants!

At the Inauguration Day, for it is written, As I live, saith the Lord, every knee shall bow to me, and every tongue shall confess to God. So then every one of us shall give account of himself to God. Romans 14:11-12 KJV

My Lord says in preparation of His inauguration: "And when I saw him, I fell at his feet as dead. And he laid his right hand upon me, saying unto me, Fear not; I am the first and the last: [18] I am he that liveth, and was dead; and, behold, I am alive for evermore, Amen; and have the keys of hell and of death. Revelation 1:17-18 KJV

In my Lord Inauguration, there shall be no more politics or diversity, hysteria or betrayal, animosity or lies, viruses or sickness, gowns or face masks, elbow kicks or hand fists, hunger or thirst, terrors or darkness as it is written: "Saying, Amen: Blessing, and glory, and wisdom, and thanksgiving, and honour, and power, and might, be unto our God for ever and ever. Amen. [13] And one of the elders answered, saying unto me, What are these which are arrayed in white robes? and whence came they? [14] And I said unto him, Sir, thou knowest. And he said to me, These are they which came out of great tribulation, and have washed their robes, and made them white in the blood of the Lamb. [15] Therefore are they before the throne of God, and serve him day and night in his temple: and he that sitteth on the throne shall dwell among them. [16] They shall hunger no more, neither thirst any more; neither shall the sun light on them, nor any heat. [17] For the Lamb which is in the midst of the throne shall feed them, and shall lead them unto living fountains of waters: and God shall wipe away all tears from their eyes." Revelation 7:12-17 KJV

My Beloved is God the Most High and no One like Him! When my Beloved comes in His Inauguration, all people not just from America but from the entire world shall attend His Inauguration! And not just the living but all the generations since the beginning of creation, the dead and living! All shall bow to My Beloved when He comes to be Inaugurated!" Revelation 1:17-18 KJV

At my Beloved Inauguration, the earth and heaven shall triumph and rejoice with archangel Michael and Heavenly angels as the dragon called the devil 😈 satan and his demons and spirits shall be firever be casted away in the lake of fire and brimstone: "And there was war in heaven: Michael and his angels fought against the dragon; and the dragon fought and his angels, [8] And prevailed not; neither was their place found any more in heaven. [9] And the great dragon was cast out, that old serpent, called the Devil, and Satan, which deceiveth the whole world: he was cast out into the earth, and his angels were cast out with him. [10] And I heard a loud voice saying in heaven, Now is come salvation, and strength, and the kingdom of our God, and the power of his Christ: for the accuser of our brethren is cast down, which accused them before our God day and night. [11] And they overcame him by the blood of the Lamb, and by the word of their testimony; and they loved not their lives unto the death. [12] Therefore rejoice, ye heavens, and ye that dwell in them. Woe to the inhabiters of the earth and of the sea! for the devil is come down unto you, having great wrath, because he knoweth that he hath but a short time." Revelation 12:7-12 KJV

At the Inauguration of my Beloved the Lord God Almighty and the Holy Lamb, —the twelve gates were twelve pearls; every several gate was of one pearl: and the street of the city was pure gold, as it were transparent glass. And I saw no temple therein: for the Lord God Almighty and the Lamb are the temple of it. And the city had no need of the sun, neither of the moon, to shine in it: for the glory of God did lighten it, and the Lamb is the light thereof. [24] And the nations of them which are saved shall walk in the light of it: and the kings of the earth do bring their glory and honour into it. [25] And the gates of it shall not be shut at all by day: for there shall be no night there. [26] And they shall bring the glory and honour of the nations into it. [27] And there shall in no wise enter into it any thing that defileth, neither whatsoever worketh abomination, or maketh a lie: but they which are written in the Lamb's book of life. Revelation 21:21-27 KJV

Now let us write the list of attendees of my Beloved's inauguration, He is standing at the door and knock and whoever hear His voice and open the door, his name shall be written and surely shall be awarded to sit with Him in His Throne: "Behold, I stand at the door, and knock: if any man hear my voice, and open the door, I will come in to him, and will sup with him, and he with me. [21] To him that overcommit will I grant to sit with me in my throne, even as I also overcame, and am set down with my Father in his throne." Revelation 3:20-21 KJV

While I was dreaming of my Beloved's Inauguration, I was told, His Inauguration day is set by the Heavenly Clock at the fullness of time January 20th in the heavenly Calendar!

Let us be ready to my Beloved Inauguration and do to be worthy saying with the Holy Four Beasts and the twenty four elders: Holy Holy Holy: And the four beasts had each of them six wings about him ; and they were full of eyes within: and they rest not day and night, saying, Holy, holy, holy, Lord God Almighty, which was, and is, and is to come. [9] And when those beasts give glory and honour and thanks to him that sat on the throne, who liveth for ever and ever, [10] The four and twenty elders fall down before him that sat on the throne, and worship him that liveth for ever and ever, and cast their crowns before the throne, saying, [11] Thou art worthy, O Lord, to receive glory and honour and power: for thou hast created all things, and for thy pleasure they are and were created." Revelation 4:8-11 KJV

At our Savior Inauguration, it shall be a pure river of water of life, clear as crystal, proceeding out of the throne of God and of the Lamb. [2] In the midst of the street of it, and on either side of the river, was there the tree of life, which bare twelve manner of fruits, and yielded her fruit every month: and the leaves of the tree were for the healing of the nations. And there shall be no more curse: but the throne of God and of the Lamb shall be in it; —

The Spirit and the bride say Come to Your Inauguration Day, please come, come soon: "And he shewed me a pure river of water of life, clear as crystal, proceeding out of the throne of God and of the Lamb. [2] In the midst of the street of it, and on either side of the river, was there the tree of life, which bare twelve manner of fruits, and yielded her fruit every month: and the leaves of the tree were for the healing of the nations. [3] And there shall be no more curse: but the throne of God and of the Lamb shall be in it; and his servants shall serve him: [4] And they shall see his face; and his name shall be in their foreheads. [5] And there shall be no night there; and they need no candle, neither light of the sun; for the Lord God giveth them light: and they shall reign for ever and ever. [6] And he said unto me, These sayings are faithful and true: and the Lord God of the holy prophets sent his angel to shew unto his servants the things which must shortly be done. [7] Behold, I come quickly: blessed is he that keepeth the sayings of the prophecy of this book. [12] And, behold, I come quickly; and my reward is with me, to give every man according as his work shall be. [13] I am Alpha and Omega, the beginning and the end, the first and the last. [14] Blessed are they that do his commandments, that they may have right to the tree of life, and may enter in through the gates into the city. [15] For without are dogs, and sorcerers, and whoremongers, and murderers, and idolaters, and whosoever loveth and maketh a lie. [16] I Jesus have sent mine angel to testify unto you these things in the churches. I am the root and the offspring of David, and the bright and morning star. [17] And the Spirit and the bride say, Come. And let him that heareth say, Come. And let him that is athirst come. And whosoever will, let him take the water of life freely." Revelation 22:1-7,12-17 KJV

Amen to the Coming of my Beloved Jesus Inauguration!!!

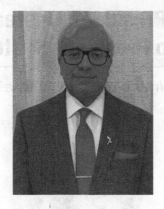

JM. AMEN

KE. Goodness Great Writing

TY RAMSIS*

BL. So very true.

DL. Amen.

CR. Beautifully said ‼️ Looking forward to my Savior's inauguration. Every knee will bow. Maranatha! 🙏🙏🙏

JM. Beautiful

CG. Your devotion to God is so inspiring. Thank you and bless you! 🖤🙏

TM. We understand, and we're ready for HIS inauguration 🖤. God bless you, Ramsis.

<u>GR.</u> AMEN !!!

Trio Presidents Instead of Unio President System!

Written by Ramsis Ghaly

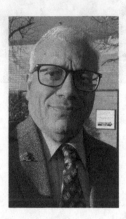

America 🇺🇸 it is the Time to have Trio Presidents and Not just one!!

The system of Uno-Leader of a nation is ancient and outdated and it is the time for a change! It is the time to abandon the old traditional system and implement a multi-sharing system of Trio-Presidents, Trio-Kings and Trio-Queens! The Uno-King, Uno-Queen and Uno-President is 6000 years old and isn't compatible with the multitudes of highly developed nations possess millions of frontier human brains 💬💬💬 well diverse and continently and intercontinentally connected!

In an era with so much views, numerous views and unlimited ethnic culture diversity and very strong believes that no longer one doctrine or one discipline ruled by one party is sufficient to address such diverse nations! Perhaps, update the government be divided into three sections and each section has an equally responsible president with his or her autonomy but not all responsibilities are fallen upon one person but instead three equally ranked leaders!!!

Perhaps the ongoing challenges in selecting the ideal president for a huge nation is simply explained by the doctrine of one president may no longer be accepted or held true by all people with modern civilized human minds! And perhaps it is the time fir a change from having Uno m-president to Trio-presidents System sharing the burden to lead the nation with all its diversities and demands!

As the Heavenly Trinity so is three presidents working together as one not competing but completing each other to meet the modern challenges and the unlimited demands!

The time of one president, one king and one queen is gone!! It was the past! The intricacies among the people, diversities among constituents and the widespread of urbanites demand much more than one president and one ruler! The time of man or woman show is over!

The world 🌐 now is much sophisticated and can't run with one president or even two presidents but three sounds ideal!

It is the Time to Consider Having Three Presidents!! It is hard to believe that one person and one brain could exist to lead the most advanced nation in the world in 2020! We aren't any longer just yes people!

Who said a hug country as America must have one president??
The modern era is all about specialization and one person can't do it all!
It is the Time to Consider Having Two Presidents!!
In fact, it is the time to assign up to three presidents as the Holy Trinity and assign the responsibility of each!

Now it is the time to rewrite history and establish updated version of our constitution and the world shall follow America!

The idea of one president, one show and one commander is over! It is the time to share talents and gifts to be able to compete with highly complex world we live in and be able to lead diversity and conquer adversities!!

Trio-Presidents Instead of Unio-President System! America 🇺🇸 it is the Time to have Trio Presidents and Not just one!!

Thank you 🙏
Ramsis Ghaly

KE. Great Doctor
AA. I prefer the Constitution as written. We have three branches, Executive, Senate & House and the Judicial.
I think that is the trinity.
CG. I would have a hard time excepting trio-presidents, except if they were all related and had same political views. 🖤🙏

Guard against the Fallen America!!

United States 🇺🇸 is moving from leading the world, free creative innovative America, the land of opportunity, ambition, dreams and achieving the impossible where MARS is it's limit in Lord Jesus Name to being a follower crumbling in a narrow angle pass, intimidated, restricted, terrorized, rioting, being told what-to-do, restrained under godless doctrine, controlled and slaved by little metallic buttons and hard drive technology, little robots and drones mastered under do calked "artificial intelligence"!!!

The movement in 1960's will be forever remembered for being the best page of American history where our brave men and women refused status quo and have transformed America from scratch to a New Free Visionary America 🇺🇸 today that made the world look up to America 🇺🇸! While those brave men and women trusted us to continue their dreams and instead, the land of brave and free, the nation of liberty and opportunity is being held captive to stubborn minds and if left alone it is going away before our eyes hiding behind the metallic brainless industry under cover of convenient interpretation of the constitution!

Ramsis Ghaly

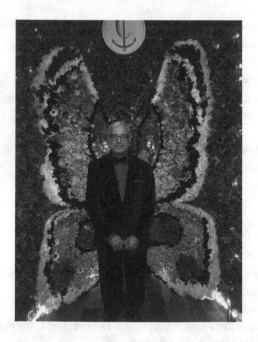

954

AV. Very well said!! And that's a great photo!! 🖤🙏

BK. God is in control

VA. We becoming the land of hate, arrogance, snobbery, lying. We wonder why God has not lifted the pestilence. With so much hate and vengeance in high places. With laws and politicians letting babies be murdered.

Hate is brewing like a volcano.

JC. Makes me fear for my grandkids, what life they will have 😫 Nice picture Dr. Ghaly 😃

RC. What a lovely photo!

CR. But God!!!

CG. This year has been a constant test of my emotional endurance and it is only getting worse. I pray to our Lord to help stop the virus and to repair our broken country. 🖤🙏

KG. Great photo!

We are broken 😟. We must continue to pray for healing 🙏

RH. I am with you doctor. We must change into something more beautiful. Now is the time. God Bless you

MH. I hope & pray that 2021 brings us much needed peace & joy. Also an end to the virus. Great picture of you.

TG. Great pictures of you. Pray God help and protect our country. Pray for democracy not sell our country to China it very difficult time for all of us. All we do is Prayers. 🙏🙏🙏

A Christian Phone Call Biden-Trump Working Together!!

Sunday column written by Ramsis Ghaly

America 🇺🇸 needs Jesus the good Shephard!! Jesus said: John 10:11 KJV "I am the good shepherd: the good shepherd giveth his life for the sheep."

Our Lord Jesus is looking at America 🇺🇸 and His heart is moving with compassion because "—they fainted, ah and were scattered abroad, as sheep having no shepherd." Matthew 9:36-38 KJV "But when he saw the multitudes, he was moved with compassion on them, because they fainted, and were scattered abroad, as sheep having no shepherd. [37] Then saith he unto his disciples, The harvest truly is plenteous, but the labourers are few; [38] Pray ye therefore the Lord of the harvest, that he will send forth labourers into his harvest."

America 🇺🇸 today is divided and the two parties are tearing each other and the people are in the middle. Darkness lead to darkness and gate feed with hate and the cycle is vicious!!! Destruction is imminent if not stopped and the hate replaced by love and authoritianship changed to for the people and not the rulers. Our lord Jesus words to Todays America 🇺🇸 politics: "And if a kingdom be divided against itself, that kingdom cannot stand. [25] And if a house be divided against itself, that house cannot stand." Mark 3:24-25 KJV

[OBJ]

The American people had enough and ready to explode 💥 between political curfew, COVID imprisonment and social isolation and no more leg to stand if any further touching words or move!
[OBJ]

My New logo to redirect the uprising in America 🇺🇸 and unrest to hang it, to talk about it and to teach it every where is:

"America 🇺🇸 America 🇺🇸 America 🇺🇸 The Land of the Brave, Unity, Prosperity and Opportunity! America 🇺🇸 America America 🇺🇸"

O my gosh how far one sincere Christian phone call between Biden and Trump will take the entire nation?? It will go so far!! It will dissolve much mistrust, apprehension and hate. It will bring both parties together and lead the country to healing, unity and prosperity! How much both will share and do that will unit and heal the people! This what our Lord Jesus want to see!

For Unity to occur, it needs a faithful Christian Phone call 📱📞☎️ well heartedly virtual communication! For God sake, talk for the good of America!!! No one cares about America 🇺🇸 except America! The outside world 🌍 is so dangerously sophisticated and the competition of powers is unrelenting!

A Christian Phone Call to begin Working Together is the only way for true healing and unity! The first step is what it takes to open the doors!

A lengthy speech, a touching poet, lady Gaga, Jennifer Lopez, Garth Brook,———— will not cut it! There are so much goodness, expertise, wisdom and skills in both parties to be shared if we love one another and come close to each other—-!

America needs an urgent Father look at all people as one! The entire staff; the congress, senate and house representatives needs to take a crash course and an urgent spiritual and professional in-service and full obligatory course on love, healing and unity!

The roots of all evil is money and ego! The White House and Oval Office needs prayers and urgent actions to eradicate ego and money!!!

I wonder who will be first to make a phone call 📞 Biden or Trump??? Compromise, sacrifice, meet have way and keep building America!!

There is so much to lose and more destruction and breakdown to do if we didn't get it together as one leading nation and our differences are huge! Please I beg you all take the first step and see how much love will follow and how far we as one nation will go!! Ease the pains and sufferings and be the exemplary nation as America always been!

America 🇺🇸 America 🇺🇸 America 🇺🇸 The Land of the Brave, Unity and Opportunity! America 🇺🇸 America 🇺🇸 merica 🇺🇸

We must speak about it! Let us face it! The true of the matter is the nation's gab is getting wider and wider and the world is laughing at America!

One administration is tearing apart the other in public and out loud disrespectful and egocentric!

Who will remove the ego and look at a country as one people and reach out to the other Aisle!

Words of unity and healing for the nation are easy but actual deeds are hard! But the first step is what it takes to open the doors!

Where are the so called spiritual leaders and professional coaches to step in and intervene between the two administrations and help bridging and cross the aisle for the sake of people!

With love, unity and healing and neither ego nor money, they will result in healthy decisions to serve the American people and not immature orders for the sake of revenge, show, ego and money!!!

This is the true spirit of our Lord Christ! Our Savior Lord Jesus said in the Aptitudes Matthew 5:8-9 KJV "Blessed are the pure in heart: for they shall see God. [9] Blessed are the peacemakers: for they shall be called the children of God."

Amen 🙏 Lord Jesus for the sake of thy people and our nation and the country You love 💜 please come and send Your Holy Spirit! Our nation is crumbling, full of hate and disgrace and each party is busy tearing the other apart while Satan and the world are laughing at us and America Politics are viewed no longer as a mature but as an immature nation!!!

A Christian Phone Call Biden-Trump Working Together!!

My New logo to redirect the uprising in America 🇺🇸 and unrest to hang it, to talk about it and to teach it everywhere is:

America 🇺🇸 America 🇺🇸 America 🇺🇸 The Land of the Brave, Unity, Prosperity and Opportunity! America 🇺🇸 America 🇺🇸 America

Let us pray Amen.

Respectfully
Ramsis Ghaly

JG. Yes !! Everyone should read this, it's perfect Dr. 🙏🙏
BT. Dr. Ramsis Ghali. Thank you for your wise and touching words in such a difficult situation.

GR. Sadly, that one call will never happen. If done, will never be accepted. We are left with prayers.

CG. You are so knowledgeable and give such solid advice. It would be amazing if they would talk for the good of America. ♥🤚

AM. Maravilha... Deus conosco sempre...

GS. No more Republicans! Now it's the PATRIOTS PARTY!

Do not you think a global warming is a better choice than the deadly and dreadful freezing cold weather?

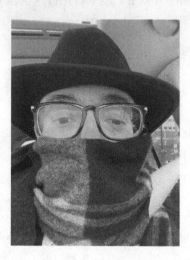

Don't you think a global warming is a better choice than the deadly and dreadful freezing cold weather across America affecting the country nationwide!!!

Electricity is out, pipes are blocked, streets are slippery and cars are climbing above each other—!!

America stay warm and please protect yourself against the freezing cold! It is deadly and dreadful to the human flesh??

Ramsis Ghaly

JBV. Dr. Ghaly. Please stay warm and safe. Be very careful, falls are so devastating!!

Scientists confused everyone when first calling it global warming. It made people think that everything would get warmer and warmer. In some places like the glaciers, and polar ice caps things are getting warmer and melting. But in other places things are getting colder. They then changed the name to climate change in an attempt to cause less confusion. What we are seeing is strange climate changes and climate shifts colder or warmer in many places in the world. Some may change permanently and others just have become erratic. Stay safe Dr. G.

BL. Brrrrr is that you under the warm scarf, Dr Ghaly? Thank you for being the wonderful person you are 🖤

KO. Be safe Dr Ghaly, and all your associates, and everyone in this frigid snowy weather

CG. Brrrrr it is so cold. Stay warm under that scarf. 🖤🙏

MS. Stay warm. 🙈

JD. Stay warm and safe Dr. Ghaly !!!

LG. Stay safe Professor.

A Puzzle with dead end no one could figure to solve Palestine and Israel!

A Puzzle with dead end no one could figure
to solve: Palestine ≈ and Israel ☲
Written by Ramsis Ghaly

Two very different parties with no similarities whatsoever and praying to two different Gods and under two radically different cultures, backgrounds and inheritance were negotiating a peace deal to coexist together!!

Both came to the same so called a "Peace Deal" and the world powers as well, arrived to the same conclusion that each party must have an independent home!

Yet both are competing for the same home!

Can both be an independent state in the same address, in the same home and the same location at the same time???

How can both share the same home, the same location, the same roof and yet each be an independent state??

The fact is over time the differences between both parties never ever been dissolved or came close but despite centuries of causalities and very significant loses atrocities between both parties continued so strong!!

If however, both parties continue to compete for or live in the same home, the home will be divided against itself cannot stand and be brought to desolation as our Teacher said: Matthew 12:25-28 KJV Every kingdom divided against itself is brought to desolation; and every city or house divided against itself shall not stand: [26] And if Satan cast out Satan, he is divided against himself; how shall then his kingdom stand? [27] And if I by Beelzebub cast out devils, by whom do your children cast them out? therefore they shall be your judges. [28] But if I cast out devils by the Spirit of God, then the kingdom of God is come unto you.

Only if —-

The same home has double faces and double personalities!

The same home in the same location can possibly exist in two places in the same time!

If each party is from different nature such as one physical and the other spiritual!!

Physically if in the fantasy world of unrealism where the law of physics permit one home occupied by two and yet considered independent home for each and it comes the time that two independent states be in the same region, in the same time under the same roof breathing the same air, sleeping in the same bed, having the same interest and governed by the same government! Only theoretically in the out space reality show

This can only occur if LOVE 💜💜 IS ABSOLUTE in this equation and no difference exist between the two parties!!!! Love not only dissolve differences and boundaries but promote transparency and break all walls and—-As it is written: 1 Corinthians 13:1-8 KJV 1] Though I speak with the tongues of men and of angels, and have not charity, I am become as sounding brass, or a tinkling cymbal. [2] And though I have the gift of prophecy, and understand all mysteries, and all knowledge; and though I have all faith, so that I could remove mountains, and have not charity, I am nothing. [3] And though I bestow all my goods to feed the poor, and though I give my body to be burned, and have not charity, it profiteth me nothing. [4] Charity suffereth long, and is kind; charity envieth not; charity vaunteth not itself, is not puffed up, [5] Doth not behave itself unseemly, seeketh not her own, is not easily provoked, thinketh no evil; [6] Rejoiceth not in iniquity, but rejoiceth in the truth; [7] Beareth all things, believeth all things, hopeth all things, endureth all things. [8] Charity never faileth: but whether there be prophecies, they shall fail; whether there be tongues, they shall cease; whether there be knowledge, it shall vanish away.

Only between a husband and wife married under One God snd became one flesh: Genesis 2:24 KJV

[24] Therefore shall a man leave his father and his mother, and shall cleave unto his wife: and they shall be one flesh.

Only between the Goid Shepherd and His sheep a one sheep for One Good Shephard as it is written: John 10:16 KJV 16] And other sheep I have, which are not of this fold: them also I must bring, and they shall hear my voice; and there shall be one fold, and one shepherd.

Israel 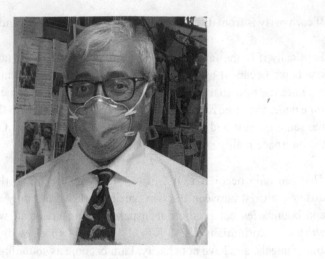 and Palestine ⌐ we pray for you both! We pray! 🙏🙏🙏

Respectfully

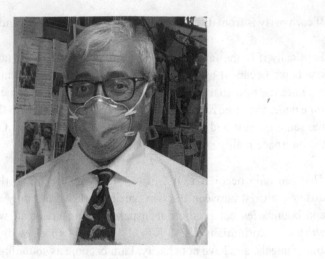

DM. Only love can solve it.
CG. Prayers for Israel! 🙏🙏🙏
NC. Heartbreaking with no easy answer.

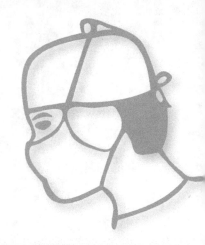

SECTION 19

With My Residents and Students During COVID 19

My two wonderful residents Brian and Shaun surprised me today!! Both bought my book: "A Christian from Egypt: a life story of a neurosurgeon and quadruple boards"

My residents decided one of the ways to learn about their mentor is to read his memoir book. So smart! So kind and thoughtful of them, so touched.

After I autographed the book, Brian and Shaun requested to take a camera picture imitating my picture in the back cover of the book 📘 and so I did! https://books.google.com/.../A_Christian_from_Egypt.html...

Thank you 🙏 Shaun and Brian. So proud of you both! I pray you find my book useful and beneficial! Much blessing

Ramsis Ghaly

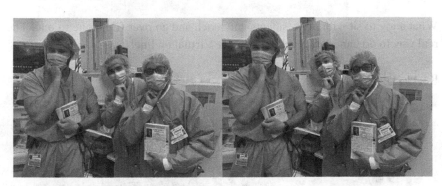

PN. Much love Dr Ghaly my friend!
KJ. So sweet! You are a mentor to many, Dr. Ghaly!!!
VK. Beautiful 🖤🖤🖤
MS. Nice 😄
TJ. So cool.
PS. Good luck Shaun and Brian ... follow the lead of Dr **Ramsis Ghaly** and your career will be most rewarding
SP. They are learning from the BEST!
MD/ Wonderful book. I read it.

With My Residents During COVID Unfolding

Teaching our residents in the midst of COVID surge and at the time of healthcare storm! Bless you all!

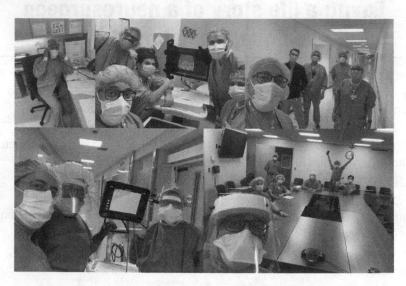

What a joy to sit with my residents and teach and go over films one to one! The real way to do hands-on teaching and not Virtual on line!

Ramsis Ghaly

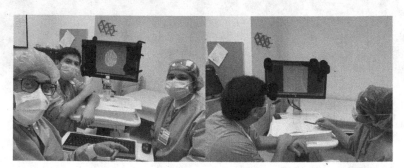

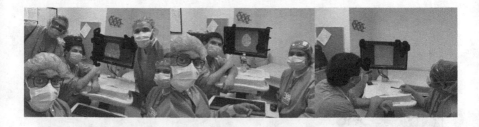

GS. They are learning from the best! I sure hope they realize how lucky they are!

CW. Show them MY brain Dr. Ghaly & see if THEY can get me to live 14 years longer than I should have + still going strong!!!

TM. They are blessed to have you teach them!

CG. You are an extraordinary doctor. They are fortunate to have you guiding them to be the best they can be. 🖤🙏

PR. Ahhh, thank you for this..

LW. You truly have the message of what working in medicine is all about,,,,i.e. the patient!

BL. Thank you for sharing this!

JM. Congrat's To In Person Teaching Dr. Ghaly. 💕

RH. Thank you. Hero's

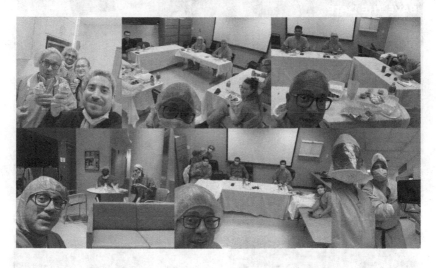

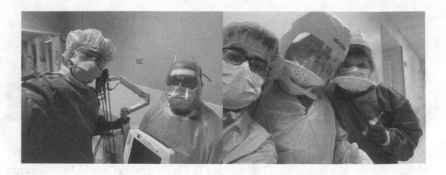

January 2021

This year has been very challenging for all of us and I am very thankful to all of my colleagues and friends who helped me make this NANS 2021 virtual meeting a big success with 1,690 participants!!!

I hope to see all of you in person at the summer NANS meeting - July 15-17, 2021 in Orlando

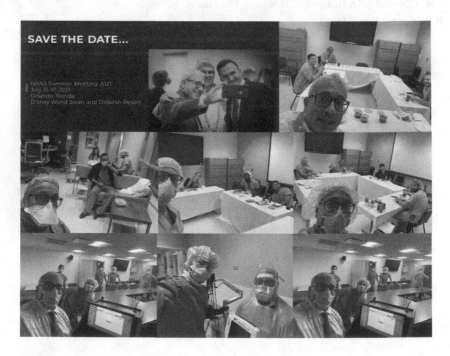

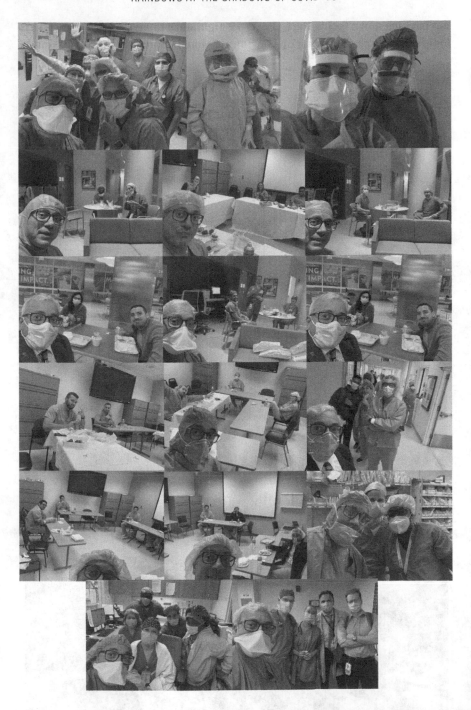

The Journey of frontline with my residents continues for the second year in the row. Thank you 🙏 all for all what you do, your sacrifice and persistence not backing down facing the COVID-19 nightmare to saves lives as you all are looking forward to moving on continuing your journey across our nation!!!

Ramsis Ghaly

The Academic Year is almost over for our residents and their graduation 🎓 🎓 🎓 is coming soon!! So many days and nights on call together to prepare them for that day!! So proud of each of them!!

Ramsis Ghaly

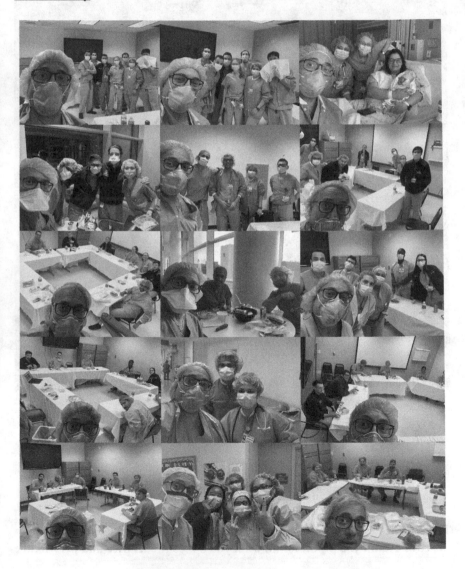

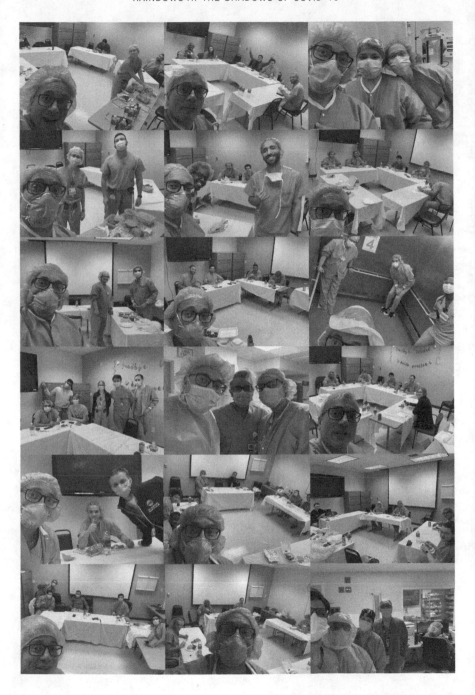

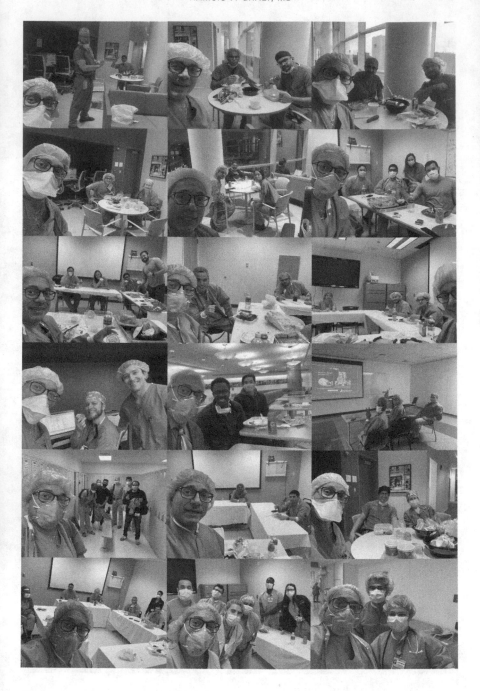

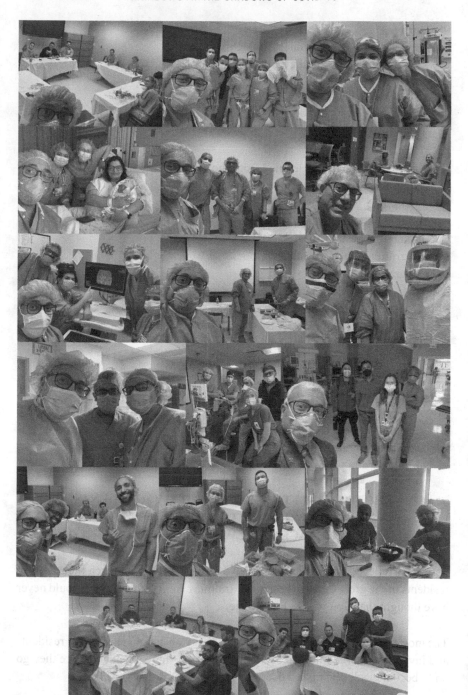

PS. family 💕
BM. Congratulations Everyone!
CR. Congratulations to all the residents!
DL. ravo!!
CG. What a wonderful achievement.
Congratulations to you all and may God guide you in your future endeavors.
Bless you all!
RR. Thanks, still teaching
JC. You young people have learned from the master.
DM. congrats you had the best mentor
AP. Looks like you eat a lot! 😜😆 Congratulations and best of luck to your
residents! I bet you are a great teacher.
HM. You're the best doctor 💜
JU. Congratulations to you all!
VG Congratulations 💜💜💜
AV. That's awesome! Congratulations! & God Bless each one! 🐵
MR. Congratulations! Well deserved!
AG. God bless you dear Dr. CG. Be safe all of you and God Bless. 🙏💜
GC. They're learning from the best.
Ed. Please stay safe and healthy
Cg. You all work so hard. Bless you all and stay safe. 💜🙏 My Trainees since
1991, so proud
MR. Congratulations! Well deserved!
AB. Congratulations to all the graduates, thank you for your dedication and
sacrifice. You have been prepared to step into your profession by the best,
absolutely and you will make him proud!!!

PHOTOS FROM THE PAST, WITH MY RESIDENTS
IN THE PAST PRIOR TO THE PANDEMIC BEFORE
THE FACEMASK WAS MANDATED.

I am So privileged and so honored to have the opportunity to teach thousands of
residents in the great Chicago best major trauma centers since 1991. I would never
have thought that God will be kind to me.

The most spectacular time is at the end of a heavy on call and gather my residents
and invite them for a dinner to eat all together and share so much before they go
on to become well established doctors in the great country of USA. ...

Thank you all students, residents, staff and hospital programs that trusted me in doing so

Thank you Lord Jesus, my Lord and Savior.
Ramsis Ghaly

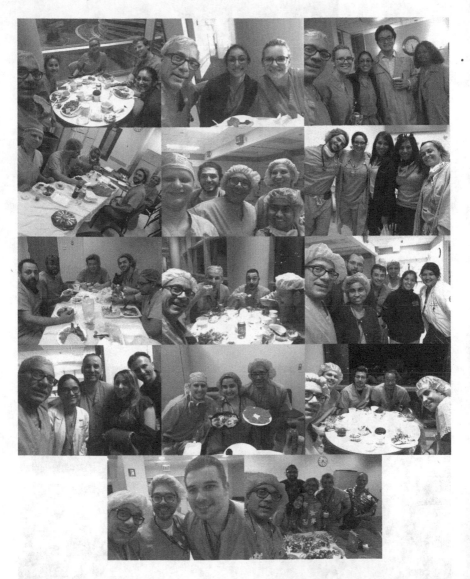

JP. Can't wait till we will all feel safe to burn our masks. In the meantime, we will follow protocol and be patient. God is in control

977

My new year Eve with my Residents serving COVID 19 Patients.

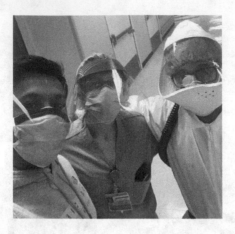

My last Intubation of COVID-19 in New Year Eve of 2020!

Let us open a New Page for 2021 to thy will in our Savior Name Jesus the Lord!

Thank you 🙏 all! Much love and blessing to you all! Happy New Year.

Ramsis Ghaly

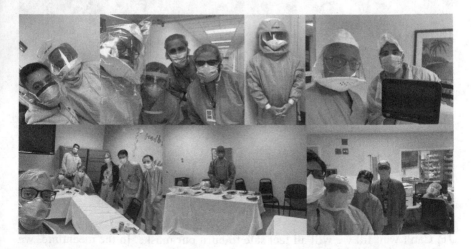

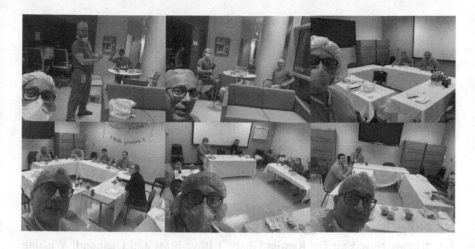

GR. DEAR RAMSIS !!! New is the year, new are the hopes and the aspirations,

New is the resolution, new are the spirits and…
Forever my warm wishes are for you
Have a promising and fulfilling New Year
Here is a wishing that the coming year is a glorious
One that rewards all your future endeavors with success…
Wishing you heartfelt and prosperous

Happy New Year !!!

ND. Happy New Year! Thank you for all you do!

VV. Happy New year Dr.Ghaly

LL. Happy New Year!!!! GOD Bless you. 🙏🙏🙏

JD. HNY my friend.. bless you for all you do!

AA. Happy new year 2021! God bless you always.

SJ. Happy New Year, Dr. Ghaly. I wish you, your residents and your family back
home blessing for a healthy and joyous New Year 🖤

YA. Happy New Year ✨🥂🎉 Thank you for all you do! 🌷

CG. Happy New Years Eve to you all. Be safe! 🖤🙏

PP. Happy New Year!

DM. happy safe new year

AB. Blessed, brother.

MB. Happy New Year Dr. Ghaly!!!!

RN. Blessings to all 🖤🖤🙏🥲

KG. Happy New Year and God Bless you and your team

KO. Lord bless you and your staff now and always for a safe and better New year 🙏🙏

KE. AMEN

KC. Thank you for all you do Dr. Ghaly. Happy New Year!

RS. Happy New Year 🎁

LM. God Bless you all 🙏🙏🙏

PP. May God blessed you all 🙏

AB. Praise God

KG. Happy New Years to you and your colleagues, Dr. Ghaly 🎉

LW. Wishing you a wonderful 2021 Ramsis with less hours treating Covid patients..... 🖤🖤

JC. Happy New Year Dr Ghaly! God bless you!

NE. Happy New Year 🍷 🎁🎉

KJ. "Happy New Year Dr. Ramiss Ghaly"! Love Starr and Diamond! Wishing you Love, Hope, Peace, Health and Prosperity!

KS. Happy New Year!! 🎉🎉

JH. Happy New Year, Dr. Ghaly.

JM. AMEN 💕 "Happy New Year 2021" 💕

AR. Happy and healthy New Year.

VW. Happy healthy New Year, Dr. Ghaly!

ED. Safety, health, love and hugs to you all

VM. Happy New Year! God bless! 🎉🎉🎆

RP. I say it all the time- Thank you for all you do!!!

SN. Happy New Year. Dr. Ghaly!!

MR. Wising you a year fill a joy and health and happiness God bless you doctor

AS. Happy and blessed new year!

SS. Happy New Year! God Bless you!

MB. Happy and blessed New Year Dr. Ghaly

BM. Happy New Year! 🌷 God Bless you!

GH. Happy new year

Gh. Happy new year

Ch. May God bless you and your team!

Mp. Happy 2021!

Ap. Happy New Year 🎁🍷 🎉

As. Happy new year! Stay safe!

Pe.r. 'm grateful for this, I'm on the frontline everyday myself, good greetings to all, may the new year bring health, love and joy for all.

Ns. Happy New Year! My God bless you abundantly!

Kg. Happiest of New Year's 2021, Dr Ramsis Ghaly. God Bless you abundantly! Love from Egypt.

Years ago with our angels

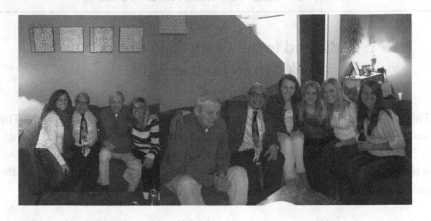

KC. Awe, one of my favorite Christmas's, loved spending it with you!
BB. Love this Dr. Ghaly!

End of the Academic Year!!

Dedicated to the Graduating Residents
Written by Ramsis Ghaly

This End of the Academic Year for our Residents and Students Nationwide! The senior class of residents and students is graduating and the new class is joining!

It is a month of celebration and joy for the great accomplishment and perhaps the best to achieve this far!

It comes in a time, the new graduates regain full Independent, maturity and ready to practice! It is that time they all have been waiting for!

It is the time full of excitement as the doors of opportunities are wide open and countless potentials about to explode!

Yet, unsurprisingly, it is joined with mixed feeling!!

Separation anxiety and apprehension in regard to a new beginning full of challenges and decision-making!!

And a chapter full of unknowns and pages to be written and title and subtitles to be determined!!

It is the first step to an endless potential: dreams to achieve, fantasies to become reality, freeways to drive through, skies to fly, walkways to step in, many doors to open and choices to make!

There is that "Learning Curve" and always learning and more new things to learn, experiences to gain and skills to acquire!

The beginning is beautiful and so is tomorrow you have earned every piece of it and you deserve nothing than the best! The love, the sacrifices, the dedication, the commitment and the list keep going—-

You aren't alone, we the mentors worry as the mother to her children! The bond is real and the emotions are high! You are our dreams and the reason of our purpose and the cause of our living! We will miss each and every one of you! You are part of us as we are part of you! You will take us with you!

For all my four decades, every year is the first year for me full of excitement and joy with appreciation and gratitude! I am so privileged and honored to be considered a mentor for you all! You are my reason to keep going and rejuvenate my soul and flourish my dreams and legacy for generations to come!

They indeed all deserve congratulations and best wishes to a bright future ahead!

You all are in our hearts and thoughts knowing we have the full trust in each and every one of you!

Stay in touch and our love and prayers always with you all Amen.

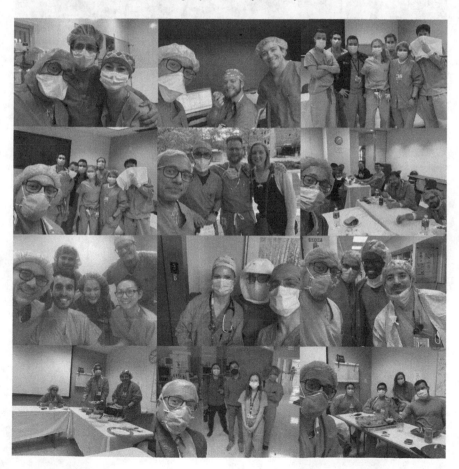

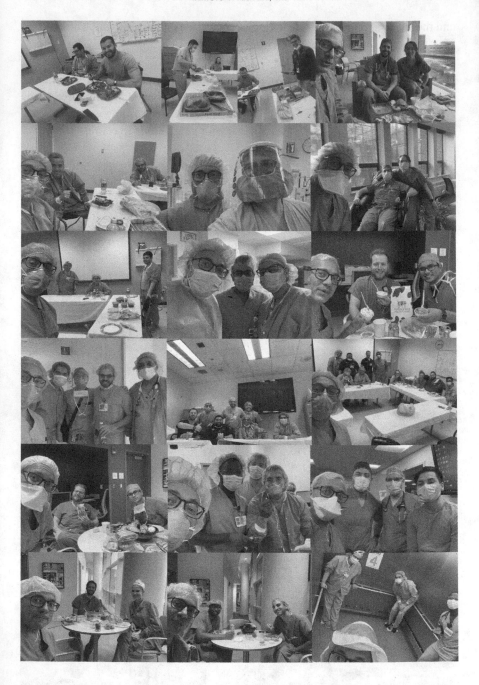

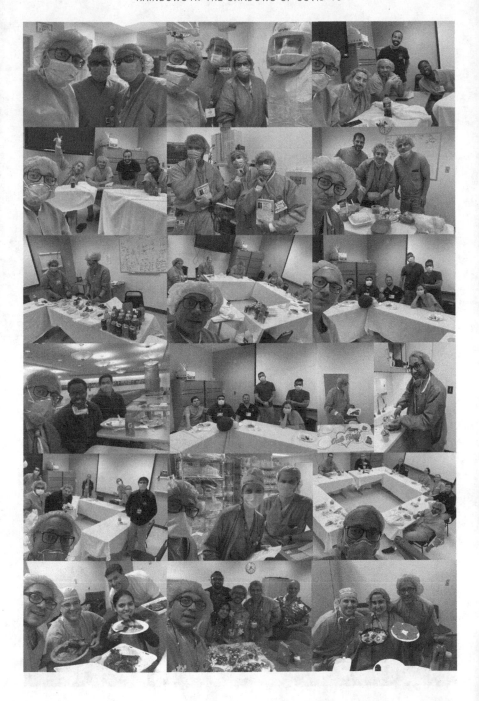

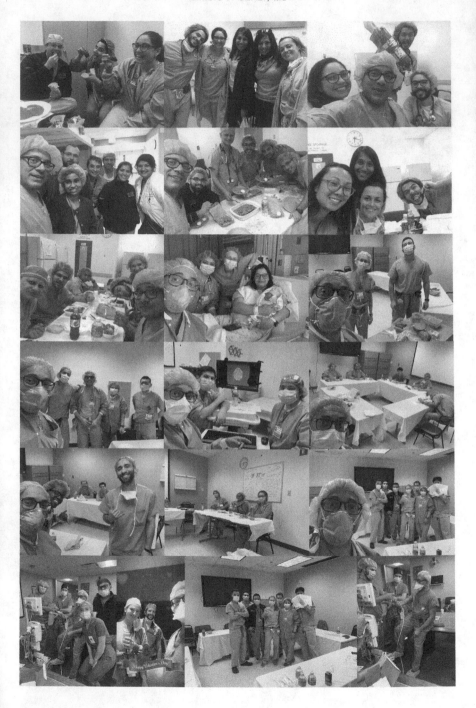

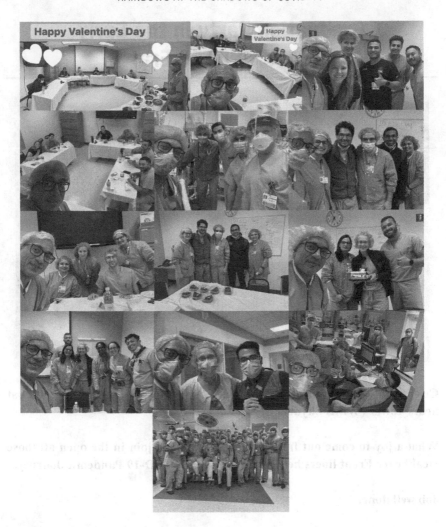

MS. Congratulations!

SK. They have learned from the best!!

KG. Congratulations!

JG. Awesome! Congratulations!

DL. Best teacher ever!

DL. That's awesome! Congratulations!

KG. So lucky to have you as their mentor and teacher, Dr. Ghaly!!!

SP. That's awesome!

Congratulations

ML. Congrats!!

CG: Congratulations to all! Good luck as you begin your new journey! Dr. Ghaly is the best mentor you could have.

Graduation Party in the Early PostCOVID-19 Era!

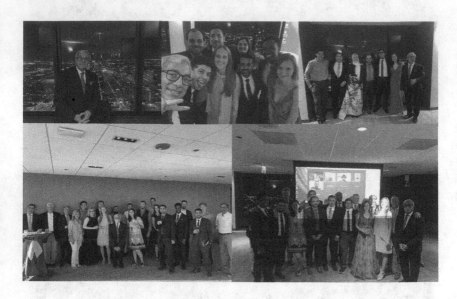

Celebrating graduation of JSH of Cook County Hospital senior Class 2021 at Sears Tower (Willis Skydeck).

What a joy to come out from social limitation to join in the open all those Healthcare Front liners heroes through the COVID-19 Pandemic Journey.

Job well done!

Full of emotions wishing the best of those spectacular hardworking residents to care for our patients nationwide and carrying along our legacy!

Can't be more proud. May our Lord keep you all safe and bless all your steps!!!

Ramsis Ghaly

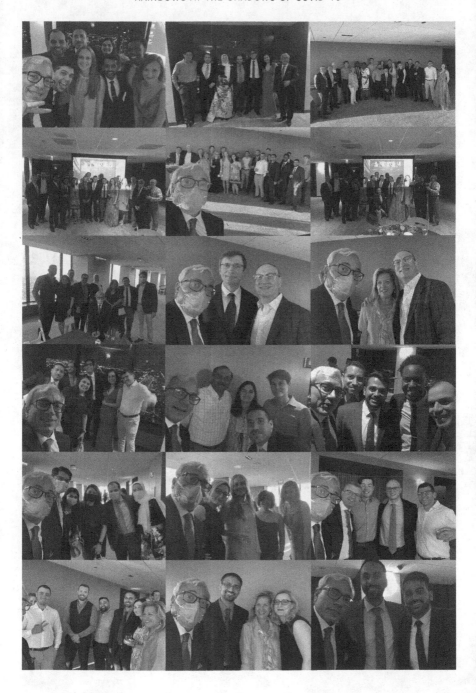

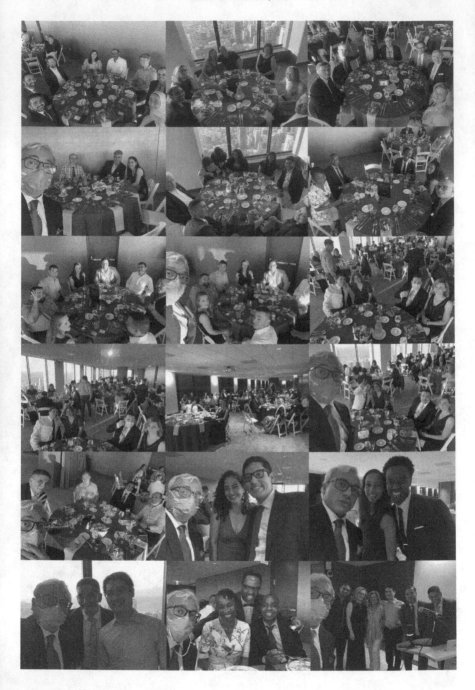

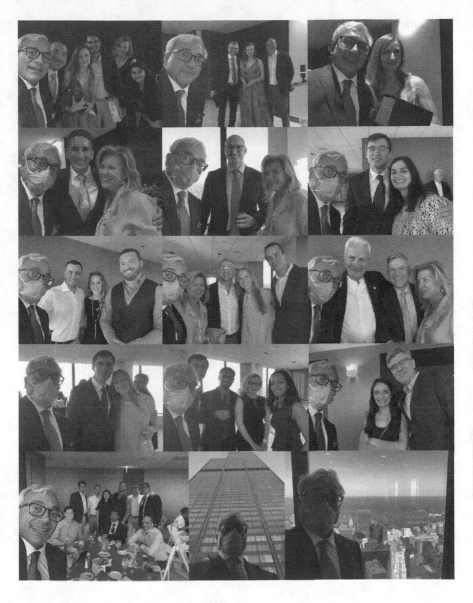

OC. Congratulations! And good luck!
BM. Congratulations Everyone and God Bless!
NE. Congrats!
AL. Congratulations graduates. God bless you all.
SM. Congratulations 🎉

SJ. Congratulations
MG. Awesome congrats!
CG. Congratulations to all the graduates! Best wishes for your next adventure.
CP. Congrats to all! 🎉🎉
AV. Congratulations
& God Bless all of u!

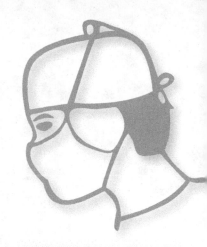

Section 20

Illness Journey Goodbye
2020 to my Patients!

My gratitude 🙏 to all my patients entrusted my device! Much blessing as 2020 is almost past and new year 2021 at the door.

The illness journey isn't easy but it is full of joy when recovery is complete!

It is a journey of suffering and aches beyond belief!

With no warning and overnight, it throws the human flesh to the floor!

Illness Journey is a life changing event and leaves a lasting painful memories!

It won't be forgotten and the both the Fallin and Rescuer are to be praised!

What a fulfillment when you see Jesus accompany the ill and reach out the sick and says to the suffering soul; "Don't be afraid I am with You"!

In fact, as a physician and surgeon, I am honored to be trusted to care for such a soul and witness, Jesus's hand reaches out to do the miracle!

The fact is, each human flesh is destined to fail and everybody must get sick! There isn't eternity in the human flesh formed from dust but life eternal in the human spirit within!

Therefore, together let us fight the good fight and go through the illness journey in courage with no fear standing strong together praying the Lord of Healing, letting it end according to God's destiny!

Carlos is going back to work. Praise our Lord Jesus!

Thank you Carlos for beautiful gifts 🎁 and best wishes! Amen 🙏

Ramsis Ghaly
Www.ghalyneurosurgeon.com

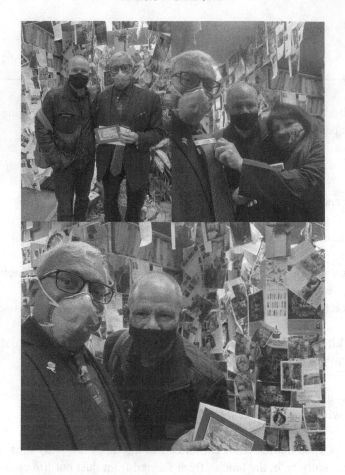

CG. Great looking tie you received.

MA. Amen in Jesus name

JP. Thank you for using your medical skill to heal my daughter in law, Amy Witte

My Patients during the Unfolding COVID

Anthony Fauci Christmas Dress
Eye shield white with crystal glass
Green N95 Mask
Navy blue gown
Pink gloves

I am okay with Fauci Christmas dress Abd virtuality but I really need real Christmas wrapped gifts 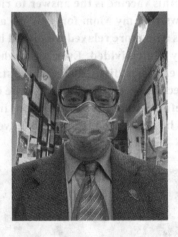 and Stimulus check! Don't you all okay with that????

Be Ready for 2021 Professional Clinic Attire!

Blue gown and blue facemask well-sealed and pink gloves with virtual reality and loneliness with NO handshakes, kisses or hugs but limited hands-on care.

Welcome aboard! I do the best I can and I never once closed my clinic to see patients that needed to be seen!

Ramsis Ghaly
Www.ghalyneurosurgeon.com

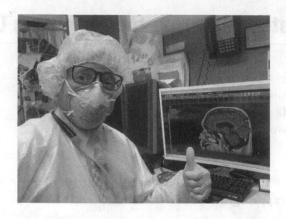

Cg. So you don't think this vaccine is the answer to ridding covid 19? 🖤🙏
Dg. We are doing elbows with my Mom for now. We are over 2 months' post
    COVID so she feels a bit more relaxed we should have strong antibodies.
    Doctors even in my clinic divided. Even some who have had the illness-
    fortunately not severe-seem divided on vaccine stance. The one who still
    thinks vaccine is necessary. Those who say maybe in few months- verified
    had antibodies. Definitely not something I want in near future. If others
    want why should I be prioritized if I already have resistance?
Ch. Hugs

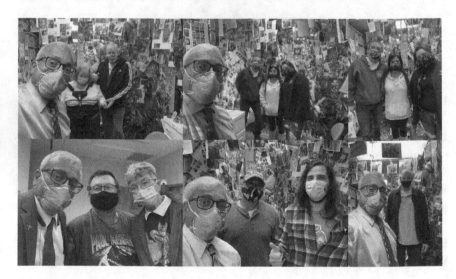

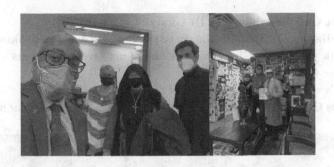

My patient Zdenek ready to go back to full duty work after my surgery three months ago. Hallelujah. Thank you 🙏 Lord Jesus. They are angels and brought me a beautiful Christmas 🎄 angel 👼 and hand written Christmas card!

Thank you 🙏 I sooo much and many blessing!

I follow Dr Anthony Fauci and CDC guidelines if my patients in my practice!

I am okay with Virtuality and Christmas but keep the gifts 🎁 coming!!!!

Www.ghalyneurosurgeon.com

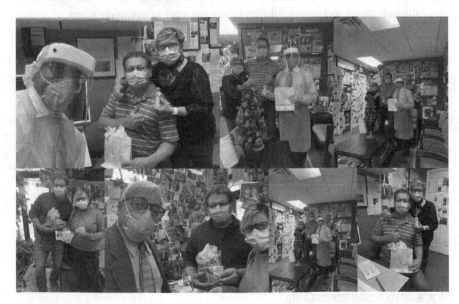

CG. Wonderful news for her. She did have the best. What a beautiful angel. 🤍🙏

AV. Praise God for helping you Dr Ghaly! 🙏

MR. Myslím na vás! Ráda slyším, že se vše povedlo a že se Zdeňkovi daří!

FA. Thank you Doctor Ghaly they are one of my favorite patients 🖤

AB. Praise God

JU. That's wonderful news. Awesome! 💕

PH. Praise GOD!! GOD works many heartfelt blessings through your hand.

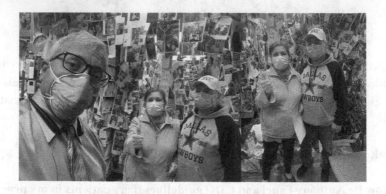

What a great honor and joy to be a Neurosurgeon for great grandchildren of my former patients in my early days. Thank you all for you your love 🖤 and trust!

My Lord Jesus has been so kind to me and merciful to give me a life to see that day of the children and grandchildren of my patients in my early years

Ramsis Ghaly

Our angel Josh is ready to go home after his surgery yesterday. Josh is in his way to speed recovery. Praise our Lord Jesus. What a talented young man. Speed recovery.

Ramsis ghaly
www.ghalyneurosurgeon.com

Early Merry Christmas 🎄 **to my wonderful patients. Jane, Debbie and Joe enjoying great recovery and new lease in life after surgery. Blessing to you all. Praise our Baby Jesus and Early Merry Christmas** 🎄

Ramsis Ghaly
Www.ghalyneurosurgeon.com

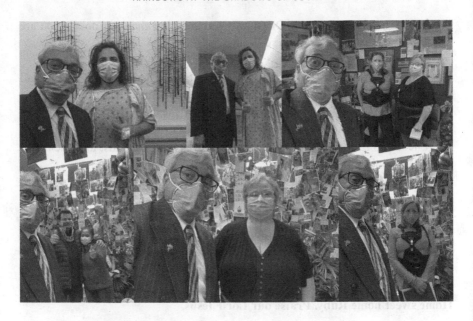

Three years later, after surgery, still with us enjoying the gift of life with his great wife Angi where their love 🖤 is going stronger and Carl condition made them both together and close to Lord Jesus.

It just. Rings tear to my eyes!! What a miracle!!! Who could have imagined!! Amen thank you 🙏

Thank you 🙏

Ramsis Ghaly
Www.ghalyneurosurgeon.com

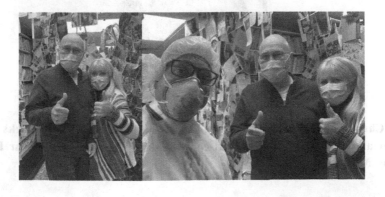

Angela J Miller We love you Dr Ghaly. You are more than our doctor you are family ♥. It was soooo good to see you.

AM. Doesn't look great! He was glad to see you too Dr Ghaly and your phone call this evening made the BIGGEST smile appear on his face!

MP. Amazing! You guys look more like you're on vacation!

AM/ honestly Dr. Ghaly visits are truly wonderful to spend time with that man! Encouraging and you know he's being upfront with you! Just love the man.

MS. Woo Hoo! Looking good!

MA. Love this!! Love y'all!!!

MP. I imagined!!! ♥♥ So thankful!

JM. Wonderful

After long day hours of surgery to reconstruct spine of the back, our terrific angel going home.

Home sweet home Ruby. Praise our Lord Jesus.

We all pray for your speed recovery, Amen 🙏

Ramsis Ghaly
Www.ghalyneurosurgeon.com

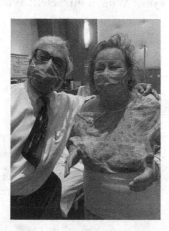

My Christmas gift, Ruby recovering from major surgery three weeks ago. Ruby and Don what a wonderful couple. Many blessing. Praise our Lord Jesus. Merry Christmas 🎄

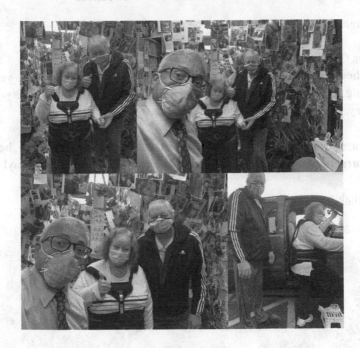

A beautiful message from a patient's husband that she was suffering from horrific pains and tremendous disability screaming day and night. I did her major Spine surgery two months ago!

"Dr Ghaly my wife is doing better everyday thank you I do everyday"

It touched my heart in the midst of difficult times of COVID

Amen 🙏 praise our Lord Jesus

Ramsis Ghaly

MN. Dr Ghaly you and God are the greatest with saving lives and fixing people and their pain. Bless you two.

FA. God bless you Dr Ghaly

CG. How thoughtful of him. It is so true how you relieve the suffering of those in pain including me. Bless you. 🙏🖤

LK. Me too!! Bless you Dr. Ramsis Ghaly

JG, Thank you for your sweet wishes! My life is so much better cause you are a part of my life. May God Bless you this new year and surround your life with Love and comfort!! 🖤🖤🖤

Our angel

Rebecca Crawley
going home after major surgery two days ago on Friday with years of suffering. Doing terrific with no more pains. Congratulations Becky. Speed recovery. Praise our Lord Jesus.

What a special person you are! What a special privilege to be your neurosurgeon! Only goodness awaiting for you! We continue to pray!

Www.ghalyneurosurgeon.com

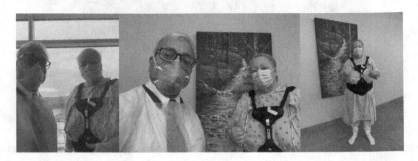

Rebecca Crawley
Thank you, Dr. Ghaly. You are wonderful! You've taken such good care of me.

Sending healing prayers. Dr. Ghaly was my daughter in laws' Dr. He did surgery and Amy is pain free. God bless him!!!

JP. Yes, he is wonderful. God bless him. 🖤
BR. Praise the Lord for good surgeons! Praying you will be pain free soon 🙏

Becky, here's to a speedy recovery! Let us know if you need anything. Love you!!!

CG. What a wonderful Christmas gift you gave her. Wishes for a speedy recovery!
RP. Wishing you all the best in your recovery, cuz! Thank you, Dr. Ghaly for taking good care of her!
EA. Oh my...what did you have done? Continued swift recovery! Hugs!
BK. Excellent work Dr. Ghaly. I'm glad she's doing great.
BK. Way to go Becky!

Praise the Lord! So glad you are on your way to a pain free life! Sounds like you got special care!

Glad your surgery went well, prayers for your recovery. 🙏🙏🙏

CP. Get better soon
CC. I'm so happy he was able to help you.
LM. Hoping for a quick recovery so u will be pain free.
BC. Excellent work Dr. Ghaly. I'm glad she's doing great.
BC. He is outstanding! Does he ever sleep? 🖤 **I don't think so. He gives so much to his patients.**

Glad to hear you're on your way to a quick recovery!

JS. Thank you! Looking forward to a girls night when I'm able and the craziness finally ends. 😊
BE. Hope your well. I have seen him several times. What a wonderful Christian man.
RC. Yes. I couldn't ask for better. 🖤
JD. Wonderful, Wonderful news Becky!!! Congratulations 🙏🖤
PS. Thanks, Jen! Looking forward to feeling good! 😊 **news Wow. Didn't even know you had a bad back. Glad the surgery is over and we will pray for continued healing and no more pain. Hugs.**

Our shining star

Rebecca Crawley
progressing well and ready to do more and more having a new lease in life and remarkable potentials. Becky and her great friends

Pam Kalafut
came and visit today. Thank you 🙏 much and to God our Lord Jesus the Glory

Ramsis Ghaly
Www.ghalyneurosurgeon.com

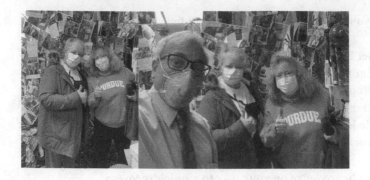

RC. Thank you, Dr. Ghaly. You've done so much for me! 😊💜😊

Early morning rounding on our beloved Scott!

Our angel
Scott Swanson
is recovering well!

It isn't a surprise Scott is doing fantastic since our Lord Jesus was present all the way! Despite it is the third surgery yet it was full of blessing to lead the journey together!

Thank you 🙏 to all your prayers!

Ramsis Ghaly
Www.ghalyneurosurgeon.com

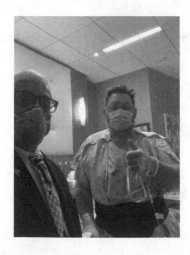

My angel

Scott Swanson

is doing fantastic and he is going hone today. Symptom free with no pains. His legs are so strong after major surgery on Friday and our Lord Jesus blessed him with second lease in life. A loving man, father and a husband.

And look at him once his wife Lynn came, he went back to bed spoiled and served!! And guess what??? Scott is working from the hospital now and reaching out his clients scheduling appointments. What a great American Hero!!

Thank you all for your prayers. Home sweet home

Ramsis Ghaly

Www.ghalyneurosurgeon.com

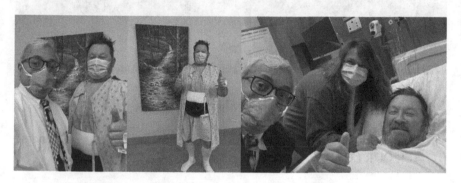

KO. hat is marvelous to hear. Stay healthy sir

AV. Praise God! 🐸🙏

LB. Wonderful news!!

MM. You go Scott. Do everything the doctors tell you. Say hi to your mom for me.

CL. On our feet that's great

BD. He is truly blessed. Good job doctor

TR. Great news

DG. Keep kicking ass Scott! 🤘

KS. Awesome! 👀

BF. Great news

Up and about already!

DS. Awesome stay healthy

LB. Awesome. He's a great doctor!!

JH. Were so glad to hear you are doing well and on your way to recovery!

DB. Great news Lynn 😸😸

SS. Wishing you a speedy recovery Scott! You're in good hands.

Our lovely Chrissy came and visit with me and her wonderful husband and mother

Annette Cozzi
much blessing and live

Stay safe

Ramsis Ghaly
Www.ghalyneurosurgeon.com

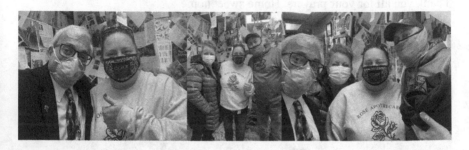

DB. Love you ALL...blessings to each other!
BV. Storming the heavens....
JG. God we are asking for Miracles- In JESUS name we pray! 🙏❤️ Sending
    ALL OUR LOVE!

Agnes Rosa
is 😇 feeling blessed with

Michal Bolkunowicz
and
Ramsis Ghaly

Yesterday at 6:27 PM ·

Today my husband had surgery on both his arms. Dr. Ramsis Ghaly

Thank you so very much for taking care of my husband and being so skilled at what you do. Every day of our lives will be better because of you. We are forever grateful 🙏❤️ This also marks 1yr since I had my back surgery and I feel great.

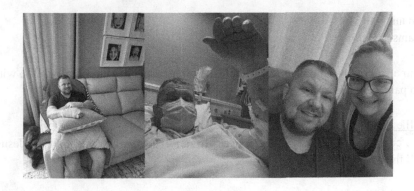

What a beautiful gift from my patient

Michal Bolkunowicz
Michal. I did his surgery last weeks free of pin and recovering well. Praise our Lord.

Agnes Rosa
Did do good to help michal. Thank you

Michal squeezing ghsly stress brain sponge to get stronger. Speed recovery.

Gorgeous Gift our Lord Jesus framed. Thank you 🙏

<u>Ramsis Ghaly</u>

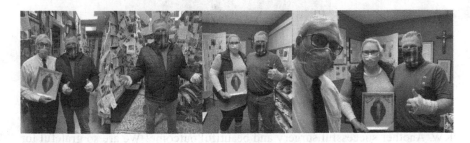

JF. A beautiful gift honoring a beautiful gift!

What a great visitor today Jillianne Renee Overman and a future Neurosurgeon Max!

Much a surprise visit after I did surgery 7 years ago on Jilliane. The children are our future and we must inspire them. Much blessing

Thank you 🙏
Ramsis Ghaly

Our angel recovering well and went home after surgery. A new lease in life with no pain. Much blessing g to you

Allie Larson
We be praying for your speed recovery to our True Gealer God the Lord Jesus. All the best! Amen 🙏

Ramsis Ghaly
Www.ghalyneurosurgeon.com

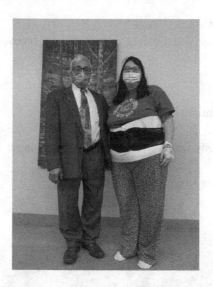

AL. Thank you again for everything. You are truly an amazing doctor and person. 💕

GL. What a beautiful thing to say Dr. Thank you so much for everything you did for my daughter she now can be pain free.

KW. Another successful surgery and beautiful outcome! We are so grateful for your gift to the world Dr Ghaly!

KS. Thanks doc for fixing for friend up! Just talking to her the night after her surgery she sounded so much better!!!

CO. Glad you're doing better Allie.

Going back to work with no pain 2 months after surgery!! What a pleasure and honor to care for you

Allie Larson
A new person with joy and great smile after horrific time with pains. Much blessing and greatness for your future!

Our Lord is a great Healer. Thank you 🙏 out Lord and Savior

Ramsis Ghaly
Www.ghalyneurosurgeon.com

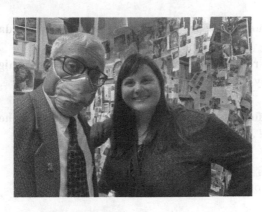

Gl. Once again thank you Dr Ghaly for taking such wonderful care of my sweet daughter
Kw. The future is bright!!!
Jm. Simply "Wonderful"!!

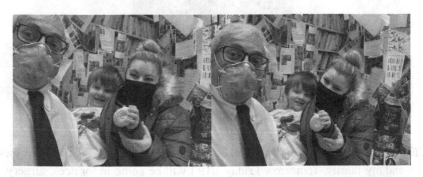

19Rebecca Crawley, Rick Malina and 17 others
3 Comments
Like
Comment
Share
Comments

KG. Beautiful 🖤🖤🖤

JO.. So great to see you today! You're the best!

DT. She only goes to The Best!!!!

BK. **Hard to believe it's been 7 years already since I had my neck surgery. Dr Ghaly gave me my life back! Thank you Dr. Ramsis Ghaly**

NE. Glory to God!

CP. Dr Ghaly God has gifted you with amazing skills and a beautiful caring heart 🖤.

Our angel Carmen Einsiedel is recovering well from yesterday surgery.

Early morning rounds blessed to see the hands of the Almighty caring for Carmen. Speedy recovery!!!

Thank you all for your prayers. Ready to be home sweet home 🏠. Praise praise our Lord Jesus!

Ramsis Ghaly
Www.ghalyneurosurgeon.com

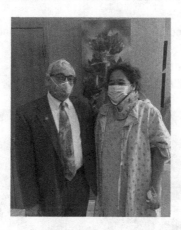

CE. Alright Prayer warriors I need all of you right now. I am asking this for myself and my family. Tomorrow Friday 3/19 I will be going in for neck surgery. I could not being doing this without the love and support from my family and friends and most of all without the help of Dr. Ramsis Ghaly

He was there for me 4 years ago when I needed him for my back surgery and is here for me again. My husband who I know has to take care of me for the next 3 months plus, my kids who will have to do everything I can't including helping with my mom and dad and to my sister who is always there to hold me and cry with me. My best friend kris who is ready to go on vacation once I'm better to make me feel better, My great friend Amy who has checked on me everyday and has brought wonderful meals to my family I can't tell u how much I appreciate u. My dear Laura for all the info u have given me and the wonderful pillow ur husband dropped off for me. My co-worker Lauren ur wonderful gift basket! All my friends for ur support and everything.. Just know it's another obstacle I have to overcome and God will be by my side but every Prayer is appreciated and received with love.

KE. Great news still praying 😊
BK. Excellent.
LD. Oh Carmen praying for a great recovery! So happy all went well!
LG. That's wonderful! Continued prayers
LH. Glad to hear! Praying for a speedy recovery!!!
RV. 👍 Praying For A Great Recovery, Still 🙏
GS. More prayers.
NC. Thank you Dr!
SE. Thank you for caring for her.
Ea. Recover soon

I love 🖤 the fashionable masks on my patients when they come for clinic visit after surgery. It tells me immediately as a surgeon they are doing well with the grace of God!!!

Look how Carmen Einsiedel doing a week after surgery in her recovery after surgery. Praise our Lord Jesus. From horrific pains to ER to recovery back home. Much blessing and Speed recovery!

Ramsis Ghaly
Www.ghalyneurosurgeon.com

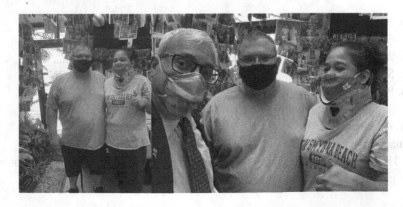

1013

CE. Thank u Dr Ghaly. I'm trying my best. Some days better than others but not what it was. I am blessed to have u as my surgeon and call u my friend. May God continue to bless u everyday!

CG. Wishes for a speedy recovery!

VG. Wishing you a speedy recovery! Many thanks to the doctor for successful surgeries, and great concern for his patients! 💜💜💜

Look at our angel. It is really great when at the end of my clinic, I saw my patient Cheri with a smile, Coming to two years from surgery, pain free with new lease in life after ten years of suffering!

And not only I received the beautiful smile and appreciation but also a gift she brought from Jerusalem a cross made of original olive tree from the holy land. Amen. Thank you 🙏 Thank you 🙏 so much.

Cheri Polich

Ramsis Ghaly
Www.ghalyneurosurgeon.com

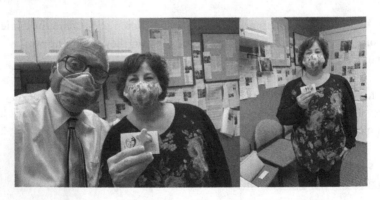

KG. Beautiful 💚

SA. Beautiful! 💛

GS. What an amazing recovery thanks to you!

RH. Smiling with you both

AB. Praise God!

JZ. Thoughtful gift. Happy you are now pain free. That is truly a gift.

EM. Awesome

So happy for you Cheri!

SP. Thank you again Dr. Ghaly! You saved me in so many ways, and I'm forever grateful. 💜 May God continue to bless you 🙏

LS. Congratulations u have a wonderful dr!!

My wonderful patient ready to go home 🏠 free two days ago major surgery with no leg pains and regain function back. Hallelujah praise our Lord Jesus

let us pray for Tricia speed recovery. Amen 🙏

Ramsis Ghaly
Www.ghalyneurosurgeon.com

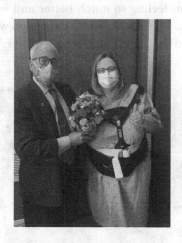

BK. Amen

TL. Praise God for her relief and prayers for her recovery! You are amazing Dr, Ramsis Ghaly

What a blessing you are to so many! Thank you and God Bless YOU!

AV. Praise God! Thank u Dr. Ghaly for sharing!! 💜🙏

MC. Amen

BK. Wonderful!

CG. I hope each new day brings you closer to a full and speedy recovery! Bless you!

JM. AMEN!!

JF. Amen!!!!!

AF. Amen

What a great joy to see AL with no more pains and aches in her clinic visit after two weeks after surgery! Praise our Lord Jesus seeing you with a smile and new lease in life!

What a blessing to see this young couple ready to move forward putting the suffering behind! Much blessing Allison and Frank! Praise our Lord and many years in health and joy!

Ramsis Ghaly Www.ghalyneurosurgeon.com

AL. Sometimes, God puts a special person in your life for a specific reason and it makes you feel truly blessed to have the privilege to be treated as such. Thank you, Dr, RAMSIS GHALY, you are simply the best and I'm so grateful to have found you. I am feeling so much better and in a few weeks, I get to return to work! 🎉🎈💕🐨 **TO JP.** you're the reason why I went to him in the first place! Thank you so much for telling me about him. He is truly an awesome person and doctor.

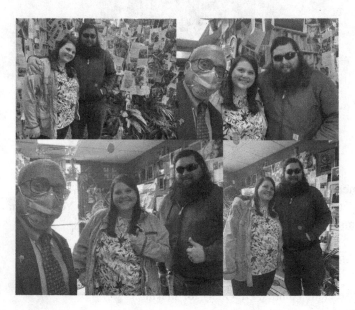

CT. My injections a week ago unfortunately haven't done their job like past injections. I may be looking him up. I love my dr but I'm in pain every day. Some days are worse than others but ughhh. What's it like to be pain free, I'd love to know lol?!!!!

CT. ugh I feel ya girl and I'm so sorry it didn't work out for you. I knew the minute I woke up from surgery that my nerve pain was gone and it was an amazing feeling. 😸

GL. Thank you Dr Ghaly for doing an amazing procedure and for your kindness to my daughter

MS. I'm so happy you're feeling good

AL. Free of pain Love you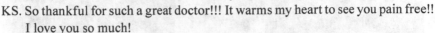
JP. He's such a wonderful dr. So thankful you are doing so well 😊
KS. So thankful for such a great doctor!!! It warms my heart to see you pain free!!
 I love you so much!
JS. Awesome ‼️

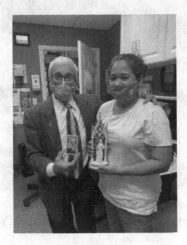

I am so touched with the thoughtful gifts my patient Carmen Einsiedel and her husband brought today fir her second visit after surgery. Incredible!!! Both searched all my office gifts and brought these three gifts I don't have!!

A Bracelet written on it The Lord's Prayer Matthew 6:9-13 KJV "Our Father which art in heaven, Hallowed be thy name. [10] Thy kingdom come. Thy will be done in earth, as it is in heaven. [11] Give us this day our daily bread. [12] And forgive us our debts, as we forgive our debtors. [13] And lead us not into temptation, but deliver us from evil: For thine is the kingdom, and the power, and the glory, for ever. Amen."

And the most beautiful of stature of our glorious Lord Jesus standing up high with bright light shining through the glass!

And the physician prayer 🙏 as our Lord Jesus guide the hand of the surgeon

Amen 🙏 and thank you soo much.

Much love and blessing

Ramsis Ghaly

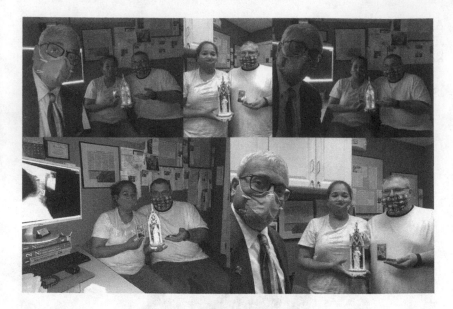

SP. You've touched many thousands of lives, God Bless You. 👀

AB. Praise God

CG. How wonderful that you are so loved and appreciated by so many of your patients. Bless you!

CE. Dr Ghaly there is in no way I could ever repay you for what you have done for me. You are a wonderful surgeon and an amazing person. These gifts were given with love from us because you are a dear friend. I will keep spreading your gift to help people to whomever needs it. May God continue to grace us with you and your healing hands 💚💚

AU. Hi Dr. **Ramsis Ghaly** You are an angel to your patients and everyone that you have helped.. God fearing Dr. God bless you!!!Shalom!

AV. Beautiful! 💝🙏

RM. OUTSTANDING.! God bless you Dr. Ghaly 🙏

Our wonderful patient Julie came for her follow up visit after surgery. What a smile and joy for No more pains. So proud of you Julie!! Much blessing and speed recovery!! Thank you Amen to our Savior!

Ramsis Ghaly

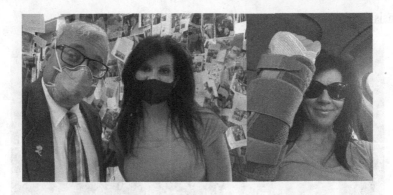

Cg. Wishing you a speedy recovery.
Tc. Hope you get better soon
Bm. Healing Prayers sent your way! God Bless!

So glad you're doing so good. Take good care of yourself. 🖤🖤

Nc. Amen
Dw. He is a great man ❗ your in good hands get well soon 👍

How do you know him?

My husband had a back surgery from him. He just did a carpal tunnel surgery on me. He's a good man yes 😊 yes I went to him 👍

tf. 🖤🙏 speedy recovery.
Jm. Wonderful!!

So happy to see my former patient

<u>Greta Paglis</u>
Greta, two decades ago after my surgery. She recovered completely and still remember me and came to visit. Hallelujah praise our Lord Jesus!

She brought flowers **that she grew in her garden: Daffodils and tulips!!**

Her husband now is my patient, Jim and Greta.

Much blessing to you both

Thank you for visiting

Ramsis Ghaly

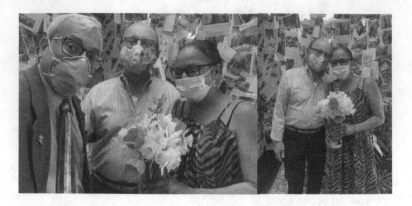

Cg. Beautiful flowers from beautiful people.
Rh. Love these wonderful healing stories. Thank you Lord Jesus
Jm. **Congratulations**

"To All 🖤🖤

Dm. you are too hard to forget by anyone...with all the things you have done

Jim's home and doing well. Thank God for His covering, Dr Ramsis Ghaly for truly being an instrument of God and using the gifts God put in his hands and heart. Thank everyone for your prayers and kind words. Blessings 😇

Jim Paglis at home

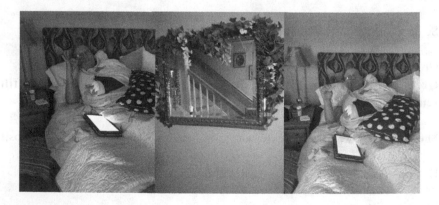

LW. Get well soon brother n law love ya
AV. Please rest and get well soon!

CM. Get well soon 🙏 Total Recovery !!!
JC. Get Well ----Your Welcome 😊😊
DB. Wishing you a speedy recovery

Jim is doing well a week after surgery with his smile. Both came from Indiana. I did surgery to his wife in 2001.

Bless you both. Praise our Lord to your recovery. Keep healing.

Ramsis Ghaly

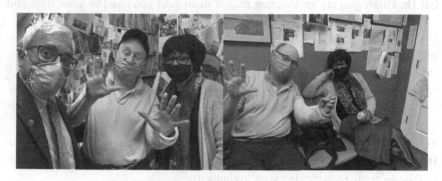

What a day in my clinic today, as soon as my first patient Renee left after bringing two beautiful plants, my second d patient Jim came for his clinic appointment with gorgeous flowers seeds and a Grow light for my garden made possible by his wife horticulture and skilled gardener my firmer patient do that the plants grow beautiful in my office. The seeds are Nasturtium and Moon Flower!

I was so excited!! I took off some of the surrounding photos immediately and I made place in my garden for the grow light. What a day and what gorgeous garden blessed with my patients and grow with their prayers and God endless Grace Jesus our Lord and Savor.

Speed recovery 💟 🩹 Jim and thank you so much Jim and Greta. Thank you thank you 🙏

Ramsis Ghaly
Www.ghalyneurosurgeon.com

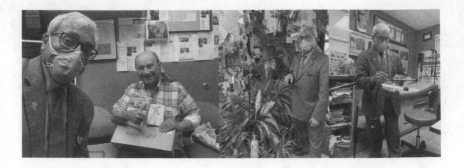

GP. Dr. Ghaly you are an amazing man. I'm so glad you like the grow light and flower seeds. Blessings

DH. You are So Loved and Appreciated. 🌷

BS. Ho wonderful!

CG. A verse came to mind while reading about your grateful patients. "Ramsis, Ramsis, how does your garden grow? With patients love and doctor care. That's how your garden grows." 🤍

SC, yay my tree of life

RC. How wonderful!

JM. What A Super Gift, Enjoy Dr. Ghaly!!

RH. Goya enjoy redecorating with loving gifts.

SC. Outstanding!!

Tricia Burkard

came today only two weeks after surgery. She couldn't walk and much of pains. Now she us much better and Doing terrific after major surgery. Praise our lord Jesus. Her wonderful mom Judy continues to care for her. Thank you. Much blessing and speed recovery. We pray!

Ramsis Ghaly

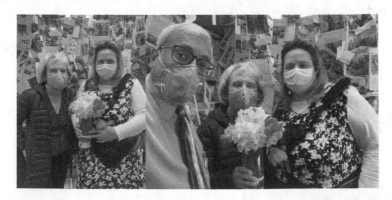

Dm. Thank you Dr. Ghaly!! Lord continues to bless your hands
Jm. "Awesome" 🖤🖤

Our angel is home after successful surgery yesterday free of pains. Thank you Michael and much blessing and speed recovery. Thank you 🙏 Lord!

<u>Ramsis Ghaly</u>

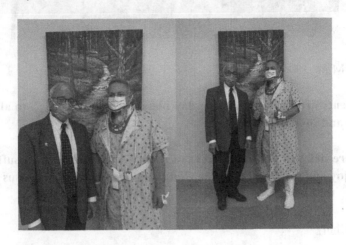

MR. Hope all went well for you Mike!!!! Proud of ya 😁
CG. Sending healthy thoughts and wishes for the fastest recovery.
RF. Is that Mike Acup from Dresden?
MR. <u>RF</u> yep....he›s another one healed by Dr. Ghaly 🙏
MJ. Thank the lord and thank you Dr. Ghaly
JV. Good luck Mike
SP. Get well soon!
AD. Sending healing hugs Mike! 🤗
DS. Looking good Mike.....
MJ. I'm happy to hear that everything went well!!
TR. Thank you Daddy God for your healing power 🕯️
JD. Wow!!!!! Glad it went well!!! Love the belt matching socks!! Stylin!!!
😄🤗🙏🤍

Hallelujah Michael came today and his wife after surgery doing well with no more horrific pains. Much blessing. Speed recovery ♡🩹 Michael.

<u>Ramsis Ghaly</u>
<u>Www.ghalyneurosurgeon.com</u>

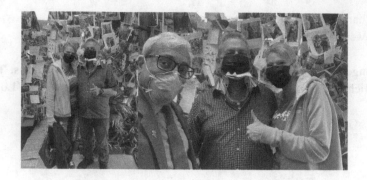

DS. Yay Mike.... looking good!

My patients are my joy and everyday blessing. Thank you 🙏 to all of my patients and those trusted.

They were sick and suffering and I saw them healed and no more suffering!! What a joy and privilege! Glory to God in highest, to our Lord Jesus Christ, Amen 🙏 thank you 🙏

Ramsis Ghaly

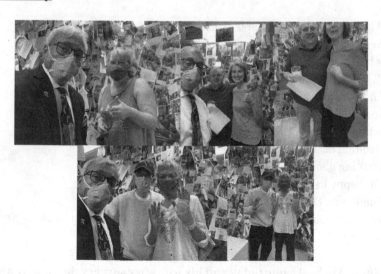

I got great visitors day, Micah and Mela kids of Nikita the daughter of my wonderful patient Ellis, a week after her surgery. Ellis is doing terrific praise our Lord and she spent the entire day yesterday buying two great plants 🪴🌱 for my office 🌱 to join my growing garden blessed with my patients names. The Lucky Bamboo and the ficus

In the mean time her grand children were exploring the human brain and tearing it apart and outing it back together. Much much better and more genius than I have ever been able to do!! I can see Micsh and Mela will be competitive neurosurgeons in the future. I pray I put the seeds in their growing brains 🧠 today and in addition they all got Ghaly brain 🧠 sponge to squeeze!!!

Ellis daughter is another hardworking well accomplished ICU Nurse. I cannot thank you all enough. You bring joy and blessing to my life and practice. Speed recovery Ellis and best wishes to grandchildren for bright future.

Thank you 🙏 so much

Ramsis Ghaly
www.ghalyneurosurgeon.com

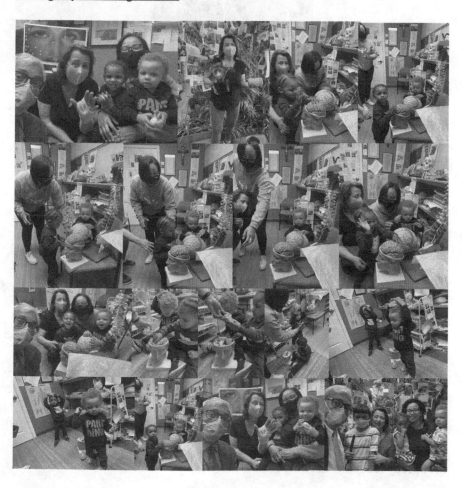

<u>Renee Colosi</u>
After years of suffering with pain I feel so blessed to have found you. I know I'm in good hands with you as my surgeon. It makes me happy to be able to add something to your beautiful garden. May God continue to Bless you and the gift he has given you to help so many. 🙏🙏

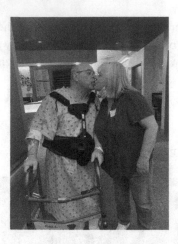

My Memorial Gift Donald is going home 🐿 today after major surgery last Friday on 5/28/2021 with no pains at all after years of horrific pains and difficulty in walking and sleeping——Praise our Lord Jesus!! Speed recovery Donald

<u>Ramsis Ghaly</u>
Www.ghalyneurosurgeon.com

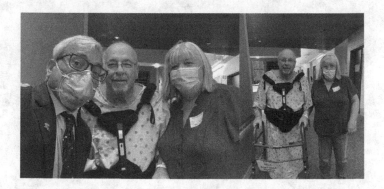

CG. Wonderful! Wishes a a speedy recovery.
BM. 💙🙏💙 Llooking good uncle love you
PP. Speedy recovery! Looking good

NP. Love to see ya up and about and am so happy recovery has begun

JS. Look good dad!!!

BL. Hope for a speedy recovery.

SG. Didn't you get a kiss Dr. Ghaly?

CG. Wonderful! Wishes a a speedy recovery.

BM. **Best wishes** and prayers for a speedy recovery!

MN. Good luck Donald with Dr. Ghaly. and Jesus performing your surgery you are on the right track to a much easier recovery take care of yourself and stay safe.

JB. That's wonderful!!!!

BL. Praise God and I thank Him working through Dr. Ghaly to do such amazing surgeries.

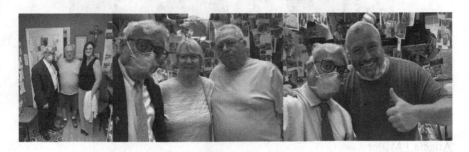

FLASHING BACK PRIOR TO COVID-19 PANDAMIC

2019! God blessed you with a tremendous gift.

Carol Nelson

and we all pray for your speed recovery. please pray for Carol, big surgery is coming. Our Lord is full of kindness and love 🖤. Thank you Lord Jesus

Love 🖤
Ramsis Ghaly
www.ghalyneurosurgeon.com

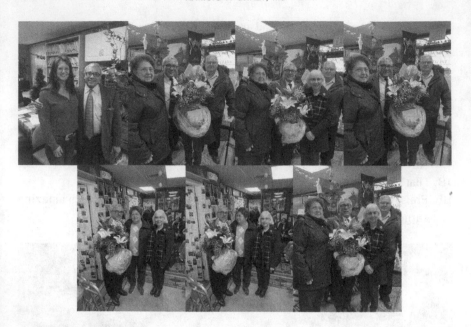

Ramsis Ghaly
is with
Angela J Miller
January 10 at 11:55 AM ·
Shared with Public

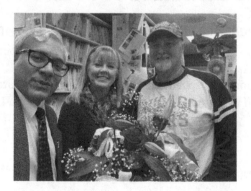

Happy new year my sweet Carl and Angi. What a blessing. We praise our Lord Jesus so much for His multitude of blessings and healings. Many more! Keep up my friend and thank you so much for blessing us

My wonderful patient came all the way to present me with outstanding Bouquets of Roses 🌷 with spectacular smell filled the entire office with blessing. Bless your heart.

Thank you

AM. We miss you Dr Ghaly! We really must come see you

Ramsis Ghaly
is with
Jack Jane Cole Duvick
and
Eileen Markusic
.
January 10 at 11:55 AM ·
Shared with Public
🌐

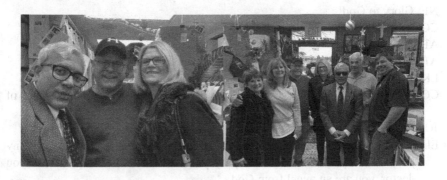

J DUVICK
My two angels visited me today and my new eye glasses just arrived. Bless your hearts 💜. Spectacular couple and family. Our Lord is full of kindness and love 💜. Thank you Lord Jesus

Love 💜
Ramsis Ghaly
www.ghalyneurosurgeon.com

JD. You are our Angel Dr. Ghaly !!!

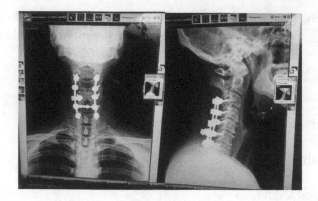

EW. Impressive.

KH. Wow! That's intense!!

DS. Looks familiar. My last surgery was 1997. Still hanging in the. I believe he assisted on my second one

KG. That's awesome 🖤

LD. You're strong wonderful women, God Bless you!

NE. Glory to God!

CG. Looking good Ruby. Bless you!

AB. Praise God!

AR. Your in good hands! The most amazing Doctor 🖤

LK. Yes such an amazing doctor 💜

CG. Prayers for a speedy recovery. You have the best doctor to take care of you. 🙏🖤

JC. You are amazing 💚🙏

ED. God Bless you Doctor. You are a wonderful person and have helped so many people with your medical JB. I pray you will feel better now. Thank you doctor, you are an angel from God. 😊💜

BM. Prayers of healing sent your way!

MY. دائما مع الرب وهو ينجح كل ما تمتد له يدك امين ثم أمين يارب العالمين ونشكرك يارب ونحمد فضلك يا ابن الله اللحى آمين

CL. Praying for a complete and speedy recovery! 🙏🙏 God is Great!!

CL. Thank you doctor for healing her. 💜😅🙏🙏

VG. Looks like another great job, doctor. Congratulations!

JK. Our Loving God is so good and Merciful

AP. Wishing you a speedy recovery

Thank you 🙏 to my wonderful patient
Charlene Mentzer Glowaty
a beautiful Christmas music nativity scene snow globe music box. Thank you so much merry Christmas much blessing!!

Ramsis Ghaly

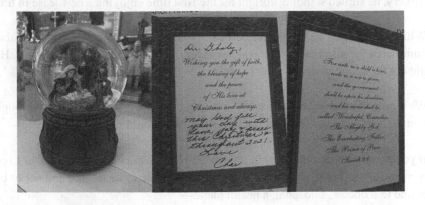

LP. Beautiful! 🖤
KO. How beautiful this is for a very deserving caring Person as Dr. Ghaly is to
all 🖤

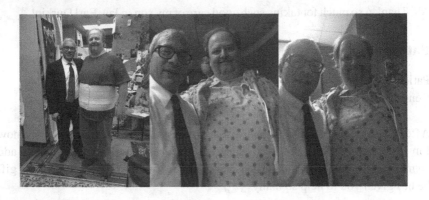

Ramsis Ghaly
January 18, 2017 ·
Shared with Public
🌐

A story of an angel
This great angel after being turned away for being overweight by his surgeon,
came to my office in crutches from excruciating pain and severe sciatica for three
months in misery since the Halloween. No minute had passed by throughout the
holidays without hurting and crying of pains and aches. What an angel!

Immediately I took him for surgery before more loss and damages. Next day after surgery, he smiled standing upright for the first time enjoying a new lease in life.

What had happen to medicine?? Not only the patient was suffering but also humiliated for his obesity??? It was not insurance issue and no other reasons. He did not do wrong to deserve but the best.

We should never deprive patients from helping them. God Jesus ask of us through Him to help and save lives but not be judges. We should never discriminate---.

If you cannot help another may be able to help and do not close the door. Our Lord is merciful--- This what America offers to all people to be treated and not to be bound to a doctor, a hospital, a health plane----

Thank you for allowing me to write briefly about you that may help many. Thank you Lord for helping this great angel: Your child

AV. Thank u so much for taking such good care of my son in law Earl Durkin!

Patient quotes

Patients quotes 42
Renee Ellis Colossi

After years of suffering with pain I feel so blessed to have found you. I know I'm in good hands with you as my surgeon. It makes me happy to be able to add something to your beautiful garden. May God continue to Bless you and the gift he has given you to help so many. 🙏🙏

Annie Gibson
One of the most humble and deserving humans I have ever had the honor of knowing. Thankful, everyday, for the man that has saved my sister Chrissy's life, 3 times.

I cannot think of anyone more deserving of the recognition. Dr. Ramsis Ghaly is a true inspiration and Devine human being. His grace and humility can help us all understand what is is to be the best version of yourself.
We love you, Dr. Ghaly

Brenda Linquest
You more than deserve this honor, Dr Ramsis Ghaly. You are a Godsend to all who know you and even so many who don't. Congratulations 🤍! You are amazing and so many lives are truly blessed due to your excellence. 🖤💜🖤💜

Margaret Halle
Well said, Love 🖤 your ideal. No wonder why you made Dr. Of the year. No man can touch you or come close to your intelligent mind. Congratulations 🤍 Dr. Your one of the Best Dr's ever.

Mischa Doyel
Congratulation to our wonderful friend and Neuro Surgeon Ramsis Ghaly in Chicago. His quotations of the Bible are great and make understand who was on his side. You can read about his fascinating life in his first book. "A Christian from Egypt". Yes, he had a very tough start and never gave up.

Jane Duvick
Just wanted to share this with family & friends. This doctor who posted this did my back surgery and has quintuple certifications as a neurosurgeon. I trust him with my life. If his advice could help save one life it is worth the share. Thank you Dr. Ramsis Ghaly for sharing your knowledge and advice!

Lma Vilches
Congratulations Dr. Ghaly. 🤍🤍 you're the BEST 🏆

Scott Aughenbagh
Congratulations!!! Thank you for the wonderful care of all my patients over past 20 years!!! Well deserved! 🖤

Kimberly McCoy
You ROCK

Jerry Walter
Keep up the amazing work Doc! Thank you for all you do!

Aeschylus Bryant
Dr Ghaly!!! You're the best!!!

Norm park
Ramsis Ghaly Thank you Dr Ghaly. When things get a little stressed you are one man I always think of. With the love poured out to me it sure gives me a great feeling. Thank you again Dr Ghaly for your Help.

Nicole Wallis
Life saver 😊 well deserved!

Kathy Everrett
Exceptional Doctor Amen

Juli Tra
I just wanted to message you and let you know I appreciate your honestly as a physician, God bless you for that and the work you do every day! God will have a special place for you. 🖤

Ronald Feeney
Mishel Rambo God works through his hands. The ones that know Dr. Ghaly and have been healed by him know that this is true.

Bart Smith
Good luck Shaun and Brian ... follow the lead of Dr Ramsis Ghaly and your career will be most rewarding

Charlene Glowaty
You are the saviour of all those who are suffering. Just look at all those happy faces. 🖤🙏

Margaret Halle
The world's best Dr. Ever!! With an amazing love 🌹 for his patience.

Barbara Harrison
What a beautiful memory honoring this mother. This was an amazing tribute to a victim of an awful tragedy. Bless you Dr. Ghaly for all you so selflessly do. Bless you for this wonderful testimony to a lost life and all the lost lives from unnecessary violence that then get forgotten with no regard to their outcome. Its a tragedy. Bless you for acknowledging this. It hurts my heart letting it all sink in. I am crying and praying for her soul, your sweet soul and all the souls having to rely on the death of another so they may live. You are an incredibly devoted, humble, loving and brilliant man. Thank you! 💚🎂

Karen McGinnis

Looks nice & so do you. I'm so thankful that you give God His credit & as the Bible says are not ashamed of the gospel of Christ & share it with your patients. Don't get me wrong, I think your one of the Best Doctors Around & your Knowledge Remarkable. You've been in a highly Covid area & have been blessed not to get it. I'm thankful that you announce the truth about vaccines & them not being tested correctly or researched like they should. Your work & work ethics are remarkable & I applaud you being an amazing doctor, your surgical results, teaching others your techniques & knowledge, etc. You're a great person & I don't see how you have any time to sleep. Thank you for all you do to help others.

James King

BLESS is those who accept Jesus, Dr. Ghaly is the one!!! He is a preying Doctor that does for the people not what the Hospital tells him to do!!

Thank you Doc. For giving me a second chance of life threw the GRACE OF ARE LORD JESUS CHRIST.!!! You are forever in my heart & mind. 😊😊😊🙏🙏🙏

Flo Andocutin

Stay safe Dr. Ghaly 🙏 God bless you the doctor with a heart of gold.

Robin Hellenberg

What will you do when you run out of walls and ceiling. You are blessed. And appreciated and loved.

Aloysius Edekara

Sherpa Thank you Dr. Ghaly, I wish you could come on June 13th, Even just for an hour. You are the Gods messenger to save lots of lives. I will keep in touch with you.

Steve Gill

Thanks Dr Ramsis Ghaly for giving me more birthdays to enjoy!

Wittney Sargent

Thank you so much Dr. Ghaly, we appreciate you more than you will ever know!

Muin Haswah

I appreciate you sir! I can't begin to thank you enough for all you've taught & given me. You'll always have a special place in my life & I will always turn to you when I'm in need of guidance.

Sallie Dede
Ramsis Ghaly Thank You Dr. Ghaly, you are our Miracle 💜 Worker with our Lords Guidance!

Dr Chantou Vongnaraj
Thank so much for training me. It's taught me safe and compassionate care. I told everyone about you!!!

Dr Piotre Aljendi
I did Dr. Ghaly.. you are the best and I cannot express how happy we are to have you with us

Mike Nutoni
Dr.Ghaly i can only imagine what you went through and saw dealing with the covid 19.you are one strong man and best doctor in your field for that job. God Bless you and stay safe.

Stephanie Spiegel
Thank you for being such a wonderful friend/Doctor to my Mom. Thank you for being such a great friend to Mark and me. My Mom loved you so 💜

Patients quotes 41

Chrissy Weinhofen
I wouldn't be alive today if it wasn't for Dr Ramsis Ghaly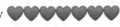

Kate Dottenwhy
Congratulations Dr Gahly! Yes you are America's most honored doctors, but most importantly, our families' most honored doctor!

Aunt of Chrissy Cozzi Weihofen! Bless you, and THANK YOU!

Carmen Einsiedel
Dr Ghaly there is in no way I could ever repay you for what you have done for me. You are a wonderful surgeon and an amazing person. These gifts were given with love from us because you are a dear friend. I will keep spreading your gift to help people to whomever needs it. May God continue to grace us with you and your healing hands 💜💜

Cheri Polich
Thank you again Dr. Ghaly! You saved me in so many ways, and I'm forever grateful. 🖤 May God continue to bless you. 🙏

Christie Loftus
You Doctor are a gift from God! You help so many people. When God created you he spent special time knowing you were chosen to help others. Thank you God and thank you Dr Ghaly. 🖤🙏

Charlene Glowaty
God did bless you. You help so many who have not been helped by other doctors. How fortunate for her she came to you. Look how you helped her. Bless you! 🖤🙏

Tiffany Lardi Wills
Praise God for her relief and prayers for her recovery! You are amazing Dr, Ramsis Ghaly! What a blessing you are to so many! Thank you and God Bless YOU!

Mark Patricoski
Dr Ghaly is the greatest human being ever. A huge heart and genius is a great and uncommon combination.

Sheri Pacewic
One of the Best Neurosurgeons I have ever met. He cares about his patience like know other 🖤

Tier Gorsak
Praise God. You are such a blessing, you have a healing hands. Gifted from God.

Dory Manlo
Jenny Cella the best dr i ever know

Jenny Celia
The best!

Anna Tzonkov
Thanks dr Ghaly. Everyone learned important points from you including myself. 😊

Jessica Pat
I'm getting published!!! None of it would be possible without everything you've done for me 💜 thank you for it all!

Dr Gwam
There is only one true Ghaly!..Inimitable!! Indeed

Taruna Waghary
No one can compare with our dear Dr. Ghaly

Leigh Anne
Dr Ghaly is the best. He did a world of good for my mom.

James King
Even tho I'm on your wall& in your book, I appreciate you for the lord blessing me for the way you I was blessed for you being there at the time I needed blessing & a God fearing Dr. That stands his ground & is bless by are lord JESUS Christ, so I say thank you Dr. Ghaly, 🙏🙏🙏😌😌😌

Thanks Doc. May the lord are God keep Blessing you with the Healing of peoples ((Mines, body, & Souls)) your old patient & friend, James S. King 🙏🙏😌😌

Robin Hellenberg
Always upfront.

Always spoken with the love of Jesus and honesty. Intelligence compassion kindness. Thank you for the truth always. God bless your doctor

Aida F Uaisele
Hi Dr. Ramsis Ghaly You are an angel to your patients and everyone that you have helped..God fearing Dr.God bless you!!!Shalom!

David Wojciechowski
He is a great man ❗ your in good hands get well soon. 👍

Margaret Hale
Your an "Awesome Dr!"

Leigh Anna
You're a great dr!

Michelle Lizette
The best Dr. ever! Love you Dr. Ramsis Ghaly. You truly are a hero.

Ronald Feeney
God works through his hands.

Scott Mitchell
The Man!!!

Kathryn Hoffman
Tenesha Brummel James Right!!!! Ramsis Ghaly is the best Dr around 💚

Dory Manalo
you are too hard to forget by anyone...with all the things you have done

Judy Burkard
Couldn't have asked for a more skillful, caring, and attentive doctor for Tricia's surgery 💛

Greta and Jim Paglis
Jim's home and doing well. Thank God for His covering, Dr Ramsis Ghaly for truly being an instrument of God and using the gifts God put in his hands and heart. Thank everyone for your prayers and kind words. Blessings 😊

You are truly the hands and feet of God. Thank you so much for You. 😊

Father Jeff Freeman
I just signed on to Facebook, and discovered these AMAZING words from my dear friend, Dr. Ramsis Ghaly in honor of our new grandson Liam. WOW!!!! Thank you, Dr. Ghaly! I must share this with everyone!!!!!!!!!!!!!! Thank you! Thank you! Thank you! Take note Cecilia Freeman, Jessica Evans, Ginny Morris Evans, Terry Lee Ebert Mendozza, Connie Reeves Cooke, Fred Ascari, Gloria Jennings, Howard Murray, Janice Moss, Martin Scott Grissom, Patty Orsini, Roger Bradford -- DR. GHALY is ABSOLUTELY PRECIOUS!!!!!!!!! (As you all know!!!!) What a wonderful gift to us!!!

Terry Mendozza
Jeff Freeman what a blessing to know Dr. Ramsis Ghaly. He is truly given his power in the operating room, by God. And how true about Liam's eyes, like sparkling pools. One can lose oneself in them. God bless Ramsis, God bless you and Cecilia, and may God bless Liam, surrounded by love 🖤

Eileen Fuesz
You are an amazing Doctor, Person and Friend. 😍

Zeneida Kapul
Congratulations! That's awesome! Your kindness Dr. Ghaly makes you the most beautiful person in the world.

Eileen Hayes
Congratulations to a superb human being!!!!

Patients quotes 40

Terry Mendozza
Thinking of you with Love, as I navigate this path back to health; all because of you, my dear friend. If I don't have to go back to Mayo Clinic, then I will plan a trip to Las Vegas in early May to see Karon Kate, and hopefully you will be there, too. May God bless you always, Ramsis. I will never forget what you did for me, and no doubt, countless other people who were lost in medical quagmires. You are the Good Shepherd. Peace and love to you always. 🖤🖤🖤

Andrea Stallworth
You're a great surgeon and I'm so glad you did my surgery.

Emily Fuesz
Linda Johnson-Smith he had a Meningioma tumor removed that was removed in full! It was large and deep. Dr. Ghaly performed a miracle through God! He is at MarianJoy

Christine Beier
Clare has a way of touching people's hearts, doesn't she?!!!

Thank you Dr Ghaly for your skill and dedication to saving people's lives. Our family loves you 🖤 Christine Fuesz – Beier

Betty Markel
How very moving the letters are, straight from the 🖤 God Bless you Dr. Ramsis Ghaly for all you the life's you have touched and healed. God has given you gifts and you are truly his Servant! 🖤

Christie Loftin
You are one of God's miracles. Thank you for helping so many people have better lives. 💃🙏😇

Jim Doyel
You are a special, gifted Doctor; my friend!

Aeschylus Bryant
Excellent service to those in need! **Congratulations**!!! Dr Ghaly you are truly a wonderful person with tremendous talent and an ability to connect with your patients! You go above and beyond!!! Forever grateful!!! Aeschylus Bryant!!! 🙏

Dr Ana Plesca
Thank you very much!
I'm grateful for all the help and support to help us get where we are today!

Dr Zinaida Perciuleax
Thank you for your continued support and encouragement!

You are a big inspiration for us!
I feel very honored to know you 🙏

Ginny Walls
Thank you Dr Ghaly for ALL you have done..U will never be forgotten 🖤

Muin Haswah
Thank you for the help yesterday, I really appreciate having you available whenever I need. I have learned so much from you clinically & in life

Carol Rambo
You are God's instrument of healing for sure 🙂

Allison Larson
Sometimes, God puts a special person in your life for a specific reason and it makes you feel truly blessed to have the privilege to be treated as such. Thank you, Dr, Ramsis Ghaly, you are simply the best and I'm so grateful to have found you. I am feeling so much better and in a few weeks, I get to return to work! 🎉 🖤💕😭

Gabbe Larson
Thank you Dr Ghaly for doing an amazing procedure and for your kindness to my daughter

Tiffany Wills
Love this! 🖤 You are such an amazing, caring and healing Surgeon.... I'm forever grateful to you, Dr. Ghaly! 🙏

Megan overcash
Not sure if you saw but you were identified as a Crane's top provider Dr. Ghaly.
Thank you for being a pillar of the medical community

Dale Christensen
Thank you for all you do. We were all blessed when God gave you to us.

Scott Mitchell
Superhero!!!!

Ihor Melnytskyy
This is my favorite 😄 👍 We love you Dr. Ghaly. Igor. Class of 2012.

Janice Hartfield
Yes a true pillar for God's work!

Cristina Rutkowski
When there are tears you are a shoulder; when there is pain you are a medicine;
when there is a tragedy, you are hope...

You are more than just a doctor, you are a friend, guide and example of love.
Thank you so much Dr. Ramsis Ghaly
HAPPY NATIONAL DOCTOR'S DAY!!!!

Allison Larson
Happy doctor's day, Dr. Ghaly. Thank you for your hard work and dedication to
your patients. You make a difference in each person's life that you touch.

Charlene Glowaty
You certainly deserve those 5 stars and more. You are a healer through Gods'
guidance and are such a caring doctor. 🖤 🙏

Sandra Crites
yes you are but in my book you are 1000000 stars

Chita Bello
You are an instrument of God with a heart full of love and compassion.

Congratulations and God bless.

Horst Henning
Doktor
Du bist der Beste
für uns Menschen.!!

Margaret Halle
You deserve it! Your one of the Best! DRS. Ever! Great teacher! You have a great gift in healing people. Thanks to you always praising the Lord & giving him the thanks for working threw you to heal his people. You are definitely someone to look up too.

Jake Duvick
Simply the best. He is in the business of helping people. That's it.

Gary Chandler
The simply the best. I'm so glad our paths crossed and that if I need your help again you are there. Thankful everyday for the help you gave me 14 years ago

Dani Toplak
Dr Ramsis Ghaly he is the dr who saved my step sisters life when she was in a head on collision. Everyone said she was gone but he never gave up and now 18 years later she has kids of her own and is alive.

Patients quotes 39

Joan Pocius
You are the hands and feet of Jesus my brother. Thank you for being you.

Maria Logan
I deeply believe our faith in GOD & trust in our good doctors, like you Dr. Ghaly is awe inspiring thank you for the many years & life saving efforts I have witnessed while working w/ you in OB/OR

Michelen Eliacin
Dr Ghaly, I thank you so much for your prayers and helping Myrna! I read your story on FB and it is so touching and humbling. Continue to pray for and with your patients is a calling from God, that is why you are an excellent and compassionate MD. God will reward you for that. God bless you Dr Ghaly

Thank you so much Dr Ghaly! God is Great and Merciful. We thank Him and glorify His Holy Name, He answers prayers. This is an uplifting and humbling story of faith and persévérance!

Toni Morgano
A beautiful account of another miracle of God right before our eyes! Thank you Dr. Ghaly for taking care of her, for praying with us & for being an instrument of Faith! May God bless you more & the likes of you who bring God's words to bedside & share them with your patients & their families as well. 💙

Carol Rambo
This story made me cry. Your faith in Jesus and His miracles increases my faith in trusting Him more. Bless you for being His vehicle of grace and healing.

Aloyuius Edakara
Beautifully written true story. Dr. Ghaly you are a true believer and I am sure you did your prayers before you intubated her and God heard your prayers and kept her alive. Thanks a million for your support and prayers. Our hearts are filled with joy.

Brenda Linquist
You are truly God's child and ambassador. You are so loved Dr Ghaly! Thank you for sharing! 🙏🙏🙏 Blessings 💕💕 I have the EXTREME privilege of knowing Dr Ghaly; he is the most amazing (and that's a huge understatement) person I have ever met!!! He has a long list of credentials, awards, accomplishments, accolades, etc and yet treats everyone as a dear friend.

He sends posts on a regular basis and they are always a faith filled lesson.

Debra Laraco
This is a true story, my former co worker (labor and delivery) and the best anesthesiologist Dr. Ghaly..

Prameela Mandela
What am amazing miracle. So glad to see Myrna active and alive. Don't even look like she has been sick and in icu for 3 months. Praise God for Dr. Ghaly, you are such a kind soul and a prayer warrior and ambassador for our Lord Jesus, May God bless you and continue to use both of you.

Sylva Cariaga Agustin
You are a true witness for Christ Dr. Ghaly who present a testimony about the truth that we have experienced and heard. God's word is a seed once it planted

it will grow and develop into the fruit the Lord intends it to become. God works in your life according to His purpose. God sent you for Myrna, and her family. Thank you Dr. Ghaly God is great, worthy to be praise. May God continue to bless you abundantly.

Glynes Roferos
God is really good and Miracles do happen. Thank you Dr. Ghaly for taking care of Myrna and for this amazing story. I am so happy Myrna is back. Glory to God.

Amelia Lucinea
True A REAL miracle of Our Lord Jesus. In Jesus name we PRAY, Thy Will be done. Dr. Ghaly you are a great instrument in the field of medicine & with the Love & faith in all you do. God bless 🙏

Norma Artenza
God Bless Dr. Ghaly for all the things that you do and most importantly your prayers - and to all those who cared and prayed for Myrna 🙏 She is a dear friend and a nursing school classmate. God is good, He answers those who believe and have faith in Him 🙏🙏🙏

Angela Larong
A very touching true to life story a Filipino American nurse who was infected by Covid and was in coma for 3months and with faith prayers and support from her Dr. Ghaly family coworkers n friends miracle happens.. Let's us pray for all those who are sick and never give up hope...Amen

Dr RK
Hi Ramsis, I sincerely appreciate your caring nature and dedication to CCH. Thanks for all you do for our patients and trainees.

Jen Viejo
Such a powerful testimony Dr Ghaly! I'm so moved by especially that it's the Lenten Season began. Thank you for sharing this story and your kindness, compassion you always give to your patients and families. God bless you 🕊️🖤

Mary Craig
🤍 Thank you Dr. Ghaly....I still consider you as being my guardian Angel.. 🤍

Debra Laraco
Best anesthesiologist I ever work with.

Charlene Glowaty
You are an extraordinary doctor. They are fortunate to have you guiding them to be the best they can be. 🖤🙏

Tiet Gorsak
You are the best extraordinary doctor they are Blessed to have you guiding them to be the best they can be prayed for all succeed everything they do. 🙏

Dianna Lynn
Best Neurosurgeon/Anesthesiologist in this country. Blessed by the Lord

Praise the Lord! 🙌 Amen! All Glory be to God!

Through Dr Ghaly's hands & the staff that took care of her !!!!!

Linda Andaz.
Gloria Gaither expresses precisely what Dr. Ramsis Ghaly refers to as the two secrets full of mystery, holiness and blessings to those taking part in both! For a moment - just for a moment the door flap between here and eternity opens and the angel dust of eternity gets on you and for a moment life gets real, and you are transformed, and you're never the same again.

Sheetal Patel
Thank you so much Dr. Ghaly for your kind words. I am glad that we got this opportunity today and was able to finish it successfully. I am also happy for the patient as her baby is doing fine as well.

Thank you for your guidance and for excellent management and follow up of the patient

Have a great day ahead.

Scott Mitchell
THE GHALLINATOR!!! 😂🤣😅

Maria Paz Logan
the savior in "full gear", keep safe Doc 😌🙏

Allison Larson
Thank you again for everything. You are truly an amazing doctor and person. 💕

Gabriel Larson
What a beautiful thing to say Dr. Thank you so much for everything you did for my daughter she now can be pain free.

Kailee wills
Another successful surgery and beautiful outcome! We are so grateful for your gift to the world Dr Ghaly!

Dr Ken Candido
That is phenomenal Dr. Ghaly! So proud of your amazing work. Keep it up and thank you for all you do for the patients and surgeons at AIMMC. You are one of a kind!

Mischa doyel
Our wonderful friend and Neurosurgeon in Chicago who helped me to get the right diagnosis when I was in pain. There is nothing more important in life than good friends. Thank you Ramsis for all you do.

Mike Nutoni
To me you are the best you saved my live Dr. Ghaly and all Ways kept in touched to see how i was. Many other doctors you don't here from on less you call there office and all you talk to is the doctor incident. God Bless Dr. Ghaly

Donita Rients Livingston
This Dr. Is AMAZING!!! IF you know anyone that needs help with ANYTHING MEDICAL CALL DR. G. He is the BEST!! WE HAVE REFERRED HIM TO A LOT OF OUR FRIENDS!! WE GOT THE HELP AND ANSWERS WE NEEDED!!!!!

Yvonne Drew Reddoch
Congratulations Ramsis Ghaly! Thank you for doing God's work. We are so blessed to have you in our lives!

Dulcinea Hawksworth
Hero isn't even a good enough word...Congrats, Dr. Ramsis Ghaly, you certainly deserve it!

Angela J Miller
That is incredibly awesome my dear friend!! I am so very happy that they recognize and honor what we, who are blessed to be called "Ghaly Patients" already know of you. I thank God daily for bringing you into our lives. May God continue to

bless you and continue working through you with each patient you touch. We LOVE you Dr Ghaly.

Gina Alaimo Svara
You're an amazing physician and teacher!

Tammy Brazeal Bedolla
You are an awesome physician 🖤

Brad Herdklotz
An angel amongst us.

Pamela Haynes
You definitely deserved that. You are the best.

Suzi Hamilton
Congratulations! You are amazing and such a blessing to so many!

Debra Severson Tarr
The Best Dr....... !!!!!!!

Kim-Connie Ellis
You are an exceptional doctor! May God bless you!

Sandi Benedict Crites
you have earned this a million times over! good things come to all that wait and now you have gotten your moment job well done dr

Liz Thomas
U r the best!

Kumar Govin
Great soul 🙏🙏🙏

Yvonne Folsom Carlson
Congratulations, Dr. Ghaly! Thank you for your tireless efforts to serve your fellow Dr. Ghaly was part of our coffee club when we lived in Illinois. He has tirelessly served during the COVID crisis and saved many lives. I'm so happy that he has received much-deserved recognition. I can't help but think of those medical professionals who don't get public praise. Last week, when we ran our Spartan race in Florida, I met a young RN from the Mayo Clinic. She's been in the

profession for just two years. Nothing had prepared her for the reality of COVID. When I thanked her for her bravery and selflessness, she cried.

This serves as a reminder to keep our first responders in our hearts and prayers. A simple word of thanks, a smile, or a meal go a long way to show that we care.

Donita Rients Livingston
This Dr. Is AMAZING!!! IF you know anyone that needs help with ANYTHING MEDICAL CALL DR. G. He is the BEST!! WE HAVE REFERRED HIM TO A LOT OF OUR FRIENDS!! WE GOT THE HELP AND ANSWERS WE NEEDED!!!!!!

Violette Sharmokh
Congratulations Dr. Ghaly

David Cheffi
Congratulations to a great and caring doctor.

Marianne Juraco Neidermann
Congratulations Dr. Ghaly. You are the best. 🙏

Youssouf Sogoba
Congratulations Dr. Ghaly 🙏 May God bless you

Marge Garbarz
Now everyone can know how wonderful you are because you are the most caring doc ever.

Charlene Mentzer Glowaty
Congratulations! You are the hero of your patients' lives, you save them from the misery of pain and you give them the best care possible. Bless you! 🖤🙏

Scott Mitchell
You need to post the picture in the superman cape!!! 😄 You're the best!!

Sharon Strons Ledbetter
Many congratulations 🎉 and may God continue to bless you and the work of your gifted hands 🙏😊🖤

Mike Nutoni
To me you are the best you saved my live Dr. Ghaly and all Ways kept in touched to see how I was. Many other doctors you don't here from on less you call there office and all you talk to is the doctor incident. God Bless Dr. Ghaly

Nina Smith
Dr. Ghaly was a resident when he took care of my husband and stood up for me A great Doctor and individual!

Flor De Andocutin
Agree well deserved the Doctor with a heart of

Sara Colwell Maiden
You are truly amazing Dr Ghaly.

John Vergo
You are a incredible Doctor. And we thank you for that

Angela J Miller
That is incredibly awesome my dear friend!! I am so very happy that they recognize and honor what we, who are blessed to be called "Ghaly Patients" already know of you. I thank God daily for bringing you into our lives. May God continue to bless you and continue working through you with each patient you touch. We LOVE you Dr Ghaly.

Diane Small-Blackman
Congratulations and thank you for your devotion to your patients.

Karen Bazzell McGinnis
You deserve this. Your belief that your skill was amplified with God's help & never take credit. You helped save my life. I'm so thankful we met & became friends. I respect you & care for you. I pray for you especially with Covid still digging in its nasty claws in people.

Jillianne Renee Overman
My neurosurgeon has been on the front lines of Covid in Chicago saving lives and innovating as he goes. Truly a man with God given talent, he's also extremely spiritual and prayerful in all of the work he performs.

Bretonya Phillips-Johnson
Congrats Dr Ghaly this is beyond deserved and sooo much more! You have no ideal how many lives you have touched let alone saved! God bless you and all that you do!

Congratulations Dr Ghaly! Proud to work alongside you @Stroger.

Scott Swanson
Ah you see this does not surprise me. Because being one of your patience and having met so many of your other patience we know one thing. You are simply the best!!! But most of all for the reason of giving your true unconditional love to everyone. You say you are just a servant but anyone who you have helped would say different. Congratulations.

Michelle Lizzethe
This is wonderful! So very proud of you! Thank you for saving so many lives.

Carol Ann De Rosa
Thank you Doctor Ghaly for all that you do, saving so many lives with such precision and dedication. 🖤🖤🙏

Patient's quotes 38
Chicago Crain's Business is nominating me for "Notable Healthcare Heroes"

Dear Ramsis,
We received a nomination on your behalf for Crain's upcoming Notable Healthcare Heroes list. We found your nomination very compelling—-

Thank you,
Notables Team

Crain's Chicago Business
notablechicago@crain.com

Sara Maiden
Congratulations Dr Ghaly. You are amazing and do gods work. I am so happy for you.

Chita Bello

Debbie Million
You SOOOOOO.....deserve this

You are The Best of the Best with a Heart of Gold

Kathy O'BRIEN
Yes you deserve it, I'm not your patient, but from all I have heard and read what you say and all the love and care you give your pts and everyone, you are very deserving of this award. Congratulations kind and giving man

Karen Boland
You ARE a healthcare hero, Dr. Ghaly!!!

Ilene Davis
Congratulations Ghaly!

You are the most worthy surgeon I know! I have seen your amazing surgical work first hand. You change the lives of everyone that crosses your path. You have been given a gift from God. The talent is in your mind and in your hands. 🖤🖤🖤

Brenda Linquist
You are very worthy and loved for being the phenomenal person you are! You are very worthy and loved for being the phenomenal person you are!

Flor Andocutin
YOU DESERVE IT DR GHALY.. THE SURGEON WITH A HEART OF GOLD 🤍

Charlene Glowaty
Congratulations on your well-deserved nomination. You are a wonderful, caring doctor who is always comforting to your patients and a blessing. 🖤🙏

Lena Waither
I cannot think of anyone who deserves it more than you....

Michelle Lizzethe
You are my Saint!

Karla Allison
I love dr ghaly. He is so passionate and cares so much for all of his patients.

Belkys De leon
A Miracle Worker

Vera Glisovic
Dear esteemed prof. Dr. Ramsis Ghaly. You are the only one in the world who consciously heals and respects human lives. God bless you all!! 🙏🙏🙏❤️

Martha Aranda
Amen Dr. Ghaly! My brother Jorge was living proof. 🙏🙏🙏

Jennifer Baxa
Thank you Dr Ghaly for all that you did for my dad and continue to do for others!!

Jonny Earles
Thank you, dear friend, for sharing your devoted work with us. It inspires us all.

Terry Mendozza
Dear Lord, Bless this good man and keep him safe. He is one of your Angels on Earth. Amen 🙏🙏🙏🖤🖤🖤💕💕💕

Janet Conger
Thank God you are on their side, thank you for caring for all lives 💕😌

Jennifer Petrucci
Thank you for all you do Dr. Ghaly!

Mara Krista
Oh your are the finest, the very light of God. Just love you Dr.

Amelia Lucinea
Medicine & the power of prayers together 🙏, their is miracle. You are a great Doc & a believer

Charlene Glowaty
You are a miracle worker. You never give up where others have. God has truly blessed you with knowledge and perseverance. 🖤🙏

Evelyn Perez
Your message goes beyond words. It gives hope to those who have family or friends suffering from COVID or any other medical condition. This message speaks very close to my family's heart. Thank you for all you do. 🙏

Charlene Mentzer Glowaty
You are a miracle worker. You never give up where others have. God has truly blessed you with knowledge and perseverance.

Micheline Demosthenes Eliacin
This is so very true Dr Ghaly! Prayers and medicine working hands I hands. Thank you Doc.

Cherie Cordero
My goodness Dr Ghaly way to represent, we are but thimble to this cup.

Sincerely, Cherie Cortez Tucker
You're awesome Doc, may God bless you and keep you safe

Cheryl Schick-Hamby
You are very courageous person Dr. Ghaly! May God keep you safe!

Lori Schlage Malczewski
You're wonderful Dr. Ghaly thank you!!!

Agnes and Michael Bolkunowiez
Today my husband had surgery on both his arms. Dr. Ramsis Ghaly, Thank you so very much for taking care of my husband and being so skilled at what you do. Every day of our lives will be better because of you. We are forever grateful 🙏 💜 This also marks 1yr since I had my back surgery and I feel great.

Carol Pasterius
Thanks to you and God, I am having another birthday. 😊

Mary Ann Cheng
Best. Attending. EVER!!!!!! 💝

Dory Manalo
The man with the biggest heart happy blessed valentine

Cheryl Esgar
Happy Valentine's Day to a wonderful man and doctor! 💕

Debbie Pawluk
Happy Valentine's Day, Dr. Ghaly. Thank you for your dedication today and every day! The world is a better place because of you!!!

Ilene Davis
Happy Valentine's Day Ghaly! You're a true saint! 💜💜💜

Elle Delacy
Happy Valentine's Day good Doctor. How very thoughtful of you to be with your residents and buy them a free dinner. God Bless You Doctor. Thank you for sharing your amazing life with us 🙏🙏

Flor Andocutin
You are amazing Dr Ghaly .. the doctor with a heart of 🤍

Sara Maiden
Dr Ghaly, you are so awesome and beyond amazing!

Susan Krohn
This is so amazing! You are a wonderful person and Dr!

Suzi Brock
Dr Ghaly
Thank you for all you do and your beautiful posts! I've been following you for a while and I'm so impressed that a doctor takes the time to reach out to people on social media!

I can't wait to meet you as I have Chiari Malformation & a messed up neck! CCI, DDD, Cervical bone spurs and possible syrinx! Once this snow and cold settle down, I'll be making an appointment!

Thank you for all you do!

God Bless you.

Kathy Manthei Sitar
Ramsis Ghaly I remembered that article. I remember that the article said that you meditated and fasted prior to doing surgeries. Also, you did surgery to remove a brain tumor on a classmate of mine. She is alive and well thanks to you!

Kathleen MacGregor Grace
Your words ever so wise, resonate with all. Thank you so much for these words of yours that lift my spirit in the darkest of times. Thank God for you! Were that the world a better place. A place where the hearts were pure. Thank God for you, Dr Ghaly. God Bless you! Blessings from Egypt

Charlene Mentzer Glowaty
You truly are a professional in the true sense of the word. You care about your appearance, you're reliable and you have ethics. You are a blessing to us all. Great photo! 🖤🙏

Ronald Feeney
That is priceless. You are one of Gods Angels walking with us and healing all you touch.

Elizabeth Tetteh
You are very sweet Dr Ghaly. Thank you for the congratulations. I owe so much of it to you and my training with my cook county family. We will catch up soon. Stayed blessed. Liz

Patients Quotes 37

Scott Swanson

You always educate us you always teach us something

Jack Duvick
You are our Angel Dr. Ghaly !!!

Scott Swanson
Getting ready for tomorrow morning the big day back surgery number 3 today I was pleasantly surprised by all my friends and customer's for well wishes thank you so much. So many have asked if I am worried but I am not. I have been blessed to have the best surgeon you can have Dr Ramsis Ghaly in my opinion being touched by him is like be touched by God. He would say he's just a servant humble he is but many of us feel different. Once again thanks and 👍👍

Lynn Swanson
Thank you for all that you do healing people. You are an extraordinary doctor and I am blessed to know you. You truly care about your patients.

Angela Miller
We love you Dr Ghaly. You are more than our doctor you are family ♡. It was soooo good to see you. Doesn't Carl Miller look great! He was glad to see you too Dr Ghaly and your phone call this evening made the BIGGEST smile appear on his face!

Lynn Swanson
Thank you for all that you do healing people. You are an extraordinary doctor and I am blessed to know you. You truly care about your patients.

Violata Morrison
Ramsis Ghaly the best Neurosurgeon at Cook County Hospital Chicago Illinois Thanks a million BFF. I always remember those happy memories we have at Chicago. Time flies my friend. Still we're so vibrant. God Blessings. We're essentials on this Universe as front liners with this pandemic. Always be safe.

Edwina Swanson
Thinking of you. I know you have THE BEST NEURO SURGEON and that you will be up and about soon. Hugs Mom ♡

Scott Swanson
Make sure you got a good surgeon the one that I have is Ramsey Ghaly don't think there's any better

Edwina Swanson
No surprise...Scott is doing well. He had the BEST neurosurgeon. We need more doctors like you. You are definitely heaven sent

Kenny O'Connell
You're the best

Angels Bullock
Ramsis Ghaly Thank you so much for the love and making my day very special!

Wishing you and yours the very best!

Thank you for who you are and all you do to bring healing into people's lives! ♥

Robin Hellenberg
Stay safe. The world is grateful for all the healing you Achieve. God's blessing to you sir

Terry Mendozza
Thank you, my friend, for calling me tonight. You did more for me in that call than all the other doctors here in months and I thank you from the bottom of my heart. God bless you, dear Ramsis the Great! ♡

Susan Harrison
Dr. Ramsis is truly a gift from God. I am pleased to know that he gave you peace of mind. You are in my daily prayers. ♡ 🙏

Charles Putnam
This is Wonderful news Terry. Thank you Ramsis Ghaly for helping a our dear friend. A man who truly has found his calling in helping his fellow man. I am honored to have you as a friend, God bless you sir and God bless you Terry for better health my friend. 🙏♡🙏

Terry Ebert Mendozza
This incredible man, this genius neurosurgeon, my friend, called me out of the blue last night, put a cardio-vascular surgeon on the line, and discussed my "case". This morning he called and had Mayo Clinic on the line. I am leaving Monday a.m. at 8:00 for

Atlanta/Minneapolis/Rochester for a 12:00 appointment at Mayo Clinic on Tuesday, to get some real answers!!! No one in Palm Beach seems to be want to address it, and they aren't seeing patients due to Covid! I am blessed beyond all to have a friend like this. Dr. Ramsis Ghaly, a TRUE friend and a true gentleman ♡.

Erika Szabo Beberman that he is. In every way. What a surprise, from Thursday night calling me, to Friday morning getting Mayo Clinic on the phone and the telling me, first appointment is Tuesday 12:00 with Dr. Long, the lung specialist who will take it from there. Shocking that my own doctors aren't seeing patients, but Dr. Ghaly got me into Mayo Clinic so soon, and I'm all set with flights and hotel and Blacklane which is the car company I use for transfers. I'm packing, and still in shock, lol.

Lilian Maycol thank you darling. I'm amazed at how fast this happened, thanks to Dr. Ghaly. I am blessed.

Derek Smith I've never been there, so I have no idea what the protocol is and I'm going alone, but I am happy to finally get some answers, and happy they could accommodate me. Imagine, our own doctors here in Palm Beach will not see patients, but I can fly up to Minnesota and get in Tuesday, thanks to Dr. Ramsis Ghaly, and see all the doctors there. It makes me shake my head.............So grateful.

Leslie Eastman
Prayers for safe travel and good results. Ramsis Ghaly is an angel on Earth.

Tom Neidermann
You're the best Dr. Ghaly

Flor Andocutin
God bless you Dr Ghaly 🙏 today and always ... THE DOCTOR WITH A
HEART OF GOLD 💚

Dotti Lopez
Best doctor ever

Joan pociòus
You are an angel of you he Lord.

Cathy Mason
My Dear Dr. Ghaly you are far from "unnoticeably". You have touched so many.
You've helped so many and no doubt that it's all been through your love of and
through God. You are truly a gift straight from God. Larry left 12yrs ago Sunday
and today is his birthday. You made such a difference in our lives and will always
be in my heart. God Bless 🤗

Michael Plunkett
Happy Birthday Dr. Ghaly, May God always be with you and in you. May your
hands, heart and soul continue to do your special work as a healer. You are very
unique in the most special ways, using your Gift of Life for the benefit of many
others. It is noticed by me and many others, and I am sure God sees what you do
every day. Amen to you, Happy Birthday, celebrate life.

KatieandDoug Salvatori
Happy birthday. You are such a great writer, so poetic. A loving child of God.

Gary Chandler
Happy Birthday Dr Ghaly!! You have and continue to impact my life. It's great
knowing a person like you. I hope you enjoyed your special day!

Aleta Finney Pavnica
Happiest of Birthdays dear doctor and thank you for teaching us and being an
example every chance you get.

Gina Alaimo Svara
Happy Birthday to the most amazing neurosurgeon and caring physician I have
ever met!

Jerry N Camille Bever

Dr. G. I think this is a milestone birthday for you!! We hope your Birthday Card arrived on time, but with the mail slow we hope it isn't late. Our Birthday wish for you is a wonderful day to celebrate you. We all celebrate you and the blessing we have of having you in our lives. Happy Birthday!

Diana Lynn Kay Happy birthday to you though you are a gift from God for so very many people and patients. You truly inspire all who meet you!! God bless you Dr Ghaly!!

Danette Meek Wishing many more blessed and happy birthdays to the most amazingly talented doctor I have had the privilege to know!! Happy Birthday Dr. Ghaly

Larry Salvatori

Happy Birthday Dr. Ghaly. May your day and life be blessed by God always. You are a great doctor, but an even greater human being.

Lma Maravilla Vilches Dr.Ghaly you are GOD send healer and I always remember how you care your Patient checking them in the middle of the night and early morning rounds. The Doctor that never sleep. HAPPY BIRTHDAY

Bart Smith

Your commitment has never waned a bit ... you rock Dr Ghaly ... going to see Sandy who turns 85 Sunday thanks in large part to you.

Carmen Einsiedel

Thank you Dr. Ghaly! Here's to another year of being able to not be in pain because of u!! May god bless u.

Sharon Ledbetter

God BLESS YOU Dr Ramsis Ghaly....we are FOREVER grateful 💜

Jana Carnalla

Thank you for taking such an amazing care of my family Dr. Ghaly! We are forever grateful to you 🌼 God Bless you 🤍

Eileen Markusic

Happy birthday Dr. Ghaly! You have truly been a blessing to us. If it wasn't for you Jim wouldn't be alive. Have a wonderful day!

Charlene Glowaty
You never gave up caring for your patients in your clinic or at the hospital. How lucky we are to have a doctor like you. May God continue to bless and watch over you. 🖤🙏

Dave Brown
Ramsis, more of your blessed successful surgeries!! Thank you for continuing to work God's miracles! Dave & Sue.

Bernie Dumyahn
Happy Anniversary Hunter..., told ya you'd be on your feet before you knew it, Dr. Ghaly's amazing beyond words, right? 🖤👌😎

Hunter Walker Bernie Dumyahn yes! 🖤 amazing, absolutely amazing. Thank you Bernie 🖤

Zoran Birovljevic
Thank you very much for your kind and thoughtful birthday wishes. You contributed so much in making my special day extra special.

Laurie Kapsalis
Miss you too Dr. Ghaly! Your kindness and compassion are one of a kind, and so rare!

Agnes Rose
Your in good hands! The most amazing Doctor 👏

Elle Delacy
God Bless you Doctor. You are a wonderful person and have helped so many people with your medical expertise, your kindness and love of our Savior 🖤🙏

Mike Nutoni
Amen Dr.Ghaly you have accompanied more than anyone young or old you have a huge heart of Gold you are the best man i know Dr.Ghaly the only man other than you is my father.

Debra Tarr
I love Dr. Ghaly he is one of the best neurosurgeons in the country......

Keith Marino
Congratulations you are one of a kind. God bless be safe and stay healthy

Piotre Aljendi
You are Awesome. The smarts person in the department and I cannot speak highly enough about you. Congratulations

Kenneth Candido
FANTASTIC! KEEP UP YOUR AMAZING WORK!!

KDC

Saran Marcus
Some people!! Just in case you felt that your 1 residency was an accomplishment, Super duper proud of you, Dr. Ramsis Ghaly! He's the only one out there like this.... And a spine surgeon. I'll never forget how you answered me when I asked you, "How did you do all that?" You're so humble....saying it's easier than remaining chaste!

You made me feel super special!!! I value all your insight and wisdom. You're one of a kind and God truly works in you! Thank you for always being there for me, whenever I needed a true friend! You're super motivational and amazing!!!! Congrats! God bless you always! 🎉

Oliver Brandt
My back surgeon..... he's the BEST. This man is a genius.... and a very skilled neurosurgeon. What surgeon waits in recovery room until you wake up? .. not many I bet

Nada Peterka Voss
Congratulations 🎉🎈 Doctor Ghaly you are the best! God Bless you 🙏

Vera Glišovic Doctor Ghaly je jedan od najboljih doctora što se jako brine za njegove pciente. On je operisao i brinio za moju mamu Zoru kad je imala stroke in 2004. Neznam da još ima takvih doctora na svetu kao je Doctor Ghaly! Vera Glišovic hvala vam, moja mama je živela 3.5 godine poslije stroke sa dr Ghaly pomoč, 2007 je imala drugi stroke I umrla od 83 Godiva 15 October 2007. Pozdrav i vama gospodga Vera.

Vera Glišovic
Nada Peterka Voss Gospođo Nado, dr.Ghalu samo divne reči, o njemu može da se govori.Veliki doktor, veliki čovek, velikog srca, posvecen pacijentima.Vašoj mami Zori želim dobro zdravlje, srecu i dug život.Pozdrav, vama i vašoj porodici, Sa velikim poštovanjem! ❤❤❤

Carol Grant
Congratulations; you are a brilliant person! Great job!

Dale Christensen
Your the best

Suzette Jennings
Praise our Lord Jesus 🖤

A well deserved recognition to our one and only Dr. Ghaly, our Earth angel who is our Gift from God.

Congratulations 🎉
and Thank YOU 🙏🖤

Billy Delrose
You are an inspiration to us all, thank you for being you, and if you didn't know is a gift to all.

Christine Bruni-Posedel
"Ramsis, you are an amazing and gifted surgeon and a person everyone should know. God bless you" 🙏

Tiffany Wills
You are a wise, talented, hard-working, intelligent and caring child of God and you are a gift to us all! Thank you for helping me and so many others! Love, hugs and prayers sent your way!

Cortez Tucker
You are a rare individual, you are brilliantly blessed, I'm so very proud of you, kudos my Friend ✨🐻✨

Lynn Swanson
Congratulations. You are truly a blessing to all.

Barbara Klemund
Congratulations Dr Ghaly!! Praise God for all your wonderful gifts. Thank you for your love and care! 🖤🖤🖤

Charlene Glowaty
You are not only a doctor who heals those who are suffering but you also heal your patients spiritually through your writings. 🖤🙏

Carol Rambo
Wish there were more doctors like you ☺ God has given you the best of gifts and yet you depend totally and completely on Him for all that you do.

Angel Schultz
You are a wonderful Dr for all that you do for people god bless you 🙏

Louise Keene
Yes, this doctor is so awesome. I will never forget he called me personally when I was in so much pain on a Friday evening. He is one of a kind.

Peter Marlo
Thanks Dr. Ghaly for keeping us grateful in the midst of this world altering event, and thank you for all your wonderful service as a medical caregiver.

Dr Subieta
We love you Dr. Ghaly for your courage and good predisposition!

Thank you Dr Ghaly for carrying out our lord Jesus Christ mission to care and love all. Through kindness and caring, we will overcome COVID and heal our nation.

Jilliane Overman
God Bless you! Stay safe and strong. Christ has appointed you to save many! Which hospital are you working now?

Patients Quotes 36

Father Athanasius Paul
Every now and then I am compelled to set my feelings to print. And now I say this to you my friend.

"God grant you increased faith, renewed wisdom, good health, much love ... ever growing in spiritual stature while deepening humility of spirit - In the name of the Father, the Son and the Holy Spirit, One God forever, Amen"

Brenda Linquist

Dear Dr Ghaly, I am grateful for your article. I believe it is needed and should be shared as much as possible.

You have treated my Brother, Larry Swarens and my niece Wendy Swarens. I am in awe of your work and your passions; thank you for sharing your talents and compassion.

I hope to get to see you some day for your medical opinion concerning my physical challenges.

Brad Herdklotz

You are the shield against the surge and the shelter in the darkest storm and we pray for the safety of you and all your brothers and sisters that rise every day to fight this evil.

Barbara Klemund

Hard to believe it's been 7 years already since I had my neck surgery. Dr Ghaly gave me my life back! Thank you Dr Ramsis Ghaly! God blessed you with a tremendous gift.

Michelle Lizzethe

Our loving Dr. Ghaly, please pray that he stays healthy so that he is able to help those seriously ill with Covid in the ICU. He gives so much of himself. 🙏❤️

Charlene Glowaty

You are amazing! You never give up hope and you care so deeply for the covid patients. I join you in prayer for those patients

Bless you and stay safe. ❤️🙏

Dr Lara Bonsara

I give thanks for your skill, energy, compassion & commitment to your patients. You are a singular, extraordinary teacher & colleague.

Dr Afshan

Dear Dr. Ghaly, One of the biggest honors of my life is being your student. Words are not powerful enough to express my gratitude for all you are doing for us. May the good things of life be yours in abundance not only at Thanksgiving but throughout your beautiful life. Dr. Ghaly you are an exceptional character that I still need to learn a lot from you. Knowing you with your genuine gold heart and kind soul was a blessing for me and I always thank lord for that.

Dr Rudi Kumapley
Happy Thanksgiving Ramsis. I am thankful for your selflessness and for all you do for our patients and trainees. Rudi

Dr Richard Fantus
Thank you 🙏 for all you do for others.

Jaime Koc
Dr Ghaly at Ghaly Neuroscience Neurosurgery. You won't find another doctor that will listen and treat you with great care like him!

Cathy Pruim
Dr Ghaly God has gifted you with amazing skills and a beautiful caring heart . R Crawley Cathy

Aardsma Pruim Absolutely he has! What a wonderful doctor and human being.

Jerry Bever
You made an incredible impact on so so many people their Dr. Ghaly. They were truly blessed to have you there.!

Shelley Sypien
Happy to see you have managed to maintain your sense of humor 😊 Thank you for risking your health to care for Covid patients. You are a hero.

I see the face of Jesus looking down at you with a pleased expression. Rhonda Lee Burgess

Suzette Jennings
Thank you, Dr. Ghaly. I am just now seeing this. You bring a bright light to an often dark world; through your talents, words and actions. Merry Christmas. I pray for the Coptic Christians.

Carlos Rosario
Thank you for helping me achieve being here today. Best person I've met in 59 years. God bless you.

Rebecca Crawley
Merry Christmas to you too! Thank you for taking such wonderful care of me and everyone! Stay safe and God bless you. 🌲🎄

Gino Spizzirri
A very classy, sophisticated, intelligent, professional, very well dressed man in a suit .!

Lol Many blessings brother

Angela Miller
Ramsis Ghaly You, Dr Ghaly, (guided by our Lord) gave us sooooo many blessings, one of them being TIME. You are the best neurosurgeon ever! We love you! Wising you a VERY Merry Christmas

Dr Fantus
Thank you for your conscientious care of our patients.

Scott Nancy Mitchell
Merry Christmas Dr. Ghaly!! Thank you for your love and compassion in everything you do!! Your truly are god sent.

Angi Perino
Merry Christmas Dr. Ghaly. Thank you for being there for our us all these years. We are beyond thankful to have you as a part of our family. We hope you Christmas is filled with all the happiness health and peace you deserve. Sending you the biggest hug and all our love! 🙏🌟❤️

Ric Malina
Merry Christmas Sir!!

Forever grateful to Dr Ghaly

Joseph Swaries
🎆🎁🎊 🌲 🌲 🌳 Merry Christmas & Blessed New Year 🌲 🌲🎆🎁🎊⛪🎄 May God Bless 🕯️✝️🍷, Protect, And Lead You & Your Blessed Family 💒💕 👭 The Way Unto His Kingdom! 📨🏘️⛪

Louise Keane
Thanks Dr. Ramsis Ghaly. Happy new year! Thanks for all that you do each and every day!

Maurice Gilbert
It is such a pleasure and a true Blessing to know you and be inspired by your teaching and devotion to our Lord and Savior. I am honored to know you. My very best wishes for a great 2021.

Tina clay
Thank you Dr. Ghaly for giving my Uncle Bob more time with Aunt Ginny! They had a love everyone wishes for 🖤🖤

Cherry Hamby
Continue to stay safe out there. You are an angel on earth to so many! Happy New Year to you.

Scott Mitchell
Ramsis Ghaly Happy new year to the Greatest man in Health Care!!!! Thanks for all you do!!!

Angi Perino
Happy New Year Dr. Ghaly! 🎉 Thank you for always helping Mom so much. Because of you she was able to spend over 20 more years with us!! 😸😸😸😸 😸😸😸😸 We hope this New Year brings you all the blessings you deserve. Sending you all our love 🙏🖤

KM. Thank you very much. You sound the same. I hope I didn't disturb you. I know your busy. 35 years' friends. Still the kind, gentle, intelligent physician, etc. May God Bless & keep you safe.

TEM. This incredible man, this genius neurosurgeon, my friend, called me out of the blue last night, put a cardio-vascular surgeon on the line, and discussed my "case". This morning he called and had Mayo Clinic on the line. I am leaving Monday a.m. at 8:00 for Atlanta/Minneapolis/Rochester for a 12:00 appointment at Mayo Clinic on Tuesday, to get some real answers!!! No one in Palm Beach seems to want to address it, and they aren't seeing patients due to Covid! I am blessed beyond all to have a friend like this. Dr. Ramsis Ghaly, a TRUE friend and a true gentleman. 🖤

RAMSIS GHALY
January 22, 2017 ·
Shared with Public

Nation----Nation
Written by Ramsis Ghaly

Before you start --- pray
Before you divide--- unite
Before you decide--- give a chance
Before you judge--- look deep inside you
Before you criticize--- listen
Before you march--- learn how to walk

The love and peace of our Father, His Son and the Holy Spirit One God Amen

TEM. Sometimes, just out of the blue, God sends you a miracle when you need one. Thank you, dear Dr. Ramsis Ghaly for calling me tonight, putting your friend the cardio-thoracic surgeon on the phone, and advising me what I should do, especially when I can get no answers from the doctors here. I am deeply, deeply appreciative of your advice, dear Ramsis. You are

Wonderful news! Know it is a relief, for you. You such a precious friend, Terry!!

LM. Wonderful, true doctors that really care.
NH. Wonderful news!! 💚🙏💚
ME. Thank you Dr. Ramsis Ghaly for helping my friend.
BS. Wonderful news!
SH. Dr. Ramsis is truly a gift from God. I am pleased to know that he gave you peace of mind. You are in my daily prayers. 💜🙏
PC. Thanks be to God!! 😭😭🙏🙏
LC. Wonderful news!!!
CD. This is good news Terry. My thank you to Dr. Ramsis Ghaly. He is such a caring man. Bob and I continue to hold you up in our prayers Terry and that God's hand will see you through this to better health. 💜🙏
CP. This is Wonderful news Terry. Thank you **Ramsis Ghaly** for helping a our dear friend. A man who truly has found his calling in helping his fellow man. I am honored to have you as a friend, God bless you sir and God bless you Terry for better health my friend. 🙏💜🙏 **Ramsis Ghaly**

I am your servant. Speed recovery our angel. Indeed the Heavenly Dove by your side. We pray

TEM. -- our precious Dr. **Ramsisz Ghaly** is the BEST!!!!!!! We need him to move to Beverly Hills!!!!!!!!! **#PastorJeff90210**

▌N ♦ £

Printed in the United States
by Baker & Taylor Publisher Services

Printed in the United States
by Baker & Taylor Publisher Services